The Healing Mission of Plastic Surgery

One Surgeon's Story

The Interrelationship of Functional, Reconstructive, and Aesthetic Plastic Surgery

Ernest D. Cronin M. D.

Copyright © 2020 by Ernest Cronin

All rights reserved. No part of this publication may be reproduced or transmitted in any form or by any means, electronic or mechanical, including photocopying and recording, or by any information storage and retrieval system, except in the case of brief quotations for use in articles and reviews, without written permission from the author.

The views expressed in this book are the author's and do not necessarily reflect those of the publisher.

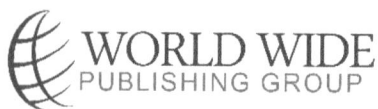

7710-T Cherry Park Dr, Ste 224
Houston, TX 77095
(713) 766-4271

Printed in the United States of America

ISBN: 978-1-68411-870-0

Dedication

I dedicate this book to my parents, Ed and Elaine Cronin, and Kathleen Kane Cronin, the love of my life and mother of our eight children and grandmother to our 29 grandchildren.

Table of Contents

Acknowledgment 1

FOREWORD Thomas Biggs and Donald Parks 3

Preface 7

Introduction 9

Chapter 1 : The Interrelationship of Functional, Reconstructive, and Aesthetic Plastic Surgery 11

Chapter 2 : Self - Image 47

Chapter 3 : The Making of a Plastic Surgeon 69

Chapter 4 : The Art and Science of Plastic Surgery 137

Chapter 5 : The best of Both Worlds 175

Chapter 6 : The Emergency Room and Trauma 199

Chapter 7 : The Cleft Palate Clinic 245

Chapter 8 : Thomas Cronin and the Silicone Gel Breast Implant 305

Chapter 9 : Breast Reconstruction after Mastectomy 325

Chapter 10 : The French Connection and the Birth of Craniofacial Surgery ... 369

Chapter 11 : Operation San Jose Mission Project 409

Chapter 12 : Unusual Cases 467

Chapter 13 : Frustrations and Joys of Plastic Surgery 521

Chapter 14 : The Place of Functional Plastic Surgery in the Healing Mission . 553

Chapter 15 : The Place of Reconstructive Plastic Surgery in the Healing Mission 643

Chapter 16 : The Place of Cosmetic Surgery in the Healing Mission 665

Chapter 17 : Development of Plastic Surgery 735

Chapter 18 : Cancer - Retirement - Legacy 767

Chronological Bibliography 785

Praise for Dr. Ernest Cronin and The Healing Mission of Plastic Surgery 793

Acknowledgment

The Healing Mission of Plastic Surgery is a reflection of my career in the fantastic field of plastic surgery. It would not have happened, but for my wife, Candy's constant support of my medical ambitions beginning even before we were married. She was a continual encouragement throughout my seven years of surgical training after medical school. She was the stabilizing bedrock of our marriage that allowed me to devote so much of my time to the "magnificent obsession" of plastic surgery. She did double parental duty at times, filling in for our children's absent dad, who was "at the hospital," or "at the office." With their mother's influence, they were also supportive of my plastic surgery career, for which I am indebted.

Benjamin Cohen and I were partners for 38years. The first ten at the Cronin, Brauer, and Biggs clinic; and the remaining 28 years with the Cohen and Cronin Clinic. He was loyal, helpful, and considerate. His comprehensive grasp of the field of plastic surgery was an inspiration to me.

I owe sincere gratitude to my mentors, especially Thomas D. Cronin, Paul Tessier, Raymond Brauer, Thomas Biggs, and Laurence Wolf, whom I recognize in chapter three.

I am also grateful to my many plastic surgery colleagues with whom I collaborated and from whom I learned so much, including Alfonso Barrera, Bruce Smith, Leo La Puerta, and Don Collins.

I am thankful for the help of several individuals who scrutinized *The Healing Mission of Plastic Surgery* and gave me feedback, including Drs. Don Parks, Donna Fox, Gary Branfman, Tom Biggs, and Hal Mentz.

I thank all the volunteers who made Operation San Jose Mission Project such a success for more than thirty years. Chapter 11 features them.

I acknowledge in chapter 7, the participants in the Cronin and Brauer Cleft Palate Clinic that made all the excellent work of the clinic possible.

I wish to thank my office staff, Janine Dubcek, Alma Lopez, and Donna McDowell, for all their support. My career would not have been possible without the expert and friendly help of all the medical personnel at St Joseph Hospital, including the nuns and especially the operating room nurses, technicians, and anesthesiologists.

This book could not have happened without the expert help and encouragement of Book Publisher Eddie Smith of Worldwide Publishing Group, and cover artist Teresa Granberry of Harvest Creek Design.

FOREWORD

Thomas Biggs and Donald Parks

***

Thomas Biggs

This is a GEM of a book

It's right for the general public; it's right for residents; it's right for established plastic surgeons. Dr. Ernest Cronin gives surgeons his perspective of thirty-eight years of plastic surgery so they can compare their own practice and consider adapting some of his concepts, techniques, and approaches.

The long and complicated path a person must take to be a certified plastic surgeon is explained. The fact that, unlike other specialties, it is not "system-based" but is surgical innovation with the human body and all its parts, which defines our system.

The author gives us a clear explanation of the broad scope of plastic surgery in his repertoire of cases, which are beautifully photographed. The challenge presented in each case is described, and the solution shown as a result. The scope of these cases ranges "from the top of the head to the bottom of the feet and from infants to octogenarians."

All of this is from his own very personal experiences, and he describes the joys and, yes, some disappointments in his own practice. This is an intimate look into his three- dozen peer-reviewed publications and many thousands of patients over thirty-eight years in practice.

All of this is done with the recognition of the fact that he was propelled and supported by his wife of fifty-one years, Kathleen, and his eight children, who were in constant awareness that his work, founded in his Catholic faith, was very strongly his effort to make people's lives better.

This book is a brilliant work of a highly skilled and experienced surgeon, an honorable and humble man trying to fulfill this Mission of Healing.

This book is a GEM.

Thomas Biggs M. D. Clinical Professor Plastic Surgery Baylor College of Medicine, ICON of the American Association of Plastic Surgeons, former President of the International Society of Aesthetic Plastic Surgery.

***

Donald Parks

Dr. Ernest C. Cronin, a true legend in International Plastic Surgery, has graced our literature with *The Healing Mission of Plastic Surgery*, a compendium and chronology of his life, his experiences, successes and failures, philosophies and dedication to his craft of plastic surgery.

Woven through the fabric of this wonderful treatise are the threads of Dr. Cronin's kindness and generosity, passion for his mission, conceptual brilliance, and surgical skills in the name of Plastic Surgery. This book highlights his professional artistry and unique innovation, particularly in the management of severe craniofacial deformities in children and adults, thousands of whom have benefitted from his personal mission as a Plastic Surgeon! *The Healing Mission of Plastic Surgery* is beautifully illustrated with Dr. Cronin's photos and diagrams, many personally embellished for instructional purposes!

Among the chronicles featured in *The Healing Mission of Plastic Surgery* are Dr. Cronin's interactions and relationships with renowned surgeons such as Dr. Paul Tessier, Dr. Thomas D. Cronin, and Dr. Tom Biggs and he provides a wonderful tribute to his colleagues at St. Joseph's Hospital in Houston, including Drs. Cronin, Brauer, Biggs, and Ben Cohen. He provides a first-hand intriguing insight into the development of the breast implant by his uncle Dr. Thomas D. Cronin and colleagues!!

Dr. Cronin has received many awards and public recognition for his numerous medical missions primarily to Central and South America, providing expert surgical intervention to needy children and a unique educational opportunity for local physicians, accompanying plastic surgery residents, and numerous other learners. His pride is clearly evident in this book as he discusses mission experiences and the patients and people that made such missions so successful.

This book provides a very personal and exciting historical perspective in the evolution of a remarkable plastic surgeon's career.

Plastic Surgery and the entire medical community should be so grateful to Dr. Ernest Cronin for sharing with us *The Healing Mission of Plastic Surgery*, a riveting chronicle of a full life of dedication, generosity, artistry, innovation, professionalism, and love of family and he is greatly admired and respected by all of us who know him.

Donald H. Parks BA, MD, FRCS(C), FACS

Professor of Surgery, McGovern Medical School, University of Texas Health Science Center at Houston, Chief, Division of Plastic Surgery (Retired)

Preface

About halfway through my 38 years of plastic surgery practice, I gave a presentation on plastic surgery at the Museum of Medical Science in Houston, which is now the John P McGovern Museum of Health and Medical science. I made a slide show that touched on several aspects of this fascinating field and intitled it, "The Healing Mission of Plastic Surgery." I received positive feedback from the audience, which was generally not medical. During the remainder of my career, I mused about writing a book that would expand on that topic. I wrote many notes and collected many photographs over the years with that in mind.

I retired on March 21, 2016, because of a sudden illness a few years sooner than I had planned. After convalescing for several months, I was delighted the Texas Society of Plastic Surgeons invited me to give a presentation reflecting highlights of my 38 years in private practice to their 2017 Annual Meeting. Preparing for that event rekindled my interest in producing a book. I have spent a considerable portion of my time the last couple of years on writing *The Healing Mission of Plastic Surgery*. I decided that it was most appropriate to develop it as my professional memoir rather than a more expansive scientific work. Hence the chronological bibliography is weighted with my publications.

I believe that I have been fortunate to have had a productive and diverse career in exciting times for the development of plastic surgery. All the cases presented, unless otherwise stated, are mine. For anonymity and convenience, I have used first name pseudonyms for patients, whom I would, in my practice, have used, Mr. Smith, Miss Jones, etc. I cropped most of the patient photographs to eliminate individual recognition. Some patient photos are of entire unconcealed faces or other recognizable parts, and I use them with permission. I also produced numerous photo-drawings to help explicate some concepts. I altered a few patient photos to camouflage possible identifying marks etc. I took many pictures with

35 mm film for slides that I later scanned and digitalized. I produced many amateur drawings, which I hope are helpful. In this book, I want to present my personal experience to a general audience curious about plastic surgery and, at the same time, leave a remembrance to my family. They might have wondered what I was doing at the hospital or the office those 38 years.

Introduction

He appeared to be an ordinary middle-aged man sitting in the first examination room of my plastic surgery clinic. The baseball cap was the only thing that seemed somehow out of place. I said, "Hello, Mr. Brown, I am Dr. Cronin; what can I do for you?". Without saying a word, he grabbed the bill of his cap and, with a little flair, removed it to expose the reason for his visit. "Can you help me, Dr. Cronin?" he said. My eyes open a little wider, and I stood a little taller as I tried to be nonchalant. The entire structure of his forehead was missing. In its place was an indentation large enough to steady a basketball. I wondered how someone with such a deformity and apparent loss of brain tissue could be such a normally functioning individual. Eventually, I was able to give him a new forehead through the art and science of plastic surgery.

This man represents only one of many intriguing plastic surgery true stories that will unfold in *The Healing Mission of Plastic Surgery*. I will highlight many of the stories with images that further bring to life the human condition of actual patients in their quests for healing. This book reveals a seemly side to plastic surgery that is transforming lives every day in hospitals and clinics all over the world. I explore the interrelationship between functional, reconstructive, and aesthetic (cosmetic) surgery. I show the scope of plastic surgery from the top of the head to the bottom of the feet, which involves patients from infants to octogenarians.

This book is a memoir of the 38 years of my very diverse plastic surgery practice. All of the cases were done by me unless explicitly stated otherwise. The book touches on the origins of plastic surgery and attitudes about it. I exemplify self-image and body image issues with case studies. I elucidate the arduous requirements necessary to become a plastic surgeon. I reveal the lack of regulation of specialists and some of the general misperceptions of the public regarding plastic surgery. I explain my early interest in medicine and my journey to become a plastic surgeon with the help of many excellent mentors.

I have had a particularly enjoyable type of practice, which combined private medicine with teaching in an academic residency program, with exposure to a broader range of cases than the average plastic surgeon. I depict exciting trauma experiences from the emergency room and beyond. I document the unique role of plastic surgery in cleft lip and palate care and breast cancer care. I disclose the development of the modern breast implant by Dr. Thomas Cronin and Dr. Frank Gerow. I chronicle the origin of the Cronin and Brauer Cleft Palate Clinic and my thirty-year experience with Operation San Jose, a cleft lip and palate mission project to Latin America.

I share personal experiences covering functional, reconstructive, and aesthetic plastic surgery. I reveal the joys frustrations and disappointments of more than 38 years of practice. I put into modern perspective innovations, which came about during my career, such as microsurgery, myo-cutaneous flaps, liposuction, endoscopic surgery, and lasers. Included are stories of courageous patients benefiting from the modern wonders of the reconstructive possibilities in the ever-evolving world of plastic surgery today. I've written a book that I hope will appeal to the curious general public through the use of case studies and anecdotes. I attempt to make plastic surgery vibrant for the reader, with before, intraoperative and after photographs, together with the many explanatory illustrations, which I have made.

Chapter 1

The Interrelationship of Functional, Reconstructive, and Aesthetic Plastic Surgery

"Clifton" appeared to be an ordinary middle-aged man sitting in the first examination room of my plastic surgery clinic. The baseball cap was the only thing that somehow seemed out of place. I introduced myself and asked what I could do for him. He smiled, and without a word, he grabbed the bill of his cap with a little flair removed it to expose the reason for his visit. He said, "Can you help me, Dr. Cronin." My eyes opened a little wider, and I stood a little taller as I tried to be nonchalant. What I saw was a horrific defect of his forehead and frontal skull. The entire structure of his forehead was missing. In its place was an indentation large enough to steady a basketball. I wondered how someone with such a deformity and apparent loss of brain tissue could be a normally functioning individual. I asked him what had happened, and he began to chronicle his saga, which had started a few years previous.

He had been a truck driver and had a flat tire. He was inflating the replacement tire when it blew out, causing severe injury to his forehead and frontal bone. He underwent emergency neurosurgery, subsequently developed a wound infection necessitating additional surgeries and, eventually, the removal of most of his forehead and frontal skull as well as much of the frontal lobes of his brain. He finally recovered and was discharged from the hospital with his mental faculties substantially intact.

For a while, he was grateful to be alive, and the last thing he wanted was more surgery. He told me that while most of his social interactions were okay, he was having trouble initiating any romantic relationship. When he took off his hat, it seemed to be a turnoff to any potential girlfriend. Eventually, he became more and more interested in having something done because he wanted a more normal appearance.

So, he went to see Dr. Wayne Hurt, a neurosurgeon who referred him to me. I told "Clifton" that I would be able to help him, but first, we needed to perform some tests and have x-rays taken. I explained the reconstruction would be a combined plastic surgery/neurosurgery effort with Dr. Hurt because of the possibility of brain exposure or injury during the case. Besides the specifics of the defect, my examination revealed he was mentally alert, coherent, and generally in good physical condition. At the end of our consultation, he was quite eager, even anxious to get started. The X-ray and preoperative photos below demonstrate his preoperative status.

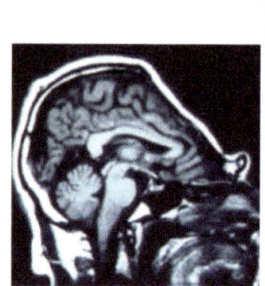 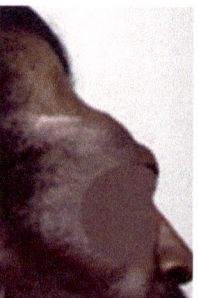 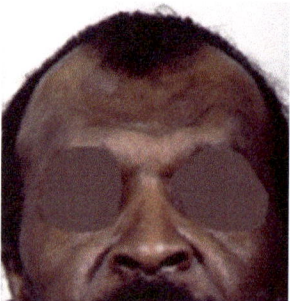 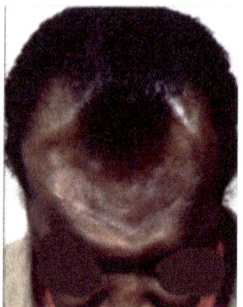

After my planning and preparation were complete, Dr. Hurt and I took the patient to the operating room for a significant reconstructive procedure. Dr. Hurt was available to attend to any unplanned penetration of the dura, which might cause a cerebral spinal fluid leak. I exposed the bony defect of the forehead and skull by going through previous scars of the forehead. I carefully lifted the skin, from the dura lining of the brain, to avoid damage to the brain and prevent any cerebrospinal fluid leak. I was also careful not to enter any remnants of frontal or ethmoid sinuses, which might contaminate the area and lead to a severe infection.

This preliminary dissection was successful, which allowed me to proceed with the actual reconstruction, which involved the replacement of the forehead and frontal bone with acrylic material. I first placed reinforcing wires across the bony defect because it was so large and then used a liquid and acrylic powder mixture, which would harden after being put into place. The wires acted to help stabilize the position and strengthen the reconstruction material as steel rebar would strengthen concrete.

I carefully molded the surface contour as the material was still in a semi-liquid state. The hardening process was an exothermic reaction producing significant heat. During the final hardening process, the reconstruction area was continuously irrigated with cold saline, utilizing small plastic catheters between the acrylic and the patient's dura to prevent overheating. After full hardening of the material, I smoothed minor irregularities with a diamond bur.

In the interoperative photos below, I have elevated a large scalp flap and turned it toward the back of the head to expose the defect. I made the incision in the previous traumatic forehead scar. In the first photo, the red line marks the area of absent bone. The dura overlying the brain is pointed out by the yellow arrow. In the middle photograph wire, "rebar" (green arrow) was placed across the defect over a dissolvable sponge pad. The third photo shows the intermediate intraoperative result after I properly shaped the originally viscous acrylic material and allowed it to harden.

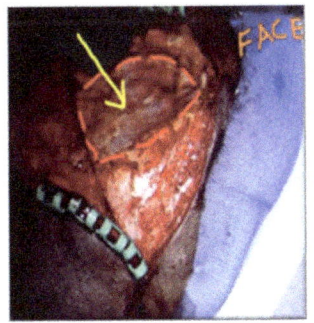 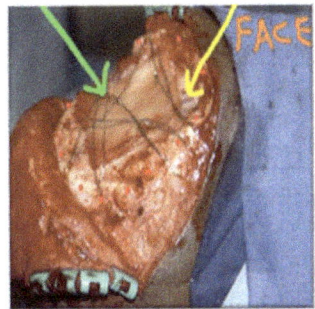 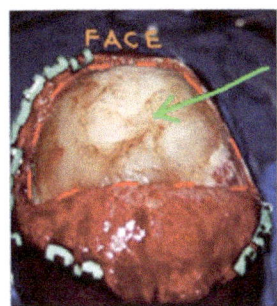

Next, I repositioned the scalp flap over the newly contoured acrylic cranium and closed the wound in layers with sutures. I could immediately tell that the reconstructive contour would be quite efficacious if no infection or other wound-healing problems ensued.

Synthetic material increases the chance of infection, which probably would require removal of the prosthesis. He did quite well, went home from the hospital the next day, and never had any healing problems. The photos below show the postoperative result about one year after surgery. He happily reported that he was married within a year of the operation. He was very thankful for our efforts.

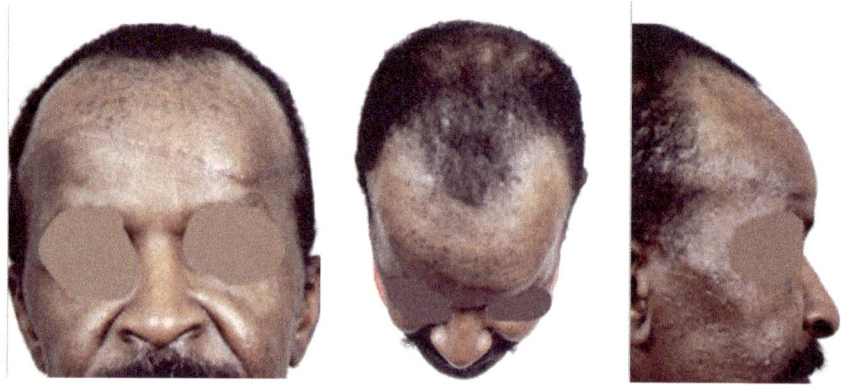

Theodore Roosevelt said, "by far, the best prize life offers is the chance to work hard at work worth doing." I believe practicing the art and science of plastic surgery enabled me to enjoy that prize. I believe we would all like to think that we have made some contributions during our brief earthly existence. I consider it a great privilege to be a physician trained in plastic surgery. It is a wonderful field of medicine that betters the lives of patients every day all over the world while giving great satisfaction to its practitioners.

I received a great deal of gratification both from ameliorating my patients' problems or enhancing their self- image as the requisite situation required. Patients go to doctors to seek relief of some discomfort. They want to eliminate their pain or other symptoms, whether physical or psychological. Patients confer with plastic surgeons because of perceived physical imperfections to which they attribute limitations to their happiness or their capacity for achievement. They anticipate the contemplated plastic surgery will improve their body image, self- image and self -esteem so they will "feel better."

Plastic surgery comprises three categories, functional, reconstructive, and aesthetic (cosmetic). Plastic surgery addresses congenital defects of the face and other areas. It deals with acquired problems, traumatic, degenerative, and neoplastic, such as tumors of the skin and more deep-seated tumors, especially of the head, neck, and hands. Plastic surgery emphasizes atraumatic, gentle techniques, meticulous wound closure, the utilization of skin grafts and flaps, and rearrangement of tissues for wound closures. A hallmark is the use of small delicate instrumentation. Plastic surgery is a field of medicine which deals with unique techniques of repair directed at restoring form and function, not of just one system or anatomic region. It involves aesthetic, reconstructive, and functional problems from the top of the head to the bottom of the feet.

Its name comes from the Greek *plastikos* and the Latin *plasticus*, which both mean moldable. It does not refer to synthetic plastic material, although sometimes such is used in plastic surgery procedures. Although there are descriptions that could be characterized as plastic surgery in ancient Egypt and India, the modern origins of plastic surgery are in sixteenth-century Europe. The western tradition of plastic surgery dates to the Italian surgeon, Gaspar Taglioccozi, who wrote in 1597, "We restore and make whole those parts which, nature or ill fortune have taken away, not so much to delight the eye but to buoy up the spirit of the afflicted." Most plastic surgeons aspire to this ideal despite the cheesy ads some practitioners produce and the tawdry sitcoms that purport to represent plastic surgeons.

I envision this manuscript as my professional *apologia pro vita sua*. I'm grateful for the opportunity I had of taking care of so many remarkable patients. I will endeavor to share some of this "prize" with you in the following pages. I include some vignettes, many pre-operative and post-operative photographs, practice reminiscences, and my clarifying (?) amateur drawings. I hope that elucidating this "prize" will be instructive, revealing, and educational to most readers and engrossing, poignant, and occasionally inspiring to some.

The following case is of a particularly courageous cleft palate patient who endured multiple reconstructive procedures. It illustrates both aesthetic and functional improvement. Hopefully, this surgery lifted his spirit in the process. Cleft lip and palate are common congenital birth defects. They present two of the most exacting surgical challenges with which plastic surgeons deal. I usually repaired cleft lips at about three months of age and cleft palates at about eight to 14 months of age. Finishing work is generally completed by 15 or 16 years of age or sometimes even later in males.

Results depend both on the inherent nature of the defect and the quality of the treatment, especially the surgery. Patients seem to have different intrinsic growth potential, and indeed, there are significant differences in clefts. Sometimes I can easily predict which cases of the same general category will be easier or more difficult. I was fortunate to have many patients referred to me for secondary (revision) cleft lip and palate surgery.

It is relatively common to see patients who have had the indicated repairs completed but have less than optimal results. Common problems are fistulae, which are residual abnormal openings between the mouth and the nasal space. Speech difficulties, distortions of the nose, or discrepancies between the upper and lower jaws are other issues with which patients frequently contend.

I also see teenage or adult patients with repaired cleft lip and palate who may benefit both aesthetically and functionally from a variety of additional standard plastic surgery procedures. Some of these patients delay seeking relief because they do not realize they can have more done for them.

"Jim" presented to me at age 15, having had multiple previous procedures to repair the effects of congenital bilateral clefts of the lip and palate elsewhere. As can be seen in the picture below, he still has significant residual deformities. The photos illustrate a deficient tight upper lip, an excessive lower facial height, and a short stub nose. He also had functional issues with residual openings between the mouth and the nasal cavity, which allowed fluid and sometimes food into the nose. Such fistulae are occasional disconcerting complications of cleft palate surgery. The first two photos below are of the patient as he first presented to me as a 15-year-old, asking if any more surgery could be beneficial for him

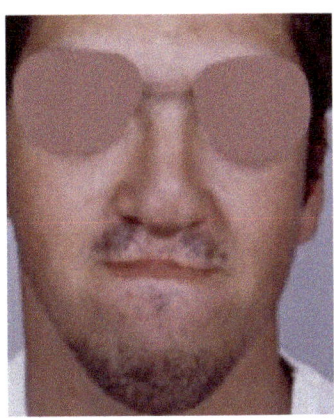 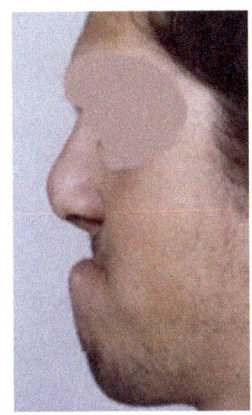

At his initial evaluation, I immediately knew that to obtain the maximum result, Jim would need several additional procedures. He did not look forward to more surgery as he had had many operations in the past. At first, Jim declined my recommendations because they seemed too extensive. Eventually, he acquiesced to my direction, and he allowed me to implement all the procedures I advocated. I performed three separate operations to obtain the results shown below. The first stage was a bone graft to the palate and repair of the residual fistulae openings. I harvested bone from the iliac crest, which is the bone just above the hip joint. Although infection and delayed healing of the bone grafts complicated this first operation, I was pleased that he did not lose hope; he persevered with the treatment plan.

In the second stage, I repositioned the upper jaw (midface) forward and moved the lower jaw backward and simultaneously moved the chin forward and up. These maneuvers involve cutting the facial bones with a power saw specifically designed for this purpose. The exact location of the cuts took into account the nerve and blood vessel anatomy to ensure minimal damage and also maintain good blood supply to the segments moved. After repositioning the bony sections, I fixed them in place with microplates and screws. There will be additional examples and explanations of orthognathic (jaw) surgery in later chapters

The third operation was a rhinoplasty with cartilage grafts and an Abbe flap. In performing an Abbe flap, I moved a portion of the lower lip into the upper lip to increase the fullness and projection of the upper lip and also to reduce the fullness of the lower lip. The Abbe flap tissue from the lower lip to the upper lip and was sewn in place, leaving a small connecting bridge of tissue with blood supply to maintain the flap. Gradually the existing upper lip produced new blood supply to the flap. After ten days, I separated the lips by cutting the bridge.

Each of the three major stages was separated by several months in this reconstructive effort, which took the better part of two years to complete. I want to emphasize that there are dedicated plastic surgeons in every major city in the U.S. and most major cities throughout the world, helping such patients all the time.

"Jim" had to bother with much discomfort to be able to get the substantial improvement that he received. He was fortunate to have a very supportive father who came to almost every office visit over the extended time needed to complete this young man's case. I'm often amazed at what patients are willing to go through to improve their body image to feel better.

The intraoperative photographs below are from his third operation, the Abbe lip switch flap. The first photo shows the philtrum area of the upper lip, pointed out in purple, and the lower lip tissue pointed out in green. The second photo shows the philtrum (purple arrow) freed and moved upward, releasing the tethered nasal tip. I used this previous upper lip tissue to lengthen the columella of the nose. Cartilage grafts were also placed in the nasal tip and columella to restructure the nose. Also shown in this photo, I incised the central lower lip tissue except for a small bridge containing the labial artery (represented as a red line). This lower lip flap (green arrow) was turned 180° and sutured into the central portion of the upper lip to make a new philtrum.

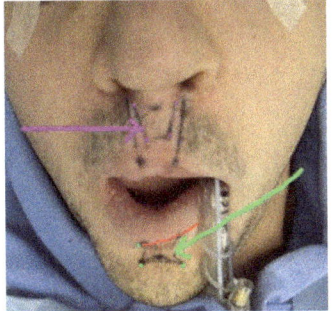 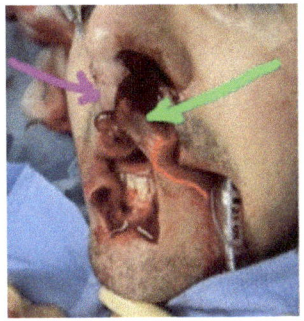

The picture below shows the now elongated columella, the Abbe flap, and the remaining lower lip segments each sutured into place. The small connecting bridge of tissue (circled in yellow) containing the blood supply from the left lateral lower lip to the transferred flap remained undisturbed for ten days. During this time, the upper lip tissue increasingly supplied new blood to the Abbe flap. The last photos are just before cutting (blue line) the narrow bridge connecting the upper and lower lip.

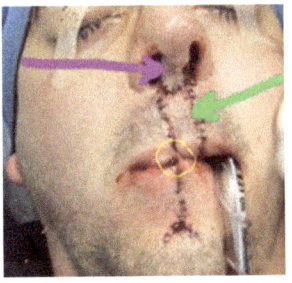 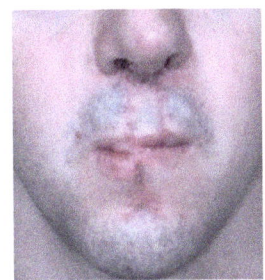 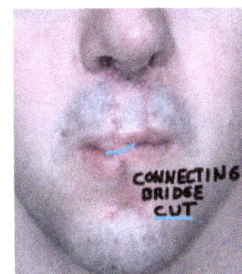

The first two procedures corrected the functional palate issues and placed the jaws in a more harmonious relationship. The final operation made the upper lip longer, fuller and less tight, released the nasal tip, and lengthened the columella. The final result is shown below after the three surgical procedures. Compare them to his before photos on page 17. I was elated with what I was able to accomplish for him. I considered it a "grand slam home run." He can now approach the world with a much more normal outlook and hopefully avoid the prejudice that he might have had to endure with his former face. "Jim's" story represents just one reason why I love plastic surgery.

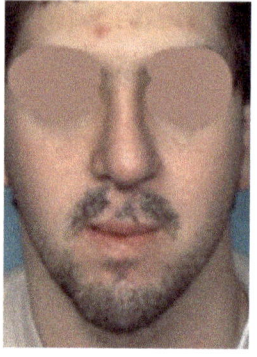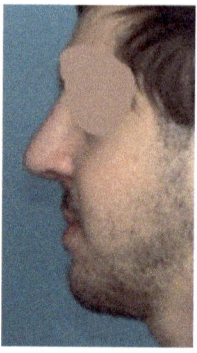

A young lady, "Dee," presented to me seeking cosmetic improvement in her appearance. Although she was not particularly overweight, she was especially concerned about her fatty neck. She wanted a "new neck." She also sought some subtle changes for her nose and chin. She represented a strictly aesthetic case, as there was no functional or reconstructive component. I explained what would be involved in the surgery and the risks benefits and alternatives.

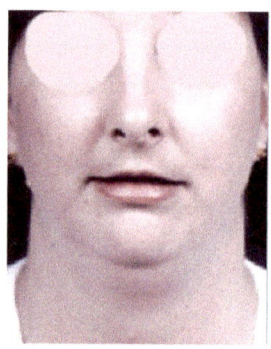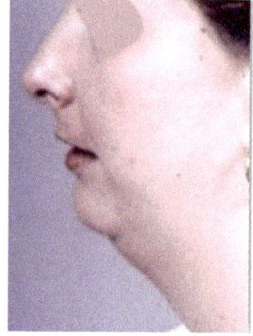

On the day of surgery, she was a little nervous but ready to proceed. I first performed a conservative rhinoplasty that reduced the bridge slightly and refined the nasal tip. I cut the chin bone and slid it slightly forward to make the chin somewhat more prominent. The most significant improvement, however, came from work on the neck. I made a small incision under the mentum and removed fatty tissue from her neck directly and tightened the platysma muscle in the neck with sutures to sharpen the angle between the jaw and neck. I performed this type of surgery as an outpatient or a one - night stay in the hospital. "Dee" had a nice recovery without complications. She obtained the excellent result shown below and was quite excited and grateful for the improvement she received.

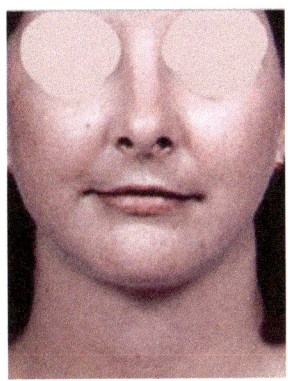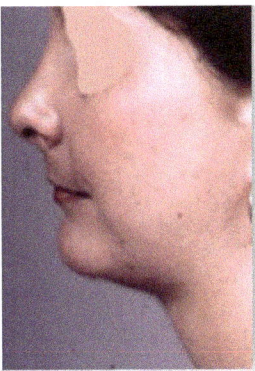

The above three cases, one functional, one reconstructive, and one cosmetic, are adumbrative examples of the broad field of plastic surgery.

Acceptance

Although plastic surgery has gradually become more accepted by the general public and the rest of medicine, it is an area that can stir up very different emotions, some not so flattering. Mainly because of the cosmetic aspect of many of the interventions, it is ofttimes rejected as vanity surgery, unnecessary surgery, interfering with nature or God's plans, not real medicine. TV sitcoms portray it as superficial and sleazy. With the advent of "reality TV," there is an excellent risk of misrepresentation of this great specialty of surgery and potential damage to the public.

However, when individuals need "plastic surgery" or could greatly benefit from it, attitudes often change rapidly. As with so many other things, it is a matter of ignorance of the details of the truth. Interestingly, support for plastic surgery was given by a leader of an institution as traditional as the Catholic Church. Pope Pius XII addressed a congress of Italian plastic surgeons as early as 1959, saying plastic surgery is "at the top of the medical profession for its beneficial work in restoring harmony and propriety to body and spirit." He also said, "Remember that your vision should go beyond tissues and outward forms and reach the soul whose interior beauty you will teach others to appreciate."

He also spoke explicitly regarding cosmetic surgery, which remains controversial even as its popularity grows. "If we consider physical beauty in its Christian light and if we respect the conditions set by our moral teachings, then aesthetic surgery is not in contradiction to the will of God, in that it restores the perfection of that greatest work of creation, man."

Gaspar Taglioccozi, the father of modern plastic surgery, understood the interrelationship between functional, reconstructive, and aesthetic surgery. "For although the original beauty of the face is restored, yet this is only accidental, and the end for which the physician is working is that the features should fulfill their offices according to nature's decree." The two patients below illustrate Taglioccozi's point. The first was a young girl, "Peggy," who had a benign growth in the caudal end of the nasal septum. This tumor distorted the nose and obstructed normal nasal breathing. It was also unsightly and certainly contributed negatively to her body image. Pre-op photos are below.

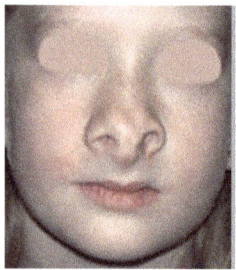 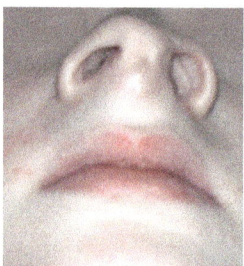 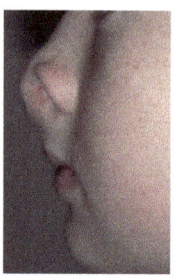 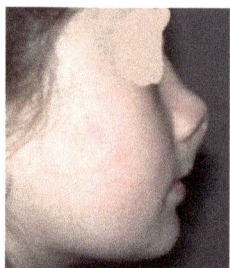

I performed two operations. The first removed the benign tumor, while the second refined the restoration of normal form and function of the nose. She was a charming girl who was appreciative of our efforts, as were her parents. The last four photos below show the result after two procedures. Reproducing normal form and function has restored her original beauty.

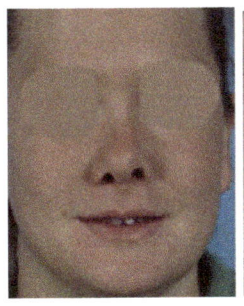 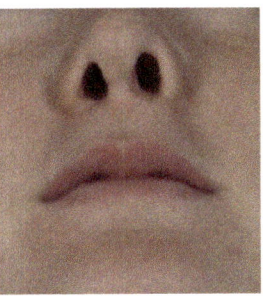 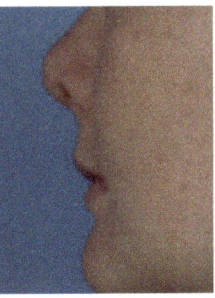 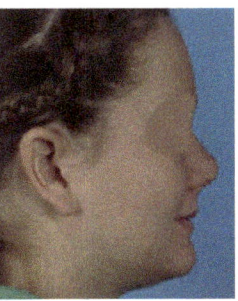

The second case below case also illustrates Taglioccozi's point. This middle-aged lady "Gloria" had an ectropion, a turned - out lower eyelid, which caused her to have excessive tearing and eye irritation. Ectropion is usually a spontaneous degenerative problem resulting from an eyelid that is too lax. I made an incision along the edge of the lower eyelid (presented in green) and elevated the skin and muscle of the eyelid. Then I removed a full-thickness wedge of the deeper tissues, including the tarsal plate (the firmer fibrous portion of the lid). The red triangle represents this wedge excision.

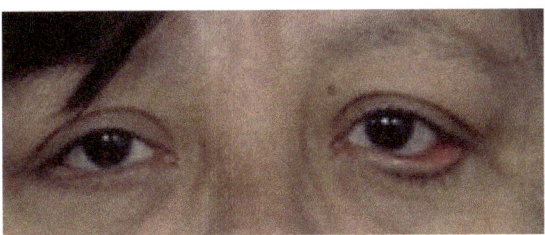 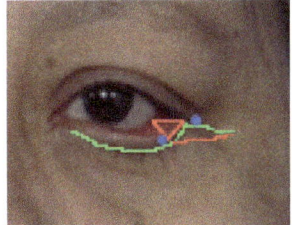

I sutured the lid, tightening it horizontally. The two blue points on either side the wedge excision came together. A small amount of skin laterally was removed to adjust the eyelid skin after the wedge excision. Correction of the ectropion allowed the eyelid to fulfill its normal function and, in doing so, restored the original beauty of the face.

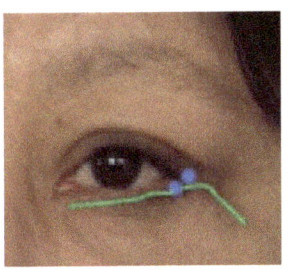 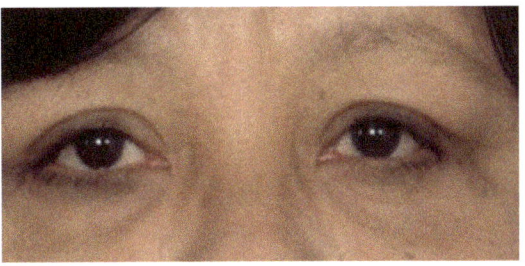

The interrelationship of functional, reconstructive and aesthetic plastic surgery

What is functional surgery?

Surgery performed on abnormal structures of the body caused by congenital defects, trauma, infections, tumors, or other diseases is functional surgery when done to improve function, cure disease, or relieve symptoms. A 35-year-old seaman, "Gregory," sustained a severe crush injury to his dominant right hand, which destroyed the thumb. The initial surgery was to repair multiple lacerations to the hand and complete removal of the devitalized thumb. The first pictures show him after healing from the initial injury. He has essentially four good fingers and no thumb. Since the thumb represents about 40% of the functional capacity of the hand, this was a very debilitating deficit. The arteriogram shows the vascular supply

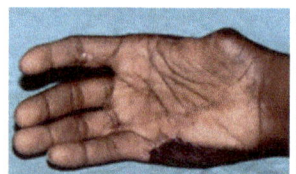
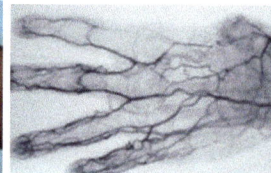
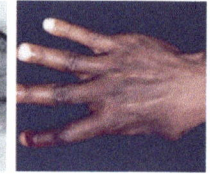
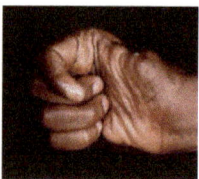

For this unusual case, I consulted with my partner Dr. Ben Cohen, and together we decided to move his index finger to the position of the thumb to create a new thumb. This pollicization procedure would give him a three-fingered hand with a good thumb, which would be about twice as functional as his existing situation with four fingers and no thumb. Dr. Cohen and I planed the operation and executed it together as a team. It was a tedious operation, which took a few hours. It involves shortening the bone of the index finger in the palm while at the same time moving the rest of the index finger of the hand and affixing it to the stump of the thumb amputation. Concurrently the blood vessels supplying the index finger needed to be preserved but rerouted with the new position of the thumb. The new thumb had to be pinned in place for many weeks until the bone healed. The photos below show mobilizing the index finger and repositioning the index finger to make a thumb.

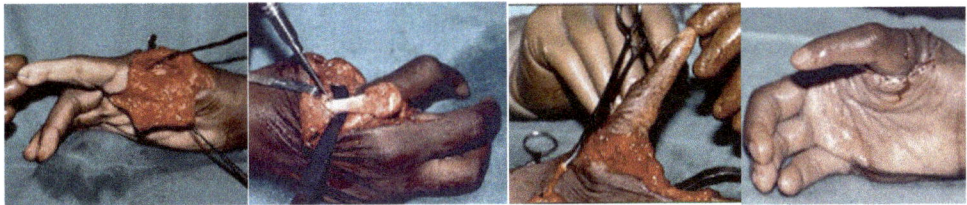

This man was a very grateful patient, as we were able to restore most of his hand function. "Gregory" obtained good pinch and grip with the new thumb shown below.

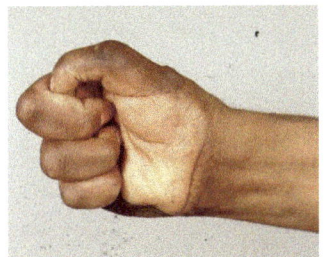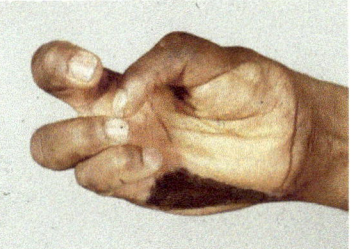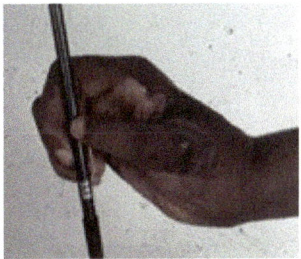

About 15 years later, he returned because of a minor injury to the left-hand sustained while working offshore. At that time, I took the opportunity to x-ray both hands. The radiologist read the x-ray of the right hand as having a previous amputation of the index finger, not noting any abnormality of the thumb. He continued to work as a seafarer with no restrictions in activities.

The gentleman below "Moye" represents another example of functional surgery performed to cure disease. He presented with a small lesion that occasionally bled. It had the appearance of basal cell carcinoma. The likely extent of the excision needed for a cure is shown in red below.

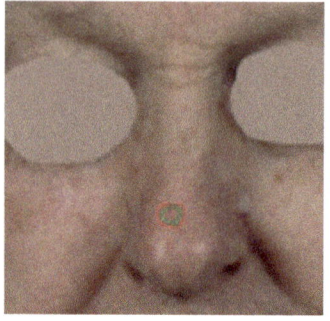 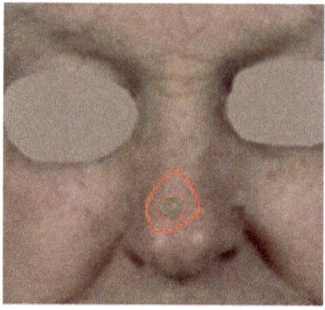

I took him to the operating room and removed the lesion, and obtaining fresh frozen section checks of the margins by the pathologist. The picture below is after getting clear margins. The blue markings outline a dorsal nasal flap based on the right cheek. This flap is a "workhorse flap" for many nasal repairs. By following the colored dots, you can understand the movement of the flap.

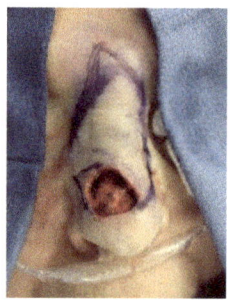 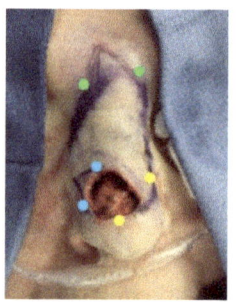

I elevated the tissue at a level just above the periosteum and perichondrium of the nasal structures, as shown below. I included the small nasal muscles in the flap; they add vascularity. The blood supply comes from the right cheek through the small remaining base of the flap, as in the second photo drawing. I both advanced and rotated the flap to cover the defect, and at the same time, I closed the glabella donor site primarily. The colored dots show the movement.

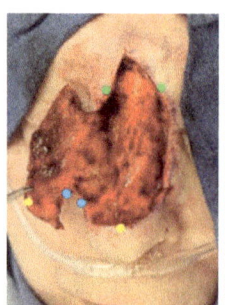 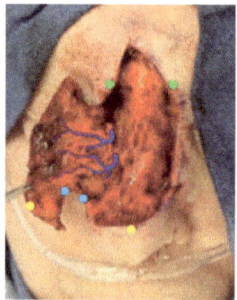 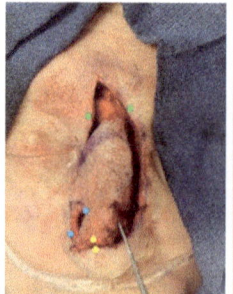 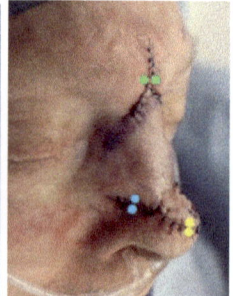

"Moye's postoperative results are shown below after several months.

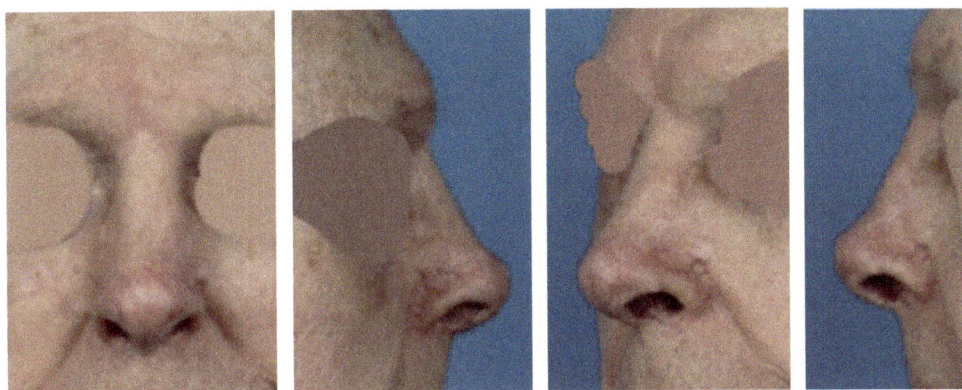

Other examples of functional plastic surgery are the closure of a congenital cleft of the palate to allow normal speech and cure of disease such as the removal of tumors. Relief of pain is also considered a functional issue. Reduction of large pendulous breasts that cause significant back, neck, or shoulder pain is a fairly standard quite successful procedure that is often functional. There are numerous other examples throughout this book. Chapter 14 is devoted to functional plastic surgery.

What is reconstructive surgery?

Reconstructive surgery is performed on abnormal structures of the body caused by congenital defects, developmental abnormalities, trauma, infections, tumors, or other diseases to approximate a more normal appearance, not specifically to improve function. An example may be a congenital absent external ear or traumatic loss of a portion of the ear. Surgery to construct the visible outer ear is an attempt to build a normal-appearing anatomic structure but will not aid in the hearing function of the ear.

Benjamin and his four-wheeler accident illustrate just such a case. His mother narrated his story. One day his family, mom, dad Benjamin, and his brother Brandon went shopping for a Massey Ferguson tractor part. However, they ended up buying a four-wheeler instead. The boys 10 and 12 years old had wanted a motorcycle for a long time, but as a safer compromise, mom and dad decided upon a four-wheeler. They set clear rules and parameters for its use; never the less the four-wheeler incident occurred soon after. It was a hot day; mom remembers they had chicken fajitas for lunch. Mom and dad were working in their office behind the house. At that time, Benjamin and Brandon decided they wanted to use the four-wheeler. Brandon wanted to drive, so he was holding the handlebars. He had Benjamin sit in front of him, holding on to the gas tank. Both kids knew the safety rules but decided they were going to do this their way. The boys didn't have their helmets on.

They drove in the tall grass by a rice field with an irregular contour. As they drove, the four-wheeler sank into a depression, and Brandon fell backward. Benjamin remained momentarily on the four-wheeler as it rolled forward, flipping him off onto the ground. Before he could get up, the vehicle then ran over Benjamin's face and head. A neighbor said he saw the four-wheeler spinning but thought that the boys were playing. Mom thought she heard laugher while working in her office.

She came out of the office, and as she got closer, she heard not laughter but crying. She also saw the four-wheeler zoom by with no one on it. Brandon ran towards Mom and yelled, "I didn't mean to kill him." She then saw Benjamin walking towards her. His face was swollen, bloody, and disfigured. She saw track marks of the tires on the side of his face and head. Benjamin said, "my head hurts." In a panic, mom got a towel and a bag of frozen peas to put over Benjamin's head. They all ran and got into the car. Mom remembers that Benjamin said he wanted to go to sleep, but she tried to keep him awake. As mom held Benjamin, she told him, "Jesus loves you, Benjamin." Benjamin said, "I know mom. He is already here."

They arrived at Katy Medical Center, where mom said the Doctor told the family that Benjamin's condition was not right and recommended that they call the pastoral services. At the hospital, mom felt lost and was in a panic. Brandon told Mom that if Benjamin dies, he couldn't live with himself, and he would kill himself. Mom, who is a nurse, was in shock at this point. She remembers going to the restroom sobbing and felt as if she was having a nervous breakdown; she was begging for her son's life. She said that Benjamin never cried. The doctors said that the CAT scan of his head showed he was bleeding and recommended transfer to Texas Children's Hospital in the medical center via an ambulance.

Upon arrival at Texas Children's Hospital Emergency Center, the doctors immediately began helping Benjamin. At this point, they had a 2nd CAT scan done; thankfully, it indicated no further bleeding this time. Mom remembers as the doctors were trying to examine Benjamin; he was calling out to her. Benjamin didn't allow the doctors to poke around in search of his eye and requested that his Mother do it. Mom finally found it. She said it turned out he had cracked his orbit, but his eye was intact.

She said Benjamin had shredded much of his left ear and was missing the top of the ear. He had 40 stitches placed to repair that ear. Mom said one of the doctors told her had he had his helmet on Benjamin might have broken his neck. Benjamin was finally stable and lying in bed. His face was so swollen he couldn't see out of his eyes. There was fluid behind the tissues; both eyes were swollen shut. After they drained some blood, you could finally see "little slits" that were his eyes.

After several days Benjamin was released from the hospital to go home. About two weeks later, mom and Benjamin were at home and talked a bit about the accident. Mom asked Ben, "you know you told me Jesus was with us." Benjamin answered, "no, Mommy, His Angels were there; two of them were in the field. They were calling for me". Mom, thinking that Benjamin was making this up, asked him, "were they dressed in purple?" Benjamin cried and said, "no, Mommy, they were dressed in white and were shiny; they were beautiful." The above is a personal recollection, Benjamin's mother, related to me regarding this frightful accident.

I first saw Benjamin several weeks after the injury. He still had a lot of swelling and bruising on the side of his head. He had a hematoma, which is a pooling of blood in a tissue space. I aspirated this with a large needle and syringe on three occasions a few days apart to get the blood out to speed the healing. The main residual problem was the upper fourth of the helical rim of his left ear was missing. The rest of the ear had healed nicely. We waited until all the injuries had healed before I began the reconstruction of his ear.

Benjamin's pediatrician referred him to me. His mother said she also knew of me from seeing me as one of Marvin Zindler's angels on TV. (Marvin Zindler was a Houston celebrity on ABC channel 13 as a consumer advocate. He would occasionally bring patients to me who could not afford the reconstructive care they needed. The well-known play, the *Best Little Whore House in Texas*, is about Marvin Zindler exposing the Chicken Ranch bordello in La Grange, Texas.)

I reconstructed Benjamin's ear by harvesting cartilage from the concha, which is the concave bowl portion of the ear. I positioned and shaped that cartilage at the absent helical rim.

I then bent the ear down and buried the cartilage beneath a skin flap behind the ear. After two weeks, I cut the flap, releasing the ear with skin from behind the ear, now covering the cartilage, thereby completing the reconstruction. This procedure was successful, and Benjamin obtained the result, shown below. I present a similar reconstruction in greater detail in chapter 6.

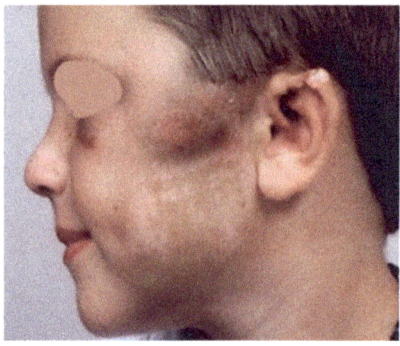 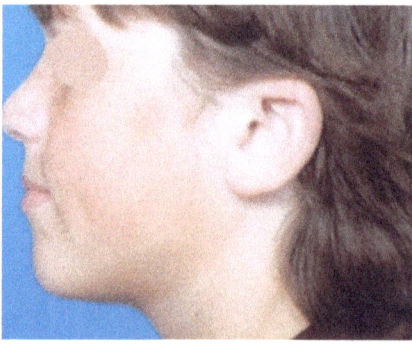

About a year later, he came to the office with his mom, and it was easy to overlook the injury because it was relatively inconspicuous. I found out that he was a model for many magazines and Blue Bell Ice Cream, a local

Texas favorite of mine. Also, last time they visited my office, Benjamin was admiring one of my medical plaques on the wall that included a gavel and asked his Mom, "Mom is he a judge too"? We all got a good chuckle out of that.

The man below, "Leroy," represents another curious reconstructive plastic surgery case resulting from injuries suffered in an automobile accident. I first saw him as pictured below after he survived his significant abdominal injuries and surgical repairs.

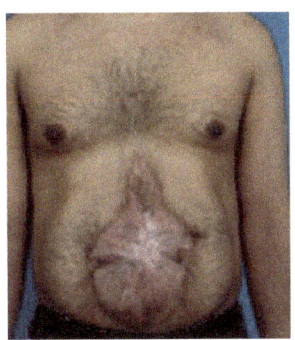

He had two reasons for wanting me to do something to improve the scars of his abdomen. First, of course, he wanted it to look more natural. Because the abdominal wall fascia was intact and stable, he had no functional defect. The second reason was that, because of a fatality associated with the accident, which he allegedly caused, he was to serve time in prison. Undergoing surgery would postpone, at least for a while, his reporting to prison. I performed one procedure for him, which consisted of cutting out the abdominal surface scars (red lines below), and then closing the resultant defect with large abdominal flaps, advanced from each side (green arrows). His result is on the right below. Last I heard, he did have to report to serve his sentence.

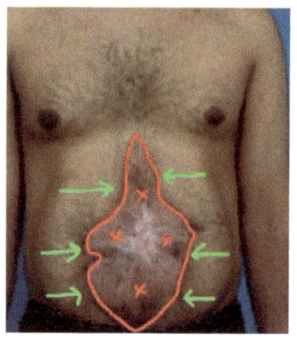 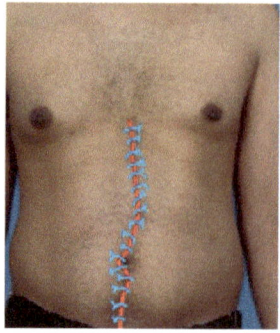 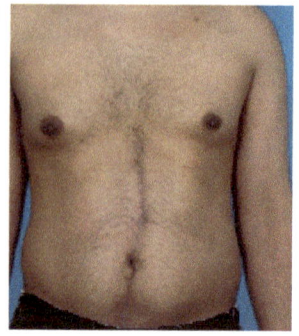

Another example of reconstructive surgery is to rebuild a portion of the nose destroyed by trauma when the patient has no problem breathing but naturally wants to restore a natural appearance.

What is aesthetic surgery?

Aesthetic or cosmetic surgery is performed on typical structures of the body to enhance the patient's appearance. Some indications for aesthetic surgery are aging changes the patient might wish to address with a facelift. Another impetus may be a typical hump on a nose that a patient wants to diminish. Often improved self- esteem results from aesthetic surgery, especially when the patient can articulate precisely their objection. In the example below, "Roger" was "normal" nevertheless, he requested changes to improve his appearance. He was bothered by his prominent nasal hump and wanted it reduced. I believed he had realistic expectations and was an appropriate candidate for rhinoplasty.

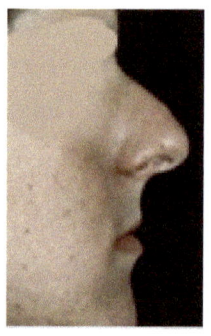 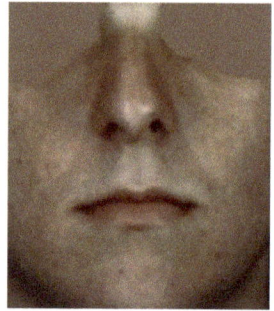

I removed a large amount of cartilage and bone from the bridge of the nose and in-fractured the nasal bones immediately to compensate. His post-operative photos are below. By explicitly addressing the problem about which he was concerned, he was able to obtain his desired result.

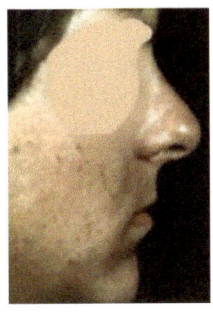 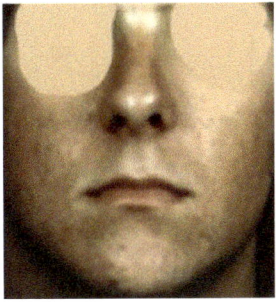

Rhinoplasty was one of my favorite operations. I exhibit abundant examples in chapter 16.

Another "normal" patient sought cosmetic surgery because of aging changes. "Bonnie," pictured below, had particularly loose, wrinkled, and sun-damaged skin, especially in the neck for which she sought improvement.

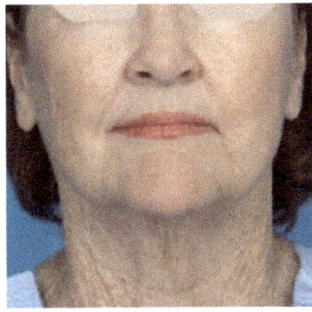 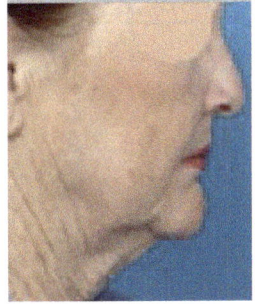

I performed a facelift with a deep tissue plication in the cheeks, which also helped the cheek and jowl areas. The skin tightening and midline neck plication of the platysma muscle has given her the desired more youthful contour in the neck and has dampened the neck rhytids (wrinkles). She was pleased by the changes which "rejuvenated" her face and neck. Sometimes helping grateful aesthetic surgery patients was as satisfying as helping patients with severe deformities. I guess we all respond to being appreciated for our efforts.

The Healing Mission of Plastic Surgery

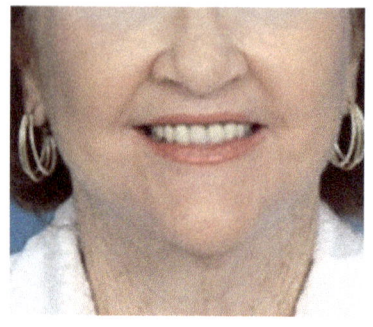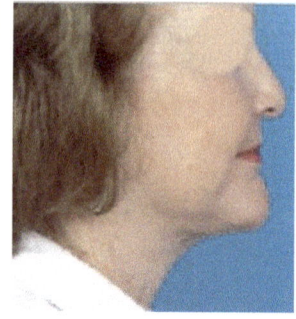

Eyelid surgery to improve appearance, liposuction, augmentation, mammoplasty, and ear pin back procedures (otoplasty) are additional typical aesthetic plastic surgery procedures. As is the case for all plastic surgery, cosmetic surgery is demanding and requires highly scientific, technical, and artistic expertise. It requires careful selection of patients who are realistic in their expectations and can accept improvement without demanding perfection. If these criteria are met, then aesthetic surgery is one of the most satisfying branches of plastic surgery for patients and surgeons alike. However, if surgery is dispensed on-demand by an unqualified or inexpert entrepreneur, it can and has led to many cases of personal tragedy.

There is a certain amount of asymmetry to everyone's face. We have all seen examples of photographs like the ones below in which two right or two left sides of the face are put together as mirror images, demonstrating minor differences in all "normal" faces. In the faces shown below, the center one below is real, while the photo on the right shows two right-sided images, and the picture on the left shows two left-sided images.

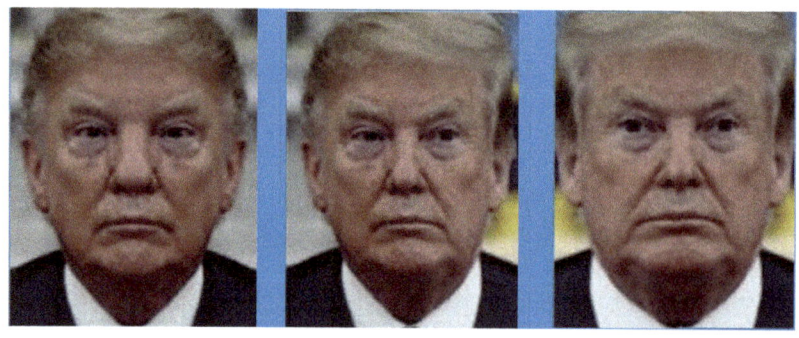

This issue comes up occasionally when a patient wants to address a minor asymmetry surgically, which is ordinarily considered a cosmetic case. The patient may erroneously think that his health insurance policy will cover the procedure as a deformity. Indubitably there are instances in which the asymmetry is so evident that it "crosses the line" from normal variation to deformity. In other cases, the issue might be some disproportion in the face rather than asymmetry. The next exciting case presented later in this chapter illustrates an imbalance in the face, which I addressed as an aesthetic issue rather than a deformity. However, the techniques needed to remedy her situation were indistinguishable from those I have used for the correction of functional and reconstructive cases.

Functional, reconstructive, and aesthetic surgery overlap

Although I have just tried to define it, the distinction between functional, reconstructive, and cosmetic surgery may be unclear in some instances. If looked upon as in set theory, elements of each of the three types overlap with each other. The illustration below indicates that some surgeries are obviously and fundamentally either aesthetic, functional, or reconstructive, but there are many instances of overlap.

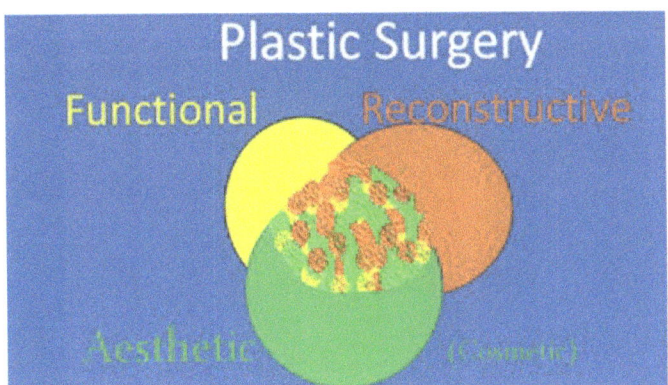

So, there are several combinations: (F), (R), (A), (F+R), (F+A), (R+A), (A+F+R). Many of the procedures depicted throughout this book are difficult to categorize singularly.

One day I received a referral from my plastic surgery partner. "Amy" was a 16-year-old young lady who felt unattractive and wanted to do something to look better. "Amy," a lovely ingenue, a good student, and an accomplished pianist thought she might need a rhinoplasty because she judged her nose was too prominent. It seemed that although a rhinoplasty might benefit her, the issues were more fundamental.

Although she was beautiful on the inside, her outward appearance and reticent demeanor did not proportionately reflect that beauty. She presented with a gummy smile, too much tooth showing at rest, straining to close her lips, all signs of a disproportionately long midface. She had been treated with orthodontic braces for five years and had a healthy bite (occlusion). I would have made her a little more attractive if I had done a rhinoplasty as she thought she wanted. However, I made the diagnosis of "Long Face Syndrome," which is a variation of normal, in which the mid-face grows excessively in the vertical dimension.

Making the correct diagnosis gave me a much better chance of formulating an appropriate surgical plan. Below are three preoperative views. There are two frontal views, one with her mouth relaxed and one with her mouth closed, as well as a lateral image. Hypertrophy of the mentalis muscle between the lower lip and the chin presents as a rounded mound in the middle photo because of the strain needed to close her lips.

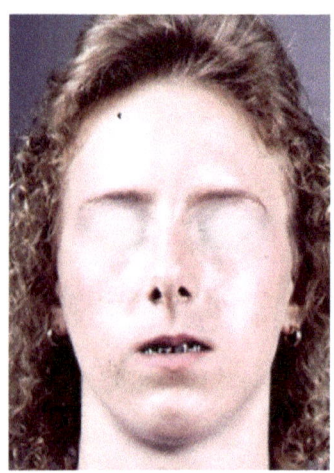
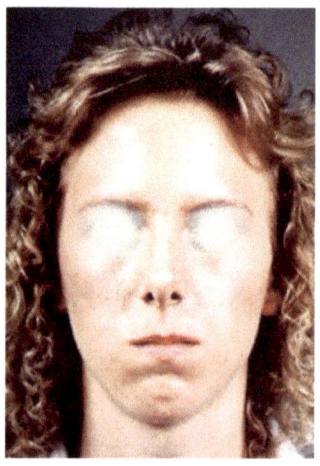
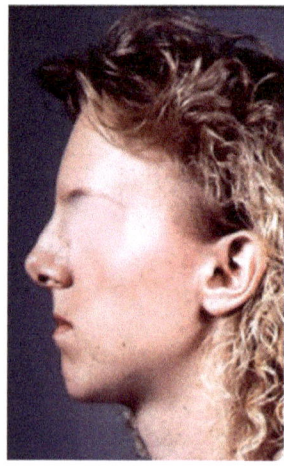

"Amy" had a "normal" appearance but had a facial disproportion, which I thought I could address to give a dramatic aesthetic improvement. I planned an operation called a Le Fort I. I planned to cut the bone of the midface above the teeth and below the eyes and nose to free the upper jaw segment, which I could then move in various directions for different effects. In her case, I wanted to impact the midface upward to shorten the face.

When someone comes in thinking they need a relatively small operation like rhinoplasty and I begin talking about cutting across their whole facial skeleton, there needs to be a lot of explanation and often multiple office visits. If the patient is a minor, the parents, as well as the patient, must be fully informed as to the risks benefits and alternatives of the proposed procedure. Even this can be tricky as some patients want a lot of detailed information, and others want the general picture without the delineation of every potential complication. This patient and her parents were quite reasonable.

I studied her lateral cephalometric - x-rays preoperatively. I then altered her cephalometric drawings to help predict the outcome based on the movement of the upper jaw. Changing the underlying bone structure would cause various changes in the soft tissues that we could anticipate.

I judged that the maximum benefit correlated with 8 mm of upward movement. Therefore, I planned to remove an 8 mm segment of bone from the mid-face, as illustrated in red in the middle picture below, allowing the upper jaw to move upwards, as shown by the blue arrows. A more balanced facial configuration would result. The lower jaw would also rotate upward and a little forward, as shown by the green arrow; this would make the chin slightly more prominent. In preparation for the surgery, I used the dental models supplied by her orthodontist and place them on an articulator. Fabrication of an acrylic bite wafer as a guide and mock surgery on these dental models helped assure that her teeth would fit together correctly after repositioning the maxilla (the upper jaw).

The Healing Mission of Plastic Surgery

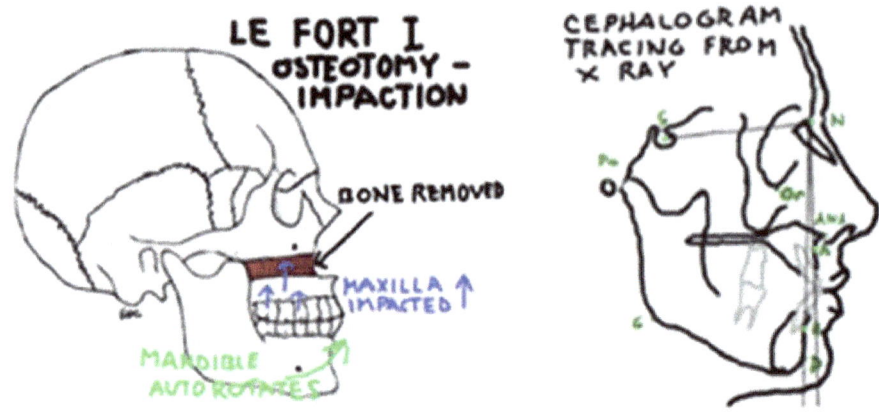
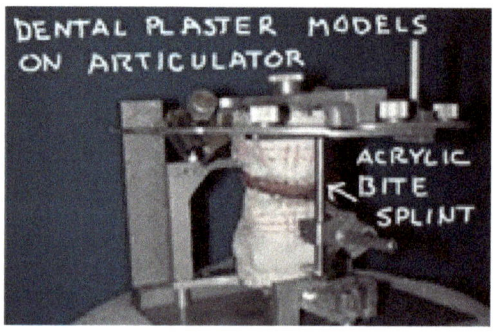
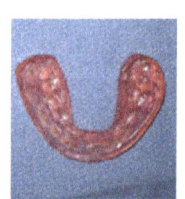

As the day of her surgery at St Joseph Hospital arrived, everyone was excited and ready. I saw Amy in the surgery holding area to identify her as the proper patient for the scheduled procedure. I marked an incision on the scalp, where I would later take bone grafts from the skull. Her mother and father said well wishes. They were understandably a little nervous as she was rolled away toward the operating room. On the other hand, Amy kept what anxiety she had hidden below the surface.

The anesthesiologist started an IV and gave her medicine to go to sleep. He then inserted a breathing tube through the nose into the trachea as it was necessary to keep the mouth free for the surgery. The anesthetic tube was secured, and the patient's position on the table cheeked. The circulating nurse then prepped for the procedure by washing the patient's face and scalp with an antiseptic solution. Meanwhile, my plastic surgery resident assistant and I washed our hands at the scrub sink right outside, operating room # 14, my standard venue. Then the surgical tech helped us into our gowns and gloves. We draped the patient with sterile sheets, and the surgical tech brought the instruments close to the operating table on her Mayo stand.

I first used an ink marker to plan the incisions and then injected a solution containing epinephrine to help minimize the bleeding. The resident assistant used retractors to expose the area under the upper lip. Finally, after several weeks of planning and preparation, I made the first incision in the sulcus under the right upper lip down to the bone. I lifted all the soft tissues from the front surface of the midface and cheek area. I then exposed the pyriform aperture, which is the opening in the facial skeleton for the nose. I controlled bleeding with an electric coagulator. The same exposure was then made on the left side of the facial bones as well. Next, I used a specific saw blade to cut through the midface from the nasal opening through the maxillary sinuses. I did the same on both sides. Using a chisel, I then separated the nasal septum from the maxilla. (upper jaw).

Now the lower facial bones were only connected to the base of the skull behind the last molars. Using a special osteotome or modified bone cutting chisel, I working around behind the last molars and made the final bone cuts on each side. This final bone separation is always a little anxiety-producing because of the potential for significant bleeding there, which could be difficult to stop because of limited access and visibility. Everything went well with slight bleeding. The next maneuver was pushing down on the upper jaw from above so that it would have complete bony separation from the rest of the face and base of the skull posteriorly.

This action often creates a cracking sound, which may be disturbing to the uninitiated. This maneuver is much more difficult in cleft palate patients because of scar tissue from previous palate surgery. Soft tissue connections preserve the blood supply to the maxilla. After removing any small bony interferences, I moved the maxilla upward to shorten the face vertically. The drawing on the left below indicates two parallel cuts through the walls of the maxillary sinuses and nasal septum, removing approximately 8 mm of bone height. On the right, I will close the gap created by removal of the bone between the two parallel cuts by impacting the lower segment of the mobilized maxilla superiorly. The blue arrows point out the upward movement of the maxilla, which obliterates the gap.

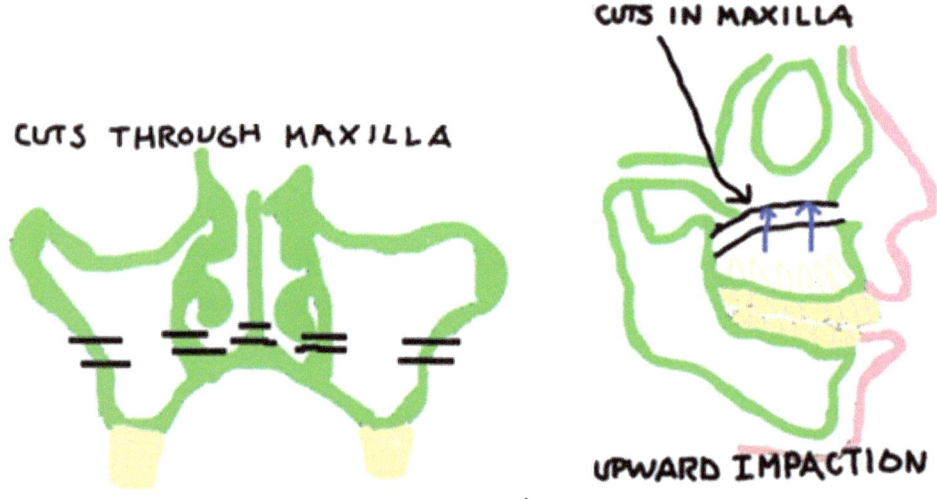

The intraoperative photo below is a view with the upper lip retracted upward. I then placed the acrylic splint, pointed out by the purple arrow below, in place with small wires to the orthodontic bands of the upper teeth and brought the lower jaw into position with elastic bands so that the teeth fit correctly into the splint. While holding the maxillary bone segment in place, I firmly secured the bone of the maxilla in its new position. I accomplished this by drilling holes in the bones and fastening them together with small titanium plates and screws pointed out by the green arrows below.

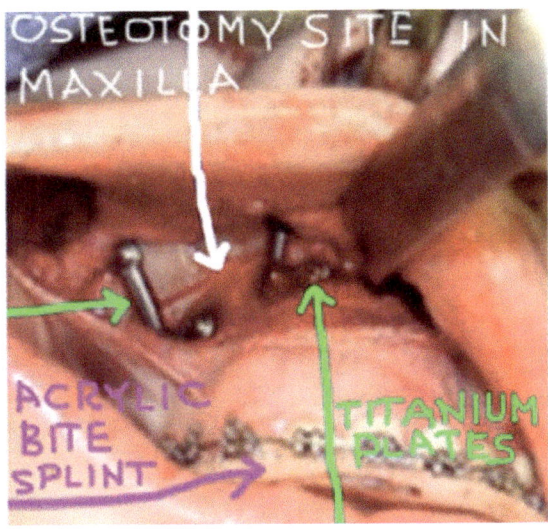

I then removed the elastics to see if the bite was still good. Opening and then closing the lower jaw placed the teeth right into the splint, so I knew the position was correct.

In cases like this, it is often helpful to place bone grafts along the osteotomy sites to aid in healing but primarily to build up the cheeks to make them a little more prominent. Harvesting the bone from the skull is less painful than the more common method of taking bone from the hip. The skull is composed of three layers with two hard cortical or compact layers and a single softer marrow layer between them. In the technique used in "Amy's" case, I removed the hard, outer layer leaving the brain protected by hard bone and with the potential for some regeneration of bone. The first photo below demonstrates this technique of obtaining outer (external) table cranial grafts on a dry skull specimen. The following drawing below illustrates the three layers composing the cranial bone, the compact external layer, the middle softer diploe layer, and the dense inner table.

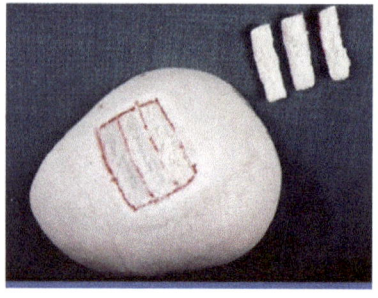 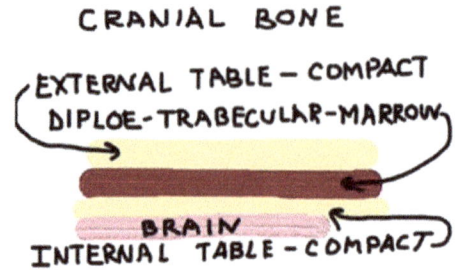

The two drawings below depict this technique. The red lines indicate cuts through the outer table into the diploe; the compact internal table remains to protect the brain. I have illustrated the harvested graft on the right.

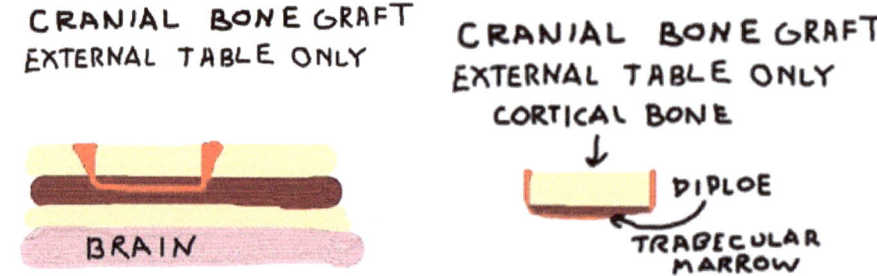

To utilize this method, I made an incision through the scalp down to the bone and exposed the area of skull needed. I used an electric burr to outline the necessary pieces. I removed the grafts with a chisel, carefully protecting the brain by remaining in the diploe layer. In the first photo below, I have pulled aside the scalp and am harvesting outer cranial table bone grafts, first outlining them with a drill down to the diploe. The second photo shows three of these large grafts turned over, ready to be shaped for use. the area of skull needed

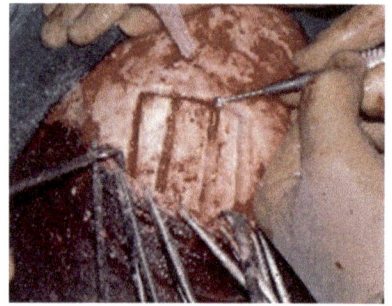 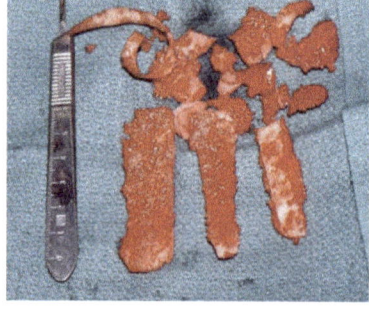

"Amy's" was a significant operation done under general anesthesia. She remained in the hospital for two nights. We kept rubber bands between

her upper and lower teeth for a few days to guide the bite. Within a week or so, the results were evident. The operation was a great success. The gummy smile was gone, her lip seal was better, the chin projected a little more, and she had generally improved aesthetics. Her parents said the surgery made an incredible difference for their daughter. One can practically discern the psychological benefit to this young lady from her postoperative photographs. I was amazed by the amount of benefit she obtained from this operation. Below are three postoperative views, first with mouth open and then with mouth closed after shortening the midface surgically. The lateral postoperative view shows some profile improvement, although nothing was done directly to the nose or the chin. Compare with her preoperative views above on page 36.

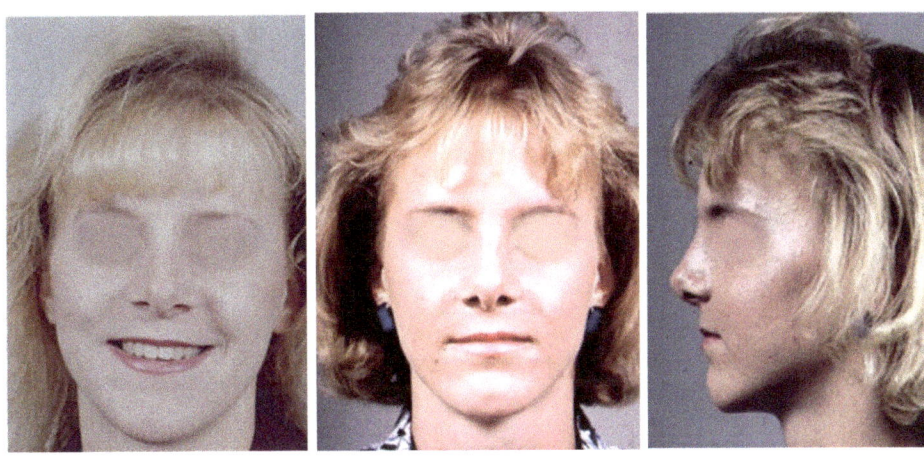

So, this young patient had an aesthetic operation that utilized several standard reconstructive techniques.

Functional, reconstructive, aesthetic continuum

The difference between functional and reconstructive and cosmetic surgery may also be indistinct in other ways. For example, a patient with a severe cleft lip and palate deformity may have initial operations that improve functions such as speech, chewing, and swallowing. However, although he may function normally, he may still have residual deformities, which leave his appearance abnormal.

Additional plastic surgery may correct these defects. Addressing such remaining distorted structures to attempt to obtain normality would be reconstructive, not functional, or cosmetic. At the same time, however, some secondary surgery may not only make the patient look better but also function better. An example is that nasal surgery to make the nose more symmetrical may also allow for improved breathing or jaw surgery to proportion the face may also improve the bite and, therefore, functionally improve mastication.

The following unique case mixes functional surgery (removal of a facial tumor), reconstruction of the defect (surgery on abnormal structures), and cosmetic surgery (for opposite side symmetry). An oncologic surgeon colleague referred a middle-aged lady to me. He wanted me to reconstruct a facial defect he was going to create when he removed a cheek melanoma. It was evident that the wound he caused by excision of her melanoma would be significant. It would require substantial tightening the left side of her face to obtain closure. I told her we might want to consider doing something on the opposite side for symmetry. She agreed, and so we proceeded with a plan to operate on both sides of her face. The first photo below shows the left cheek melanoma the oncologic surgeon was to remove. The second photo is after he has removed the tumor. The third photo is after I have partially closed the wound to help me see what additional adjustments would give the best result.

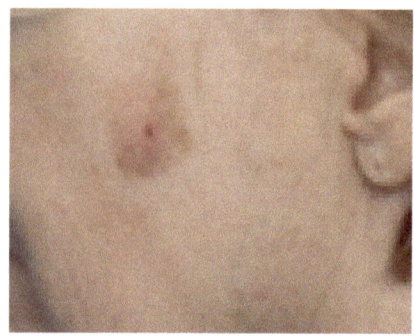 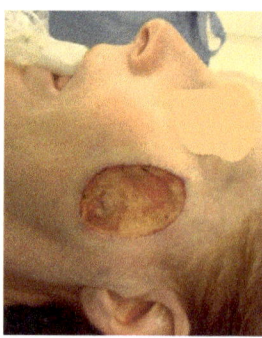 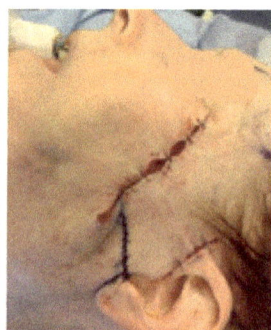

The picture below shows the final closure of the opening left by the excision of the lesion. The repair also produced a facelift type tightening. Concurrently I also did a lateral brow lift; the incision is at the frontal hairline. The photo on the right shows the patient after a compensatory facelift and lateral brow lift on the right side done for symmetry.

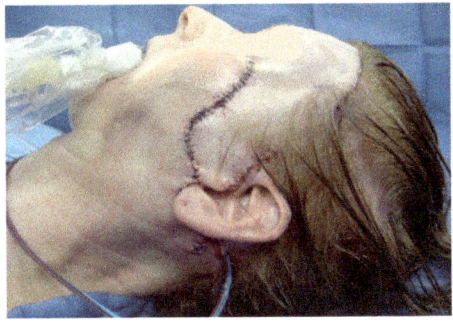 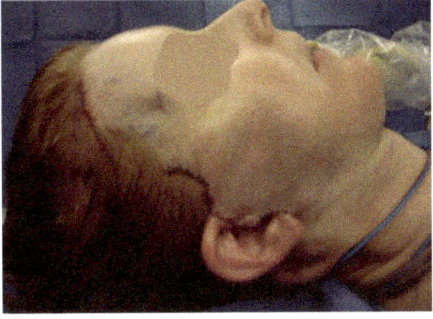

Below are her pre and post-operatively photos. I was pleased with her result in this unusual case, which had elements of functional, reconstructive, and aesthetic plastic surgery.

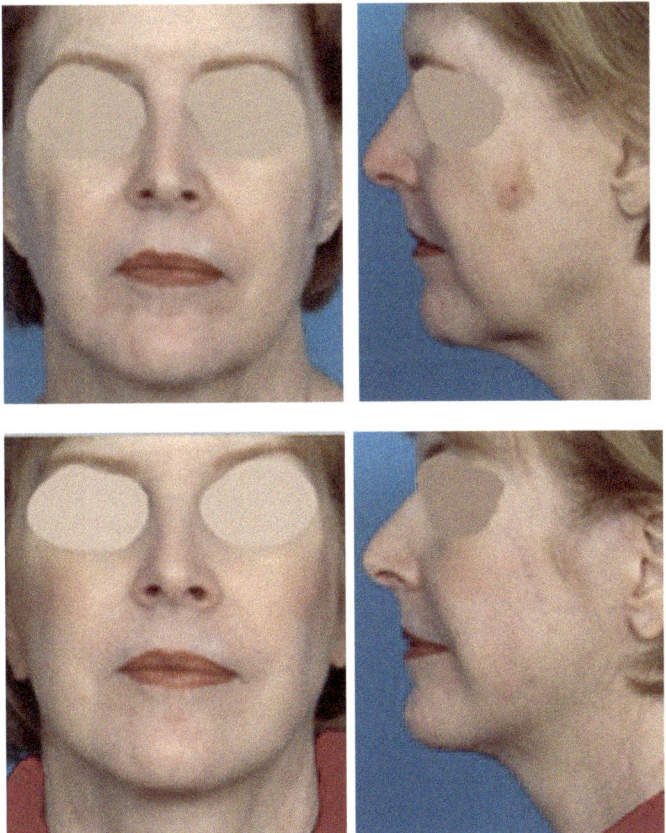

Chapter 2

Self - Image

Why do patients go to doctors? It seems to me they go to seek relief of something disagreeable. It might be because of pain; sometimes, it is a functional disorder; perchance, it is something about their body image, causing distress. Plastic surgeons are often called upon to address such discomforts. Because plastic surgery deals with psychological beings, some interesting interactions do occur. Every plastic surgeon must be an amateur psychiatrist of sorts even though he may not have formal training in that field.

Descartes' universal doubt leads to his assertion that only one thing cannot be doubted, doubt itself. So, he gives us the succinct "cogito ergo sum." "I think therefore I am" is a kind of recognition that human existence is entwined in self- awareness. The self - image probably begins in some nascent way even before we are born. I feel, therefore, I am. I hear, therefore, I am. I taste, therefore, I am. I smell, therefore I am. I see? We require a self- image to differentiate ourselves from non- self, and others. The better we understand and accept ourselves, the better we can relate satisfactorily to others.

Since we are beings of body, mind, and spirit, this self - concept, this feeling of personal identity must include an image of our own body. To varying degrees, body image is essential to us all. We appreciate our physical characteristics with different levels of accuracy through our mental picture of our bodies. Our attitude toward our body may reflect past experiences, some of which we are not consciously aware. By listening to each patient's description of his or her physical concerns and using photos of the patient to determine how the patient views himself or herself, it is often possible to learn to what extent the patient's self - perception is realistic or distorted.

There is no clear line of demarcation between normal and abnormal appearance. Much depends on one's psyche, peer pressure, social demands, cultural context, and even current fashion. The person who is embarrassed about a deformity may be motivated to seek improvement to become inconspicuous and more accepted as he tries to find his way in this sometimes, churlish world. The movie star or model archetype represents a small percentage of the population. Stunning beauty is rare. Normal is common. Even natural aging signs are becoming less and less tolerated as youthfulness becomes associated with ability. Thus, erroneously," bags under the eyes" become a sign of debauchery; a small chin becomes incorrectly a sign of "weak character," a flat or crooked nose inaptly signifies a pugnacious individual, while prominent ears may mistakenly signify someone with limited mental capacity.

I saw the occasional captious narcissist who acted like they were the only creature of consequence in the universe. However, vanity, the desire to be more beautiful than others, or frivolous self-indulgence is not usually the driving force for plastic surgery. But instead, a desire to be accepted and unmolested is often the impetus. "Your ears stick out" or "you have a big nose" are familiar phrases that some people never want to hear again. Some are better able to handle deformities of appearance than others. This capacity pertains both to patients and parents of children with deformities. I remember a patient I first saw as an infant with severe facial abnormalities. I recognized the loving facial expressions which radiated from her mother. She obviously could see past the external appearance to that interior beauty of the soul of which Pope Pius XII spoke in the earlier quotation. Would surgical intervention help that inner beauty to reveal itself?

A Mother's Love

"Beauty is truth, truth beauty, that is all ye know on earth, and all ye need to know." This quote from John Keats's poem, "Ode on a Grecian Urn," reminds me of the profound love demonstrated by the mother of one of my patients. "Rebecca" was born with a severe congenital deformity of

The Healing Mission of Plastic Surgery

the face and skull. These included a frontal encephalocele, with an abnormal opening in the forehead and upper face, which allowed protrusion of intracranial contents. She also had three rare clefts through the face: one through the right upper lip, one through the right side of the nose, and one through the right orbital area. She also had a vestigial but duplicated lacrimal apparatus in front of the right eye. Also, she had a complete cleft of the palate. Her mother was able to see past these severe deformities and appreciate Rebecca's true beauty as a child of God. Her motherly love, attention, and support were with this child throughout her ordeal of multiple reconstructive surgeries over many years.

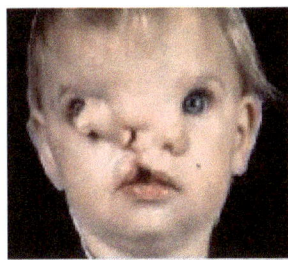

This patient was seen in our clinic by the visiting craniofacial surgeon Dr. Paul Tessier. (See chapter 10) For more than 20 years, she underwent multiple surgeries. Dr. Tessier operated on her four times during his usual yearly visit to Houston from Paris. She was initially a patient of my partner Dr. Raymond Brauer. He worked on her multiple times. After his retirement and when Dr. Tessier no longer visited Houston, I "finished" her reconstruction by operating on her on two more occasions.

Although each step of the way had been an improvement for "Rebecca," there is always a significant price of physical and psychological discomfort for the individual and family, loss of time, not to mention the financial burdens. Rebecca represents the type of case for which there is no set endpoint. We could continue to recommend possible surgeries for improvements in her situation as long as she is willing to accept the risk-benefit ratio for that procedure. Probably due in large part to the beautiful, supportive care of her mother and other family members, she became a very well- adjusted young woman, working full-time and maintaining appropriate inter-personnel relationships.

The following pictures illustrate the last operation I performed for her. It involved surgery on the jaw, eyelids, and nose. The first picture is the preoperative view before the last operation. The second photo shows a cut I made across chin bone. The third picture is a drawing of the bone I moved forward and up.

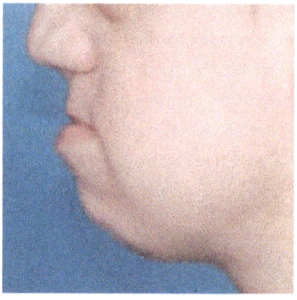 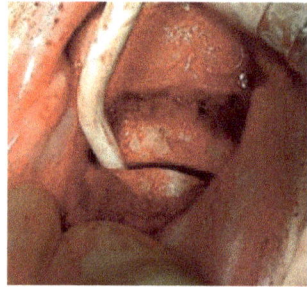 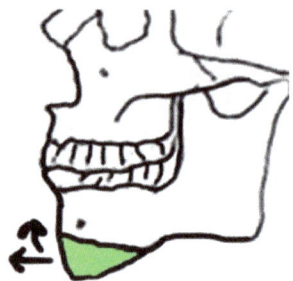

The illustration below illustrates the chin in its new advanced position. I secured the repositioned bony segment with a plate and screws, as shown in the middle picture. The final picture below shows the lower face profile view after my last operation on "Rebecca."

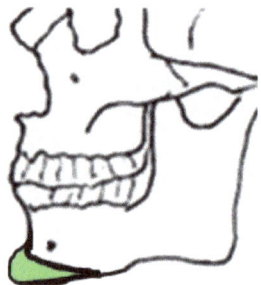 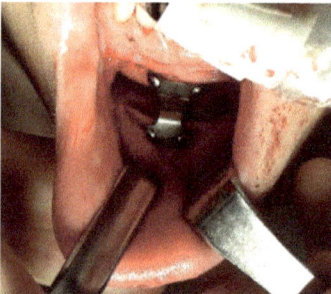 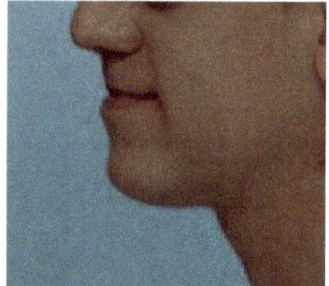

The three photographs below show a revision of her entirely reconstructed nose using a cartilage graft to elevate the nasal tip and to define the columella better. This surgery also helped to open the right nostril a little.

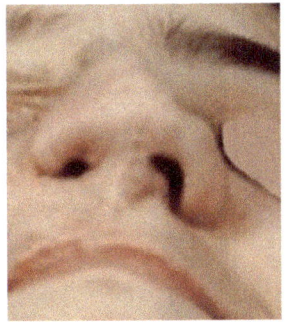 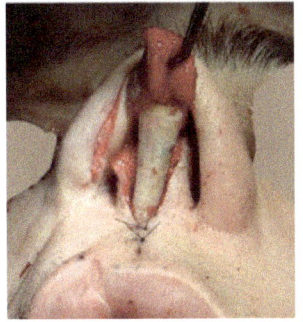 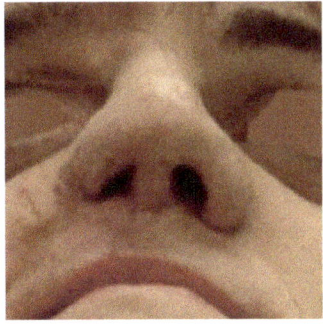

The problem which brought this reluctant patient in to see me for her last operation was that she had developed a mass of the right lower eyelid. This cystic mass grew from a remnant of the abnormal lacrimal system with which she was born. I removed this cyst outlined in yellow in the first photo below. I then placed a drainage tube from the eyelid punctum into the nasal cavity to reconstitute a tear drainage system. The postoperative result is on the right below.

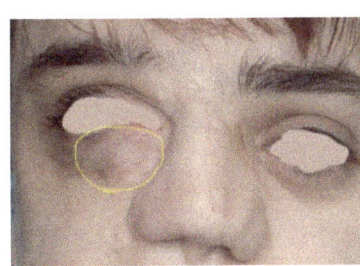 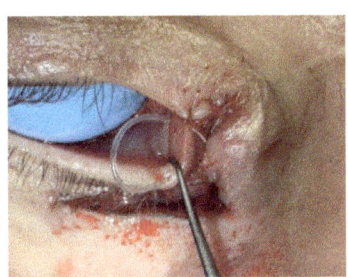 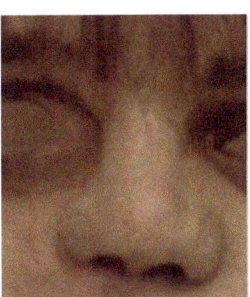

Through multiple operations, by Dr. Tessier, Dr. Brauer, and lastly, by me, she went from having a severely distorted face to one close to the range of normal variation.

I feel sure that her self-esteem much benefited from her mother's radiating love and support throughout the many stages of her reconstructive saga.

A new profile

This 20 something psychologically stable secretary felt her nose was too large for a face and that her chin was too weak on profile. She sought to act straightforwardly on her perceptions. After consultation and making recommendations to her, I performed a rhinoplasty and chin augmentation with a silicone chin implant. These procedures corrected her perceived problems, and she was happy with the result and more content with her body image and self-image. The two photos on the left are before, and the two on the right are after.

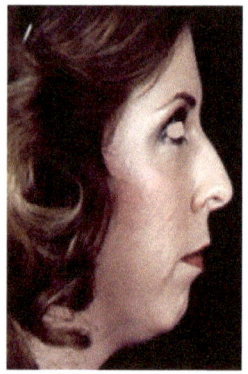 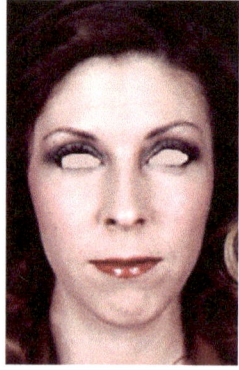 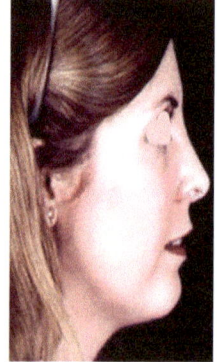 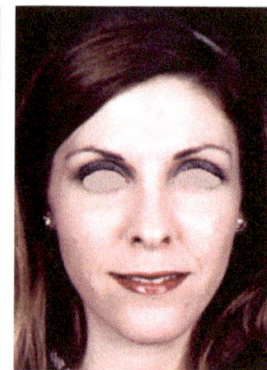

Most patients who seek plastic surgery are psychologically healthy. If surgery is done and is successful, the patients' sense of deformity is reduced or lost, and they gain a more robust feeling of physical integrity and acceptability. There is an improved body image, with increased self-esteem. Patients may now enjoy fewer emotional barriers in relationships with others and feel purged of anxiety. Being happier, they sometimes even state they are "proud" of their surgery.

Malocclusion and facial asymmetry

This teenager below presented with malocclusion and asymmetry of the lower face. The midline curved towards his left, as seen in the preoperative photos. He has a malocclusion with his upper teeth behind the lower teeth and a slant of the occlusal plane from low right to high left.

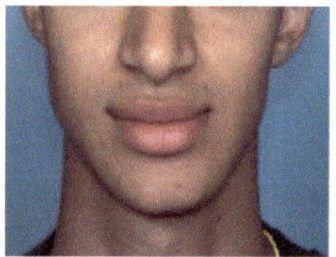 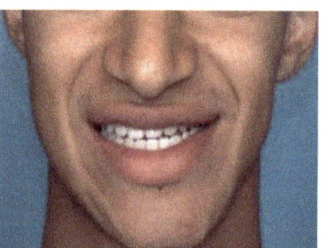 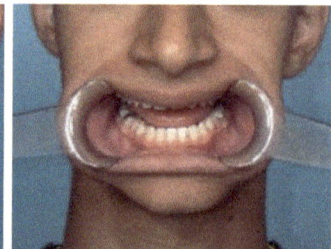

His profile is below. The middle picture shows a face bow with an orientation to the patient's ear canals and intraoral bite plate to allow proper planning of the movement of the bone of the jaw and midface. Model surgery and splint fabrication, done on the articulator, assured predictability of the operative results. An intermediate splint, as well as a final splint, is needed when repositioning both the upper and lower jaws.

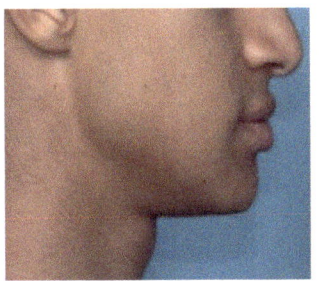 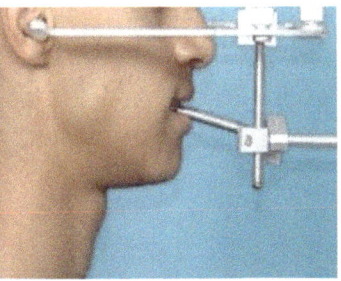 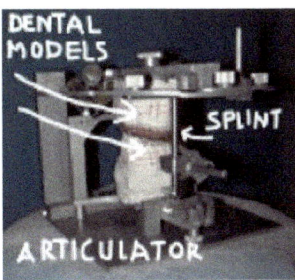

The first picture below shows osteotomies or bone cuts on the lower jaw and the maxilla. (black). I rotated the maxilla on the shorter left side down., and I turned the mandible from left to right. With the splint as a guide, I placed the teeth into their new occlusion.

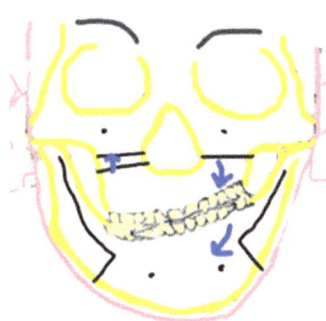 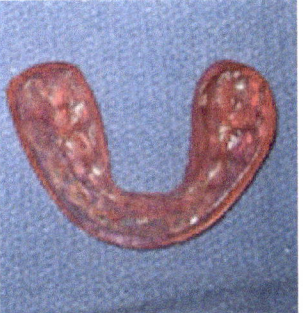 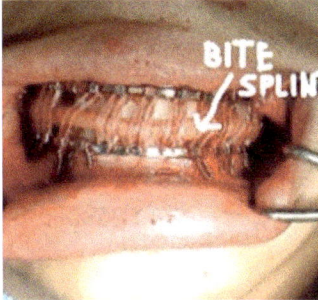

The jaws are realigned and secured in their new proper position with plates and screws made of titanium. The rubber bands holding the jaws in occlusion may remain from a couple of days to a few weeks depending on the situation.

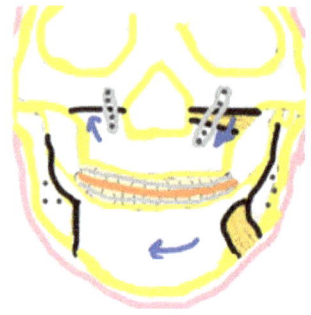 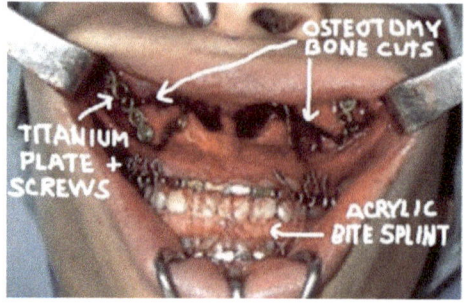

This operation resulted in the correction of the malocclusion and improvement in the lower facial symmetry.

The post-op results are below.

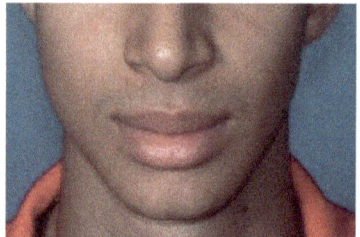 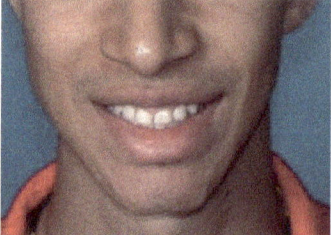 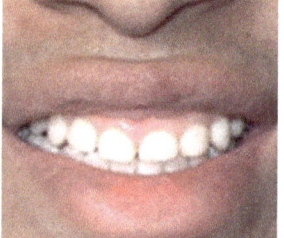

New Chin

"Pete," a 22-year-old emergency room technician, came to see me at the urging of an anesthesiologist who knew him because she sometimes worked in the same suburban hospital. She had noted that he was very self-conscious about his appearance was rather shy and somewhat withdrawn. "Pete's" preoperative condition with asymmetric underdevelopment of the lower jaw and malocclusion is demonstrated below.

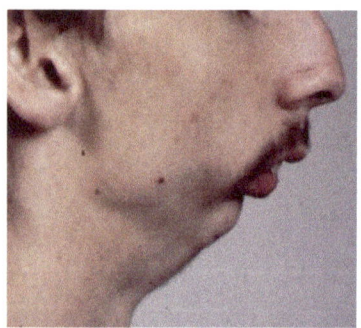 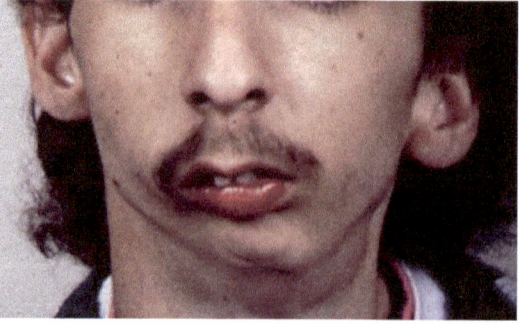

On examination, I noted he had an underdeveloped lower jaw, which was considerably more prominent on the left than the right side. He had a malocclusion with the lower teeth coming together, markedly behind the upper teeth. We arrange to get some x-rays and also to have him come to our facial reconstruction clinic. There he was evaluated by our orthodontist and our speech therapist. After completion of the workup, I decided he would benefit most from a mandibular distraction technique, as introduced by Dr. Joseph McCarthy. I show this technique diagrammatically below. The purple line represents cuts made in the lower jaw bone cortex but sparing nerves that run through the bone. The metallic pins on either side of the bony cut are attached to an external bar that can be adjusted to spread apart the two segments of the jaw on either side. The distraction is very slow so that as the bone spreads apart, new bone (red) will form in the space. In this way, the jaw bone can be elongated.

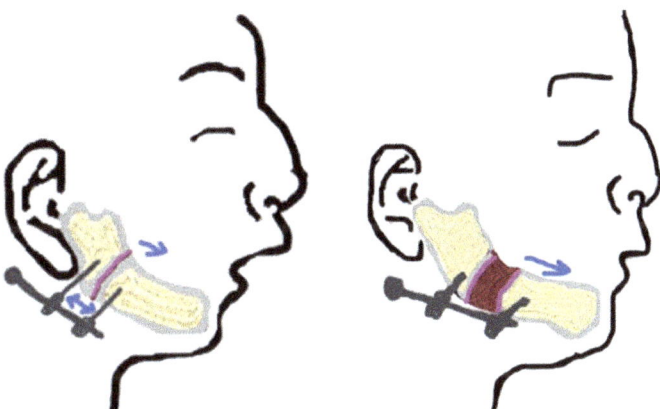

As I evaluated him for surgery, it was clear that it would not be easy to place an anesthetic tube through his mouth into his windpipe. Therefore, a somewhat sophisticated technique using a flexible fiber-optic tube was used by the anesthesiologist to guide the anesthetic tube into the trachea so that the surgery could begin. The operation itself went quite smoothly as I made cuts in the lower jaw bone via incisions made inside the mouth. I inserted metal pins as planned and applied the external distraction device to them. Because of the specialized equipment needed by the anesthesiologist to insert the breathing tube, we decided to remove it when we were still in the operating room to be sure that our patient could breathe well without it.

When the anesthesiologist removed the tube, "Jim" did seem to have quite a bit of difficulty breathing. We, therefore, felt it necessary to put a temporary breathing tube directly through the skin into the windpipe. This tracheostomy assured our patient could breathe well during the recovery phase of the surgery. Although this was unpleasant for the patient, it was temporary and necessary for his safety. Several days later, when his swelling had subsided, I ordered the breathing tube removed from his neck. He immediately began to breathe normally.

He was able to leave the hospital a couple of days after his surgery. About a week later, in the office, we began the distraction process. We instructed our very cooperative patient on how to use a special small wrench to make incremental turns to spread the pins apart. He did this daily, and we checked him back in the office every week. This process went on for six or eight weeks. New bone was being made naturally by the body to fill in the gap produced by the distraction device. We lengthened the bone about 35 mm on the right and about 31 mm on the left to obtain the optimum position.

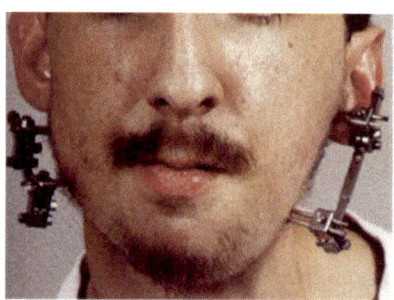
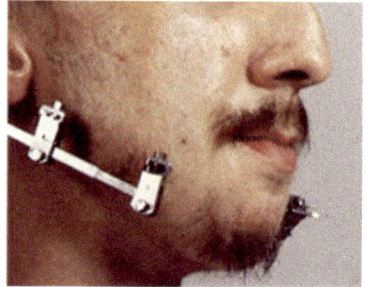

We then left the device in place for an additional couple of months to allow for complete healing and solidification of the bone so the result would be stable. I then removed the external device as a minor office procedure with local anesthesia. "Jim's" appearance improved significantly over his preoperative condition (page 55), and his speech became more intelligible. He was able to live much more comfortably, as eating was more natural. He was happy with and "proud" of his surgery. His self- image was undoubtedly improved. He declined surgery on his nose and other refinement procedures, which I recommended for him. His final result is below. His improved self- image was a boost to his general demeanor and his ability to interact with his associates.

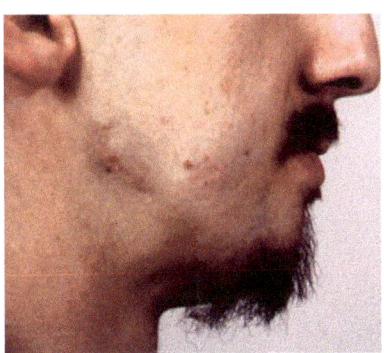 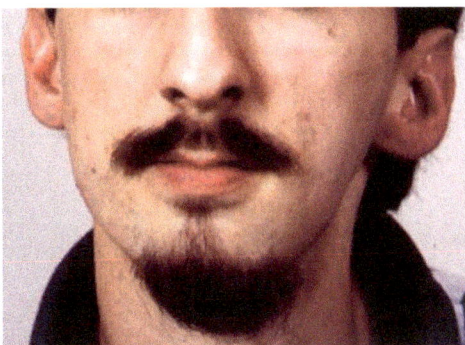

A person who seeks surgery to meet the desires of others or to solve difficulties in interpersonal relationships is a weak candidate. The young woman who comes for breast augmentation because her boyfriend is going to leave her deserves extra screening and perhaps should be discouraged from rushing to surgery. An insecure individual who feels inadequate is likely to be dissatisfied with the result of cosmetic surgery.

I may ask questions such as, "why surgery now?". "What do you expect the surgery to accomplish?" The severity of any psychological anxiety does not necessarily correlate with the magnitude of the deformity, nor is any amelioration directly proportional to the improvement accomplished by surgery. Cultural aspects complicate the picture. Poor candidates are neurotics who retreat behind a deformity or who attribute all of their troubles to it. The deformity may seem minor to an impartial observer. However, to such a patient, the deformity may assume a magnitude out of proportion to reality. The successful repair of even major traumatic or congenital malformations is not necessarily curative. Deeply embedded psychological disturbances may persist.

Patient selection is so important. How can one predict who will benefit the most and whether the risk is worthwhile at the same time weeding out the psychologically unstable? Indeed, as a surgeon, I believe that experience and common- sense judgment covers most situations. However, when red flags are waving, it may be prudent to send a patient to a psychiatrist or refuse to operate.

Even though we teach our children not to judge a book by its cover, the physically attractive person is just that; attractive. It seems to be part of human nature to move toward the beautiful and away from the ugly. Although certainly not universal, many physically attractive individuals tend to have higher self- esteem and a better sense of well-being than their more homely counterparts. Cultural factors complicate the picture. As in *Molly Brawn,* "beauty is in the eye of the beholder." At times adornment can take a turn toward mutilation. In our society, anything other than pierced ear lobes for earrings would have once been considered excessive. Now on our streets and in our stores and restaurants, we see noses or lips pierced, multiply pierced ears, even tongues pierced and occasionally exposed pierced belly buttons. My old Latin teacher might say "De gustibus non disputandum est" (there is no accounting for taste). In primitive cultures, scarification of the skin in set patterns has been a method of adornment. Distortion of lips or ear lobes by extraordinary stretching of the tissue with successively larger devices was an adornment technique of some African and South American tribes. Incidentally, now a standard modality in reconstructive surgery is tissue expansion, which takes advantage of the exact principles that were used by these primitive tribes.

"Suzzy" was born with the absence of a large portion of her scalp and cranial bone, a rare condition called congenital aplasia cutis. There was only a fibrous covering of the brain to protect it. Apparently, at birth, the sagittal sinus, a large blood vessel of the brain, was exposed to the air and in danger of causing severe bleeding and death. Initial attempts to cover the defect by shifting adjacent scalp tissue only partially repaired the skin defect as part of the flap skin died. A second attempt to elevate more adjacent scalp skin to cover the area failed and became necrotic.

At that point, when she was three months old, she was transferred to the neurosurgical service of our hospital, and Dr. Hirshberg referred the patient to me. The neurosurgeon took her to the operating room for the removal of dead flap tissue. At that same time, I harvested and placed skin grafts on the dura lining of the brain to obtain healing. At this point, as in the photographs below, there was no longer any open wound of the scalp. However, there was a large central area lacking bone. There was only the skin graft on the dura, a fibrous layer that covers of the brain. Of course, these skin grafted areas had no hair.

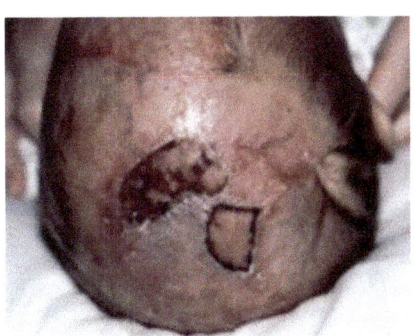 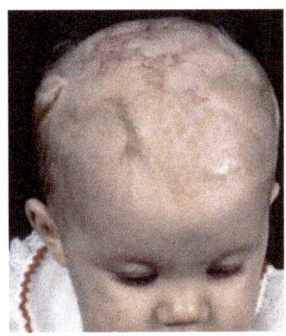

Without any bony protection for the brain, the parents had to be particularly protective of the child. They helped customize her protective headgear. The child was left alone for a couple of years to allow her to grow. Interestingly sufficient bone was formed from the underlying dura so that I never had to graft any bone.

Now the reason for reconstruction was to restore hair to the scalp and to make the skin more durable. After consulting with the parents, I decided to use what was then a new method of reconstruction called the tissue expansion technique. This method involved placing special silicone balloons under the portion of the remaining healthy hair-bearing scalp. Then weekly, I slowly added fluid to this balloon so that it would stretch the scalp. Later I excised sections of the previous skin grafted non-hair bearing areas, and I pulled the newly expanded hair-bearing scalp over to replace the skin grafted areas. I repeated this sequence several times. The first picture below shows the starting condition before tissue expansion. The second photo shows an example of a non-inflated tissue expander balloon.

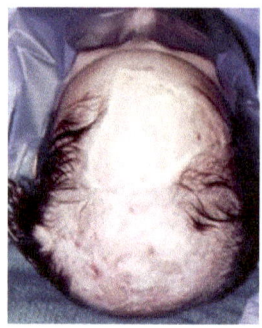 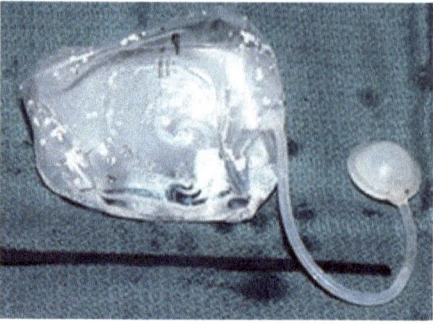

Below, I show several intermediate photos after partial excision of the non-hair bearing areas of the scalp. The last picture below shows the tissue expander before removal after the completion of the final stage.

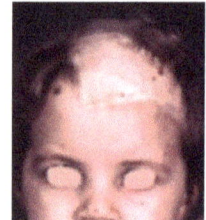 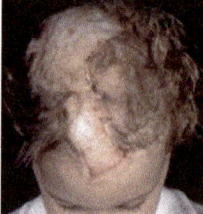 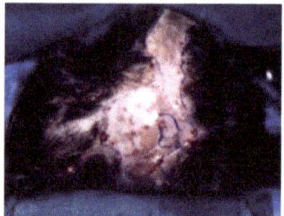 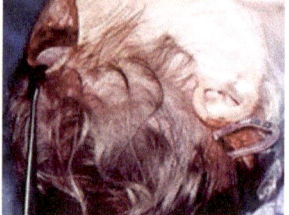

Below are photos of the final result after multiple expansions and stretching of the remaining scalp. This young patient was very much a trooper throughout this sometimes, painful ordeal. I remember her mother and father being very cooperative, helpful, and supportive during this protracted reconstructive program. We were all pleased by the results and happy to hold in reserve any further procedures. I believe the reconstruction, which gave this child the result shown, likely prevented significant body image problems that might have come up by the age she was in these final pictures.

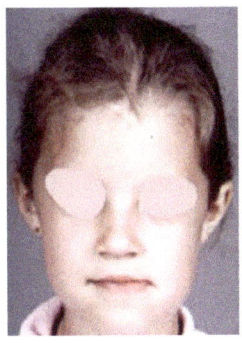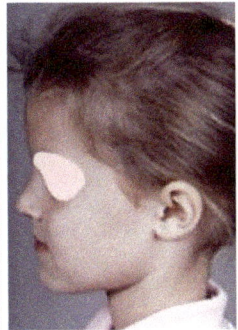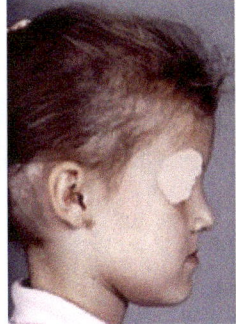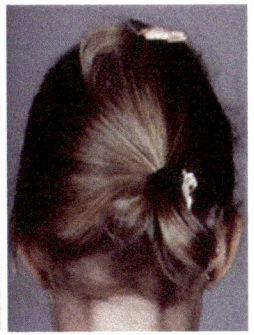

Rhinoplasty

The patient below "Harriet" had always lived with a large hump on her nose. Nevertheless, she decided to make her nose smaller because she was still bothered by its prominence. Self-image is an active psychological component of our makeup. So, even though she was in her sixth decade, she was still interested in improving her self-image by altering this facet of her body image.

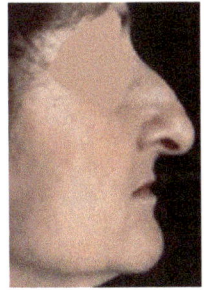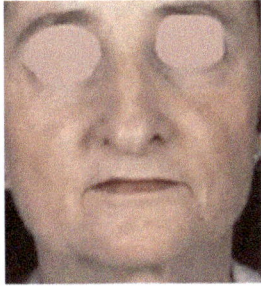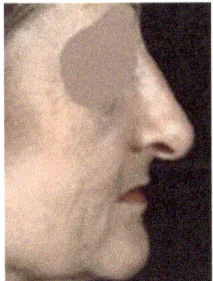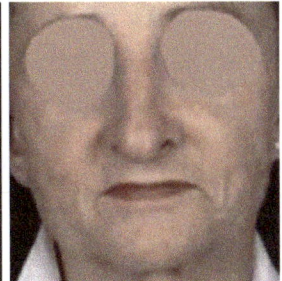

"Joshua" shown below was unhappy with his facial profile. I slightly reduced the size of his nose and augmented his chin with a moderate-sized solid synthetic implant. Relieved of his discomfort, his self-image improved so that he was able to go about his activities with more confidence.

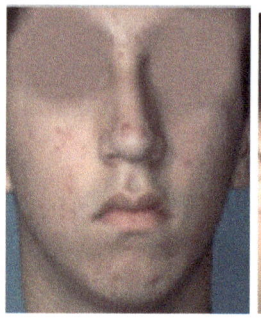 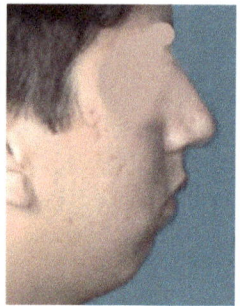 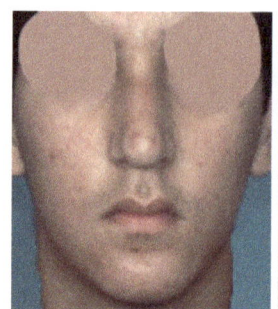 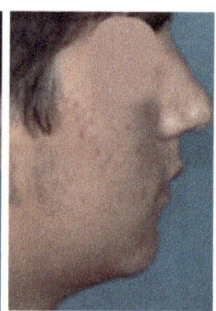

Otoplasty

The adult patient below, "Minerva," decided she wanted something done about her prominent ears. She was probably bothered by this throughout her childhood. This type of surgery is most commonly done at age six or seven but occasionally much later. Perhaps she did not have the opportunity to address this issue earlier in life. I believe she did this because she thought she would feel better about herself if her ears were less conspicuous. This relatively minor body image concern was important enough to her self-image, that she decided to go through this surgery as an adult. I performed a pin back otoplasty, which brought her ears closer to the side of her head. The procedure accentuated the underdeveloped anti-helical ear fold (green arrow). This anti-helical fold is now visible from the lateral view in the last photo. I will describe more about this type of surgery in chapter 4.

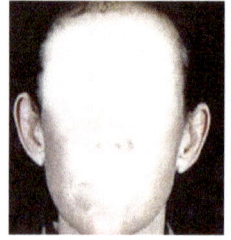 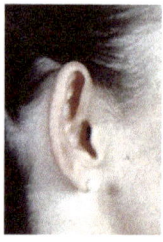 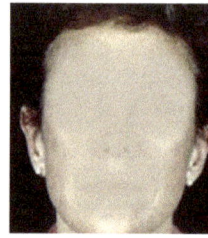 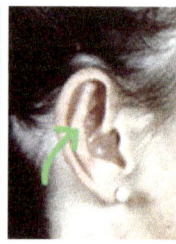 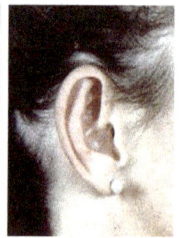

The adult cleft lip and palate patient shown below 'Oscar" had a satisfactory result from his many reconstructive and functional procedures on the lip and palate. However, he again sought plastic surgery to help improve his body image. I advanced his chin (genioplasty) and did a lipectomy of his neck with a platysmaplasty (tightening of the neck muscles). So, this patient who had previously benefited greatly from functional and reconstructive plastic surgery now sought out aesthetic plastic surgery to make him feel better about his self - image. His before and after pictures are below.

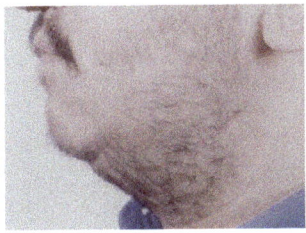 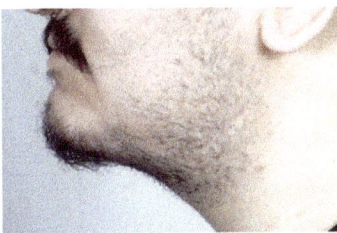

The patient "Roberta" below complained that she always looked tired and even hungover. She wanted to improve her self image. Sometimes individuals who have puffy lower eyelids from excess fat are falsely thought to have overindulged in too much alcohol or excess partying behavior. I removed tissue from all three lower fat pads and a minimal amount of skin. She had some removal of the medial upper fat pad and a small amount of skin. The most notable improvement has been in the lower eyelid contour. This surgery offered a practical solution to her psychological discomfort caused by the puffy lower eyelids. More details about this type of surgery are in chapter16.

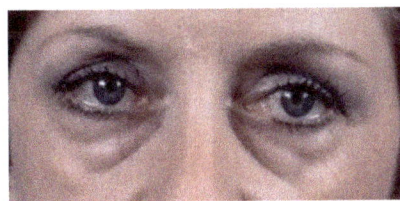 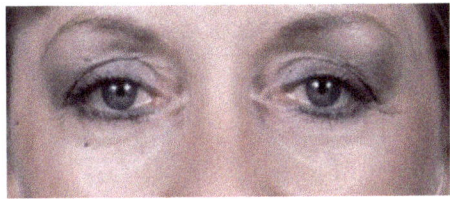

Breast

The developed breast is a sign of femininity. It is vital for body image, self-image, and self-esteem. Chapter 9 is devoted to breast reconstruction.

Of course, there is no procrustean answer to what is a standard or desired breast size.

A particular self- image problem that is relatively common is the young lady who regards herself overly endowed with breast tissue. She feels conspicuous and may think she is the object of lascivious jesting. Perhaps she has been the victim of unwanted and unsolicited catcalls or worse. Some of these patients are shy and withdrawn as a result. A patient like this seeks surgery not to be more attractive or beautiful than others but rather to become inconspicuous.

Occasionally I have seen a patient as young as 13 years of age for this problem. Ordinarily, I would operate on such a patient only if she were at least 18 years of age for two reasons. One is so that the patient can give informed consent on her own. The second is that the patient's breasts may still be growing, and such surgery should usually wait until growth has ceased. There is one exception to this.

There is an entity called Virginal Breast Hypertrophy, which is characterized by rapid breast growth during puberty that may require breast reduction or even mastectomy when exorbitant. I have had patients as young as 16 who have breasts that have not gotten larger for a couple of years and request a reduction of their breast size. Of course, they would need the permission of their parents to receive surgery before they are 18. Such a patient, the young lady "Pam," pictured below, was uncomfortable with her fulsome breasts.

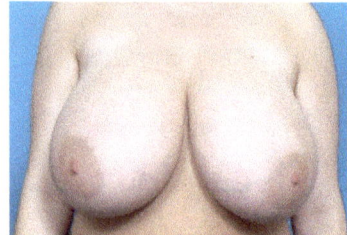
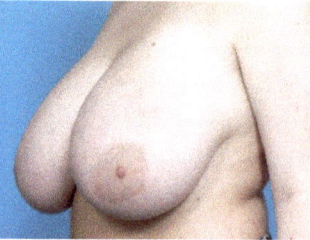
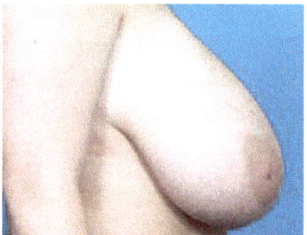

I performed a bilateral reduction mammaplasty upon her. She did well. Because she received a more acceptable body image, her self-esteem improved. She was happy with being less endowed as she felt less conspicuous and more comfortable.

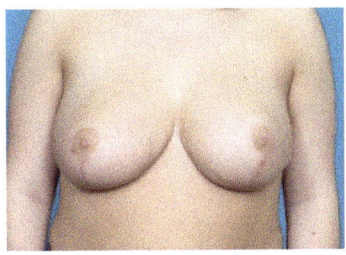 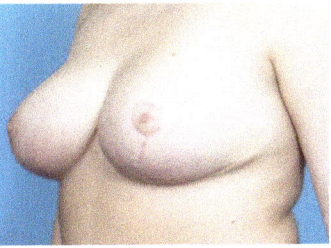 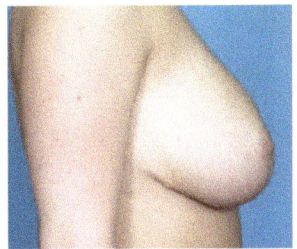

Another type of patient who also does not seek to be more attractive than others, but simply wants to feel normal and inconspicuous, is demonstrated by the patient below, "Catherine." She never developed much breast tissue and had limited self-esteem. She related her feelings of inadequacy to her exiguous breasts. She sought to improve her self-image by obtaining an augmentation mammaplasty. She felt no external pressure from anyone but wanted this for herself. Her preoperative and postoperative photos are below. She was satisfied with her result, which seemed to improve her self-confidence as is usual in such situations.

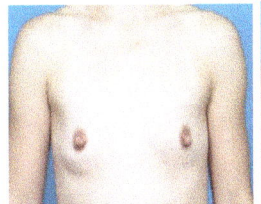 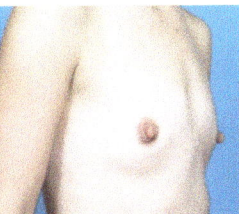 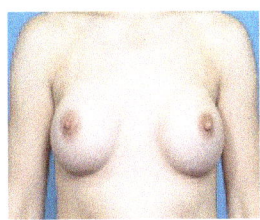 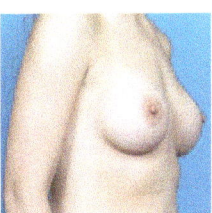

Risk/ benefit ratio

The risk-benefit ratio is a universal concept we can apply to any endeavor in our everyday lives. It is especially important to consider this when contemplating surgery. A common cliché among surgeons is that the only surgeon without complications is the surgeon who does not operate. All operations have potential complications.

If someone has a trauma such as a broken leg with exposed bone or a severe injury of the hand with lacerated tendons, the necessity and benefits of surgery outweigh the risks involved. However, in instances where the patient has had multiple operations, for example, for a congenital facial deformity, the likelihood of additional surgery, improving the situation is perhaps less certain. Therefore, patients need to discuss the pros and cons thoroughly with their plastic surgeon.

The same thing holds for cosmetic surgery done on healthy structures. The patient with abnormal features may be more willing to take increased risks for possible improvement than the patient with essentially normal appearance might be willing to risk to improve his/her looks.

When I turn down a patient for surgery, I often use the concept of risk-benefit ratio to explain why I have decided not to recommend surgery for that patient. Posilutely, these are not mathematical decisions. Sometimes we might judge that the psychological condition of a particular patient would be less tolerant of failure than that of another patient. As the surgeon, I also must live with the results of the surgery, as does the patient.

So, I need to make the judgment that the patient has a good chance the surgery will be genuinely beneficial. Surgeons may be very individualistic in this regard. For example, in plastic surgery, some operations are somewhat on the fringe. The surgeon may be fully capable of technically doing a procedure but, because of previous experience does not like the results. Examples of this might be pectoral implants in male patients or calf implants for cosmetic purposes. Individual surgeons might avoid some types of cases such as sex change operations because of the psychological complexities or ethical concerns.

Of course, some surgeons are, by nature, more cautious than others. Some individual surgeons are willing to accept higher risks in introducing new procedures into their practice. Unfortunately, sometimes the economic aspect of surgery comes into play more than it should. For example, as managed care has become more sophisticated, it can influence the type of surgery done on patients by the reimbursement offered for procedures. One example has to do with breast reconstruction after mastectomy. Some patients may be particularly good candidates for reconstruction with abdominal tissue, which is an operation that is quite complex and time-consuming and involves several nights of hospital stay. However, once healing is complete, the patient should have virtually no ongoing maintenance costs.

An implant only procedure may have lower initial costs but more potential for higher later costs related to periodic replacement of the implants. However, because insurance contracts are yearly, the insurance company wants whatever is cheapest in the short term. Therefore, managed care companies may pay the surgeon no more for the more difficult and time- consuming procedure than for the simpler one. Therefore, many surgeons will not do more complicated procedures because they cannot justify it financially, and the risks are more significant, even if it is best for a particular patient.

There is potential for the reversed circumstance to be a problem also. For example, if the insurance company pays higher reimbursement for a microsurgical free flap technique breast reconstruction compared to a pedicle flap or an implant reconstruction, there is an incentive to perform the more sophisticated technique when a lesser operation is best for the patient. All this boils down to the fact that a plastic surgeon should be a professional who is honest with his patient and keeps his patient's best interests at the forefront at all times.

The risk-benefit ratio also applies to older patients. Sometimes the patient's fragile medical condition does not warrant surgery, which might benefit a healthier patient. For example, a patient may have a chronic sore of the lower leg that could be cured by a massive operation. However, because of a history of strokes, this may not be warranted when simple bandaging of the wound will allow the patient to have comfort and continued ability to go about his routine activities.

I recall a particular patient had a long history of squamous cell carcinoma of the scalp. He had significant radiation therapy to the scalp previously, which caused the necrosis of some of the soft tissue and even cranial bone. I ended up treating him in an extremely conservative manner; that was with antibiotic ointments and dressing changes. So, for a couple of years, he had an open wound with exposed bone on the top of his head.

He might have benefited from an extensive operation, which would have been several hours under anesthesia and a few days in the hospital. However, he had such severe heart disease that his cardiologist did not want him to undergo any significant surgery. Such benign neglect was not an ideal situation; on the other hand, he was able to go about his daily activities, and the only drawback was an inconspicuous bandage on the top of his head. I illustrate a variety of other methods of treatment of scalp wounds in chapter 4.

Sometimes a cancer patient has an advanced disease for which radical surgery would be futile. The surgeon must always act in the patient's best interests, even if it is to turn down the patient for surgery.

Another patient I saw illustrates the risk-benefit ratio. She was an elderly lady who previously had a partial mastectomy and radiation on one side. A local recurrence now dictated a complete mastectomy. Although she was 70 years old and generally not in the best of health, she was quite interested in reconstruction. I steered her away from the use of abdominal tissue because I felt it would be too hard on her. Instead, I advised her that a latissimus flap from the back would give an excellent reconstruction, and she would tolerate it more easily. If she had been younger and a little less fragile, I would have used the generous abdominal tissue which was available.

Sometimes patients for breast reconstruction come with the preconceived notion that the use of abdominal tissue will offer them not only a reconstructed breast but also the benefits of an abdominoplasty or tummy tuck at the same time. I often needed to tell my patients that a TRAM flap that uses abdominal skin, subcutaneous fat, and muscle to make a breast is an arduous way to get a tummy tuck.

Chapter 3

The Making of a Plastic Surgeon

My first recollection of things pertaining to medicine is quite unclear. However, I remember as a small child going to my pediatrician Dr. Qualtrow on Montrose street in Houston with my mother. It was a large old house converted into the doctor's office. When we opened the door, it smelled of rubbing alcohol. The usual reason for going was to get a shot. The first thing I remember was getting my head stuck between the wooden poles of the stairs and everyone getting excited. The nurse came out and told my mother to make me pull my head out. I remember her saying, "you tell him." When I finally was able to squeeze my head back out from between the bars, it was quite anticlimactic. I still had to go in and received a shot in my upper arm.

Another time, I had a bad sore throat, so my mother took me to see doctor Qualtrow. He painted my throat with an iodine swab. It was quite an unpleasant experience. I tended to keep sore throats to myself after that. I also have a vague recollection of Dr. Qualtrow coming to our house because I was quite sick when I was probably about six years old. I remember my mother putting me in my parents' bed, which was quite unusual. I think I had a considerable fever and was somewhat weak. I overheard the doctor talking to my parents and hearing the word "polio" and saying that if I did not get better soon, he would put me in the hospital. In a few days, I got better; it must've been the flu.

Polio was a real menace at that time in the early 1950s in our city of Houston. Even as a small child, I remember hearing about discussions of the yearly summer polio epidemic. Also, a few months before, my best friend who lived around the block from me, Denny Allison, had become sick and was soon diagnosed with polio. There was talk that he might need an "iron lung." That was a primitive breathing machine in the form of a cylinder in which the patient's whole body would lie except for his head. They had become common because of the frequent polio epidemics.

Denny got much better but had a considerable residual weakness. I remember going with him on a few occasions to a physical therapy clinic and vividly remember helping him to do the prescribed exercises at his home during the next year are so. He and I have remained friends. He lives in California now; we play chess on the internet frequently.

A couple of things happened about this time. The Salk vaccine came out, and my first -grade class at St Anne School was taken "en masse" to a nearby public school, Woodrow Wilson, to receive vaccinations. We were probably in a pilot study; this was about 1953. A year or so after that, we went to the same public school but received the Sabin vaccine on a sugar cube. All my classmates liked that better than the shot.

The next significant medical involvement I remembered had to do with playing football in the fifth grade. At that time, the parochial school system in Houston had a good sports league. Most of the Catholic schools had a fifth and sixth-grade football team and a seventh and eighth-grade football team. My sports career started quite strong, as I was asked by our coach to join the fifth and sixth-grade team while I was only in the fourth grade! That year I played cornerback and was proud to get a starting position after a few games. The following year I played halfback. Toward the end of the season, I was tired of our quite grueling practices. I had a few daydreams about how much sympathy I would get if I broke my arm. I learned to be careful about what I wish!

One of our last games was with St. Theresa grade school. As I was carrying the ball around the left end, I was hit simultaneously by two tacklers from my right side. I heard a loud crack that sounded like a one -inch tree limb breaking. My thigh bent unnaturally and, for a moment, felt numb and rubbery. Then it began to hurt big time. Those fellows broke my femur, the large bone of the thigh connecting the hip to the knee.

My coach came on the football field and straightened and splinted my leg with a board. It seemed a little like a dream. I remember all kinds of people coming on the gridiron and looking at what was going on. After a few minutes, that seemed like an hour; an ambulance came and took me to St. Joseph Hospital. I remember being quite scared as I was only 11 years old. Little did I know what was going to happen?

At that point, I thought I would have a cast put on my leg and that we would go home, and I would sleep in my own bed that night. Then I met Dr. Michael Donovan, nicknamed "Iron Mike," from military service in World War II. He placed my right leg in traction. It was raised at about a 45° angle with a pulley with weights placed on the end of a stout cord. I remember asking my father, "when are we going to go home?" It turned out I remained in the hospital in traction for about six weeks. The purpose of the traction was to reposition the bones, which were overlapping, into correct alignment.

It was an exciting experience to spend six weeks in the hospital as an 11-year-old boy. I read a lot of books, mostly Hardy Boy books. It was commendable that one of the Sisters of Charity of the Incarnate Word nuns visited me at least once a day and sometimes read to me. I appreciated that a priest would come periodically and bring me communion. I remarked to my mother that every time Dr. Donovan came in, it seemed my leg later started hurting.

Eventually, I learned he would slip additional weights on the traction for my leg while he was talking to me, and that was why it bothered me. At the end of six weeks, Dr. Donovan removed the traction. Immediately, it seemed there was a lot of pressure on my leg as if it wanted to shorten by itself. I remember that was one of the worst moments for pain. Next, Dr. Donovan placed me in a body cast that went from the upper chest down to the toes of my right foot, and I was discharged home with crutches.

At first, I slept downstairs in the den, where my parents had brought my bed. Later I became mobile enough with my crutches to move back upstairs. My parents arranged to have a teacher come from the public-school system to tutor me at home. She was great, and it was easy to make excellent grades with virtually a one-on-one tutor for a teacher. After a few months, I went back and had a shorter cast placed from my toe to my groin. This one also stayed for several months. After that, it took the better part of a year for me to bend my knee fully.

In school, I was always interested in science and somewhat interested in all of my studies.

In the seventh grade, we had a big science project for Mrs. Barlow. I made a detailed drawing and exhibit on the human ear, which was quite interesting to me. I won a blue ribbon for this at school. Later our school's best exhibits were entered in a regional tournament, but my work only got honorable mention there.

My parents had always spoken admiringly about my paternal grandfather, who was a general practitioner in Houston. He died before I was born. His picture below in his home office reminds me of Norman Rockwell paintings

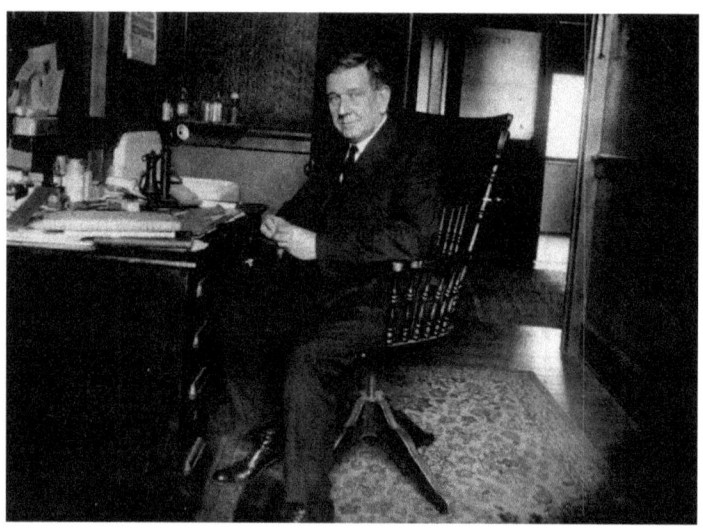

There were many stories about him. When he was a young man on a trip around the world, his father called him back prematurely when his father's railroad business had a huge financial setback. My grandfather was sent to Tulane Medical School in New Orleans so that as a

professional, he would be able to support himself. I learned that during the great depression, he brought home all kinds of barter in payment for his services as a general practitioner in Houston. He did a lot of obstetrics and often went to an out-of-the-way part of town and delivered "Syrian" babies. Maybe we had Syrian immigrants back in the 1920s in Houston. I don't know. That story always seemed strange to me.

I do know that during the earlier part of my medical career, I ran into several patients who said that my grandfather had delivered them. More recently, a friend of mine found out and told me that his mother had been born in Houston, and Dr. Philip Cronin delivered her. Also, when I was a resident in plastic surgery, I did a chart review on cleft lip and palate repair cases of my uncle Thomas Cronin. Some of my uncle's earliest charts indicated his father, Phillip, gave drip ether anesthesia for his procedures.

As I was growing up, I knew that my uncle was a doctor, a plastic surgeon, and perhaps even famous. He had visited me with Dr. Donovan when I had been in the hospital with my broken femur. Otherwise, I would see him once or twice a year at large family get-togethers. One summer, I remember playing in the backyard with my younger brother Pat as he was teasing a small neighbor's dog. Sure enough, the pup jumped up and bit him close to his eye. He had a laceration of his upper eyelid, which bled profusely. My parents took him to my uncle's office so that Pat could have the eyelid repaired.

One day I was helping my older brother Clint and a neighbor boy named Jimmy Lyle put strings on rolled-up newspapers in preparation for delivery. I accidentally stepped on a sharp piece of metal, cutting the sole of my foot. It bled a lot as I walked home. My mother cleaned and bandaged it and then took me to my uncle's office. He gave me a shot in the foot that hurt a lot for a short time, and the nurse gave me a tetanus shot as well. My uncle then sutured my cut and told me not to bear weight on foot for two weeks. We had some crutches at home and probably a souvenir left over from my broken leg episode. The next time I went down the street to Jimmy Lyle's house, he and my older brother Clint razzed me as being a sissy for using crutches for something as slight as a cut foot.

Another time, when I was in high school, I went by car to pick up my younger brother Pat from his grade school. As I arrived, I noticed the coach looked rather severe and called me over. My brother had been high jumping and hurt his arm, he said. It looked like his arm just above the wrist was quite bent, obviously broken. The coach said he thought I better take him to the doctor. Being a young teenager, I was not sure what to do. My parents were not readily available, as this was before the advent of cell phones. So, I took Pat to my uncle's medical office. I did not know him well at that time but knew he was a doctor and would help us. He saw the arm and said he would have Dr. Donovan take care of it. He had his office personnel make the logistic arrangements. I was very relieved that I was able to get help for my brother Pat. Dr. Donovan applied a cast and said we could go home. I did get some points with my parents for being able to help handle this situation. Pat soon recovered completely.

I remember being very impressed by watching two short filmstrips about medicine as a sophomore at St. Thomas high school. One of these showed a couple of operations. I was intrigued by them. By today's standards, these films were primitive. At that time, we did not have things like Discovery Medicine TV to watch. One of the operations was an amputation of a leg. I believe the other activity was the removal of an inflamed gallbladder. I do know that day I decided to become a physician. I soon began finding out what was necessary to go to medical school etc.

During my junior and senior years in high school, I was a voracious reader. Two particular novels I read reinforced my desire to become a physician. One was Arrowsmith by Sinclair Lewis. I was impressed with Martin Arrowsmith's passion for selfless patient care, medical science, the scientific method, and intellectual honesty. At the same time, I was dismayed by his propensity to fall prey to universal ethical flaws relating to family loyalty, fame, and mammon, the very failings the nuns and priests taught us to avoid.

The other persuasive novel was A. J. Cronin's The Citadel, which starts with highlighting the inequities and shortcomings of the medical situation of coal miners in Wales. In this story, Andrew Mason begins by doing everything he can to improve the lot of these workers. He devotes his research efforts to help the coal miners afflicted with lung diseases. Later, he is enticed by a perceived, more comfortable, and more prosperous life as a private practitioner.

However, this hoitytoity environment spawned discontent and led to separation in his marriage. A surgeon's incompetence resulting in the death of his patient so disillusions Mason that he abandons his private practice and resumes his investigations into the treatment of lung disease, but not before denouncing the surgeon. Having returned to his altruistic ideals, he and his wife reconcile, but their reunion is spoiled when she dies in a bus accident. In a retaliatory action, the accused surgeon charges Mason with unethical conduct for working with an unlicensed practitioner to treat a tuberculosis patient. In a fierce and persuasive presentation, Mason vindicates his actions before a medical board, absolving himself of wrongdoing. Again, this novel caused me to want to contribute to society in some way by pursuing a medical career while being watchful not to be seduced by selfish goals.

My first experience with cosmetic plastic surgery was minor but significant to me. I had a common mole develop right in the center of my forehead when I was about 13 years old. For a few years, it did not bother me, but then one of my friends began to tease me about it calling me Cyclopes. After that, every time I looked in the mirror, I saw this bump, which, although trivial, was an issue on the front burner to me as a teenager. After I summoned enough courage, sometime before high school graduation, I made an appointment to see my uncle. He took the offending bump off in his office for me in a few minutes under local anesthesia. I was much relieved. This experience has helped me to understand that even little things can be significant to my patients at times.

Sometime later, also when I was a senior in high school, the same younger brother Pat cut his foot on a large sliver of the glass while playing sandlot football in the vacant lot next to our house. It bled quite a bit, so we got a clean towel and wrapped it around his foot and put some pressure on the wound to minimize the bleeding. I went with my father to take him down to the emergency room at St. Joseph hospital, where my uncle Dr. Thomas Cronin met us. He led us into a small examination room where he had Pat lie down on the treatment table.

To my surprise, my uncle had me wash my hands, put on gloves, and assist him in sewing up my brother's laceration. He instructed me to cut the sutures as he finished tying the knots in them. It was exhilarating for me. It went a long way in confirming my desire to become a doctor. That kind of thing really couldn't happen today in our era of excessive regulations.

So, I decided while in high school that I would like to become a doctor. My wife reminds me that we double dated in high school. Not with each other, but with mutual friends. I went to excellent all-boys high school, St. Thomas, run by the Basilian order of priests. The motto was *Bonitatem et disciplinam et scientiam doce me*. Teach me goodness, discipline, and knowledge.

I have great memories of those four years, which were decisive in my formation as a Catholic Christian. I indeed graduated with the conviction that one should attempt to become a contributing member of society and the church. My wife went to an all-girls school St. Agnes run by a Dominican order of nuns. She says that one evening, on such a double date, we had gone to the annual football bonfire on campus at St. Thomas High School. On our way home, my high school girlfriend and I and my future wife and her date were talking about what we would like to do when we "grew up." Her friend, Eddie Prince, a classmate of mine, said he wanted to be a race car driver. My wife Candy whimsically said she would like to be a Broadway star and mommy. My date said she would like to be a ballet dancer. My wife says she remembers I was quite sincere when I said I plan to become a doctor.

The first real step in my goal was to enter the premed course at Tulane University in New Orleans as a freshman. It seemed like half of my classmates were in the same situation. The first "weeding out" class was freshman chemistry. I naively thought that my high school chemistry would put me way ahead. Although I did study for my first test, I made a poor grade, as did the majority of students in the rather large class. Many students dropped the class immediately because it was just before the deadline to exit without penalty. I was shocked but determined to recover. I talked with the professor, who gave me some recommendations for additional self- programmed texts. I redoubled my efforts and made up most of the lost ground finishing with a B plus. My grades that year were good, but not all A's. This timeframe predated the grade inflation occurring a little later related to the Vietnam war.

Because of financial issues, I needed to transfer to the University of Texas in Austin the next year. I decided to go to The University of Houston for summer school to get ahead. I took about 15 hours of credit and did exceptionally well. I did run into one problem upon transferring from Tulane to the University of Texas. I had taken a calculus class at Tulane, which was four credit hours. The University of Texas wanted only to give me three hours of credit because the freshman calculus course there was a 3- hour course. I didn't think this was fair, so I decided to write the chairman of the mathematics department at Tulane and explained my disappointment that Texas did not consider their four-hour course was worth four credits. Well, this had the desired effect. I believe the chairman of the mathematics department at Tulane must have persuaded the powers that be at the University of Texas to give me the full four credits for this course.

However, when I registered at UT and was assigned an advisor, I did not get any encouragement. The single theme of my councilor was that I needed to decide what I was going to do when I did not get into medical school. I took umbrage at that and determined I would show the "jerk" that he was wrong about my abilities. Even though I transferred to UT after my freshman year at Tulane, I was able to finish my premed courses and complete a degree in Zoology in just two more years. So, I was ready to begin medical school after only three years of college. But was medical school prepared for me? My grades were good, but the competition was intense.

I consider myself very fortunate that during the summer of 1966 between sophomore and junior year in college, I serendipitously reconnected with my future bride. Although Candy and I had double-dated in high school a few times, we had never had a date with one another. She had gone away to school in Iowa for freshman and sophomore years. I had gone to Tulane for my freshman year, then transferred to the University of Texas at Austin, where I spent my sophomore year. I had broken up with my high school sweetheart sometime during my sophomore year in college.

It just so happened that a couple of my high school buddies, Eddie Prince and Paul Speck, call me during the summer after the sophomore year. They wanted to get together and go out and have a beer. Paul attended the University of St. Thomas and wanted to go to a student hangout, Griff's, near the school owned by a former St. Thomas University student named Mike Griffin. That night probably changed my entire life. Griff's was a pub where one could get sandwiches or other light foods, but most people came to drink beer or play pool. When we arrived, there was a large rectangular table filled with many St. Thomas university students.

A blond girl at the other end of the table caught my eye. Although it'd only been a few years since I had seen her, I could not place her name. I knew that both Eddie Prince and Paul Speck knew her, and I kept nudging them, asking for her name. She remembered me and realized I could not remember her name. She said hello and pointedly called me by name from the far end of the table. Later that night, I got her name and number from my friends.

Within a few days, I had called her back and was able to talk her into going out with me. Our first date was to a Rice University versus University of Texas football game at Rice Stadium in Houston. And get this, I wore a suit and tie to the football game and was not out of place. My date, my future wife, wore a business suit. Things have decidedly changed since then. During that summer and the following year, our relationship blossomed. Although Candy now attended the University of St Thomas in Houston, I was about 150 miles away in Austin, finishing at the University of Texas. Every few weeks, I would drive to Houston to see Candy. Interestingly, she was involved in music and drama at the University of St. Thomas, as was my previous girlfriend. They remained casual friends.

Candy even helped me fill out applications and type letters to numerous medical schools in Texas and throughout the country. She was always very supportive of my ambitions. I sent applications to several schools and prepared to take the Medical College Admissions Test. I never received the scores; only the schools I requested did. A waiting game for responses from the various schools came next.

Some flat rejections were very disappointing. However, there were also some invitations for interviews. I traveled to several schools for these, usually nerve-wracking experiences. It seemed there were always other applicants who were so smart or knowledgeable or accomplished that no one would want me. We were generally in a group of applicants for tours of the facilities and general orientations, but the interviews were private, usually with one professor at a time. Most of the interviewers were pleasant and noncommittal, but some gave me the impression they were not sure how I got this far.

On the other hand, one doctor at The University of Texas Medical Branch at Galveston commented that my score on the section of the MCAT dealing with general knowledge was impressive. That was the only compliment I remember getting throughout the interview season. Then the waiting began again. If I remember correctly, I soon received a few "you are on our waiting list," replies. Finally, UTMB (University of Texas Medical Branch) sent me an acceptance letter, and I felt vindicated. I wanted to convey that discouraging UT (Austin) councilor a note. My next real step toward becoming a doctor was at hand.

Medical school

Acceptance into medical school was so exciting. Toward the end of the summer, I began to receive information on upcoming orientations and also about the medical fraternity system, which was prominent at The University of Texas Medical Branch in Galveston. I was not involved in fraternity life in undergraduate school and therefore was unfamiliar with it. I think it was probably unusual to have such active fraternities in medical school. There were many invitations for parties in Galveston. Some were beach parties; some were water skiing parties on rivers or lakes, and many were dances at the various fraternity houses. I attended some of these parties, usually with my future wife, Candy, who was much more socially adept than I.

She recalls one party where we were water skiing on Dickenson bayou. She told me to take off my glasses before skiing. I had an elastic band on them and told her I would not lose them. Well, you guessed it. I lost my glasses. I am very nearsighted; Candy had to drive us back to Houston that evening.

As the rush week came to a culmination, the fraternities extended offers, and I needed to make a decision. I vacillated between two fraternities whose houses were situated right next to each other, Phi Beta Pi and Phi Rho Sigma. At that time, most of the single medical students lived in the fraternity houses, which were immediately adjacent to the campus and within walking distance to the classes. At that time, I had been dating my future wife for about two years. She had come to several of the fraternity parties in Galveston with me. She already knew some of the people that we saw during some of these parties. Both Candy and I liked many of the people in both fraternities.

On the final day to decide on joining a fraternity, I had spent time at both houses and was having a hard time. Candy could tell it would be difficult. About 30 minutes before the deadline, I told Candy I wanted to get away so I could decide. We walked about two short blocks to sit down and relax where we could have a soda.

As the clock was ticking down to the wire, we walked back toward the adjacent fraternity houses. Groups at both fraternities were out in the front yards partying and celebrating with their new members. As we got closer, some of the members of both houses noticed us. They each began yelling encouragement for me to join immediately. As Candy and I got to the first house, a friend came forward and talked with us for a minute. I told him we were going next door to Phi Beta Pi. We shook hands, and for a few seconds, the house next door became quiet. But in the next moment, as we walked onward toward Phi Beta Pi, a cheer rang out. In retrospect, it could not have been more melodramatic.

I found that medical school was quite hard but a lot of fun. Since Galveston was a small city on an island, the fraternities were a major social factor for most medical students. I lived in the fraternity house for the first two years. There was great diversity in the study habits of the "inmates." Some seem to read their notes every waking hour, which would extend until 2 a.m., while others seemed not ever to cram. I thought I studied quite a bit but could not keep up with the hours of some of my classmates.

My roommate David Simons was a great help as he also spent a lot more time studying than partying. Most of my classes were quite enlightening. The first year was pretty much classroom work, except for the dissections in the cadaver lab, which I did enjoy very much. As freshman medical students, our uniform was a white short-sleeved smock. We were all quite proud to begin our medical studies. It seemed I spent most of my waking hours at the fraternity house studying. I would usually get tired and go to bed at 10 or 11 o'clock. However, some of my classmates would burn the midnight oil to one or two o'clock in the morning, and yet they were able to get up and go to class at the same time I would. Most of the relationships between the medical students were quite collegial. Those fraternity brothers a year or two ahead gave excellent advice to the lower classmen about the various courses. Living in a fraternity house was quite convenient. During those first two years, most of my breakfasts, lunches, and dinners were at the fraternity house.

The inter-fraternity sports program was quite good. It created some healthy rivalry between the various fraternities. It was a competitive way to get some good exercise. I remember mostly playing flag football and basketball in the fraternity intra-mural system. It is worthy to note that as a junior playing intramural flag football, there were some very accomplished players, including four college quarterbacks. My fraternity, Phi Beta Pi, had a player named Jim Halla who had quarterbacked for SMU. That was impressive enough. However, the KA's team had two former college quarterbacks. Walter McReynolds, a former quarterback at Rice University, amazingly did not make the quarterback position, so he played center instead! Another college quarterback from Oklahoma State, Rick Parker, was their fraternity's regular quarterback.

Because I was very serious about my girlfriend, who lived in Houston, I made frequent weekend trips from Galveston to Houston. Often, I would meet her at the library at the University St. Thomas Friday evening, where we would study until the library closed. We would then go to the movies or get a late ice cream treat or something like that. I would then take her home as she was living with her parents. If there were a Saturday night party at the fraternity in Galveston, we would often go; however, I would always have to take her home to her parents in Houston after the party, so we often left early. We were very traditional.

Stress

Medical school

Nicolas Clayton was the architect of the beautiful 1891 Old Red building. I had only a few classes in this building.

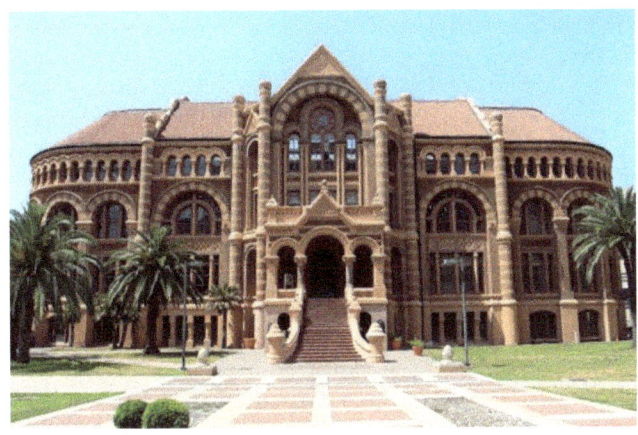

Medical school was quite stressful. Candy and I met some couples who were already married as freshmen but divorced by the time of graduation, or we later heard about their breaking up during residency training. Then there was the charismatic genius, with the photographic memory, who graduated from college at age 16, flew through medical school in three years, hardly studying at all. Everyone was jealous. I later found out he had committed suicide.

Most of the first two years in medical school consisted of didactic classroom courses with some laboratory experience and were very difficult but engrossing. Biochemistry, gross anatomy, neuroanatomy, and physiology were all rigorous. Additional subjects were pathology, pharmacology, immunology, cell biology, microbiology, and genetics. However, I did have a little trouble staying awake in one class, an introductory course in interpreting X rays, which the powers that be, decided to have right after the lunch break. I vainly tried to focus my attention on the x rays projected on a large screen in an otherwise utterly dark auditorium.

My neuroanatomy professor had a thick German accent. The scuttlebutt was that he first saw Galveston Island through the periscope of a U-boat he captained during World War II. He was a no-nonsense type teacher who later became head of the anatomy department. The only lecture where there was some rowdiness was professor Blount's famous lecture on the embryologic rotation of the gut. This class was always very theatrical. He waved his arms to demonstrate the embryologic movement of the intestines. This lecture was in an ancient lecture hall that had very vertical rows of seats, making it seem like a miniature opera house. It was similar to the one below in the Old Red building. When the professor got particularly dramatic, the students would throw coins down to the lectern area!

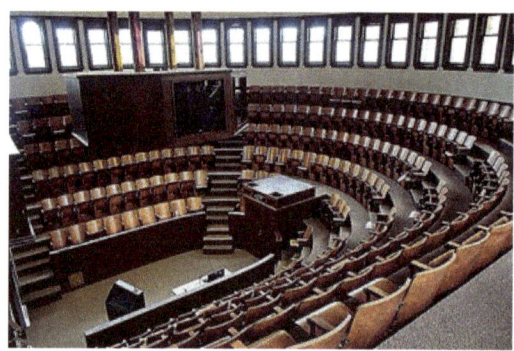

During this lecture, Dr. Blount was unintentionally struck by a coin on his forehead but just ignored it.

I think most Physicians have a profound memory of their first gross anatomy lab dissection sessions. Only a few students had any qualms about the necessary hands-on instruction. At UTMB, we had a particularly interesting gross anatomy lab. The first picture below is from an earlier class gathered in the lab for a class photo. The second picture is the view of the lab I experienced with rows of tables each with a full cadaver ready for the first session of the year. As you can see it was one large room with rows of dissecting tables each with a full cadaver. There were skeletons hanging from pullies near the ceiling, which could be lowered for inspection.

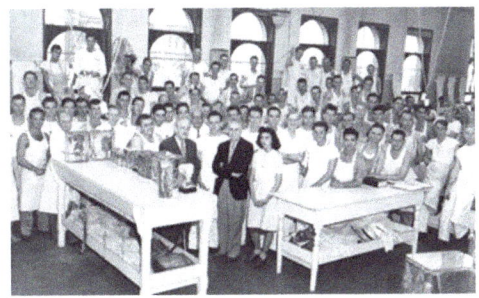 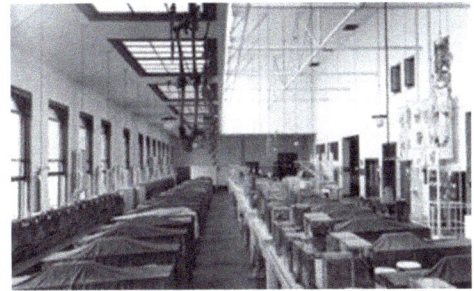

Scattered throughout the lab were glass encased cadaver dissections of every conceivable human body part, some quite ancient as shown on the left below. As we were carrying out dissection assignments, we would sometimes refer to those previously dissected specimens on display for insight. The final picture is of a modern gross anatomy lab.

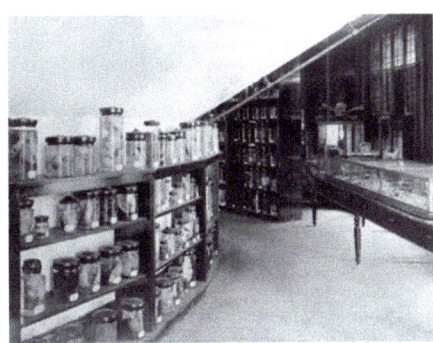 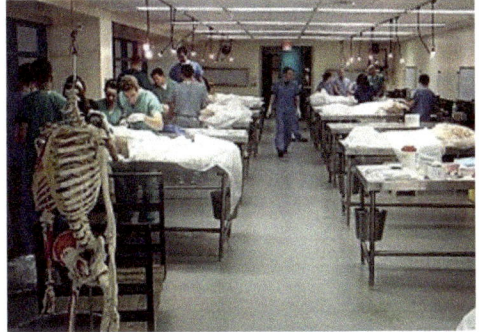

My anatomy chief Donald Duncan PhD. was a soft-spoken, pipe-smoking professor who was both admired and liked by almost all the students. After I had completed my anatomy course, I wanted to get a job as a prosector the following year. This job entailed helping the medical students with their dissections of the cadavers in the gross anatomy laboratory.

The third and fourth years of medical school were more oriented to clinical skills. Students learned to take medical histories and perform physical examinations. There were rotations on various services. Before I went to medical school, I thought I would probably like to be a general practitioner. I had always heard great things about my grandfather, who was a general practitioner at St. Joseph Hospital. He died before I was born, so I never knew him personally. I probably romanticized the idea of being a general practitioner.

During medical school, I seem to be always changing my mind with each new rotation. If I had an OB/GYN rotation, I would think that might be a very agreeable specialty practice. Delivering babies is such a happy occurrence. Some exposure to orthopedic surgery was also intriguing. It seemed so practical and even mechanical. One could see the results of one's effort much more directly than in a field such as internal medicine.

I had particularly informative exposure to ENT (otolaryngology) as a medical student and was quite interested in that. There were several impressive faculty members. In the back of my mind, I believe I always had some idea also of plastic surgery. It was about this time that the American Board of plastic surgery became more liberal in its prerequisite requirements. It became possible to use ENT residency as a prerequisite to plastic surgery. ENT was more appealing to me than general surgery because I felt I would be happy practicing ENT if I didn't continue to plastic surgery. The usual route, training in general surgery, then plastic surgery was less appealing because, if I were unable to finish plastic surgery, I felt I had less interest in general surgery compared to ENT.

At the end of my sophomore year, I had an elective opportunity, and I chose to go to M.D. Anderson Hospital in Houston. Rotating on the surgery service was quite an eye-opening experience for me. I first learned how to scrub and gown for surgery. I learned how to tie knots and assist in operations. I saw a great deal of pathology. I also observed that some surgeons seemed to have much more skill than others. I was somehow surprised by that. I guess I thought that at a prestigious institution like M.D. Anderson, all of the surgeons would be of the highest quality.

Candy graduated from the University of St. Thomas with a degree in education. She did student teaching at St. Anne grade school in Houston and then taught at Holy Ghost grade school in Houston. Candy and I married between my sophomore and junior year of medical school. The best thing that I ever did was marry Candy. I have learned so much from her example. She always treats everyone with the dignity a child of God deserves. She could have been the model for Mr. Rogers! (My wife and I recently saw the movie starring Tom Hanks, which was delightful.) We were married at St. Anne's Catholic Church in Houston, which was my local parish. We liked St. Anne's better than St. Vincent's, which was her family's parish. The best man was my childhood friend Denny Allison.

We are still friends. He and I frequently play chess on the internet together as he lives in California. Denny devised a way that he would take us to our car after the reception so it would not be garishly decorated. However, we made a mistake stopping at a local Japanese restaurant for dinner. My brother Clint and his wife Sharon happened to be driving by on their way home after the reception and saw our car pull into the parking lot even though I parked it in a spot one could not see from the street. Near the end of our dinner, the restaurant manager said someone left us a note. With that, we knew we had been had! There were "Just married" inscriptions and other decorations on our car when we went outside.

Candy and I didn't have any money for a glamorous honeymoon. We drove about three hours to a relative's cabin near Wimberley, Texas, a picturesque area in the hill country. It was dark when we were driving the last stretch down a dirt road. We saw several deer which were illuminated by our headlights. The cabin, located on a little creek, was perfect and even had a small waterfall right by the house. We spent a few days there on our honeymoon. We were indeed impressed with the starry nights out in the country, which are very different from those we in Houston. We were such babies then.

We rented a furnished apartment in a brick quadruplex on Broadway in Galveston, which was close enough that I could walk to the medical school, and we could walk to the beach, usually in the evening. To help a little with our finances, I had been able to talk Dr. Duncan into giving me the job as a prosector. I was also able to walk to that job on the medical school campus. Candy was always very supportive of my work.

After we married and moved to Galveston, she taught first grade at Goliad Elementary school in the Galveston Independent School District. She was very good with children. Even though Goliad was in a poor neighborhood with most children coming from socially deprived backgrounds, Candy did enjoy her work. Candy became pregnant, and we expected our first child in November of my senior year. She contracted rubella early in her pregnancy. Vaccination for rubella was not yet available. We had a lot of people praying for our unborn child and us. November 8, 1970, Erin was born with no defects despite her mother's rubella infection.

Another of my medical school rotations took place at Breckenridge Hospital in Austin, Texas. I was on the obstetrical service and was able to "catch" some birthing infants. Placing a baby in a new mother's arms was a happy experience for everyone. At the time, it made me think; perhaps OB/GYN would be a good specialty for me.

Another surprising encounter during medical school was attending an autopsy. The patient had been a smoker, and the lungs had emphysematous blebs and contained a large amount of black soot. The most striking thing was observing the pathologist light up a cigarette immediately following the autopsy. Fortunately, I never had much desire to be a smoker. When I was a child, my mother, who was a three-pack a day smoker, would have me light up her next cigarette so she would not have a hiatus between smokes. Although she eventually gave up smoking, she suffered a lot, being on constant oxygen during the last ten years of her life. She died of pulmonary failure in St Joseph hospital. Our family was so fortunate to have gathered at her bedside and recited a rosary together with Chaplin Father Ben Meyer shortly before she died.

As medical school progressed, I needed to begin planning for postgraduate training. At that time, most medical students spent the first year after graduation in a one-year internship program and, after that, separately sought residency programs to follow the internship year. Now, most medical students apply directly for residency programs, the first year of which constitutes the "internship."

I looked into various internship programs at different hospitals in different cities. The selection is through a matching program in which the medical students make a priority list of the programs in which they would like to participate. Likewise, the various hospitals make a ranked list of the potential interns they would accept. On the designated day, almost everyone found out where they would be going after graduation. Occasionally someone would not match. For those few students, there was a clearinghouse, which linked the graduate with a hospital that still had positions. In preparation for the internship match, I applied to several hospitals.

Internship

Upon completion of medical school, I matched at Kansas City General Hospital for a rotating 2 (surgery) internship. Probably not coincidentally, that was where my plastic surgeon uncle had done an internship. The hospital consisted of old buildings from 1908. The west front of the main hospital building included decorative stone gargoyle rain spouts. There was an impressive frieze over the primary entryway, which quoted a portion of Portia's speech in Shakespeare's *Merchant of Venice* "the quality of mercy is not strained it droppeth as the gentle rain from heaven upon the place beneath."

When I interned at Kansas City General Hospital, the old building was nearing its final days. The top floor had once housed the "interns and residents" but now served as on-call rooms and break rooms for the interns and residents. The second and third floors contained large wards. The general surgery ward was one huge room with rows of beds on either side with curtains available to partition off the bed for privacy. It certainly made making rounds for the doctors convenient and rapid but offered little privacy for the patients or visitors. The first floor housed the laboratory, x-ray, and record room. The basement area contained the ambulance entrance, emergency room, and various consultation and waiting rooms. Soon after my departure, new buildings of Truman Medical Center replaced that building.

Kansas City General Hospital was the public hospital that received a lot of trauma, such as the proverbial knife and gun club participants. One of my first rotations was in the emergency room. As an intern, I was the initial doctor for all the trauma cases. My backup was general surgery residents, who were immediately available 24/7 in the hospital. The emergency room rotation was 12 -hour shifts each day for a month at a time. After arriving home following my first rotation, my wife said I looked almost as white as the white uniform I wore in the emergency room. I came home and immediately collapsed, telling her I had three patients with gunshot wounds that first night in the emergency room. So, I thought medical school was stressful? Internship transformed that stress to a new level! Although, as an intern, you have the least experience, you are often on the front line of care for either very sick or seriously injured patients. Yes, there are always backups. When you needed to, you could call on residents a year or so ahead of you to help you with the problems you encountered. I am also indebted to many of the nurses I worked with that year.

I seriously considered various fields of surgery and thought I wanted to go into ophthalmology after having a very enjoyable and exciting rotation near the beginning of my internship. So, I applied for a residency position in the ophthalmology program at Kansas City General Hospital. During the rotation, I had enjoyed studying the anatomy of the eye. I had become at least somewhat proficient at using a slit lamp to examine the eyes. I learned how to do refraction for common nearsighted and foresighted problems. I enjoyed assisting at surgeries such as cataract removal and lens replacement.

The only surgical procedure I did as an intern on the ophthalmology rotation was an orbital enucleation on a recently deceased organ donor patient. I did this under the supervision of the ophthalmology resident on the service. An enucleation removes the entire globe of the eye. I don't know what happened to the specimen; I assumed at least one patient received a corneal transplant.

When I thought I wanted to go into ophthalmology, I signed up for a military draft deferral in the Berry Plan. Of course, 1971 was during the Vietnam war. The deferment would allow me to complete the ophthalmology residency before going into the service. Later during the internship, I decided there was not enough surgery to satisfy my interest as there seemed to be more clinic time in the ophthalmology specialty as compared to some surgical specialties.

Therefore, I relinquished my upcoming position in that ophthalmology program. By turning down the ophthalmology residency, I was no longer eligible for that deferment. Consequently, I was again available for the draft. However, I was assigned a high number, which never came up.

Recently my wife reminded me of one small episode she said she would never forget. One evening I was scheduled to finish my duty at about 6 PM. She had brought me to the hospital with our only car two mornings before. I'd worked all day, then been on call overnight and again worked all day until 6 PM. It was never sure that I would be actually on time, so rather than remain in the parking lot, she came through the front entrance and waited by the telephone operator's office. While there, she remembers the telephone operator announcing over the hospital intercom "gunshots fired in the surgical ward." She was especially concerned because she knew I was rotating on the surgical service. As it turned out, I was in another area and did not witness anything. I found out later a security officer disarmed the shooter without incident.

I was fortunate to be able to have a one-month rotation on the plastic surgery service. I saw a variety of cases, including tendon lacerations of the hand, facial fractures, hair transplants with large circular plugs (an older technique now superseded by micro hair grafting). At a regularly scheduled plastic surgery weekly conference, I met Dr. Fred McCoy, who was a friend of my uncle, Thomas Cronin. They worked together in the army plastic surgery service during World War II. Years later, I would see him at national plastic surgery meetings.

During my internship year, my wife stayed home to care for our first child, who had her first birthday in Kansas City. She and the baby saw a lot more of Kansas City than I did. It seemed I was always at the hospital. I do remember enjoying a few things about the city. Once, we went to a performance at an outdoor theater under the stars at Swope Park. Once or twice during that year, we were able to have dinner at a restaurant in the Country Club Plaza, which was an old but very fancy retail shopping area.

On a few occasions, we would go to a popular local hamburger joint called Winstead's, which was good. Also, I remember enjoying sliced brisket sandwiches from Gates barbecue, which was probably the most famous barbecue place at that time in the early 1970s. I remember accompanying my wife and daughter to the Nelson art museum. I remember they had a significant Egyptian collection. The museum was not too far from our house, and Candy was able to go several times.

General surgery residency training

While further considering what to do, after turning down the ophthalmology residency, I arranged to do a second-year of general surgery training back in my hometown of Houston at St. Joseph Hospital. At that time, there was virtually no hiatus between finishing my internship and starting the residency. Candy and our little daughter flew back to Houston. As soon as I finished my last day of internship, I drove straight through overnight from Kansas City to Houston so that I could report on time for my general surgery residency position at St Joseph Hospital.

My general surgery year at St Joseph Hospital was excellent for me from the standpoint of having great mentors and obtaining a lot of experience and skills in surgery. Dr. D.L. Moore, a general surgeon, was in charge of the program. He was very supportive of his residents. I remember being very impressed with the way the nuns ran the hospital. There seemed to be one in charge of every ward. I was amazed that even as a resident doctor, the nurses would stand up and greet me if I came to the nurse's station. Those were the days? I recollect my first paycheck from St Joseph Hospital was for one dollar and 13 cents. It was so small because the timing reflected only one day's pay but included the withholding of insurance and taxes, etc.

Nevertheless, I was pretty disappointed; I never cashed that check. At Kansas City General Hospital, we would receive our paychecks in our mail slots, open 24 hours a day in the medical education office. One Saturday early in my general surgery residency at St Joseph, I went by the medical education office to get my check, which was issued the day before. I had been unable to get it because of constant resident duties.

The office door was locked. Candy and I were undoubtedly living paycheck to paycheck at that time. I knocked hard on the door, and finally, the director of medical education came and opened it. I did not have regular contact with him as he related to the interns and the internal medicine residents, and I was under the auspices of Dr. Moore. The medical director was, by all accounts, a great teacher who was revered by many of his students. However, that morning he was unpleasant. He asked what I wanted. I said I just want to go to my mail slot and get my paycheck. He said, "the office is closed; come back next week." I was livid. I told him I need my paycheck then. All he had to do was let me walk ten paces and pick up the check. I don't know what I said, but it was apparent that I was irate. I had to restrain myself deliberately, or I would have slugged him right there, which would have been to my fortuneless downfall. He finally relented and let me get my check but continued to be very acerbic until I left.

I learned a lot about anesthesiology on a one-month rotation with some very good anesthesiologists. I particularly remember Lectoy Johnson teaching me how to facilitate placement of the endotracheal tube through the patient's mouth into the trachea at the induction of anesthesia. My skills improved considerably during his time. Dr. Charlie Williams, another anesthesiologist, was also an excellent teacher. From him, I learned quite a bit about the physiology involved in general anesthesia, as well as taking care of surgical intensive care patients after surgery. However, after the rotation in anesthesia, I was not inclined to make a career in that specialty.

General surgery was enjoyable, but I thought the field was narrowing because of inroads by various surgical specialties. B.V. Williams was a prominent general surgeon who taught me a lot about the essential practice of general surgery. I assisted him in many cases, especially intra-abdominal cases such as gallbladder surgery, bowel surgery, splenectomy, etc. I was fortunate enough to spend some time with Dr. John Bardwill, who was a general surgery trained, head, and neck surgeon. He had formerly been at M.D. Anderson Hospital and Cancer Institute. I did a lot of thyroid surgery with him, as well as other head and neck cancer surgery, such as resection of intra-oral cancers, radical neck dissections, and laryngectomies. He was an old-time hard-core surgeon who was very serious and did not put up with any frivolities.

Dr. Richard Hirshberg was another influential surgeon. He practiced neurosurgery. I assisted him in many intra-cranial procedures, as well as many spinal operations. He was a very meticulous surgeon from whom I learned many good technical points. I spent a couple of months on rotation at Breckinridge Hospital in Austin, Texas. Even as a junior resident, I got to do a lot of surgery at this public hospital.

I remember being impressed with a particular surgeon, Dr. Riley Ross. He was the fastest operating surgeon that I have ever seen. He moved very quickly and had a few wasted moves. It appears he must have been from an era when anesthesia was a lot more "shaky," and one would like to get the surgery over with as quickly as possible. Dr. Ross guided me through my first gallbladder removal case. I was also pleased to be able to spend a month on the plastic surgery service at St. Joseph Hospital. There I began to appreciate the delicate nature and extensive range of cases dealt with by plastic surgeons.

I needed to make arrangements for the next year and decided that I would apply for an otolaryngology (ENT) residency. Its recent designation as a prerequisite for plastic surgery meant that if I were unable to go on to a plastic surgery residency, I could practice ENT, which appealed to me more than general surgery. During that time, I applied to ear, nose, and throat residency training programs, and the University of Texas Medical Branch in Galveston accepted me for otolaryngology training. I had been influenced quite a bit during medical school by Dr. Richard Lawrence, one of the professors in the otolaryngology department. He was undoubtedly one of the reasons why I went the route of ENT training. Later I found out he had gone back to train in plastic surgery. That further encouraged me to continue the possible ENT then plastic surgery training route.

ENT Residency

UTMB had an outstanding ENT residency program. We had a nice mix of academic learning and surgical experience. My chief, Byron Bailey, was the consummate academician. Our residents always did well on in-service examinations. During the next three years, I learned how to diagnose and treat diseases and injuries of the ears, nose, and throat, and head and neck region. I collected a small sample of foreign bodies. I removed insects and beans from ears, a fishbone from a tonsil, a peanut from the trachea, and a penny from the esophagus. Once a child came to the ENT clinic because of a small bean in the ear. After I removed that, I did a routine exam and serendipitously found a plastic tiddlywink in the same child's nose!

I had quite a good ENT residency experience of operating as well. I particularly liked doing parotid surgery and other head and neck surgery, such as radical neck dissections. I performed extensive surgeries like laryngectomies and maxillectomies, also rhinoplasties, and some other facial cosmetic surgeries. The most momentarily stressful and intense elective surgery was stapedectomy for otosclerosis. This surgery involves the removal of the stapes, one of the three small bones in the middle ear, which helps to conduct sound. Sometimes the stapes becomes sclerotic, making it immobile and no longer able to transmit sound properly. Removing this small bone while not penetrating the thin membrane separating it from the inner ear is necessary.

One small overactive move might penetrate the inner ear membrane and render the patient deaf in that ear. A substitute stapes, either synthetic or of bone, is placed to reestablish the bony chain between the eardrum and the inner ear. I was fortunate during my ENT residency to have a rotation at Houston with a Doctor Edward Maddox. He was the best stapedectomy surgeon I ever saw.

He also was involved early on with the development of cochlear implants for deafness. During that rotation in Houston, I lived in the "temporal bone lab." I had a bed and bathroom and stayed there during the week, and if I was not on call went home on weekends to Galveston. This "bone lab" had multiple temporal bones available for practice for stapedectomies and drilling out the facial nerve within the bone with the electric drills.

Upon finishing my ENT residency, I could have put out the proverbial shingle and begun ENT practice. I felt like I had been quite lucky to have the mentors Drs Byron Bailey, Thom Love, and Caruso and others. During my ENT residency, I enjoyed all of the activities except dealing with dizzy patients and those with nosebleeds. Therefore, during the last year of my ENT residency, I looked into the idea of going on to training in plastic surgery. Throughout all of this training, my wife Candy was so supportive and was always encouraging me to continue to learn so that I would be able to be most beneficial to my future patients.

Plastic Surgery Residency

Today, about half of the residencies are using a shorter tract known as an "Integrated Program" that mixes general surgery and plastic surgery and other subspecialties in a six-year continuous residency in the same institution beginning immediately after medical school. The impetus for introducing this tract was fundamentally financial. The federal government pays for training residents by subsidizing hospitals and universities, and it wants to limit the number of years of training for which it will pay. Theoretically, the experience could be more specifically related to plastic surgery during a more limited six-year residency.

One drawback is residents are selected directly out of medical school with no residency track record with which to judge their performance or likelihood of success. Our program continues for selecting residents with approximately five years of prerequisite training. We then have three additional years to train them in the art and science of plastic surgery.

Toward the end of my ENT residency, I was thrilled to be accepted into the plastic surgery residency program at St. Joseph hospital in Houston. So, it was at this point that the proverbial "two roads diverged in the woods" moment hit me. "I took the one less traveled by, and that has made all the difference." I am sure I would have enjoyed an ENT career if I had chosen that road. I was particularly interested in this plastic surgery program because of the preceptor nature of the teaching. During various one-month rotations, I shadowed and assisted a particular surgeon in the office and operating room. I saw his private patients with him in consultation.

With this type of preceptorship program, I learned about the real world of plastic surgery. Two of my mentors, Dr. Thomas Cronin and Raymond Brauer, were world-renowned plastic surgeons and had a tremendous amount of knowledge and wisdom to impart. Another mentor, Dr.

Thomas Biggs, had an extensive aesthetic practice and would become a well-known, world-renowned expert in the area of cosmetic plastic surgery. Finally, Dr. Lawrence Wolf was the youngest member of my teaching staff. He was also exceptionally bright and eager to teach and impart knowledge. The two years of training with these gentlemen flew by rapidly. Besides learning from them, I read every plastic surgery book that I could get my hands on. The vast educational opportunities the internet offers were not yet available.

ENT BOARDS

I was able to sit for my ENT (otolaryngology- head and neck) board certification exam six or eight months into my plastic surgery residency. I had to double up my studies to prepare for the ENT exam while continuing my plastic surgery reading. The ENT exam had both written and oral sections. The written exam did not frighten me too much as I had done very well on previous in-service tests. I took my oral exam in a hotel. I had several examiners, one each in individual rooms along the corridor. The examiner asked questions about the practice of otolaryngology. They were all reasonable.

I also remember there was a pathologic microscopic slide examination in one of the rooms. I remember there was a basal cell carcinoma slide that was straight forward. But, for fear of some trick, I was not able to spit out the answer as quickly as I wished but ultimately got it right. Fortunately, I did well enough to pass both parts of the exam and become board-certified in otorhinolaryngology.

Mentors

Dr. Thomas Cronin

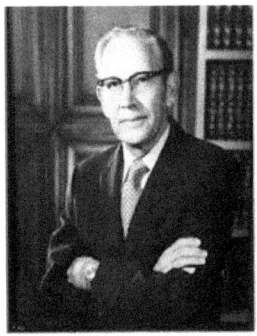

During my plastic surgery residency at St. Joseph Hospital in Houston, Dr. Thomas Cronin, my uncle, was in charge. In Houston, we have had many contributors to the field of plastic surgery. I have been fortunate to have many as my mentors. Dr. Thomas D. Cronin, an internationally known and respected plastic surgeon, was one of the pioneer plastic surgeons in Houston. I was so lucky to have him as one of my mentors.

He trained under Gordon New at the Mayo Clinic, but the relationship was somewhat strained and challenging. Later, when he was the mentor, he made a point of treating residents with respect and was always eager to listen to their ideas and consider them colleagues. He was generous with his time and was always willing to explain his thoughts to his residents. Dr. Cronin served in the U.S. Army medical core during WWII and spent three years in Great Britain, treating patients with war injuries.

He returned to the United States and worked under Dr. Truman Blocker, a prominent military plastic surgeon and great administrator, Wakeman General Hospital. Later in Galveston, Dr. Blocker became famous for triaging and organizing care for hundreds of burn patients from the Texas City disaster of 1947, which was the deadliest industrial calamity in US history. The SS Grandcamp caught fire, and its cargo of 2100 metric tons of ammonium nitrate exploded. That was the first in a concatenation of explosions, fires, and detonations of nearby ships and other oil storage facilities that killed at least 581 people.

It was also in the army that Dr. Cronin met and worked with Raymond Brauer, who had previous plastic surgery experience with Dr. George Pierce in San Francisco. After discharge from the military, Dr. Cronin returned to practice in Houston in 1946. Dr. Brauer joined him in practice in 1948. The relationship was mutually agreeable, and they began a 40-year partnership and collaboration in plastic surgery.

Dr. Thomas Cronin was a pioneering plastic surgeon in Houston who published more than 100 articles on an impressive array of topics. Promethean, throughout his career, he is considered one of the ten most influential plastic surgeons of the 20th century. Besides being the inventor, with Frank Gerow, of the modern silicone breast implant, he did innovative work in many other areas.

He wrote the first article on cross finger flaps for repair of traumatic finger injuries. He wrote extensively about innovative cleft lip and palate repairs and rhinoplasty for correction of cleft lip nasal deformity. He authored numerous articles on breast reconstruction after mastectomy. He wrote about burn reconstruction, including cervical burn scar release with pressure splinting therapy of split-thickness skin grafts to prevent recurrent cervical skin contractures. He also wrote about burn alopecia treatment with hair grafts. He and Tom Biggs described the T-Z plasty for male "turkey gobbler" deformity. He performed many congenital microtia (inchoate ear) reconstructions with a flexible silicone ear framework and reported his results. He described a syndactyly (webbed fingers) repair with zigzag incisions and double triangular webspace flaps, a unique blepharoplasty (cosmetic eyelid) approach, and various flaps for nasal reconstruction. His work involved almost every area of plastic surgery.

Dr. Cronin was actively interested in the education of plastic surgeons. He made a point of teaching residents with respect and was always eager to listen to their ideas, considering them colleagues. He was generous with his time and willing to discuss all areas of plastic surgery with his residents. Incidentally, his first resident at Jefferson Davis Hospital was

Ralph Millard, also considered one of the ten most influential plastic surgeons of the 20th century.

Dr. Cronin was a perfectionist who emphasized the need for excellence in plastic surgery and was always looking for innovative solutions to problems. A tireless worker, he spent most weekends in the office preparing slide presentations and writing papers. He was always ready to stop what he was doing and take time to discuss any plastic surgery case or subject. He could not be rushed either in the office seeing patients or in the operating theater. Excellence was his goal. Routinely, instead of finishing the office consultations at 5:00 pm, he would usually finish those patients who had a 5 o'clock appointment at 6:30 or 7:00 pm. Dr. Thomas Cronin was a prolific writer, as noted above.

Dr. Thomas Cronin operated very slowly. However, he was very meticulous, and on many occasions, after having put in numerous sutures in a wound closure, I saw him take them all out and start over again because he did not like the result. He always treated residents with respect. Something he felt was not the case during his residency at the Mayo Clinic. He often asked residents their opinion about a surgical problem or what they would do with a particular operative situation, and it was not unusual for him to try out something suggested by his resident. He was always an innovator.

I remember assisting him in a particular case during which he was looking for tissue to make nipples for a patient who had had bilateral mastectomies. At that time, it was fairly common to use labia minora. However, in this case, he decided to use external hemorrhoids that were visible when he was looking for the routine graft. When he was with a new resident, he would often say, "If I drop dead now, you have to finish this operation; how would you do it?" He was also fond of saying, "just because you know how to do operation does not mean you should do it" He was a strong proponent of the preceptor method of teaching. He felt it was essential to learn how to do an operation correctly by helping a very experienced surgeon rather than learning to do a case from a resident one year ahead of yourself.

Through his influence, he brought scores of visiting plastic surgeons to Houston, whom he thought could teach new ideas and techniques to the Houston plastic surgery community. For example, Dr. Cronin saw Dr. Carl Hartramph's presentation on the TRAM flap, and about two weeks later, at the invitation of Dr. Cronin, Dr. Hartramph did the first the TRAM flap done in Houston. Perhaps the most notable visitor was Dr. Paul Tessier. After attending a demonstration of Dr. Tessier's craniofacial work in Paris, Dr. Cronin was so impressed that he invited Dr. Tessier to come and operate on patients of the Cronin Brauer Biggs clinic. He visited Houston for a week or two every year from 1972 to 1989.

Dr. Cronin was a member of all the national plastic surgery organizations. He served as president of the American Association of Plastic Surgeons, the Texas Society of Plastic Surgeons, and the Houston Society of Plastic Surgeons. He served on the editorial board of the Annals of Plastic Surgery and received many individual awards for his outstanding scientific contributions to the development of plastic surgery

In 1987 the Thomas Cronin Chair of plastic Surgery was established at the University of Texas Health Science Center in Houston, along with Thomas D. Cronin Burn Fellowships in plastic surgery by the Dunn Research Foundation to honor Dr. Thomas Cronin. The Dunn Research Foundation and the Sisters of Charity of the Incarnate Word funded an endowment in 1987 for the advancement of plastic surgery at the former St Joseph Hospital Foundation.

Dr. Cronin had a particular interest in the repair of children with cleft lip and palate problems, feeling they deserve the best care possible. He did much pioneering work in the field of cleft lip and palate deformities. He wished the endowment to support a cleft palate clinic. The Christus Foundation for Health Care (formally the St. Joseph Hospital Foundation) now helps with funding the Cronin and Brauer Cleft Lip and Palate Clinic at Shriners Hospital for Children in Houston.

Dr. Thomas Cronin's plastic surgery legacy lives on in additional forms: the further development of surgical techniques he originated and the work of the many plastic surgeons he trained. He will long be remembered by his many patients, colleagues, and friends for his quiet manner, open friendliness, willingness to listen, and his innovative approach to solving problems and his pursuit of excellence. Chapter 8 has more information about Dr. Thomas Cronin and the development of the silicone gel implant.

Dr. Raymond Brauer

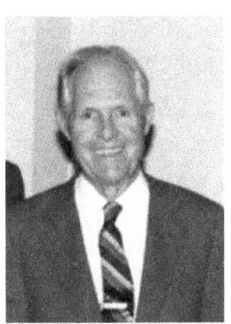

Dr. Raymond Brauer was Dr. Thomas Cronin's partner for 40 years. He was a very meticulous surgeon as well, who had many interests. Surgically Dr. Brauer was much more conservative than Dr. Thomas Cronin. He did not want to do any risky cases, whereas Dr. Cronin would take on almost any situation if he felt he could be of help. Dr. Brauer also had a great interest in cleft lip and palate surgery, hand surgery, and most of plastic surgery. I particularly appreciated his precise and exacting skills when he was working on intricate hand surgery cases such as the release of Dupuytren's contracture. He was also a master at cleft lip repair, and I learned a tremendous amount from him about that subject. Dr. Brauer was a wonderful mentor, from whom I learned many reliable lessons.

He had a healthy reticence to operate. For example, he would not be persuaded by the patient to return to the operating room too soon for revision surgery. He seemed to have a sixth sense in being able to tell which patients to pass up for an operation because they were not correctly predisposed, psychologically. He was quite precise in the operating room and worked at a steady pace.

He would usually carry on a light banter with all the personnel in the operating room, making working with him a pleasure. He had quite a repertoire of jokes and was ready to share new sententious variations with his coworkers. Even years after his retirement, his former residents still speak of "Brauerisms" from the operating room. They might be a small truism or a little rhyming phrase or some alliteration pertinent to work in the operating room, all of which were in good humor and none more than minimally risqué.

Dr. Brauer was quite an outdoorsman. He liked to play golf, enjoyed fly fishing, and loved to go snow skiing each year. Dr. Brauer would periodically remind everyone to 'stop and smell the roses." I was decidedly impressed when he bought himself a new pair of skis for his eightieth birthday! When ski season approached, he wore weights around his ankles even in the operating room to build up his leg strength. He would also challenge the residents to match his ability to squat and lean against the wall for several minutes. He usually outlasted the much younger residents.

Dr. Tom Biggs

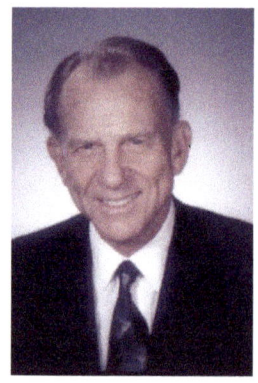

Another influential mentor was Tom Biggs. I remember he told the residents that at Ben Taub hospital during his residency training, he did dozens of tendon laceration cases and never saw one of these patients back in the clinic for follow-up. He reveled in participating in the preceptor type residence training. Dr. Thomas Biggs was a master at interpersonal relations with his patients and colleagues; he had an outstanding bedside manner and seemed to instill confidence in his patients. He was a very skilled surgeon known for rapid dissection in the operating room.

Dr. Biggs was particularly active in facial aesthetic surgery and breast surgery. He enjoyed an extensive cosmetic practice. Dr. Biggs was quite interested in classical music when I rotated on his service as a plastic surgery resident; so, we listened to great masterpieces throughout the surgical day. He was a hard worker and had a very busy practice. I learned a lot about how to deal with patients from him. After my residency, when I joined the Cronin Brauer and Biggs plastic surgery group, I found Dr. Biggs to be fair and generous. He had some favorite sayings for which he was known. "No key fits every lock" was used to good effect on numerous occasions when I was a resident to explain the various surgical options for particular plastic surgery problems. He was not dogmatic but rather quite ready to embrace new techniques. Another favorite saying was, "youth is the capacity for change."

On several occasions, I've heard him tell former residents if they are still doing particular cases the way he taught them, then they are behind the times. After his retirement, he continued to be involved with organized plastic surgery. It seemed like he was friends with every prestigious plastic surgeon around the world.

Dr. Paul Tessier

Dr. Paul Tessier was another mentor from whom I was fortunate to learn copious valuable lessons. I was especially happy that he invited me to visit and work with him in Paris in the summer of 1987. Chapter 10 is devoted to Dr. Tessier.

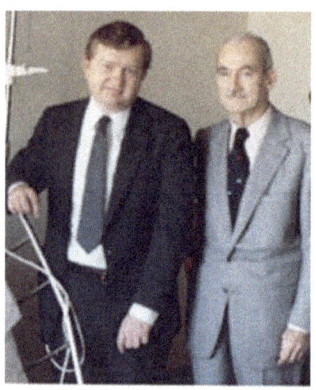

Dr. Robert Wise

Dr. Robert Wise is an example of a mentor of mine that I will never forget even though I only had relatively few interactions with him. His name is known to every plastic surgeon and every plastic surgery resident because of a breast reduction or breast lift incision pattern he developed. This "Wise pattern" is still commonly used today for breast reduction and mastopexy procedures. See chapter 14.

I first met Dr. Wise under somewhat unfavorable conditions. I was a first-year resident in plastic surgery. My two senior residents and all my immediate supervising staff went out-of-town to a national plastic surgery convention. The only plastic surgeon on staff at our hospital, not a regular part of the teaching program, was on call for the emergency room. I was to call him for any problem I might have with our service. As it turned out, a patient came to the emergency room with multiple severe facial lacerations from an automobile accident. The patient was a teenager accompanied by his mother. For some reason, there was a sharp fall out between this patient and the plastic surgeon on call. Therefore, I received a call from the Chief of Staff of the hospital, who briefly told me the situation and said to "take care of it." I examined the patient, who was already in a regular hospital room. Fortunately, his condition was not at all critical. The main problem was innumerable small lacerations of the face. I told them I would make arrangements for taking care of the patient.

The Harris County Medical Society roster listed about 30 plastic surgeons. Today there are well over 100. I knew many were at the same meeting my staff surgeons were attending. I started to make phone calls. I reached Dr. Robert Wise, whom I had only heard of but had never met. I told him who I was and explained the situation to him. I didn't know what to expect, but I was pleasantly surprised by his kind manner and his quick positive response.

I told him that the Chief of Staff would give him immediate emergency privileges as he was not on staff at our hospital. He told me to get the patient ready for surgery and that he would meet me outside of the surgery area in 45 minutes. I was happy to see him. We examined the patient and made a plan for surgery, and then the anesthesiologist brought the patient into the surgical suite and put him to sleep. We worked together for several hours on these multiple lacerations. He taught me several small tricks that have been useful to me on many occasions. This minor emergency turned out to be a great teaching experience for me. Incidentally, after that episode, better arrangements were made for backup staff coverage.

During my residency at St. Joseph's Hospital, there was a citywide journal club that met in a faculty member's house to go over the monthly plastic and reconstructive surgery journals. On one occasion, the journal club was to meet at Dr. Wise's home. My directions to his home were easy to follow, and I reached it more quickly than I had expected. I noticed only two cars in the driveway. It seemed like there should be several more, but maybe I was a little earlier than I thought. I went to the door and rang the bell. Dr. Wise answered the door and welcomed me. He said, "I guess you're here for the journal club." I told him I was. He said, "you are the first to arrive, and you are a little early- about 24 hours".

I was quite embarrassed. Dr. Wise said they already had dinner but were getting ready to sit down at the kitchen table for some dessert and insisted that I come in. I met his wife, and we proceeded to have a long discussion about plastic surgery as we had desert. I felt quite blessed by the whole event. The next day when I came back for the journal club, it was not nearly as exciting, nor did I learn as much as I had a one-on-one with Dr. Wise.

On the third occasion, I was quite pleased by Dr. Wise's response a few years later to an article that I had written about breast reconstruction. The report was in the St. Joseph's Hospital Journal, now defunct. He told me that it was one of the best articles on breast reconstruction he had seen and that he had frequently consulted it when planning breast reconstruction procedures. I was very grateful to him for these comments. He is now deceased. He was a great example of a caring, righteous plastic surgeon.

Dr. Melvin Spira

Dr. Melvin Spira became head of the Baylor plastic surgery residency program after Baron Hardy retired. Dr. Hardy and Dr. Thomas Cronin originally started the Baylor plastic surgery residency at Jefferson Davis Hospital. They would rotate the supervision of the residents every six months. He was a great gentleman. He would always come to the surgical demonstration when Dr. Tessier was visiting us in Houston. I never had the pleasure of directly working with Dr. Hardy.

Dr. Spira was always interested in research and how plastic surgery procedures could be improved. He always seemed interested in his patients and in doing the right thing. He was always very supportive of his residents and was an outstanding teacher. My exposure to him was mainly at conferences. During my residency, we had some meetings in common with the Baylor residents, such as a dermatopathology conference as well as conferences with visiting professors who would come to Houston to speak at the Houston Society of Plastic Surgeons. Dr. Spira was a great contributor to the field of plastic surgery. He continued to teach even after he retired from active practice.

Walls Unit rotation

One common overlapping aspect about both my ENT residency program at UTMB and the plastic surgery program at St. Joseph Hospital was a rotation at a nearby prison located in Huntsville, Texas, about 70 miles north of Houston. It was nicknamed "the walls" because of the impressively high walls surrounding the complex. Going to this prison for the first time was a somewhat scary experience. After first checking in at the information area and getting a badge, one faced the main entry hall, which was mostly brass gates and brass barred sidewalls.

As one approached, the first big brass gate would open, and you would walk in surrounded by a brass barred enclosure. The big brass gate would thunderously slam shut behind you, and another would open in front of you. I appreciated the nickname "the slammer" after this experience. On either side of this hallway, only bordered by brass bars, was a holding area for prisoners transferring in or out. So, as a visitor to the prison, I felt conspicuously like a fish in a glass bowl with prisoners checking me out as I walked in. After going through about three sliding brass gates, a few more steps took you into an enormous courtyard with the prison buildings all around.

The hospital building was on the far side of the yard. As I walked toward the hospital building, I saw prisoners in one corner playing basketball, in another area, lifting weights, and in another area simply milling around. Several guards were conspicuous in the courtyard. I observed several guard towers high around the periphery of the walls with officers peering down.

The hospital itself was Spartan. There was a clinic area on the first floor, where we would see our patients. Some of these patients were from other prison units. Upstairs there was a surgery suite with two operating rooms and a couple of wards of inpatient beds. In the plastic surgery clinic, we would see patients with broken noses, various hand injuries, lumps and bumps, and skin cancers. Besides that, we were able to operate upon a small number of cosmetic cases. The rationale was that improving the inmate's appearance would strengthen his self-esteem and perhaps make him more suitable for employment and overall success upon discharge from prison incarceration. An example was the patient who had always been made fun of because of large protruding ears. I pinned back his ears, and he was quite pleased with it and said maybe he was less likely to get into a fight now.

We also had very many cases of fractured noses. A man with a very crooked nose gives the impression of a pugnacious individual, whether true or not. Fixing such a nose in a prisoner may give him a better outlook on life. For me, as a resident, these were usually quite arresting cases, and generally helpful for the patients as well. A few years later the practice of allowing such cosmetic surgery on prisoners was eliminated either for budget-cutting reasons or more likely because prisoners getting cosmetic surgery for free was looked upon as bad publicity for the prison system

During the summer of 1974, in which I had I weekly ENT rotations at "the walls" prison hospital, there was a notorious attempted prison breakout. Thankfully I was not there on the day of the hostage-taking, but I did return the week following the end of the siege. A drug lord named Fred Carrasco, who was serving a life sentence for the attempted murder of a police officer, had pistols smuggled into the prison. He and two other prisoners, all armed with handguns, forced their way into the prison library and took 12 hostages. An 11 - day siege ensued, which lasted from July 24 to August 3.

During that time, negotiations took place between the convicts and the Texas Department of Corrections, FBI agents, and the Texas Rangers. The convicts made many demands, including walkie-talkies, bulletproof helmets, tailored suits, dress shoes, and pointedly an escape vehicle. At approximately 10 PM on Saturday, August 3, an armored getaway car rolled into the prison courtyard.

Next, a makeshift tank consisting of library books taped to blackboards slowly meandered out of the library toward the waiting vehicle. Eight hostages were tethered outside the tank while inside were the three convicts and four hostages. When they came out into the open courtyard, the prison authorities directed a stream of high-powered water hoses on them, which knocked over the tank. However, the hose ruptured, giving the convicts time to execute two women hostages. A shoot - out began; Carrasco and one of his accomplices were shot dead. The official report states that Carrasco committed suicide. The state executed the surviving convict in 1991

I was back at the prison hospital a few days later after things had calmed down. It was fascinating that the story I received from some of the prisoners in the hospital ward was a little different. They said that they had been able to watch the escape attempt from the third floor of the hospital building, which looked out onto the atrium. The prisoners said they knew this escape attempt was going to fail when they saw a Texas Ranger coming out into the courtyard after the waterspouts ended. They told me that the Texas Ranger shot dead the ringleader Carrasco with a big revolver.?

Another rotation I had for two months during the plastic surgery residency was at M. D. Anderson's Cancer Center. I worked with Dr. Ballantine, a prominent general surgery trained, head, and neck cancer surgeon. He was very engaging, quite innovative, and was an outstanding surgeon. The Cancer Center attracted patients with unusual and severe pathology. During this rotation, I received a lot of new experience in both the ablation of tumors and head and neck reconstruction.

At the end of the plastic surgery residency, the graduating residents from all the area programs presented a series of cases representative of their plastic surgery experience to the Houston Society of Plastic Surgeons. I think everyone enjoyed this great experience. After I completed my residency, I immediately went to work in the Cronin Brauer and Biggs Plastic Surgery Clinic. A handshake sealed my verbal contract agreement.

The four years of medical school are just a necessary background for what follows. The majority of plastic surgeons in practice today went through a five-year residency training program in general surgery as a prerequisite to plastic surgery training. The next most common alternative route taken by plastic surgeons was completing a five-year residency in otolaryngology (ear nose and throat surgery) as a prerequisite to plastic surgery residency training. This prerequisite training requires the individual to learn how to operate, think like a surgeon, and learn to fine-tune surgical judgment and technique. Residence programs choose the best candidates interested in plastic surgery from this eligible group to enter formal plastic surgery residency training.

In the program with which I was most involved, we have had almost 200 qualified applicants each year for two positions. This final training now consists of three years of concentrated study and practical work limited to the field of plastic surgery. Therefore, most plastic surgeons in practice today have had approximately seven years of post-M.D. degree residency training. Many more recently trained plastic surgeons will have graduated from 6 - year Integrated Programs mentioned above.

Plastic Surgery Boards

There was still one more hurdle before I would consider myself a real plastic surgeon. That was passing my Board Certification Examinations in plastic surgery. Although I had been reading and studying throughout my residency years, I began an extensive review and study of plastic surgery in preparation for my board examinations. For example, I read the previous ten years of standard plastic surgery journals. I learned from cover to cover the most comprehensive seven-volume textbook in plastic surgery. I went to two exam preparation courses, one for the written and one for the oral examination.

At that time, the written examination included a test on anatomy and physiology, an evaluation of the theory and practice of plastic surgery, and a test on pathology, including the reading of microscopic slides. To prepare for that, I obtained a series of slides from the Armed Forces Institute of Pathology. These were typical glass slides. I photographed these microscopic slides and turned them into 35mm slides for viewing, all done in preparation for the written examination. I remember taking the review course for the written exam and hearing my uncle Tom Cronin's name repeatedly mentioned in various areas of plastic surgery as a significant contributor and innovator. I was pleased to pass my written examination and immediately began preparing for the oral part. I was now ready to take the oral exam in Palm Beach, Florida.

Dr. Benjamin Cohen

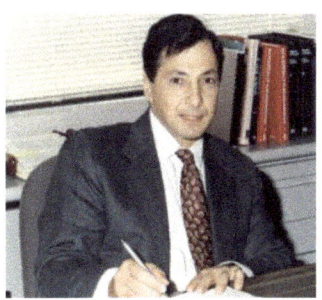

Dr. Benjamin Cohen joined the Cronin Brauer and Biggs clinic at the same time I did. We flew together to take the oral examination in Palm Beach. A tropical storm a day or so before dropped 17 inches of rain on the area. The grounds adjacent to the drive into the Breakers Hotel, still covered with water, looked like a lake.

The oral examination process was much more stressful than the written examination. Each candidate was required to pass two oral exams, one on the theory and practice of plastic surgery, and the other on a series of cases that each examinee had prepared. In the first instance, two examiners showed pictures of some defects or plastic surgery problems and then asked questions. In the other examination, two examiners asked questions about our selected cases. At that time, we needed to have eight of our cases that demonstrated at least six different categories of plastic surgery. We might have a congenital case of a cleft lip or palate and a cosmetic example such as a rhinoplasty or a facelift. We would likely have a hand surgery case, a traumatic injury example, and a breast case.

The evening before the examination, we had a meeting to go over the format for the next day. We were required to turn in our set of eight cases for review; if they did not meet the prescribed criteria, we would not be able to take the examination the next day. If our performance was borderline, examiners could require us to take a third examination. Conversely, if we felt that our performance was not as good as it could have been, we were allowed to ask for a third examination so that our performance might improve. We had to request this before knowing the results of the first two examinations.

The next day we went to a particular assigned room in the hotel and told to stand outside the door and wait. The long hallway soon filled with apprehensive inchoate plastic surgeons standing outside of every room down the hall. I was also very nervous at this point. The fellow who was standing outside of the room immediately across the hall from me struck up a conversation

He said, "Is this your first time taking the oral exam?" I said yes. He said, "I took it last year. Let me give you some advice. If they asked you to take a third exam - just go home. That happened to me last year, and what I endured was the worst experience of my life." Well, that little episode did nothing to help alleviate my anxiety. However, both examinations went quite well. Later I was so pleased to find that I had passed the oral exam and had earned my Board Certification by the American Board of Plastic Surgery. I will always remember it as one of the most significant accomplishments of my life. I was now a "real" plastic surgeon.

Because I was fortunate enough to join the Cronin Brauer and Biggs clinic immediately after finishing my residency, I was able to take further advantage of learning from these great mentors even after completing my residency. In retrospect, I would have to say that in the year immediately following my residency, I probably learned as much as I did during my formal residency.

It was also during that year that I came to know and appreciate Dr. Ben Cohen, who would be my partner for 38 years. I have been very fortunate to be associated with such an outstanding, perspicacious plastic surgeon, colleague, and friend. Ben graduated from Columbia University in New York and Harvard Medical School in Boston. He did his residency training in general and plastic surgery at Massachusetts General Hospital in Boston.

Dr. Cohen is both an erudite academician and a dexterous clinical plastic surgeon. Especially during the first years of our practice, we did many notable microsurgery free flap cases together. In the first photo below, Dr. Cohen (back left) is harvesting a latissimus muscle as a free flap from the back while I am preparing the recipient vessels near the defect in the lower leg (front right). Traumatic tibial fracture cases with open wounds and exposed bone often need free tissue muscle flaps. Skin grafts are not applicable, and often there are no local flaps appropriate for coverage of these wounds.

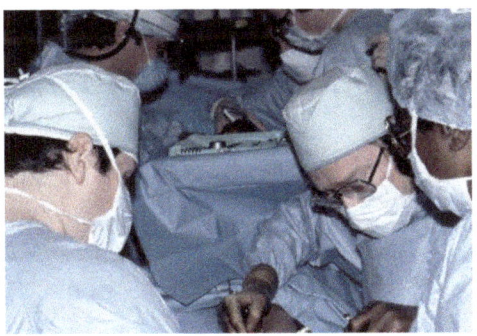

The blue stripes below outline the proposed size of the latissimus muscle flap together with a small elliptical skin island in solid blue. The second picture shows the muscle elevated and the divergent blood supply. The third and fourth pictures show the nerve and vascular supply entering the muscle from the axilla.

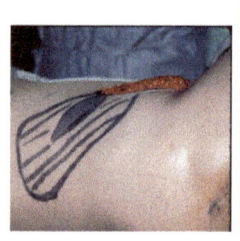 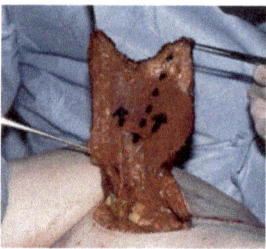 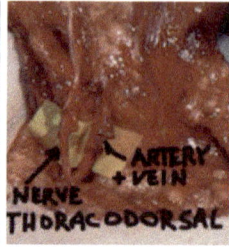 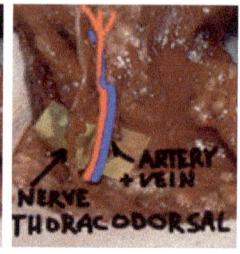

Below, the latissimus muscle is being thinned from the external surface safely as the blood supply runs on the deep surface. We did this thinning to assure the proper amount of tissue for the wound on the leg. A split-thickness skin graft resurfaces the muscle. The small skin island is an indicator of assessing the blood supply. It is easier to tell if there is adequate blood supply to that skin island than where the skin graft will be covering the muscle. If the skin island lost blood supply, we would have to explore the wound and check the anastomoses to the muscle. In the middle, Dr. Cohen and I are working together under the microscope on such a case. We connected the thoracodorsal artery and vein from the latissimus muscle to the recipient vessels in the leg to re-establish blood supply to the muscle flap.

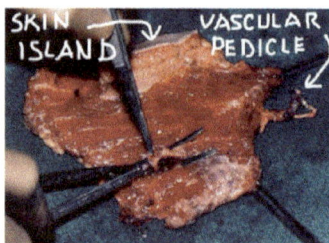 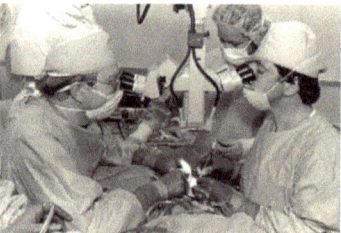 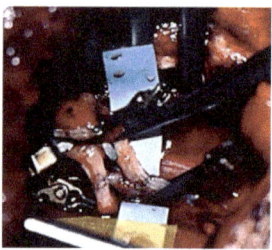

Below, after anastomosing the vessels, we placed the flap to cover the wound in the leg just above the ankle. We gained additional access by temporarily removing the external orthopedic fixation device. In the last photo, the orthopedic external fixator is back in place.

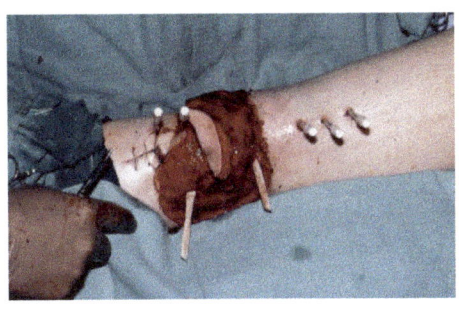 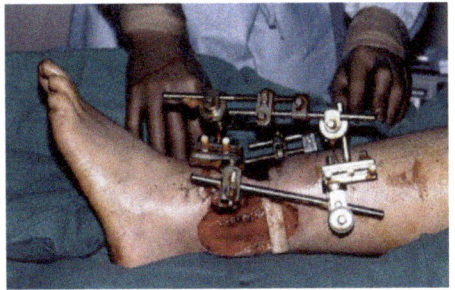

Will the real plastic surgeon stand up?

Sometimes I am flabbergasted by the lack of understanding some patients have about medical specialists, particularly in my field of plastic surgery. On many occasions, I've seen a patient after she had some operation with which she is unhappy. When I ask her who did the procedure, sometimes I recognize the doctor's name as not a plastic surgeon. I might say oh, Dr. Blank, the dermatologist. Most likely, she will reply, "no, he's a plastic surgeon."

Some patients won't believe the truth. In our state, there are virtually no restrictions on advertising by doctors. Often you will see ads that say that the doctor is board-certified. However, the board referred to may be a fictitious board, that is, one not recognized by the National Board of Medical Specialties. Individual people have created other medical boards without specific qualifications. But they may sound impressive to the public. In Texas, a mountebank may complete medical school and do a one- year internship and hang up his shingle calling himself a plastic surgeon. There is no law to prevent this.

Years ago, if a physician ever advertised to the public, he was ostracized by the medical societies. However, because of the Federal Trade Commission and the influence of lawyers and the courts, medical organizations can no longer restrict their members from advertising. Legitimate medical societies might be able to discipline doctors who have gross false advertising. However, now many physicians do advertise. Ersatz plastic surgeons and some real plastic surgeons are guilty at taking self - aggrandizing adds to the extreme. One may look in various sports magazines and see numerous gaudy ads with extravagant claims and tacky pictures.

In the past, the general public would've avoided anyone who advertised, especially in such a forum. Since medical practitioners are now sometimes looked upon as vendors rather than professionals, it seems much of the public thinks the practitioner with most advertisements must be the best doctor.

I consider it a tremendous privilege to be a plastic surgeon. It is a remarkable field of medicine that can emphatically benefit patients and give great satisfaction to its practitioners. My advice for someone seeking a plastic surgeon would be to confirm his credentials and check with the American Society of Plastic Surgeons to be sure he is a member, as board-certification is one of the criteria for membership. Indeed, asking one's family doctor or a knowledgeable doctor friend can also be helpful, but occasionally they are also ignorant of the necessary distinctions.

I have seen some perplexing things, such as a patient who had an augmentation mammaplasty by an oral surgeon. Another patient had an augmentation mammaplasty by an ENT doctor. I have seen facelifts by dermatologists, liposuction by gynecologists, facial cosmetic implants by a general surgeon. I remember a particular lady who came because of difficulty after some aesthetic surgery. She had had cheek implants on both sides and a chin augmentation with an implant. One cheek implant was too high, and the other was too low. The chin was very asymmetric, as well. Her original photo is below. Malposition of an implant can undoubtedly happen with an excellent plastic surgeon, but it did seem extreme that all the implants were mal-positioned.

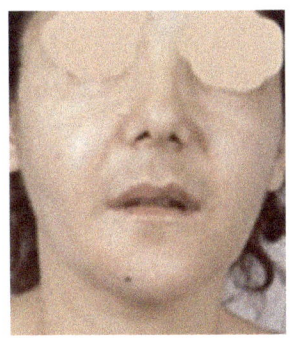

After talking with her awhile, I found out that she had gone to a general surgeon of her same ethnic background for social reasons. This surgeon did not qualify by training for this kind of surgery. He may have ventured outside of his expertise for financial reasons. I had to redo all her implant placements. It was of particular interest that there were actually two chin implants, one folded upon itself and the other not centered at all. In the first photo below, I am holding the chin implant folded abnormally on itself as it was in the patient. That chin implant, the blue one, may have been a sizer implant. The sizers are usually blue, while the permanent implants are either clear or white. The middle photo below shows the other three mal-positioned implants. Her post-operative photos are on the right below. She was pleased with her result and sent me several patients. This patient did well after her revision surgery, but her experience points out the importance of seeking out a qualified plastic surgeon for this type of surgery. Chapter 16 is devoted to Aesthetic surgery.

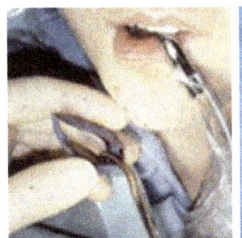 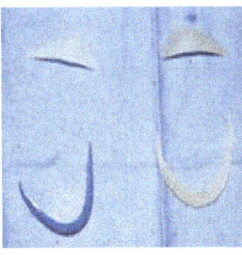 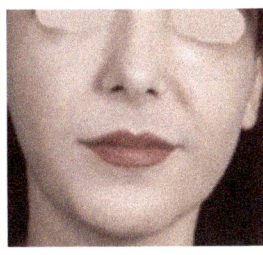 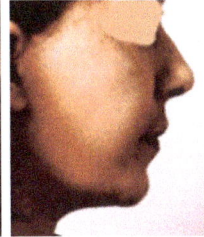

It would be one thing if these patients knew they were getting plastic surgery by individuals who are not plastic surgeons. However, some of these patients think they are having surgery done by a plastic surgeon. Misleading advertisements often fool the naïve or inexperienced public.

I recently reviewed a local fitness magazine for cosmetic plastic surgery ads. Note these are for plastic surgery, not for skincare procedures. There were seven plastic surgeons, three in ENT surgeons, three general or family practice doctors, three dermatologists, one general surgeon, one vascular surgeon, one emergency medicine doctor. Also, there was one physician for whom I could not identify a specialty. To the casual perusing public, all of these doctor's advertisements would seem to be those of plastic surgeons.

Turf battles

Turf battles between various surgical subspecialties are frequent. For example, rhinoplasty, an operation on the nose, is done by most ENT doctors and most plastic surgeons, which is fine. But what if the doctor is a dermatologist or dentist instead? Most plastic surgeons and probably the general public would object to an ENT doctor doing an augmentation mammaplasty. However, some non - plastic surgeons who get patients through advertisements will perform such procedures.

It is also amazing how pseudo technology can mislead people. I have had several patients come to see me after seeing a "plastic surgeon" who purports to do all of his surgery with the laser rather than scalpel and scissors etc. For most areas of plastic surgery, this is just a marketing gimmick that sounds high-tech but is not a better way to treat patients. There's no question that lasers have a significant role in many areas of medicine. They have revolutionized the treatment of myopia or nearsightedness by ophthalmologists. Lasers are beneficial in the treatment of various vascular lesions and some congenital birthmarks. I have also used lasers to resurface the skin for conditions such as wrinkles or certain scars or removal of tattoos. There will be many new areas ware lasers will be beneficial in the field of medicine.

As I related earlier, my background and prerequisite training were in otorhinolaryngology (ENT), and I certainly don't want to denigrate this medical field. Many ENT specialists do excellent plastic surgery in the head and neck region. Also, many ENT specialists do skilled aesthetic rhinoplasty surgery. Also, some ophthalmologists, with extra training in oculoplastic surgery, do both reconstructive and cosmetic surgery of the eyelids and orbital region. Neither the plastic surgery establishment nor I have any problem with these surgeons.

It seems that, for good or for bad, whether real or not, there is a mystique about plastic surgery. Sometimes a doctor wants to be a plastic surgeon but does not want to or cannot fulfill the requisite training requirements. In general, most plastic surgeons think if you are going to call yourself a plastic surgeon, you should do the plastic surgery residency training.

One of the reasons I decided to write this book was to defend the reputation of the vast majority of plastic surgeons who are ethical and hold paramount the best interest of their patients at all times. As in any field, there are outliers who, either because of serious character flaws or professional pressures or pursuit of fame or fortune, crossover ethical lines. Alcohol, drugs, greed, lust can all play their role in the corruption of individuals.

Professional life issues

I had a few female patients that I only knew professional, asked me to lunch, sometimes repeatedly. Although innocent-sounding, I always turned down these invitations.

I remember very distinctly seeing a young woman in follow up a few months after I had performed an augmentation mammaplasty on her. She was doing fine. After I finished the exam, she asked the nurse if she could see me for a minute in my office. The nurse asked me, and I said sure. She came into my office as I got up from my chair. She closed the door and literally threw herself at me, encircling her arms around me, saying she was attracted to me. I was startled but gently brushed her away and told her I was happily married and was not interested. She accepted my attitude, and that was the end of that.

I am sure many plastic surgeons have had similar experiences. Plastic surgeons see women unclothed for exams related to breast surgery or for body contouring or liposuction procedures, which could produce temptations to stray from the straight and narrow. The Hippocratic oath and professional ethics require plastic surgeons to resist such temptations emphatically. Most plastic surgeons are good family men who are contributors to society. They are involved in their communities and churches etc. A significant percentage of plastic surgeons do charitable plastic surgery either at home or in underdeveloped countries.

As a plastic surgeon, I have my prejudices regarding plastic surgeons in general. I think most are regular gentlemen, and ladies, who remember their Hippocratic oath, are trying to do well for their patients honestly and straightforwardly. However, there is a small percent whom I do not trust.

It is relatively common to have patients come in having had surgery done by other plastic surgeons. Sometimes the patient wants a second opinion or just some reassurance. Most of the time, I would give my opinion and try to send the patient back to the first surgeon. I am always inclined to provide the surgeon with the benefit of the doubt regarding poor outcomes. There are several reasons for this. Every surgeon has poor results some times. Often, I do not know the starting point. So sometimes there may have been significant improvement with a procedure, but because of the extent of the original problem, there is still substantial deformity or opportunity for progress. The patient may have received 100% improvement but wanted 200%. Perhaps 100% enhancement was all anyone would have been able to accomplish in one procedure.

Every surgeon has complications and unsatisfactory results occasionally. I think we have to be careful not to let our egos get out of hand. It may be easy to look askance or even openly criticize the results of our colleagues, leading to unnecessary and unjust litigation. I clearly remember receiving notice of being sued by a patient for whom I had cared since she was an infant. She had severe multiple congenital anomalies. Over the years, I operated on her many times. She did exceptionally well and had an excellent result. One of the procedures I performed for her was a partial jaw reconstruction by using one of her ribs. She was missing one side of the jaw from birth.

She moved and went to another plastic surgeon in another city about 250 miles away. A few months later, I get a notice of a suit. The allegation was that I had put her new jaw in "backward." I was more hurt than frightened by this. I knew I had done nothing wrong. I was very disappointed with the family and the patient. But also, I can imagine that someone in the other surgeon's office said something that implied they could have done a better job with her case. I have seen patients from that office over the years, some of whom have had difficulties that I treated.

This suit was quickly dismissed, I assume, because they could get no one to agree that I did anything incorrectly. In retrospect, I remember that this patient's family sued the pharmaceutical manufacturer of a medication called Bendectin, which was an anti-nausea medicine used in pregnancy. It was one of the only drugs that seemed safe for pregnant women for morning sickness. There were many suits alleging Bendectin caused congenital birth defects. The manufacturer won most of these suits because there was no clear evidence to support the allegations. However, it became so costly and risky to defend against these suits the manufacture pulled this drug off the market. So, what was probably a safe and effective medication with few substitutes was no longer available for patients.

Sometimes as a plastic surgeon, I felt like I lived in a glasshouse; therefore, I am hesitant to criticize my colleagues without reliable information. One episode illustrates the sensitive nature of seeing patients for second opinions. A set of twins came to our cleft lip and palate clinic. They had previously been seen and were being prepared for surgery by another cleft palate team in town. They wanted a second opinion.

They saw all the members of our team and received input from each. I consulted with them and told them of my high opinion of the plastic surgeon with whom they had been working. The parents later called back and decided they wanted to change the teams, not because of anything against the other group, but because they were more comfortable with our team. I decided to accept them as patients in our clinic. It may have been the wrong thing to do. Perhaps if I had been more forceful at encouraging them to stay with their first group, they would have. I had unintentionally created some ill will with the other surgeon who expressed his displeasure directly to me. I did tell him that in this circumstance, I did treat him as I hope he will treat me in the reverse situation. I was very sorry we had this confrontation. Afterword, in a written note to him, I did try to explain my dilemma. We still have a good relationship that I value. I am sure that he occasionally takes care of patients who perhaps became disenchanted with me.

There are many local plastic surgeons in Houston, and I am sure all over the USA who do volunteer work in plastic surgery to help their communities. Examples are legion. Throughout the USA, there are numerous programs sponsored by plastic surgeons to help the needy both here and abroad. In a large city like Houston, with well over a hundred legitimate plastic surgeons, it is not surprising that I would not know everything about everybody. I would certainly give the benefit of the doubt to any plastic surgeon about whom I did not know anything negative.

Another occasional dilemma arises from hearing negative rumors about this or that surgeon, which may be completely unsupported. Because I was involved in the Houston Society of Plastic Surgeons for many years, I was able to get to know a large percentage of the surgeons in our city. The vast majority are honest and try to do an excellent job for patients.

Menaces

However, within our community, we have had a few examples of malfeasance by plastic surgeons. One reprobate attempted to murder his wife and tried to make it look like suicide, but she survived. This execrated surgeon was convicted of attempted murder and sent to prison. Another surgeon evaded federal income taxes for which he spent time in prison. One perfidious surgeon committed Medicare fraud and also spent time in prison. Every large group of human beings has a few scoundrels. The local authorities accused Dr. John Hill of *Blood and Money* fame, of killing his wife Joan Robinson Hill, the adopted daughter of Ash Robinson, a wealthy Texas oilman.

John Hill, although never convicted, was eventually murdered, perhaps at the instigation of his persevering and trenchant former father in - law. A few years ago, a local plastic surgeon ran over two women with his car and failed to stop. He was soon arrested and charged with driving under the influence of drugs and alcohol and leaving the scene of the accident. He lost his license and went to prison for a time. I believe he may be subject to Mark Anthony's observation "the evil that men do lives after them; the good is oft interred with their bones…".

A different place and time

Toward the end of my plastic surgery residency, which ended in 1978, I began to look for practice opportunities in some suburban areas of Houston. I guess this became common knowledge among my mentors because one day, they asked me to step into an office and sit down. They asked if I would like to join the group in a provisional capacity for one year with a salary of about twice what I made as a resident. I had been hoping for such an invitation because this group practice seemed to have the best mixture of private practice plus academic endeavors and resident teaching opportunities. Drs. Cronin, Brauer, Biggs, and Wolf was a very prestigious group, and I felt privileged to join them. A series of handshakes was the contract for that first year. When discussing future practice opportunities with residents thirty years later, I realized the world had changed a lot. I think none of them would join a practice without having their attorneys go over in detail the specific written employment contract.

The Cronin, Brauer, and Biggs clinic was the premier plastic surgery practice in Houston at that time. The clientele included old-time Houston patricians and hoi polloi alike. Patients came from all over Texas and neighboring states. In 1988 the Cronin Brauer Biggs Clinic split apart. I will not go into any of the reasons but would like to note to the credit of all concerned the legal costs were zero. Dr. Cohen and I began a practice together at a new professional building, while Dr. Thomas Cronin and Dr. Brauer reestablished their practice next door, and Dr. Biggs moved his practice on the other side also next door to us. We continued to staff the residency program and to work closely together. Abrogating the Cronin, Brauer, and Biggs Clinic created some wistful contemplations, but change is inevitable.

Helpful Colleagues

I received many blessings by working with many trustworthy plastic surgery colleagues during my many years of practice. Below with me are Drs. Leo Lapuerta, Tom Biggs, Ben Cohen, Don Collins, and Bruce Smith. I am thankful to all of them for many years of friendly comradeship.

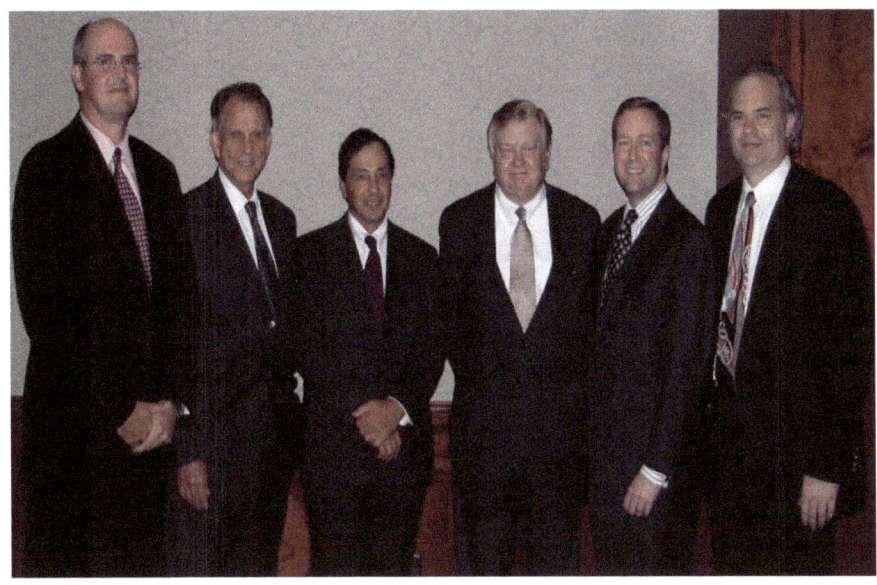

Residents

I have felt approbative about almost all of our residents. They were all highly qualified and well-trained surgeons before they came to us, eager to assimilate all they could learn about plastic surgery. There has been a lot of discussion about the generational differences between the greatest generation of WWII, baby boomers, Generation X, and Millennials, etc. Having been born in 1945, I consider myself in the baby boomer generation. My mentors were of the greatest generation. Most of the applicants we interviewed and accepted for our residency program were in their late twenties' or early thirties. I first saw baby boomers, then those representing Generation X. Now we have moved into the millennial generation. Another curious aspect of working with residents is the appreciation of these generation gaps. As I proceeded through my residency training, I readily accepted the existing educational system. I admired and idolized my teachers. I was optimistic that if I was dedicated and worked hard and tried to do the right thing that I would be successful and find validation. I was dedicated to pursuing a career but craved support from my family. I was probably typical of the baby-boomer resident in training. Books were central to learning for me. Now, less learning comes from books, and more knowledge is from the internet.

Generation X residents seemed to have less respect for authority and generally were more skeptical. They were less driven to a professional career and sought a more balanced division between their job and their personal life. They tended to be self-starters, who relish getting things done on their own. They thrived in a more frenetic, sometimes discursive environment. Rather than delve profoundly and read extensively to become erudite on a subject, they adumbrated. It seems they would instead learn by technologically scanning for the inside tips and bottom-lines of many topics.

The internet readily supports this approach. Generation X is more technologically savvy than their baby boomer teachers. Millennials are even more facile in the digital world. They sometimes think they can do anything, not always considering the experience prior generations went through to find the current answer to the problem. As George Santayana wrote, "those who cannot remember the past are condemned to repeat it." The newest generation of residents may not be as interested in institutional history. Their knowledge of the development of plastic surgery may be exiguous.

Conversely, Gen Xers and Millennials may be more open to new ways of doing things than the boomers. I have seen no Luddites among them. I think another quality of more recent residents is they are less likely to join traditional organizations; this, unfortunately, may result in less cohesion and less professional camaraderie.

It is an exhilarating experience to participate in plastic surgery resident training. These nascent plastic surgeons are eager to learn. They come from all over the country and so have varied experiences in their surgical training. This diversity can help build new, more sophisticated understandings of plastic surgery from different viewpoints. I learned a great deal from my residents.

When I was a resident, and for several years afterward, there was excellent attendance at the Houston Society of Plastic Surgeons. There was quite a high percentage of plastic surgeons in the city who would come to these monthly meetings. They were instructive meetings, often with visiting professors from all over the United States and even foreign countries who would give a lecture after a nice dinner. More recently, although the number of plastic surgeons has dramatically increased in the Houston area, the number of attendees is probably similar to what it was a few decades ago. The reasons are probably complex and a sign of the times. There is less professional cohesion among plastic surgeons today, possibly related to the fact that advertising has turned the profession into a marketplace service. Plastic surgeons may look upon their colleagues more as commercial competitors rather than comrades in the healing mission of plastic surgery. Unfortunately, this fact is something with which organized plastic surgery must contend.

Usual and Customary Basis

Early in my medical career, insurance companies paid doctors for operations on a "usual and customary" basis. The system had worked very well for many years. When I performed surgery in the ER, I would try to bill appropriately. I had no guidelines except what I had seen my teachers do, and they always tried to be fair. Of course, there was an occasional outlier who overcharged patients. However, years ago, the county medical society could censure such a physician. Having learned from the group that trained me, I became used to the usual and customary billing.

However, because of the need for standardization and also abuse, a CPT (Current procedural terminology) code system superseded the old method shortly after I went into practice. The CPT system assigned a relative value to all the procedures. Billing became more organized but created a new level of bureaucracy as medical practices needed to hire coding specialists. It is not a perfect system, but it now seems indispensable.

Insurance payments to surgeons radically changed with the onset of managed care. The system facilitated ratcheting down payments by insurance companies. Rather than being an amount that was usual and customary and had some relationship to the difficulty of the procedure and the amount of training necessary to obtain the skill, it became a matter of what the insurance company wanted to pay. Restraint of trade laws restricts physicians from discussing their fees with other physicians. Therefore, individual physicians or small partnerships of physicians had to deal on a one on one basis with large insurance entities. These companies did not seem to have anything except lowering fees as their aim. However, premiums did not go down correspondingly.

The rate of premium increases may have slowed down for a few years, but eventually, they began to rise again. Physicians either accepted contracts brought by insurance companies or rejected them and thereby lost the opportunity to care for groups of patients covered by those insurance companies. For a few years, most doctors continued to care for their patients no matter the reimbursement. After a while, the goodwill of the doctors wore thin, and many began to make business decisions and reject plans that paid less than the cost of caring for patients.

Even if I could have limited my practice to self- pay cash patients, I would not have done it, as taking care of a broad range of plastic surgery problems is very compelling. Also, if every plastic surgeon did, there would be an awful lot of patients who would not receive the appropriate care they needed. There is no legal way physicians can collectively bargain for equitable fees. So, over the past couple of decades, while medical insurance premiums have been rising sharply, reimbursement for reconstructive and functional surgery to the surgeons was drastically reduced to about 25% or 30% of previous usual and customary. That is even without adjustment for inflation, which would make it even worse. However, I doubt the general public believes this, but also if they did, they would not be sympathetic to "rich doctors." Everyone has his problems!

Early in my practice, which began in 1978, I occasionally had some dispute with an insurance company about a particular surgery fee or our coverage thereof. But we considered the insurance companies to be legitimate businesses trying to do a service for their customers and with the best interest of patients in mind. However, after the onset of managed care, it became apparent that the insurance companies cared nothing about the patients and only about the bottom - line financial situation. We had innumerable instances in which insurance companies would deny that they ever received information from us, even though we had a return receipt that they had received the data.

Managed Care

Managed care is like having car insurance that requires you to get your transmission fixed at shop A or B only and get routine car maintenance done at shop C or D only.

For several years into the age of managed care, I think the goodwill of physicians towards their patients blunted the magnitude of the problem. Many physicians continued to care for their patients even though they were not reimbursed equitably for their work.

Frustrated by the unethical conduct of so many insurance companies, physicians became worn out, and many retired early. Also, under the old system, with most people covered by ordinary indemnity insurance, there was some fat in the system to help care for uninsured and indigent patients. However, with managed care, insurance companies had no interest in this societal issue. The hardship for caring for an increasing number of uninsured fell both to not-for-profit hospitals and to physicians who still cared for these patients.

Another area that has completely changed is care in the hospital emergency room. It used to be that a plastic surgeon on the medical staff would be required to share ER calls with the rest of the plastic surgery staff. For many years this was regardless of the patient's ability to pay. Most surgeons were ok with this when insurance reimbursements were adequate. When indemnity insurance reimbursed physicians for the majority of their patients, they were willing to deliver a reasonable amount of such charity care.

However, after managed care ratcheted down reimbursements, the goodwill of most physicians was exhausted. They balked at coming to the ER to care for no pay patients. The analogy is that of a person going to the grocery store filling his bag with groceries but expecting to walk out without paying. This does not compute! Physicians have to pay staff salaries regardless. As physicians became resistant to answering such calls to the emergency room, hospitals had to change their system.

The situation finally broke down. Many hospitals now pay on-call specialist doctors to care for no pay patients in the emergency room who cannot be handled by the emergency room physician. These changes paralleled the development of hospitalists, which took the place of the patient's physician coming to the hospital to care for him.

The delivery system for emergency care has radically changed in the last decade. There are urgent care facilities on practically every corner that see many of the insured patients who used to go to hospital ERs. Now, hospital ERs continue to see more severe cases and a higher percentage of the uninsured population. Change is inevitable. When things do not work well, people demand evolution, which is from time to time favorable.

The area in which I noticed the most significant change in reimbursement was for large reconstructive operations, which might involve 5 or 6 hours of surgery, attendance for several days in the hospital, and include several weeks of post-op care office visits. In the early 1990s, insurance payments for such large reconstructive operations might be $5,000. By the early 2000s, the amount likely was $1500, a dramatic change. There was less adjustment for small office procedures such as removal of minor skin cancers.

Unfortunately, slow and low pay was not the only problem with insurance companies. We saw various entities go out of business, leaving massive amounts unpaid to the doctors while the executives ride their golden parachutes. Some larger companies have engaged in the unethical activity of withholding payment for inordinately long periods. The Texas insurance commissioner for a while helped improve such slow-pay practices after suing insurance companies.

Another problem had to do with large self-insured companies that contracted with third-party administrators. The doctor may have a contract with a third party. He deals with that company and gets approval for a proposed reconstructive operation. Then after the doctor has done the surgery and bills for the surgery, the self-insured company says that it will not pay for the procedure. After complaining to the Texas insurance commission, we found out self-insured companies do not have to answer to the state insurance commission. In contradistinction, the physician must abide by the contract with the third-party administrator.

These self-insured companies fall under the federal ERISA law, which is a gigantic loophole for large companies.

Slamming, analogous to telephone company tactics, also occurred. Sometimes an insurance company said we were participating in a contract with them, i.e., taking reduced fees. When we checked into it, we find out we had no contract, and they should have been responsible for usual and customary fees. They were challenging to deal with without becoming cynical. So, where has all the money gone? There are multiple executives of sizeable medical insurance companies making obscene salaries and profit through excessive stock options and other unethical practices. It is bad enough when there are examples of medical insurance executives making hundreds of millions of dollars. A while back, the chief executive for United Healthcare had a compensation package that was over $1 billion in one year. At the same time, many surgeons receive a rate as low as $50 an hour for taking care of patients under the global fee system.

Medical politics

Plastic surgeons, like other physicians, are involved in grassroots medical politics. For most, this consists of participating in the section or department of plastic surgery in their local hospital or hospitals. It may involve other local groups, such as a city or county plastic surgery group. In my case, we have had an active Houston Society of plastic surgeons. I spent time as an officer in this organization and am a past president of the Houston Society of plastic surgeons and the Texas Society of plastic surgeons. Their primary purpose is to promote excellence in plastic surgery in Houston and the State of Texas. Also, there are several national societies of plastic surgeons, and a significant percentage of the membership gets involved with the running of these organizations. Occasionally members from the ranks of plastic surgeons are involved in local politics such as the state legislatures. Plastic surgeons have been elected to state legislatures and even to the United States Congress.

Many other plastic surgeons are like your neighbors and are involved in community activities, little league baseball, schools, sports clubs, etc. Most plastic surgeons went into medicine because they wanted to make a difference in society and, in some small way to contribute to its betterment.

After being in practice about a dozen years, I became chief of the plastic surgery section in the surgery department at my primary hospital, St Joseph. A few years later, I was elected Secretary of the then vice chief of staff, and finally, chief of the medical staff. There is a whole culture dealing with the medical staff and the interface between the medical staff and the hospital administration. As Chief of Staff, one gets to observe all the dirty laundry of the medical staff and administration that otherwise would be unnoticed or brought up via innuendo or rumor. Some of these interactions were with petulant or querulous physicians who seemed to enjoy every kerfuffle.

Most large hospitals are very complex bureaucracies that are difficult with which to deal. As doctors in our plastic surgery section, we would often joke about trying to "find the wizard," meaning we often had difficulty finding who was in a position to make decisions about hospital problems or topics decisively. Like many other hospitals and healthcare institutions, our hospital repeatedly merged with other systems, turning an already complicated bureaucratic situation into an imbroglio.

Chapter 4

The Art and Science of Plastic Surgery

Living tissue

Plastic surgery is surgery which molds or shapes a part of the body to improve function or form. A fundamental difference between the art of plastic surgery and other artistic disciplines that mold or form three-dimensional works are that the material used is living tissue. Therefore, the surgeon must consider blood supply and innervation with every rearrangement of tissue.

As a result, hallmarks of plastic surgery are its use of delicate instrumentation, meticulous, and gentle handling of tissues. It is replete with numerous innovative methods of grafting, transfer, or rearrangement of tissues to repair or restore diseased, injured, lost, or deformed features. Various tissue flaps, such as those depicted below, are used. To understand flaps and grafts, one must have some idea of the blood supply to the skin.

There are several different ways that blood gets from deeper dominant arteries to the surface. In the drawing below, skin section one on the left receives blood from its major supplying vessel that traverses between muscles and enters the subcutaneous tissue to supply the skin. Section one is septocutaneous. The second skin section obtains its blood from a major vessel that first penetrates a muscle and then via perforating arteries, supplies the skin. It is musculocutaneous. The third skin section shows an axial blood supply in which the major vessel sends a branch directly to the fascia. The blood supply then runs parallel for a distance under the skin before reaching the surface. It is axial. Finally, the random section four, farther from large perforating vessels, has only small blood vessels to the skin in every direction.

The Healing Mission of Plastic Surgery

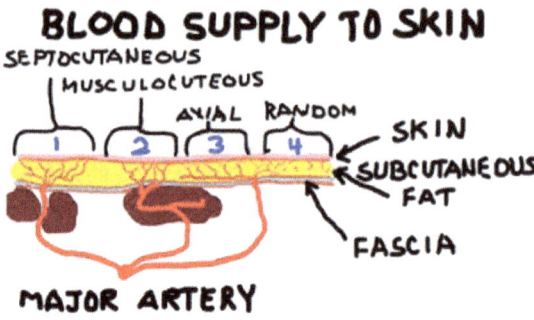

In the following drawings, I will show the creation of flaps utilizing the differing anatomic blood supply.

Random Flaps

A random skin flap contains skin and subcutaneous fat. It does not have any large blood vessels within the flap itself. It gets its nourishment through its base, which remains connected. Because of this limited blood supply, there is a length to width ratio, which must be respected, or the distal part of the flap will not survive. The two drawings below represent a random skin flap with appropriate length to width ratio of 1:1, producing a health flap

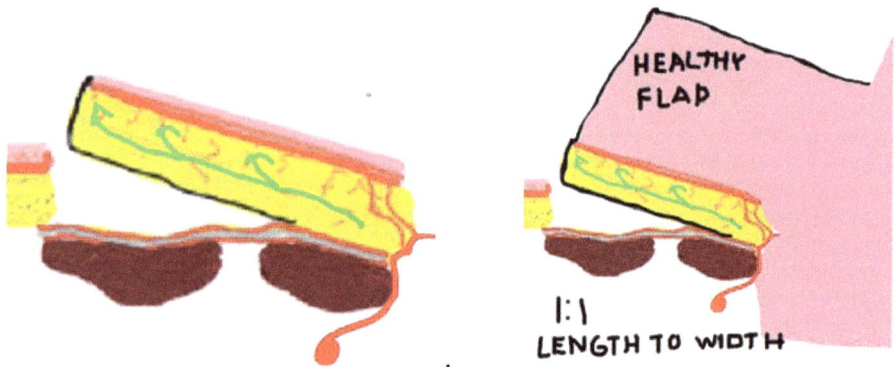

This length to width ratio is different in various parts of the body. It is most favorable in the facial area. This mathematical length to width ratio (1:1 on extremities, to 1: 5 on the face) is approximate. It takes experience and judgment to apply this principle in individual cases depending on the patient's medical condition. The first drawing below shows that as the length to width ratio increases, the chance of compromise or failure of the distal end of the flap increases. The second drawing indicates a flap that is too long for the width of its base. The distal portion of the flap died because of inadequate blood supply. This occurrence would necessitate additional surgery to remove the dead tissue and some other solution for the original problem. The plastic surgeon must take into account This type of practical concern about blood supply when planning any flap.

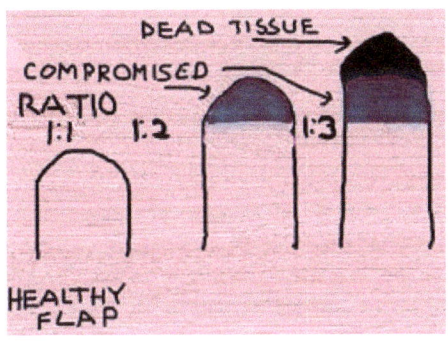
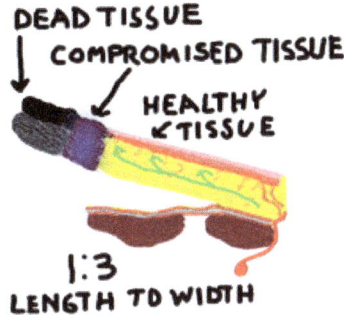

Random flaps come in many shapes and are most frequently used in the head and neck area, especially to repair defects such as those after excision of skin cancers. Four diagrams of conventional skin flaps used for closure after removal of skin lesions are below. All of these are random flaps, meaning their blood supply comes from tiny vessels in the subdermal and fatty tissue at their base. The colored dots show the movement of the flap components. Specific clinical examples are in chapter 14.

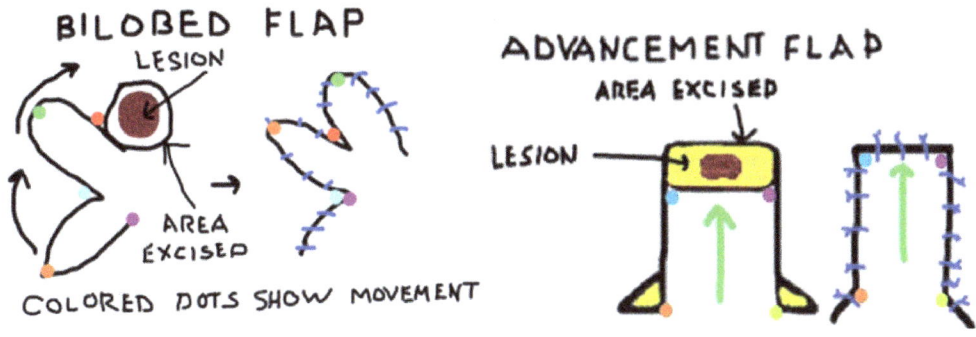

The Healing Mission of Plastic Surgery

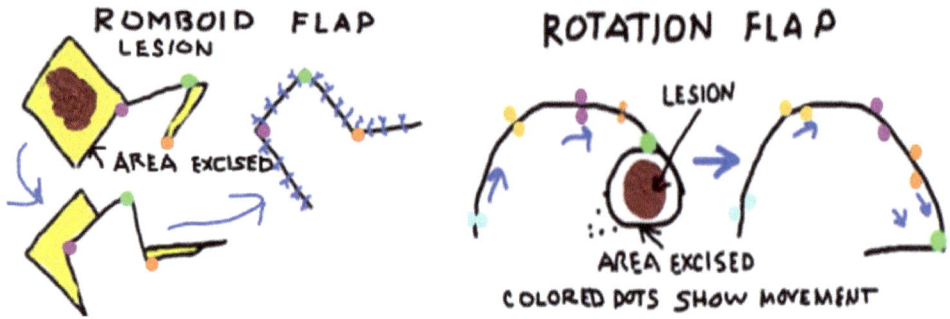

A Z-plasty uses two random triangular flaps, which can be very useful in numerous plastic surgical applications. All the limbs of the Z are the same length, but the angles between the limbs can vary considerably. It is often used in the management of facial scars to change the direction of the scar to place the scar in a more favorable position on the face. The first Z-plasty drawing below shows two triangular flaps elevated and then transposed, thus changing the direction of the scars.

One can appreciate the movement by observing the progress of the small green and orange dots. In the second drawing below, the green indicates a scar crossing the natural nasolabial fold shown in black. If this scar is prominent, a Z-plasty to rearrange the direction of the scars can effect an improvement. In this illustration, eliminating the scar crossing the nasolabial fold and placing the scar in the fold should produce a scar that will blend in better. The movement of the colored dots shows the transposition of the tips of these flaps.

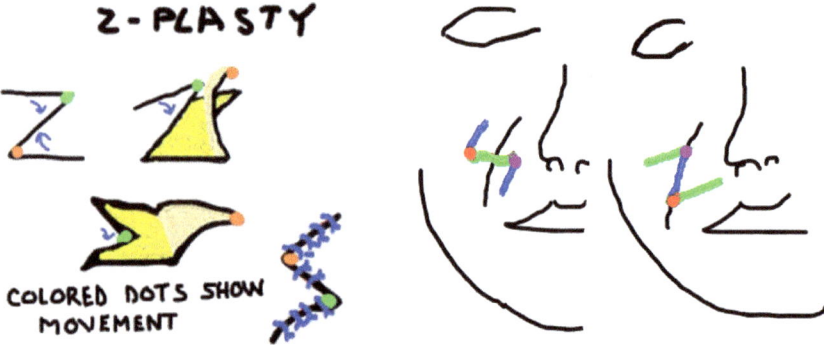

The second Z-plasty drawing below shows the benefit of lengthening a scar contracture represented by the green line. The distance between the

140

red and dark blue dots represents the length of the scar. In the first example, 45° angle flaps transposed produce a 50% lengthening or separation of the red and blue dots. The second drawing showing 60° angle flaps produces 75% lengthening after transposing the flaps. This principle is instrumental in burn scars and other traumatic scars. The length of the scar is the distance between the red dot and the blue dot. You can see how the Z – plasty has moved these dots farther apart, thereby lengthening the scar contracture.

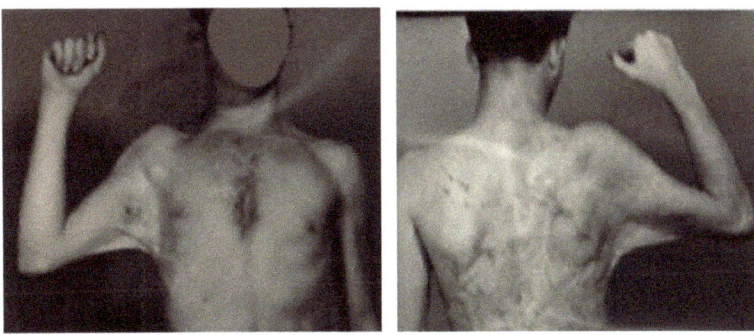

The burn axillary contracture case below was Dr. Thomas Cronin's patient. He has a severe limitation of movement, which results in a significant functional deficit.

I have used it as an example of how Z-plasties can release the scar contracture by lengthening the green line of the tightest part. I have marked the two ends of the scar with blue dots. This procedure consisted of two separate large Z-plasties, which I have color-coded to explain the movement. After the transposition of the four flaps, the blue dots have moved much farther apart, relieving the contracture.

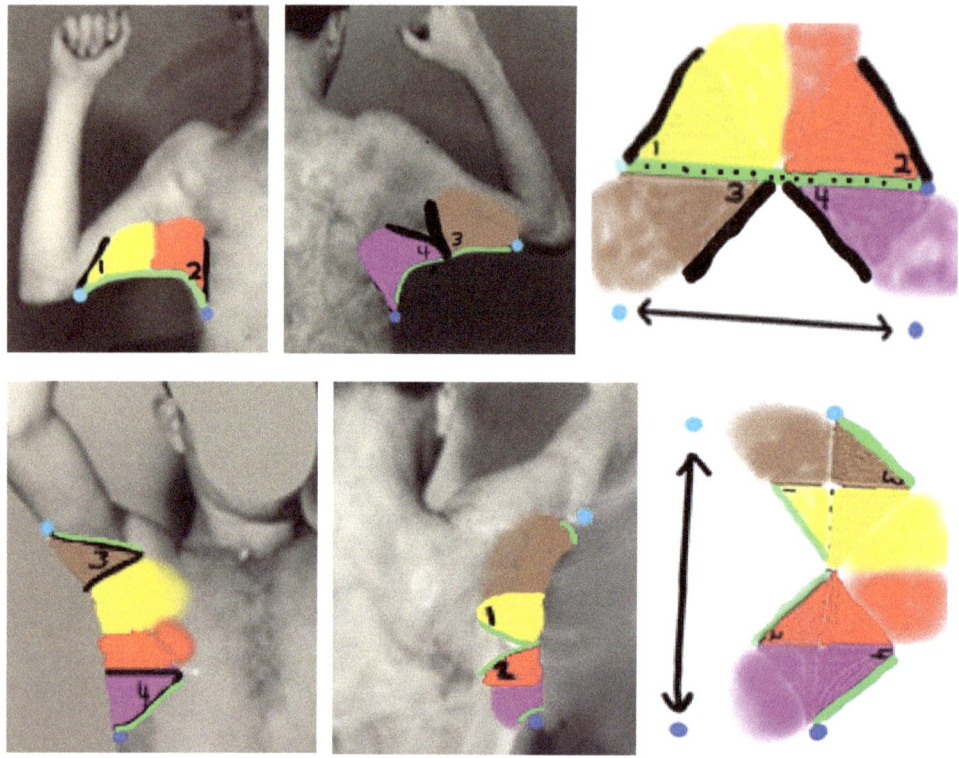

Dr. Thomas Cronin obtained the much-improved range of motion as shown in the result below.

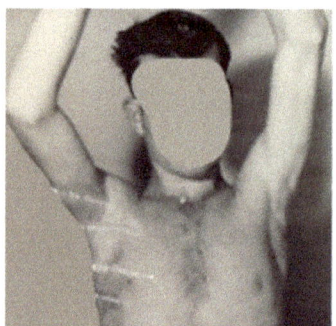

Axial Skin Flaps

Axial skin flaps, like random flaps, also have a skin pedicle base. Additionally, a significant vessel continues parallel to the skin partway toward the distal end of the flap. There are several specific anatomic areas for axial flap reconstructions. One example discussed in Chapter 5 is the thoraco-epigastric flap used for breast reconstruction. Another example is the paramedian forehead flap used for nasal reconstruction presented in chapter 14.

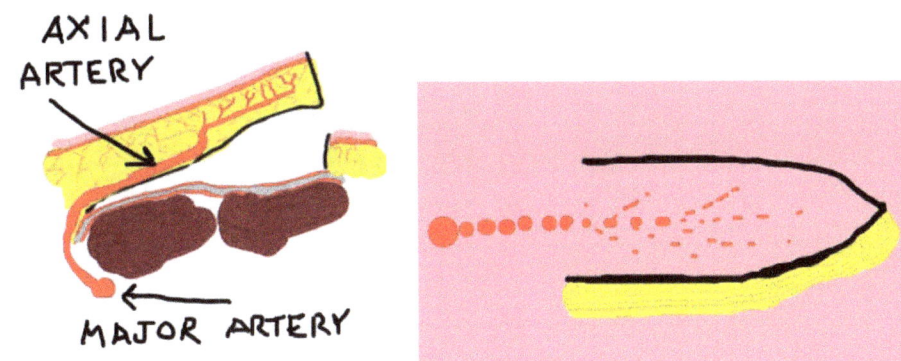

Myo-cutaneous Flaps

Myo-cutaneous flaps contain skin either as part of a pedicle or as a skin island. The skin portion is supplied by perforating vessels coming through muscle tissue. These flaps provide not only skin and subcutaneous tissue but also muscle, which may help in the reconstructive purpose. Examples of myo-cutaneous flaps are the latissimus dorsi myo-cutaneous flap and the transverse rectus abdominis myo-cutaneous flap. These flaps have multiple uses in breast reconstruction. Many cases of reconstructions with these flaps are in Chapter 9.

The diagram below demonstrates the skin island receiving blood from perforators coming through the subcutaneous tissue and the underlying muscle. The muscle gets blood supply from a major vessel that perforates the muscle. These flaps can be used as pedicle flaps if the muscle remains partially attached to the body. Or as free flaps by separating the entire flap from the body and re-anastomosing the blood vessels in a recipient area. Chapter 15 has several examples of free flap tissue transfers.

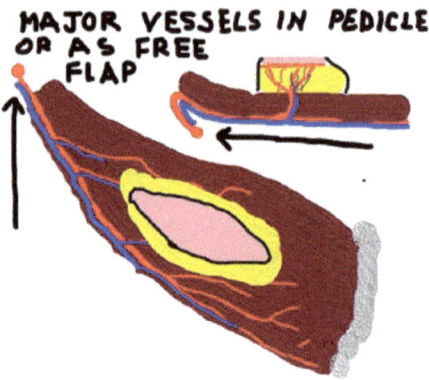

Septocutaneous Flaps

Septocutaneous flaps receive significant blood supply via a vessel coming between muscle bellies and perforating the fascia, bringing blood to the skin island. The drawing below illustrates this relationship. There are many specific anatomic areas where pedicle flaps with this type of blood supply are available. Septocutaneous flaps are free flaps if separated from the body and then placed where needed. That requires connecting the flap vessels to recipient vessels in the area of reconstruction. Examples are the scapular and para scapular flap. Chapter 15 has clinical cases.

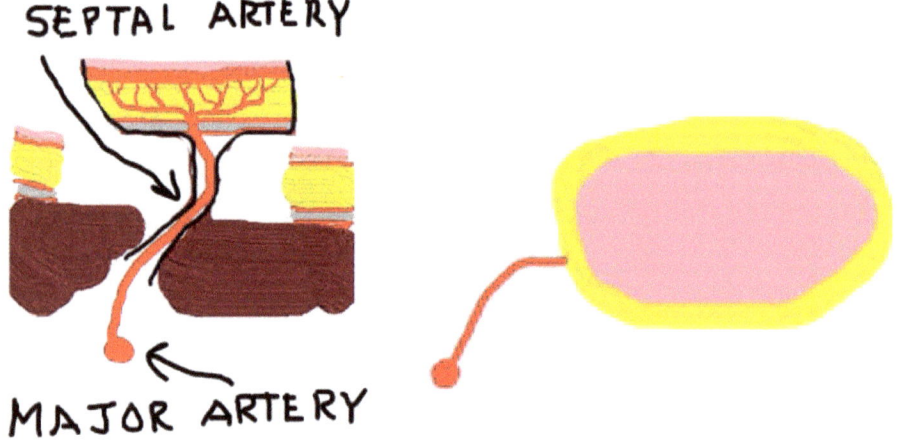

Random skin flaps have existed for centuries, and the Indian method of nasal reconstruction used the paramedian forehead axial flap. However, myo-cutaneous and septal and free flaps have only been popularized in modern times, beginning in the 1970s. I was very fortunate to practice plastic surgery when many of these developments and new techniques were coming into everyday practice.

Split Thickness Skin Grafts

Another common technique for plastic surgery reconstruction is grafting. Three common types of graphs are split-thickness skin grafts (STSF), full-thickness skin grafts (FTSG), and composite flaps. In contradistinction to the flaps previously described, all of these grafting techniques rely upon the recipient bed for blood supply. A split-thickness skin graft removes the epidermis and a portion of the dermis. Specialized instruments are available to harvest such graphs. They are analogous to a wood plan device.

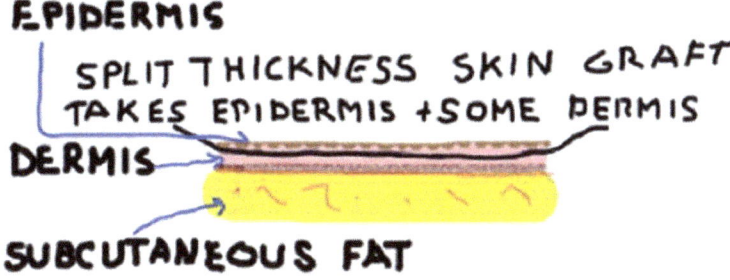

STSG's must depend on a moist raw surface on the body from which it can imbibe fluid nutrients. Within a very few days, tiny blood vessels will connect the bed to the graft for its ongoing blood supply. Therefore, it is essential to avoid friction or motion at the level of the skin graft. The drawing below diagrammatically demonstrates a STSG.

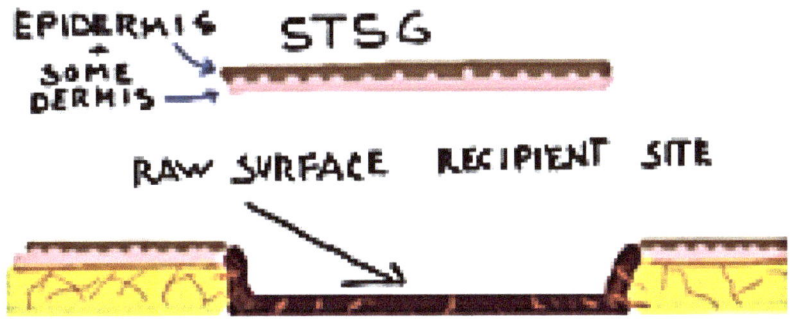

The Healing Mission of Plastic Surgery

One of the functional areas of plastic surgery is the treatment of acute burns, as well as treatment of their sequelae such as scar contractures which limit motion. This patient "Jonathan" was a worker in the kitchen of a restaurant and suffered acute burns from spilled grease on his left upper extremity. He had mixed deep second and 3rd° burns.

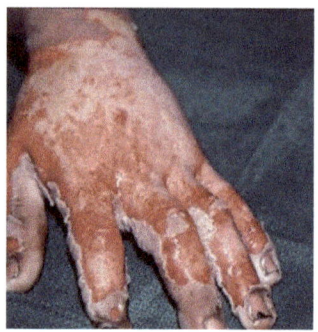 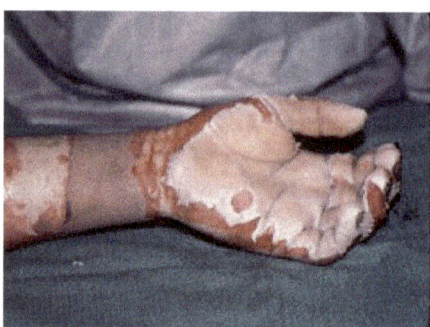

He had early debridement and skin grafting of the deeper burns on the back of the hand and wrist. The first picture below shows the skin grafts applied to the deeper areas. The second picture shows elastic compression therapy to the skin grafts and burn scars. Also, there is a small splint on the ring finger to counteract potential scar contracture, which could limit the range of motion.

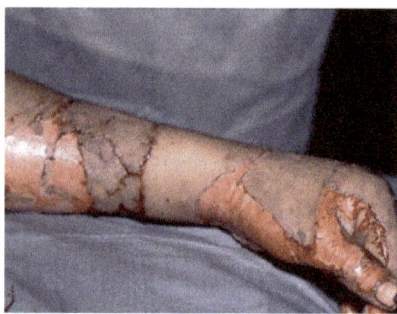 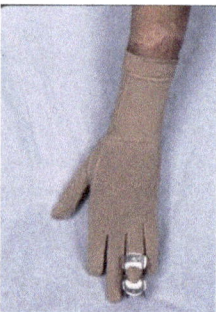

The last two pictures show he has a good range of hand motion after healing of the skin grafts. He was back to work at this point. The areas of skin graft are relatively hyperpigmented.

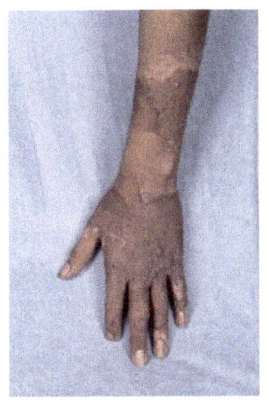 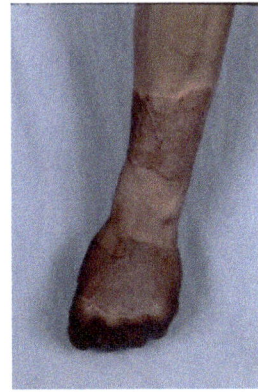

Full-thickness Skin Grafts

A full-thickness skin graft (FTSG) takes epidermis and the full thickness of the dermis at a level just above the subcutaneous fat. This graft also relies on nutrition directly from its recipient bed. Again within a few days, small blood vessels begin to grow into the graft from the bed. Because they are thicker, full-thickness skin grafts take a little longer to establish a blood supply and are somewhat less reliable to "take" as compared to especially thin split-thickness skin grafts. The drawings below diagrammatically illustrate the FTSG.

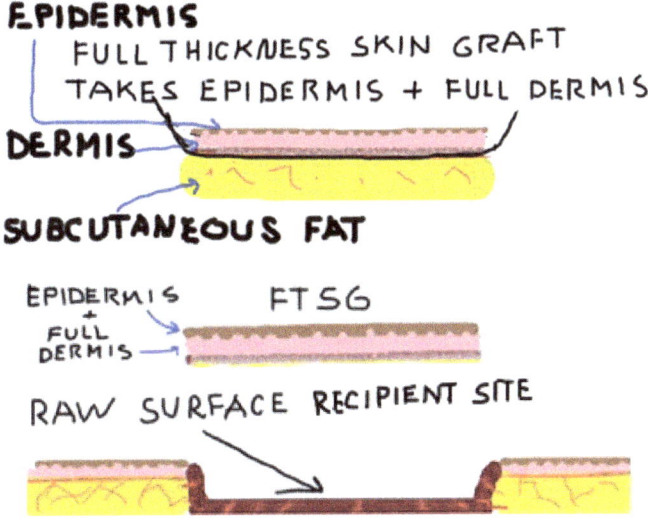

FTSG's are preferred in some instances because they are less likely to shrink or contract as compared to split-thickness skin grafts. Therefore, they are commonly used for facial grafting rather than split-thickness skin grafts. "Jane" below had a congenital pigmented nevus, which is unsightly but also has some possibility to degenerate into a malignancy. I excised the lesion and replaced it with a full-thickness skin graft from the abdomen, as shown in the middle two photos. The next photo on the right is several months later. The last photo is several years later. There is an acne blemish on the left cheek.

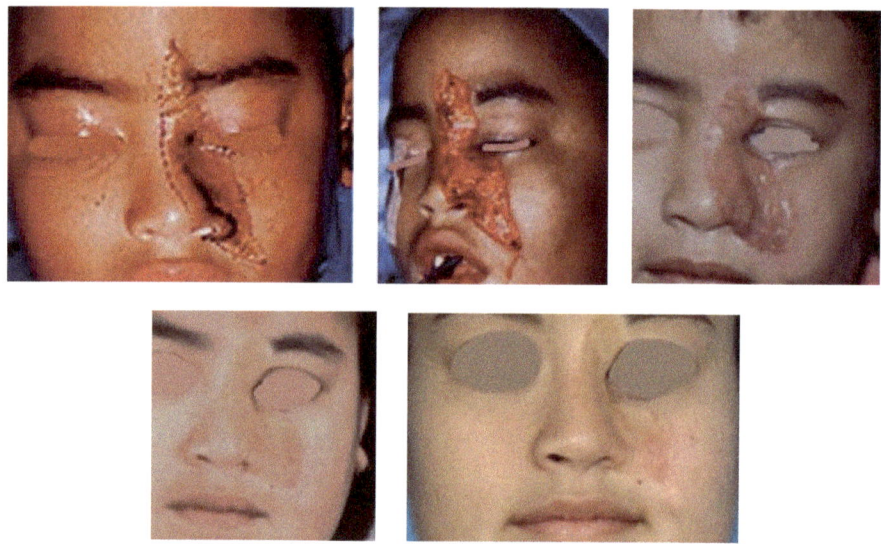

Composite Grafts

Composite graphs are grafts that contain more than skin. The most common composite graft contains both full-thickness skin and cartilage.

An example is skin and contiguous cartilage taken from an ear for partial nasal reconstruction. These graphs are less reliable than split-thickness or full-thickness skin grafts. They often look very compromised for several days before they obtain enough blood supply to be successful. They must be accurately sutured to the surrounding skin to promote the uptake of blood supply as soon as possible. Nourishing blood comes from both the underlying bed and the edge of the surrounding skin.

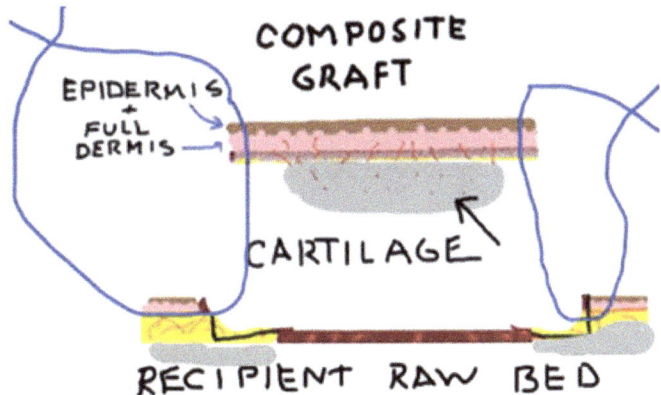

The following patient, "Robert," suffered a partial amputation of the tip of his nose because of a dog bite. He initially went to an emergency room where a nurse cleaned and dressed the wound as there was no severed piece available to sew back on. The first photo shows the injury when I first saw him in my office a few days later. He lost skin mostly but also a small portion of cartilage from the nasal tip. The second photo shows the wound as it looked when I took him to the operating room.

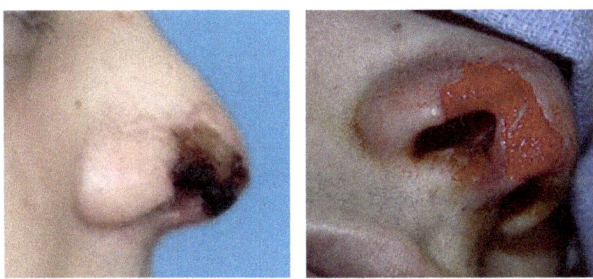

The first photo below shows an outline in ink of a "composite "graft donor site, which contains both skin and cartilage. The middle photo is the donor defect after removal of the graft, and the third is the ear after the closure of the donor site. The cartilage in this "composite" graft was needed for support to maintain the shape of the nasal tip and the nostril opening. If I used skin alone had the area would have contracted to distort the contour of the tip and nostril opening.

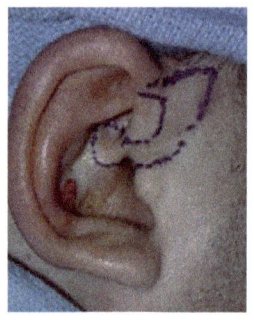 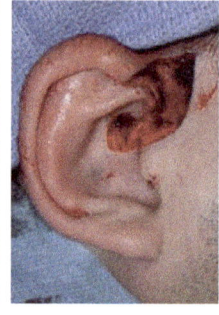 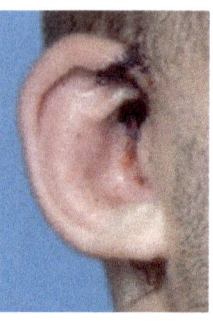

The three photographs below show the composite graft in place at the end of surgery. The middle picture is a few days after placement. The graft looks very red not because of infection but because of limited blood supply; it is just squeaking by to remain alive. The graft first receives some nutrition through serum imbibition from its bed, but only after several more days does it begins to look healthier as in the third picture, which was about three weeks after surgery. The graft has produced good contour for the tip and right nostril. This graft will blend in and become less and less conspicuous over the following several months.

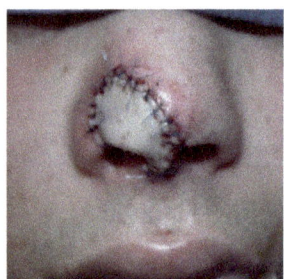 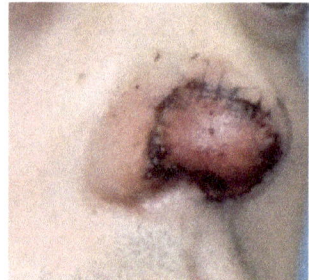 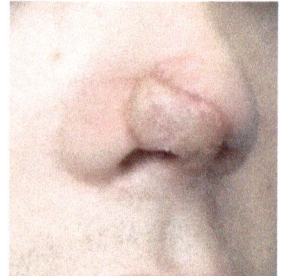

The scope of plastic surgery

Plastic surgery is not isolated to any one system or anatomic region but involves the entire body from the top of the head to the bottom of the feet. It deals with functional, reconstructive, and aesthetic problems. It also treats patients of all ages, from newborns to geriatric patients. It emphasizes the meticulous technique and gentle treatment of all tissues involved. I am indebted to all my mentors for helping me in my quest to master the art and science of plastic surgery. In this chapter, I will present a range of cases that illustrate both the art and the science of this fascinating field of medicine. I must credit my teachers, who helped me acquire the skills and insight to appraise these patients from an anatomic, historical, textbook, and scientific approach, but also, with a studied personal and artistic hand.

From the top of the head to the bottom of the feet

Scalp

The curved contour and the tightly adherent tissue of the scalp make treating wounds in this area particularly demanding. In treating significant scalp wounds and lesions, the surgeon must not only draw on his/her artistic experience but be cognizant of the scientific literature in this area. The scalp can be a challenging area in reconstructive plastic surgery. Three very different scalp cases follow.

The first patient below, "Gwendolyn," had a history of squamous cell skin cancer of the scalp. She had a previous excision with repair via a rotation flap and a skin graft of the donor site at the left posterior scalp. She presented to me with recurrent skin cancer, as in the photos below.

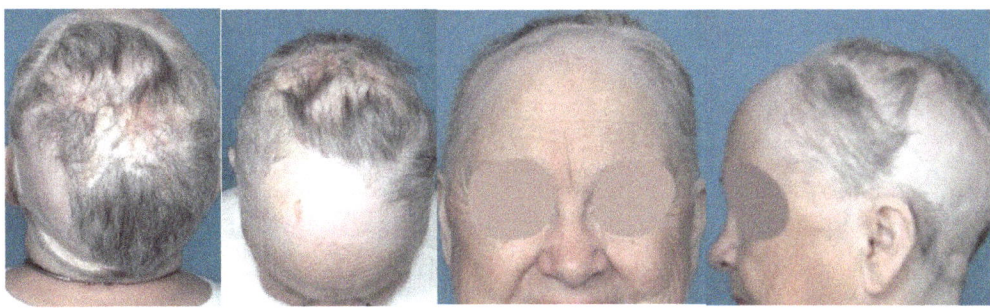

She needed the excision of a large area of the central scalp, as outlined in the first below. I closed the large defect with a large rotation scalp flap and closed the donor area with a split-thickness skin graft, which appears pinker that the older previous skin graft in this early postoperative state.

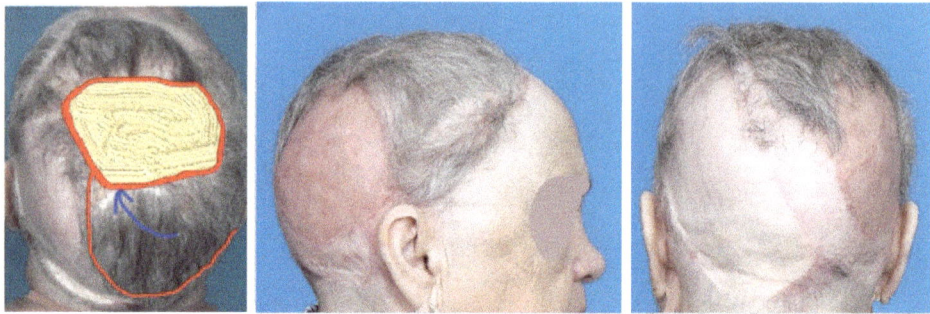

By placing all the hair-bearing scalp forward, she is now able to comb over the skin grafted areas to good effect, as shown in the final postoperative images below.

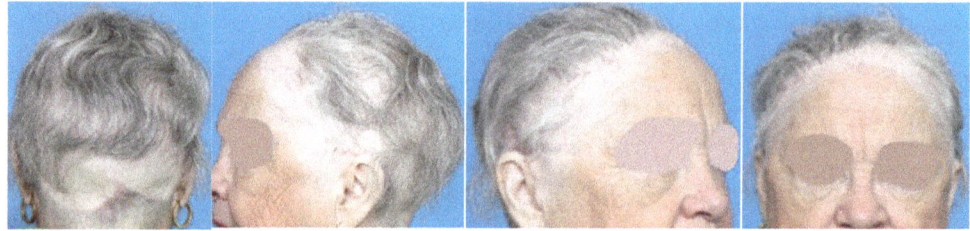

When she goes out, she likes to wear a wig, as shown below.

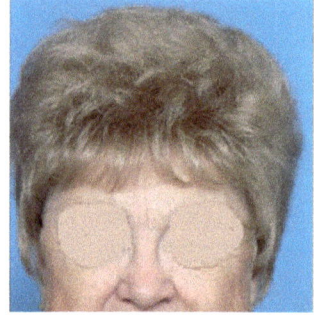

This teenage boy "Jason" suffered a traumatic motorcycle injury. The first picture below shows the white exposed cranial bone. I plan to rotate the proposed large scalp flap outlined in blue in the direction indicated by the green arrow.

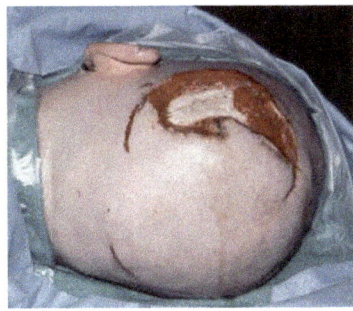 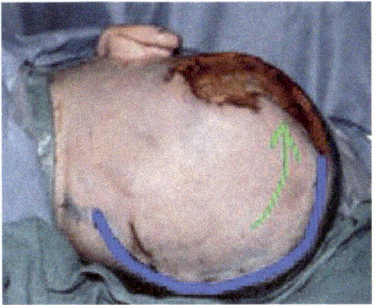

In the first photo below, one sees this large flap lifted at a level just above periosteum, which remains over the bone except for the original traumatic area. This flap continues to get its blood supply through its base from the left upper posterior neck area. The surrounding scalp was also undermined and stretched at the same level so that it could also help close the resultant donor area. The purple arrows indicate areas of the scalp which have been undermined and stretched. So, unlike the first scalp case, both the original defect and the donor areas were closed with the full-thickness scalp flap. The last two pictures show his early postoperative result.

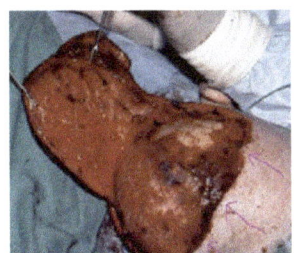 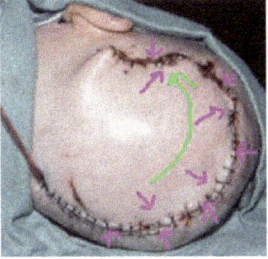 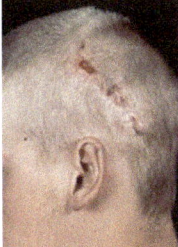 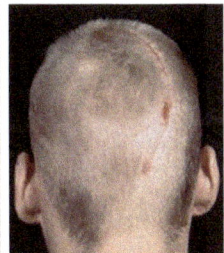

"Cassandra," shown below, had previously suffered a scalp avulsion injury that repaired with split-thickness skin grafts to the periosteum. She came to see me because she suffered chronic nonhealing sores, which were aggravating and precluded her use of a wig. She needed a more stable, healed scalp to support the wearing of a hairpiece. Her preoperative status is below.

The Healing Mission of Plastic Surgery

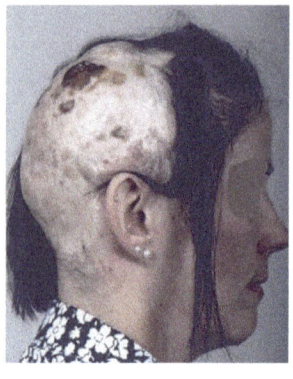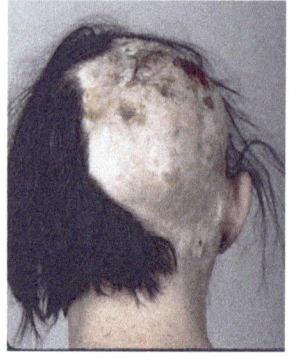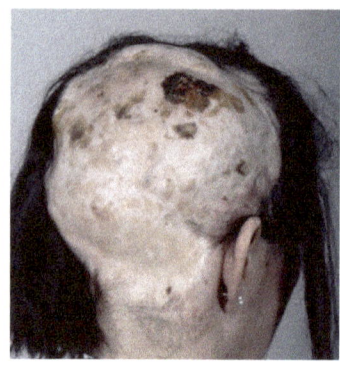

After a discussion of the pros and cons, I recommended the excision of the troublesome skin grafts. I proposed replacing them with a latissimus dorsi free muscle flap from "Cassandra's" back, as in the photo drawing below. The photo on the right is after I excised the chronic sores and removed a large amount of the previous skin grafts.

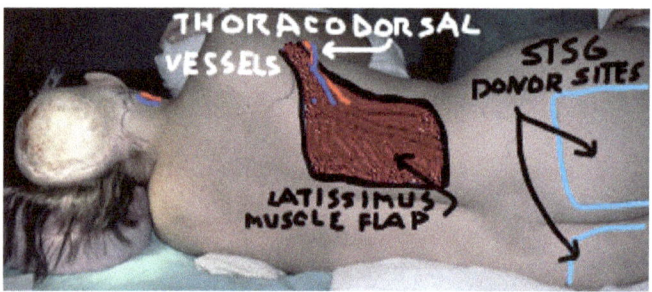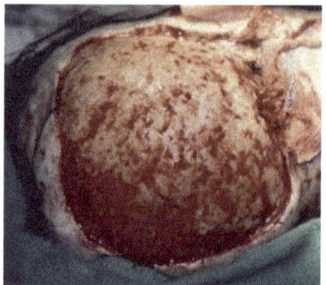

The photo-drawing on the left below demonstrates harvesting the large flat latissimus muscle from the back with its sizeable thoracodorsal blood vessels. I placed the latissimus muscle over the newly created scalp wound. The muscle added thick healthy tissue and padding needed for the skin grafts taken from her buttocks, which I subsequently placed to cover the muscle. The third image is a photo-drawing, which shows the area in "Cassandra's" neck where I connected the blood vessels from the flap to blood vessels in the neck to re-establish blood supply to this sizeable flat muscle.

The Healing Mission of Plastic Surgery

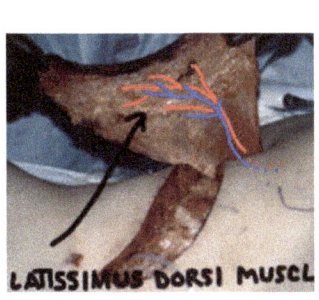 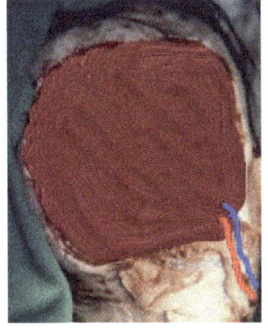 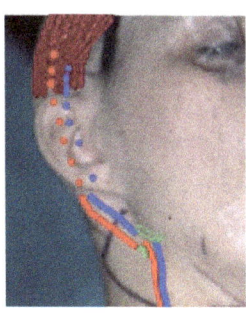

After the skin graft and muscle healed, she had thicker, stable soft tissue coverage of the calvarium, as shown below. She was now pleased she could wear any wig she wished.

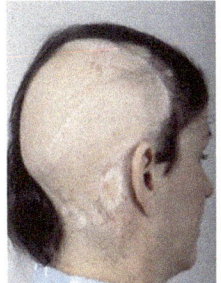 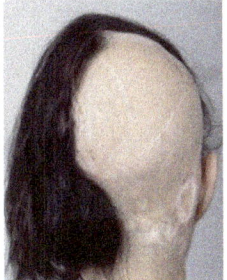 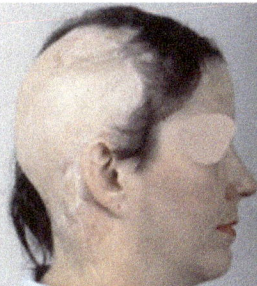 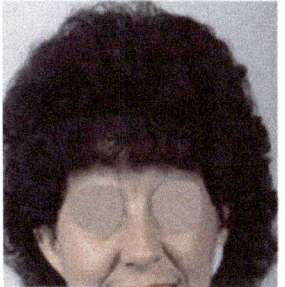

A fourth scalp reconstruction case follows later in a geriatric patient.

From infants to geriatric patients

Craniosynostosis

I saw a two weeks old baby in the neonatal ICU with an abnormal triangular-shaped anterior skull. The forehead and frontal bone had a keel shape, caused by early fusion between two portions of skull bones, which generally should have grown for a much longer time before fusing. This phenomenon of premature fusion of growth lines or sutures is known as craniosynostosis.

A preoperative photo of the child is shown below with a central prominence to the forehead. The drawing I made illustrates an infant's skull with metopic suture stenosis or premature fusion in the forehead area shown in orange. Several standard suture lines are in blue, indicating they have not fused but are still producing new bony growth. These are areas that will continue to grow, making the skull larger to accommodate a rapidly enlarging brain. When sutures close prematurely, distortion of the cranium results. Any cranial suture may be involved in craniosynostosis.

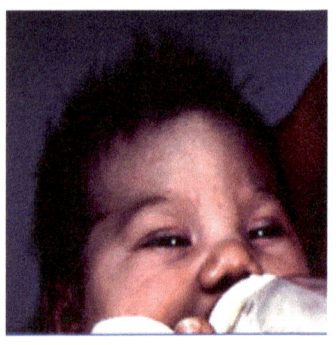
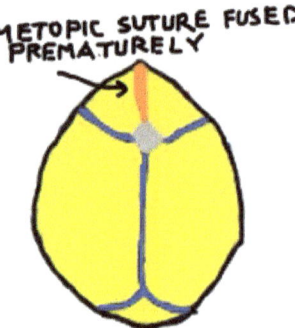

A neurosurgeon and I coordinated on this case. The cranial bones are soft at this young age. The neurosurgeon and I took the baby to the operating room when she was six weeks old. The first photo below shows the planned incision marked in purple, which I made through the scalp from ear to ear. The next picture shows that scalp flap elevated and "flipped" forward over the face, exposing the top of the skull and forehead down to reveal the keel-shaped fusion of the metopic suture. Following this, bone cuts were made, represented in the diagram below by the purple lines. The fused metopic suture is colored orange. The frontal bones are represented in yellow while the super orbital bar is green. Removal of large portions of the frontal bone (yellow) allowed access to the area immediately above and between the orbits. Removal of large pieces of the frontal bone (yellow) permitted access to the area directly above and between the orbits.

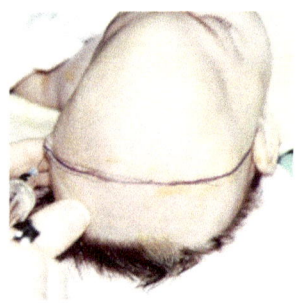
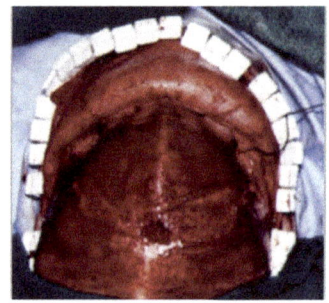
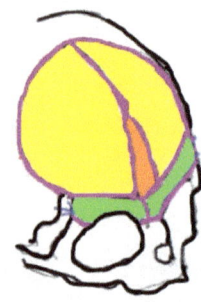

We removed the bony upper half of the orbits called the super orbital bar and placed it aside. Green arrows show it below. I reshaped it to be less pointed and more rounded, as in the middle diagram below. I returned this reshaped supraorbital bar and fixed it with titanium plates and screws. The intraoperative photograph on the right below demonstrates the stabilization of this bone. Now, most of these cases use slowly dissolvable plates and screws.

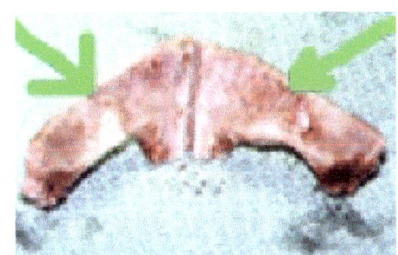 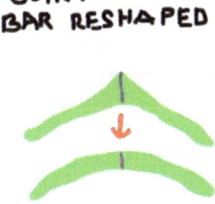 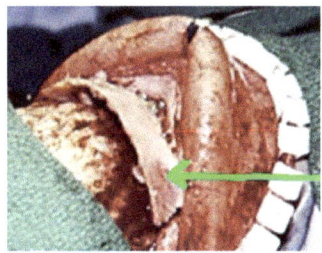

Next, I replaced two large portions of the frontal bone (yellow) just above the super orbital bar (green), as in the diagram below and the intraoperative photo. Again, the green arrows indicate the supraorbital bar; yellow indicates the replaced frontal bones. The gray arrow points out the area purposely left with no bone. This open area allows the brain the freedom to grow and to drive the shape of the skull. Within several months new bone generated by the dura forms throughout that area.

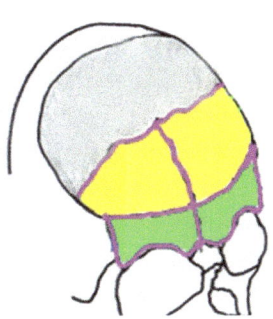 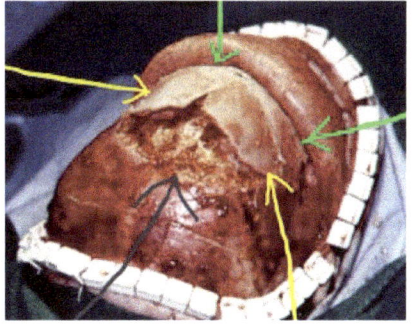

The child did very well postoperatively without any complications. The first three pictures below demonstrate her one-year postoperative result. A postop view a few years later is shown on the right.

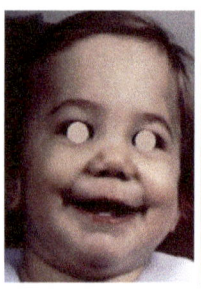 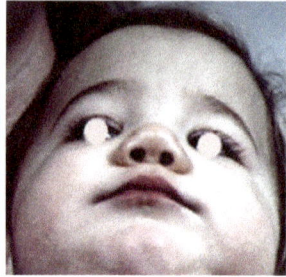 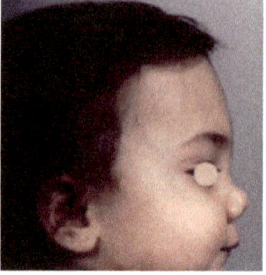 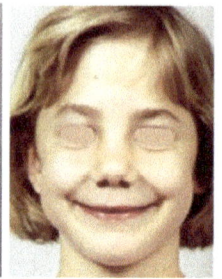

This patient's family moved out of state. Still, I received follow up information from the mom about six years later that she continued to have healthy development and was doing very well.

Eyelid Switch.

A young child presented to me with an unusual congenital deformity, which consisted of the absence of a large portion of the upper eyelids. This rare cleft deformity sometimes involves deeper structures of the eyeball itself. Fortunately, this patient's problem only involved the eyelid itself. The defect was similar on both sides. The clefts of the upper eyelids were more extensive than half the lid width. I could not pull the edges of the cleft together for a primary repair, as illustrated in the second photo. Therefore, I planned a two-stage procedure to move a wedge of tissue from the lower to the upper lid. Blue ink outlines the lower eyelid wedge for the right side in the third photo below.

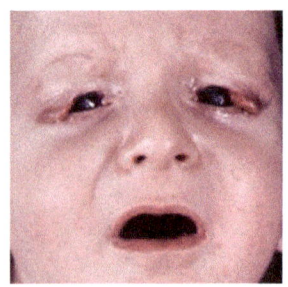 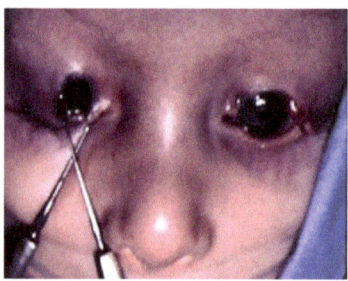 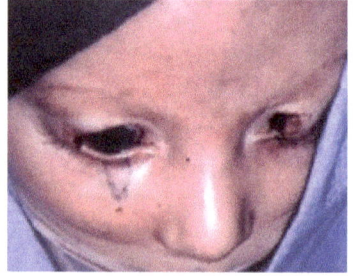

With sharp dissection, I freshened the edges of the defect in the upper eyelid. A pie-shaped portion of the lower eyelid was cut free except for a tiny pedicle on one side along the lash margin. The pedicle contained a small blood vessel, which continued to nourish the wedge until new blood supple entered the wedge from the upper eyelid. Hence, the pie-shaped lower eyelid tissue could be rotated into the defect and sewn there to replace the deficient upper eyelid. The child was able to see as through a peephole on either side of the bridge. The eyelids remained sutured to each other for about eight days to allow the new blood supply to come into the wedge from the recipient area of the upper eyelid.

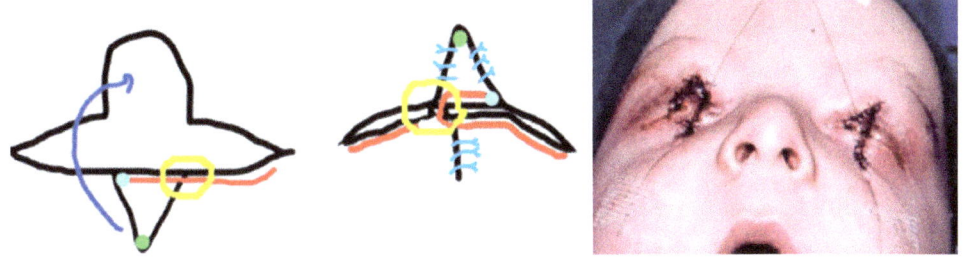

Then the small bridge of tissue was then sharply separated. The transfer of lower eyelid tissue to the upper eyelid defect was now complete. The eyelids could again open fully.

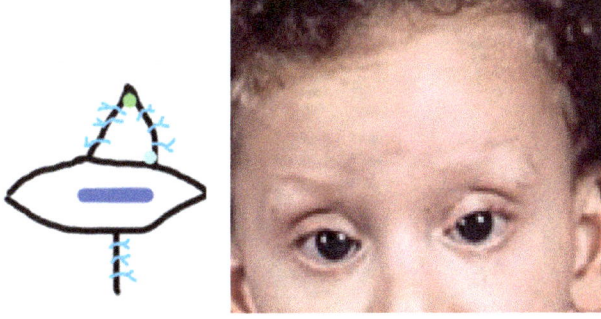

This unusual procedure was able to restore function to his upper eyelids and give a satisfactory aesthetic result. Again, this is an example of "features fulfilling their offices according to natures decree." I did this case in collaboration with my mentor Dr. Thomas Cronin.

Otoplasty for prominent ears

There is a reason for the Walt Disney animated character Dumbo. This small elephant is teased mercilessly because of his enormous ears. An erroneous assumption is that large or prominent ears equate with stupidity or ignorance. Various anthropomorphic studies have included prominent ears as associated with multiple ethnic groups. There is no relationship between prominent ears and levels of intelligence.

Nevertheless, some children may be teased by their classmates if their ears are more noticeable than average.

"Johnny," a boy 16-years-old and well adjusted, came to see me with his mother because of his concern about his prominent ears. He had a classic situation, with the absence of a standard anti helical fold resulting in prominent ears. The underdevelopment or lack of this anti-helical fold was first pointed out by a surgeon named Luckett in 1910 as the cause for most excessively prominent ears. The first drawing below shows an ear with the absence of an anti -helical fold. The second photo is of an ear with a typical anti-helical fold pointed out by the green arrow. The red arrow points to the standard helix of the ear, while the blue dots and blue arrow point out the concha or bowl in the middle portion of the ear.

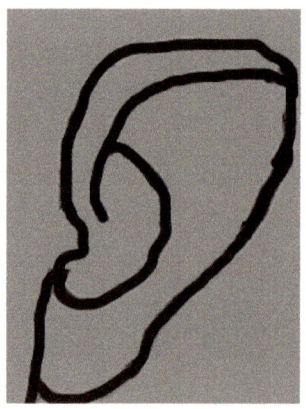 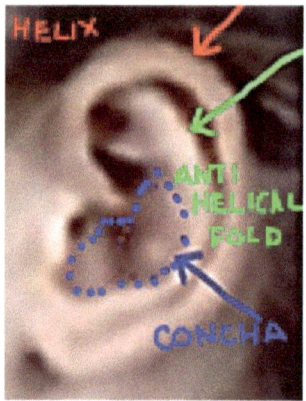

I discuss his case with him and his mother, generally explaining where I would make the incision and how I would do the procedure. I discussed the possibility of excess scar formation and failure of the operation due to the recurrence of ear prominence. Other potential complications were covered. I thought he was an excellent candidate for a "pin back" of the ear or otoplasty.

I scheduled surgery for about one month later. Because of "Jonny's" age, I used only intravenous sedation and local anesthesia. A general anesthetic was not necessary. An incision behind the ear gave access to the pertinent cartilage. The photos below from another patient show a needle with methylene blue ink inserted in the proposed position of the new anti-helical fold anteriorly. The ink shows on the surgical side in the second photo. The ink marks help guide, where I will place the sutures to create the anti-helical fold in the right position. The drawing shows the placement of permanent sutures on the posterior side of the ear cartilage in red.

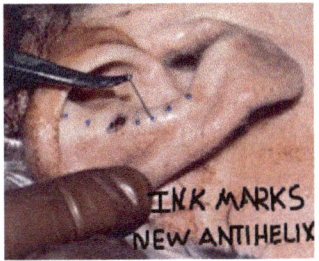 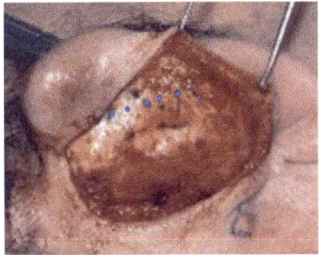 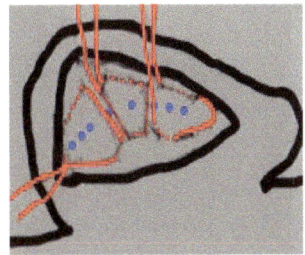

When tightened, these sutures will bend the cartilage to re-create the anti-helical fold, as demonstrated in the two drawings below. The photograph is an intraoperative photo showing the newly created anti-helical fold along the previously marked dotted lines. Again, the green arrow points out the freshly created anti-helical fold. The red pointer indicates the helix, and the blue arrow points out the concha.

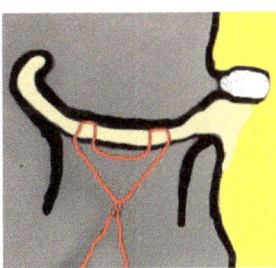 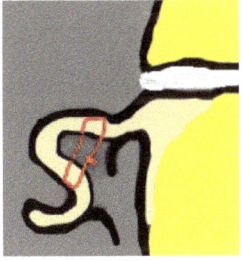 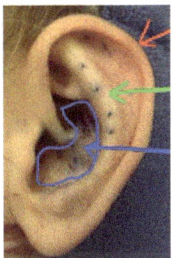

Although the most common prominent ear deformity is lack of development of the anti-helical fold, another common problem creating prominent ears is over-development of the concha or concave bowl of the ear. Another common maneuver for correction of prominent ears is suturing the concha closer to the side of the head or actual removal of part of the concha cartilage and suturing the remainder to the soft tissue over the mastoid process behind the ear.

The first photo, from behind the ear, below shows the proposed excision of concha outlined in red. Intraoperative ink marks were made with a needle to plan the amount of the reduction of the concha cartilage. In the second intraoperative photo, I am using a scissor to cut out a portion of the concha held by the forceps. The third photo below is after the removal of part of the concha. Sutures are in place, which, when tightened, will move the concha closer to the side of the head, making the ear less prominent.

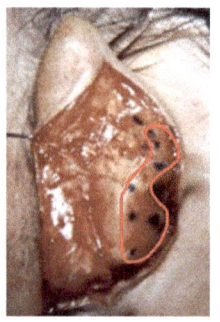 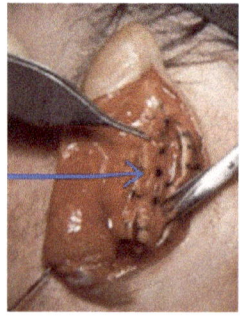 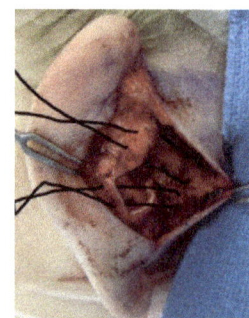

In this case, I reshaped the ear folds, which brought the ear was into a more normal position. The patient went home within a few hours of surgery with a bulky dressing around the ears. A few days later, he came to the office for the removal of the bandages. The operation was quite successful, as demonstrated in the photos below.

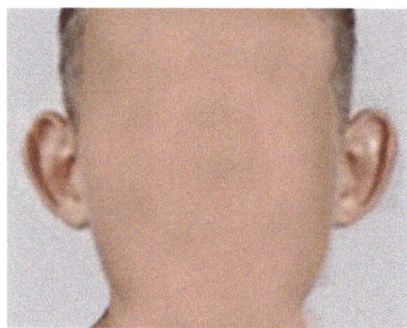 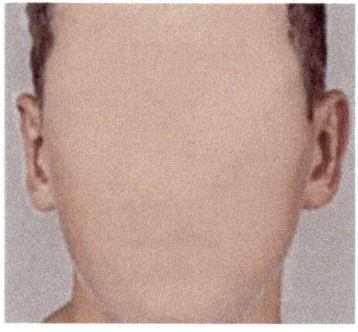

Several months later, I received a note from his mother, stating that he was doing well and was so happy and confident about himself since his ear surgery. His response was a typical response to this type of surgery. I was pleased to hear it.

There are few complications associated with otoplasty. Of course, infection is possible but unusual. Occasionally there may be some degree of "recurrence" that might need some secondary "tweaking." I only recall one patient upon whom I did such a pin back otoplasty with a significant complication. That was a young boy, probably six or seven years old. He developed very prominent scar tissue at the wound, closure behind his ears. I wanted to wait about a year and reevaluate the scar to see if a revision would be helpful. His parents never brought him back for that, however.

Ear Helix Reconstruction

"Emily" shown below has the absence of the helical rim of her right ear. The left ear as a minor "cup ear" deformity.

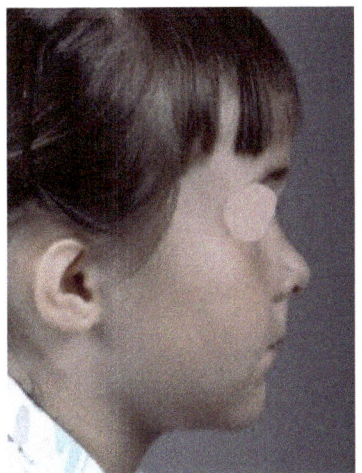
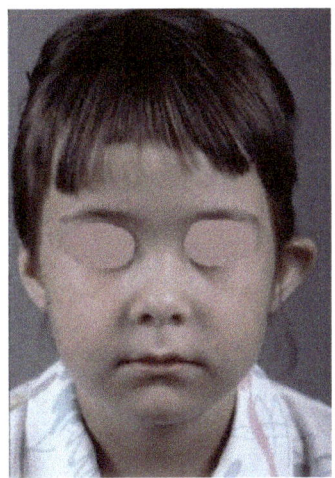

The first picture below shows a close-up of the right ear with the absence of the helical rim. The second picture shows two parallel lines drawn, where I will make incisions for the construction of a tube. The third picture shows the tissue tube healed with tissue still connected at either end.

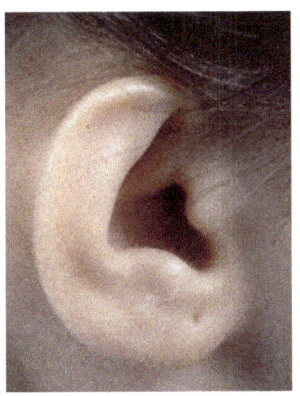
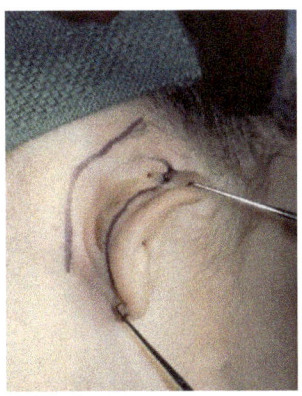
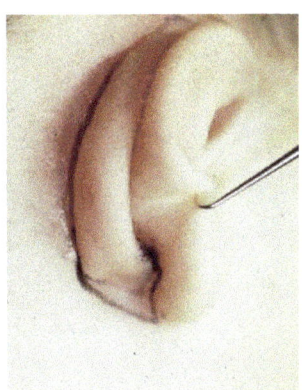

I performed two additional small procedures shown below. I sutured the superior end of the tube to the top of the ear, as in the first photo-drawing below. After allowing that to heal for two weeks, I disconnected the inferior end of the tube and sutured the rest of the flap to create the new helical rim. The third and fourth pictures are after the three stages.

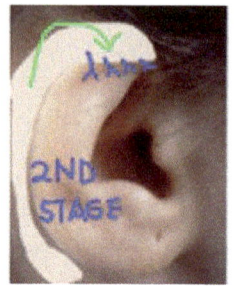 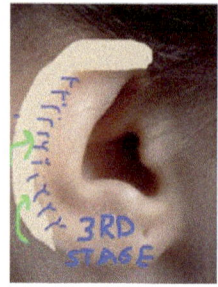 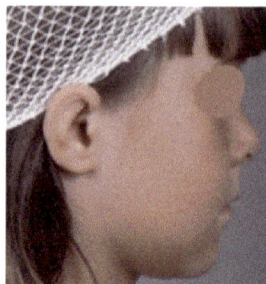 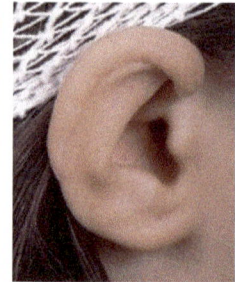

The photos below show the preoperative cup ear deformity of the left ear and then the postop result after repair by reshaping the cartilage with suturing techniques similar to the ones shown earlier in this chapter.

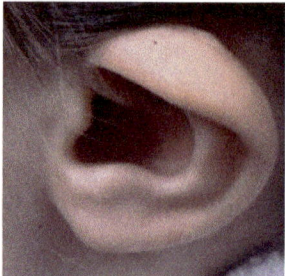 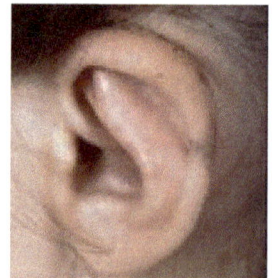

Macrostomia or large mouth

Birth defects (differences?) come in an unbelievable assortment. One afternoon as I was working in the office with my uncle, a patient arrived with an unusual congenital anomaly. The baby "Joshua" was a few weeks old and, despite a visible deformity of the mouth, was healthy and gaining weight. The baby had an enormous mouth. The muscle connections at the corners of the mouth did not occur properly, leaving an opening on both sides that extended into the cheeks. There was no family history for any congenital deformities. Preoperative photographs are below.

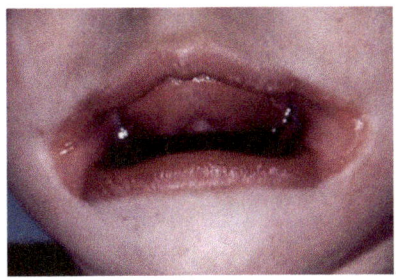 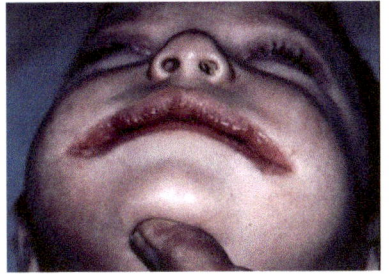

My uncle, Thomas Cronin, and I worked together on this case. We checked the plastic surgery literature to see what others had done for similar cases. I found a wonderfully illustrated case study in a book by a well-known Swedish surgeon named Tord Skoog. After going over that several times, we felt confident that our approach was reasonable and would be successful. The risk-benefit ratio was quite favorable.

When the operation day arrived, we were ready and anxious to begin. First, we tried to ascertain what structures were present and what was missing. By carefully inspecting the lip, we discerned the "intended" corners of the mouth. We marked them with ink because such landmarks can become obscured during surgery. Beginning at that point and extending laterally towards the cheek, we separated with sharp dissection between the skin and the mucosa. We identified the orbicularis muscle at the upper lip and the lower lip. This muscle was dissected for a way so that we could suture it together to reconstitute the sphincter action of the lips. We then repaired the mucosa inside the mouth and, finally, the skin.

We decided to alter our operation a little from Dr. Skoog's. His technique broke up the potential straight-line scar of the cheek by making a Z in it. We decided to leave a shorter straight-line scar, knowing a Z-plasty could always be done in the future if the scar contracted.

In the first picture below, the blue line marks the border between skin and mucosa. The blue dots indicate the lateral extent of the proposed new oral commissure. On the patient's right side, I have already separated the junction between the skin and mucosa. The mucosa has retreated towards the inside of the mouth. The yellow circles identify the two sides of the cleft orbicularis oris muscle. In the second photo, a black suture defines the orbicularis oris, on either side of the cleft, ready for being sewn together. The repair of both sides restored the sphincter action of the orbicularis oris muscle. The third photo shows immediate closure. The blue dots have come together at the new oral commissure.

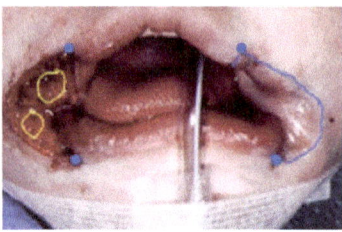 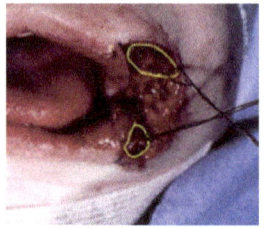 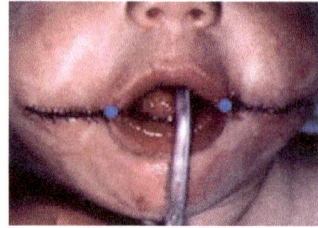

The child healed well and was restored permanently to normal. So, we were glad we made our slight modification. "Joshua," pictured below, is shown about six months after the surgery. During 38 years of plastic surgery practice, I treated a few more patients with this condition on both sides of the mouth and numerous patients with this problem on one side.

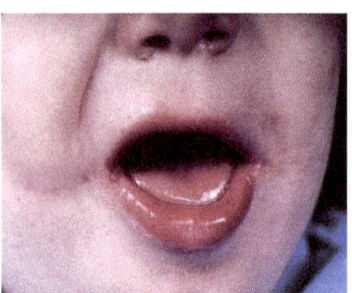 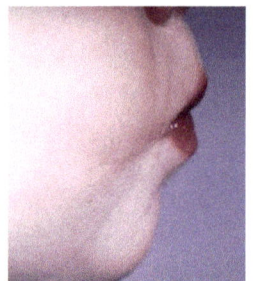 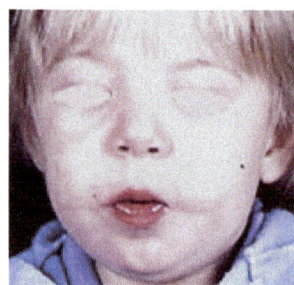

Webbed fingers

A relatively common congenital anomaly found in infants and young children is webbed fingers. These can range from simple webs of soft tissue between fingers to complex bony fusions that make the hands seem like a mitten or even a cup. If one made a direct incision straight between the fingers and then sutured each incision, over time, the fingers would curve toward each other because of straight-line scar contracture. The drawings below represent this complication.

The Healing Mission of Plastic Surgery

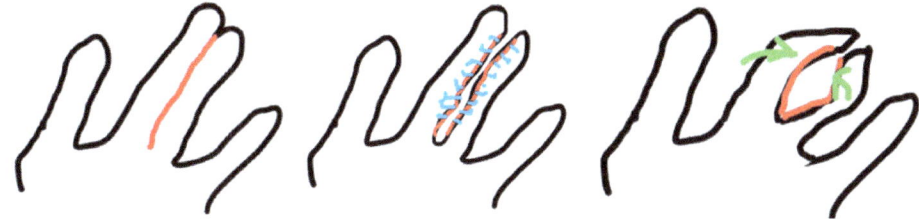

The child below demonstrates simple webbing between the long and ring fingers with no bony fusion. The incisions planned are outlined in blue ink first on the palm side and then the back of the fingers. The third picture below shows the fingers separated after those incisions before suturing the flaps.

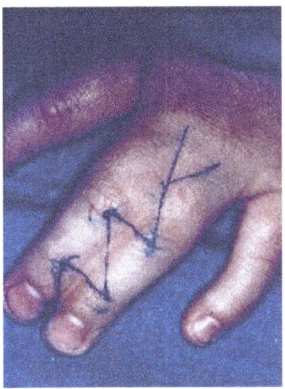
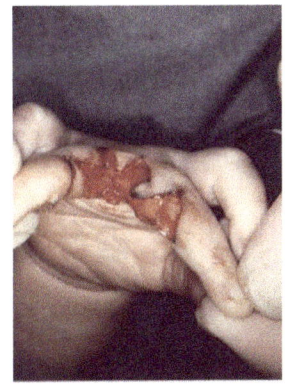

The following two pictures below show the flaps sewn in place together with small skin grafts to complete the closure. This type of zigzag closure breaks up the line of the incision so that healing will not distort the fingers. The last picture shows the final result with the long and ring fingers now separated.

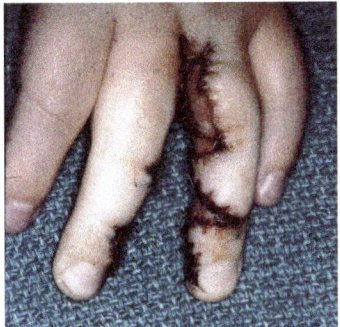
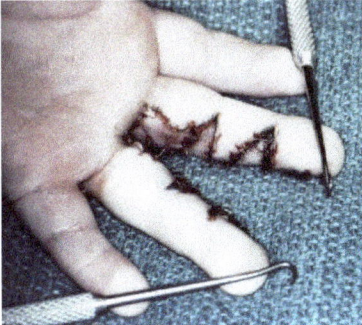
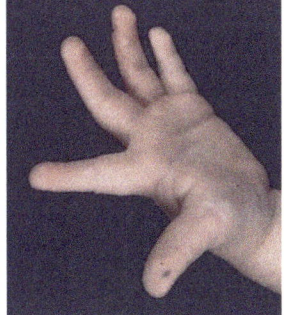

Hypospadias

Hypospadias is a congenital problem that occurs in approximately one in 250 newborn boys. In this condition, the urethra does not extend to the tip of the glans penis as usual. The urethra opens somewhere on the underside of the penis. It may open near the tip or proximal all the way the back at the base of the penis. This malposition of the urethral opening causes abnormal urine flow and later can interfere with fertility.

I was fortunate that early in my plastic surgery career, working with my uncle Thomas Cronin, I obtained some experience in treating the congenital problem of hypospadias. These cases were usually referred by urologists, who made the diagnosis or had been sent these cases from pediatricians. Over the years, the subspecialty of pediatric urology developed, and urologists referred these patients to their pediatric urology colleagues. Therefore, referral sources to plastic surgeons dried up, and as a result, hypospadias repair is no longer considered a standard area within plastic surgery.

Below is an example of a hypospadias repair from early in my surgical career.

In the first photograph, the urethral opening is at the base rather than at the tip of the penis. In this child, "Herbert," the repair uses the existing local tissue. So, it is crucial, he does not have circumcision, as the prepuce is part of the skin utilized for repair.

The second photograph shows a proposed reconstruction via the yellow and blue lines. I made an incision between the yellow and blue lines. In the third photo, I have folded the tissue between the blue lines over the red rubber catheter to form a tube and sutured the edges together. This skin tube effectively elongated the urethra from its original opening to the tip of the glans penis where it belongs.

The last photo shows I protected that raw internal repair by elevating and suturing together the lateral skin edges pictured in yellow, completing the reconstruction. The white tube shown below the scrotum is a temporary urinary diversion tube that I placed at the beginning of the surgery so that urine would not be flowing in the area of the repair for several days to allow for healing. The urinary diversion helps prevent a fistula, which is an opening in the urethra because of the failure of proper healing. Such a fistula would result in urine leakage from the urethra. A fistula is one of the most common complications of hypospadius surgery. After adequate healing, this corrective repair resulted in normal function.

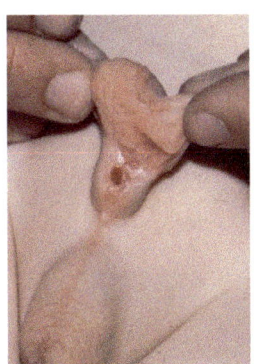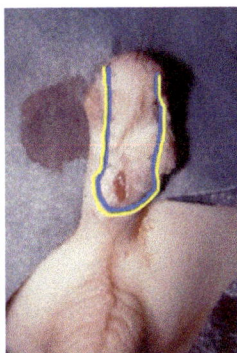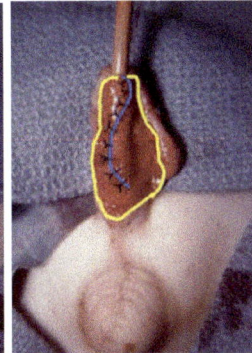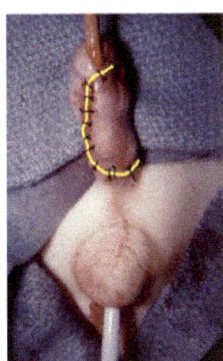

Meningomyelocele

The next case involves a newborn with meningomyelocele and spina bifida. This neural tube defect results in failure of the spinal cord and backbone to close during intrauterine development. The cause is not known. Symptoms vary greatly but commonly include partial or complete paralysis of the legs and diminished control of bladder and bowel function.

The neurosurgeon, who planned to close this abnormally exposed spinal cord, called me because he wanted help with soft tissue closure over his spinal cord repair. He wanted help with the soft tissue and skin coverage over his surgical repair. The middle view shows the closed spinal cord after the neurosurgeon finished. I elected to raise bilateral muscle and skin V to Y flaps, also visible in the central photo. The final view shows the skin and muscle flaps after I brought them to the midline to complete the closure.

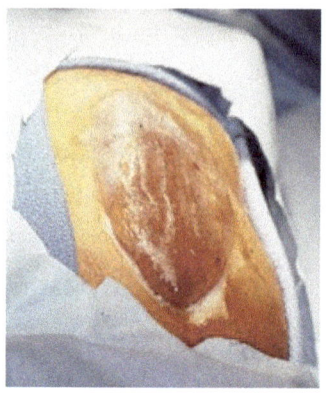 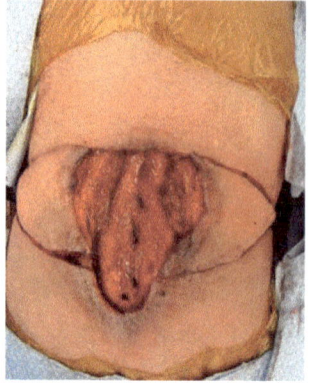 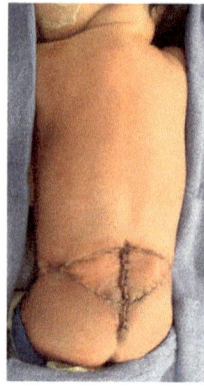

The pictures below show another meningomyelocele case. The first picture shows the spinal cord exposed because of the failure of the bony spine to close. The second picture shows the result after the neurosurgeon has closed the dura over the previously exposed spinal card.

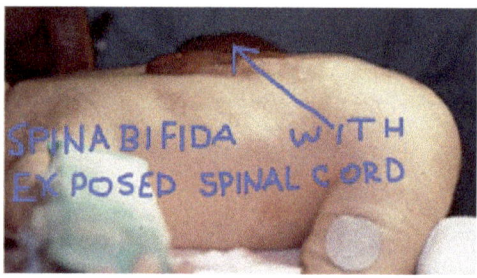 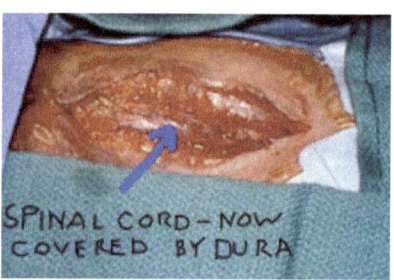

The next picture below shows a skin and muscle flap raised latterly. The wound is closed by I advanced these muscle and skin flaps from each side to produce sturdy coverage over the spinal cord in the midline of the back. The fourth picture shows the postoperative healing wound.

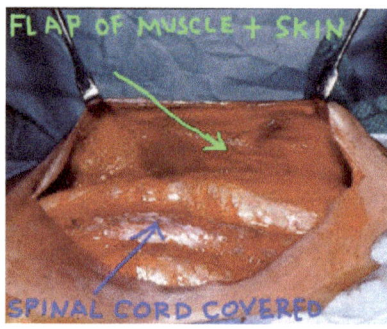 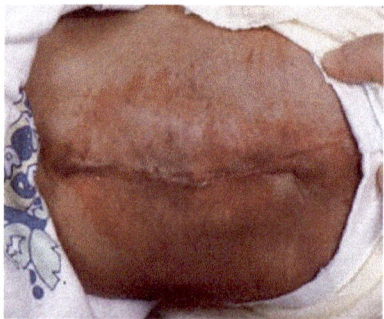

To the Bottom of the Feet

The next patient was a middle-aged lady with melanoma of the heel. She was referred to me by a surgical oncologist who recognized the difficulty of reconstruction of the heel. He planned excision of the lesion and wanted help with closure of the wound he would create.

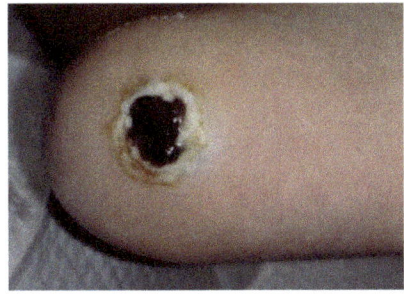

Because the heel is weight-bearing and sensation is vital for the regular gate, I felt it was essential to have a sturdy sensate flap for reconstruction rather than a non-sensate skin graft. Therefore, I decided to do a medial plantar flap procedure. In this procedure, I selected non-weight- bearing but full-thickness tissue from the instep to reconstruct the defect at the heel after removal of the melanoma. I developed this tissue as an island flap. The proper amount of instep tissue was incised and carefully kept connected to the body only by the neurovascular pedicle as a leash (blue arrow below). The photo-drawing on the right diagrammatically shows the neurovascular pedicle.

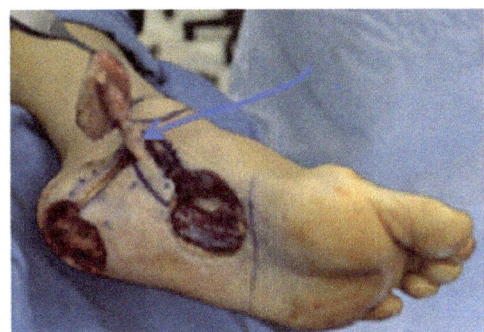 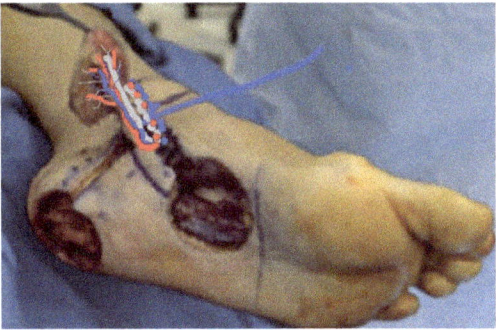

I transferred the island flap to the heel, where it would later allow the patient to feel normal pressure on the heel to aid in normal gait. The photograph below shows the flap moved to the heel still on the pedicle leash outlined in blue. The photo -drawing on the right highlights the pedicle.

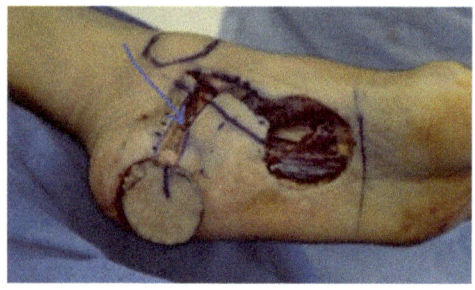 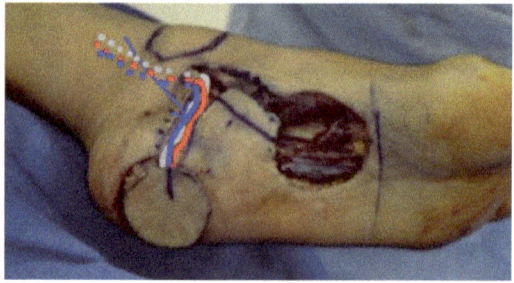

I then was then placed a skin graft on the non- weight-bearing instep wound and dressed it with a tie over bolster in yellow gauze. The final picture shows the sensate flap (red arrow) and the non-weight- bearing instep split-thickness skin (green arrow). At this point, the patient had begun walking with this reconstruction. Her case is an example of functional plastic surgery.

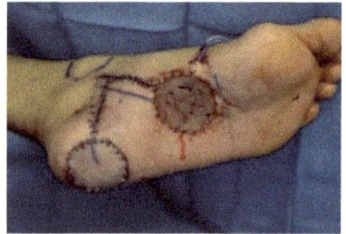 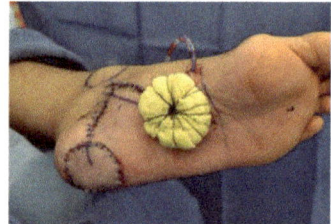 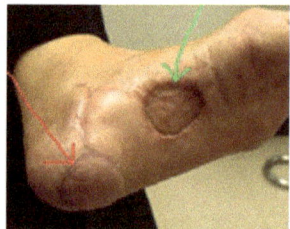

Geriatrics

"Juanita" was a lady octogenarian who had a neglected basal cell carcinoma of the scalp. She insisted nothing was wrong. Denial is so powerful at times! She is an example of a patient who denied the existence of the lesion to herself. Finally, at the instigation of her daughter, she agreed to have treatment for this large fetid basal cell carcinoma of the scalp. This cancer was slow-growing but eventually could be deadly from the local infiltration of vital structures.

I treated her by total excision of the lesion, removing all the soft tissue from the underlying calvarium, including the periosteum, leaving the bare bone exposed. The microscopic frozen section examination of the specimen by the pathologist revealed clear margins. The base of the wound was bone uninvolved with the tumor. If cancer had been more superficial and had not required removal of the periosteum, I could have placed a simple split-thickness skin graft on the periosteum to obtain a healed wound.

As in the young man with the traumatic scalp defect shown previously, I treated her with a large rotation scalp flap elevated above the periosteum of the skull. However, because of the nature and large size of the defect (outlined in red), the result is very different. A broad rotation flap was needed to cover the surgical wound, which was down to the bare bone. In her case, this left the large donor area where I had carefully preserved the periosteum over the cranium. This periosteal layer, just external to the skull, is capable of sustaining a split-thickness skin graft. So, I then grafted the donor area to complete the surgery. Although not a favorable cosmetic result, this was a practical reconstruction. She was rid of this noisome cancer and had total wound closure. Pre-and postoperative photos are below. This example of reconstructive surgery is also functional because it cures the disease.

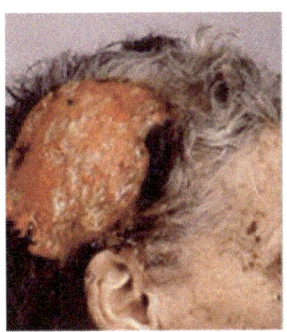
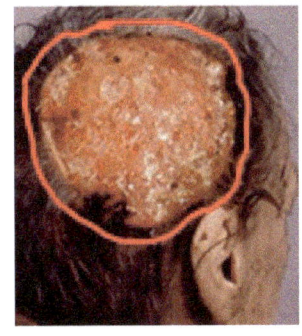

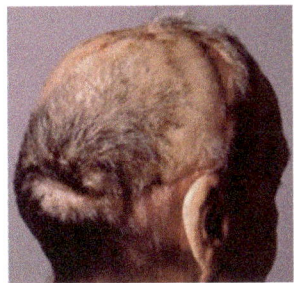
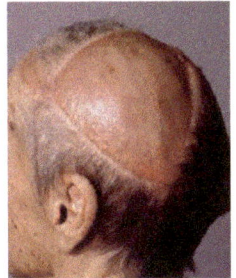
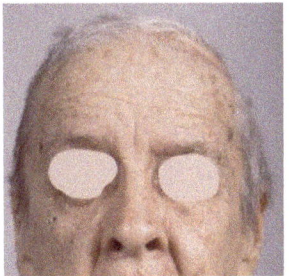

This case illustrates the necessity of using quite large scalp flaps to close scalp wounds. That is very different from some other areas of the body where flaps even slightly smaller than the original defect might be sufficient for closure.

Chapter 5

The best of Both Worlds

Throughout my career since finishing my residencies, I have had a practice that I think incorporates the best of both the private and academic worlds. After completing my residency in plastic surgery, I joined the Cronin Brauer and Biggs Clinic, a large group of six plastic surgeons, all in private practice. This group also was in charge of the plastic surgery residency program at St. Joseph Hospital. After I practiced with the group for ten years, it split up into three private practice groups.

As an aside, when the subject occasionally comes up of the breakup of any group, the assumption is, it must have been a contentious and costly process. I'm happy to tell people that all the partners were gentlemen, and with the help of our accountant, the split incurred not one dime for attorney's fees.

The members of these groups continued to participate in the plastic surgery residency program, which now is sponsored by Houston Methodist Hospital. St Joseph Hospital continues as a significant part of the residency training. The program remains attractive and very competitive. Each year two new residents are brought in for a two-year training period while two senior residents finish their training and go off into private or academic practice or perhaps to some particular fellowship training position.

The training has increased to three years of plastic surgery after completing the prerequisite training. Each year as we prepared for interviews, we received applications from almost two hundred surgeons, most of whom would have completed five years of general surgery or other surgical (ENT) residency training before applying. One of the questions that I frequently asked applicants during the interview is what kind of practice they would like to end up with after they finish all their training. About 90% say they want to have a private practice, but they want to be involved on a day-to-day basis with residents in a teaching capacity for that enjoyment and also to keep their skills up to date.

I am fortunate that was the kind of practice that I had for 38 years. Another thing I enjoyed was having a very diverse practice, which includes both reconstructive and aesthetic patients and children as well as adults. Few plastic surgeons have had, and even fewer will have such a diverse practice in the future.

We had regular conferences with the residents and staff every week in which I routinely participated. We all benefited from the ongoing, almost continual friendly, and constructive conversation about the ever-changing discipline of plastic surgery. Some lectures were didactic about a particular topic presented either by a resident or a staff member. These meetings were always relatively informal, so that a continuous discussion and dialogue about plastic surgery could occur. Some were indication conferences in which we discussed unusual cases not yet done or engaging patients already postoperative. We presented complications (i.e., morbidity) at traditional morbidity and mortality conferences to try to prevent them in the future.

Other meetings dealt with preparing the residents for the yearly in-service examination, as well as for their written board examinations, which they usually take after the first year they are in practice.

Our teaching staff was always collegial, so we avoided many of the rancorous meetings that we sometimes hear about elsewhere. No one, it seems, tried to step on other colleagues to get ahead. We discussed presentations made at medical meetings, either large national conferences or smaller meetings dealing with one topic. The staff or residents came back from meetings and reported to the whole plastic surgery section what they learned. Innovative new plastic surgery procedures characterized the late 70s and 1980s. I was fortunate to practice during this dynamic and exciting time in the development of the field of plastic surgery. I outline some of these dynamic plastic surgery developments in chapter 17.

I took advantage of belonging to a large group with prominent partners who had a history of multiple publications and contributions to the field of plastic surgery by participating in such endeavors. During 38 years in practice, I was able to author or co-author more than three dozen articles or book chapters in the field of plastic surgery. Several essays were on breast reconstruction after mastectomy. I also wrote several papers concerning cleft lip and palate issues. Others addressed miscellaneous topics such as endoscopic forehead surgery, augmentation mammaplasty, the innervated cross finger flap, removal of road debris tattoos, et cetera. The remainder of this chapter reviews some examples from this experience I had contributing to medical literature.

The first example is that of an unusual case of breast asymmetry. Miss "Wendy" was a twenty-something young woman who came to see me because she was unhappy with the asymmetry of her breasts. She had an unusual situation. Most of the time, when we see a young woman with asymmetry, one of the breasts is ptotic or sagging while the other is more nubile or normal for a young woman. However, in this case, "Wendy" had an attractive and normal-appearing breast on each side. They were just very different from each other, as shown in the first photo below.

Sometimes when discussing breast asymmetry with my patients, I talk about healthy breasts being sisters, not identical twins. In her situation, it seemed like her breasts were "cousins." To help decide what to do, I showed her three images, beginning with her actual condition. In the second image below, I superimposed the mirror image of the right breast onto the left. In the last photo, I superimposed the mirror image of the left breast onto the right. After studying these pictures, she decided she would like me to strive to make the left breast more like the right breast, even though this would necessitate leaving a scar in the upper portion of the left breast. It is quite common to elevate the nipple because of sagging breasts or breast reduction surgery. It is quite unusual to lower the position of the nipple on the breast, as I did in this case.

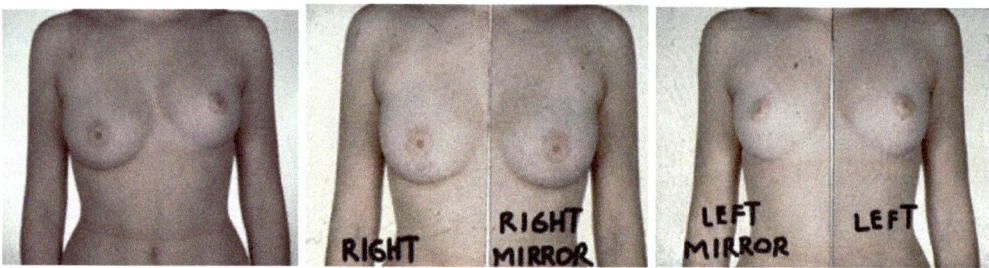

The first intra-operative photo below shows the nipple on an inferiorly based pedicle, which I de-epithelialized. The nipple thus retains its blood supply from this de-epithelialized tissue when it is folded on itself to move lower on the breast. The old nipple position is outlined with a green circle while the green arrows show the direction and extent of its movement. The middle intraoperative photo shows the former nipple position in green while the new nipple position is now lower to correspond with the right nipple-areola. There is an upside-down, lollypop shaped scar pattern. She also wanted fuller breasts, so I placed a silicone gel implant through an inframammary incision to augment each breast. The last picture below is the postoperative result, which shows improved symmetry compared to her preoperative status depicted in her first picture above.

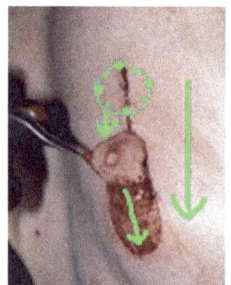 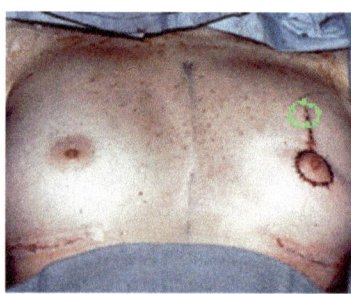 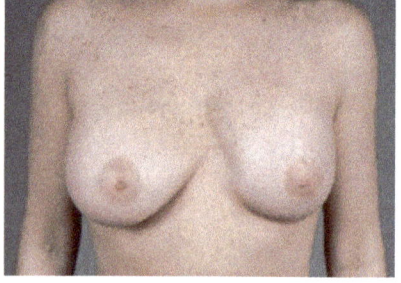

When I went into practice in 1978, breast reconstruction was in its infancy. I saw many women who had had radical Mastectomy seek breast reconstruction. Although, by that era, the most frequent Mastectomy done was a modified radical mastectomy. Also, I initially performed all restorations secondarily, often years after the Mastectomy. Today most mastectomies are of the skin-sparing variety, and some even spare the nipple-areola complex as well. That makes breast reconstruction much easier. Also, I now initiate most repairs primarily, at the same time as the Mastectomy. I co-authored several papers about breast reconstruction during the era of radical mastectomy surgery at a time in which our armamentarium of breast reconstruction techniques was much more limited than it is today.

I reported on some breast reconstruction cases with Dr. Thomas Cronin, which used silicone gel breast implants without additional skin or muscle flaps. One example from that work is the patient below, " Lynn," whose preoperative photo is one year after modified radical Mastectomy. She had an intact pectoralis major muscle under slightly tight skin. We reconstructed her right breast by placing a silicone gel implant under the pectoralis major muscle. We first split the pectoralis to gain submuscular access and created a large pocket (orange) for the implant.

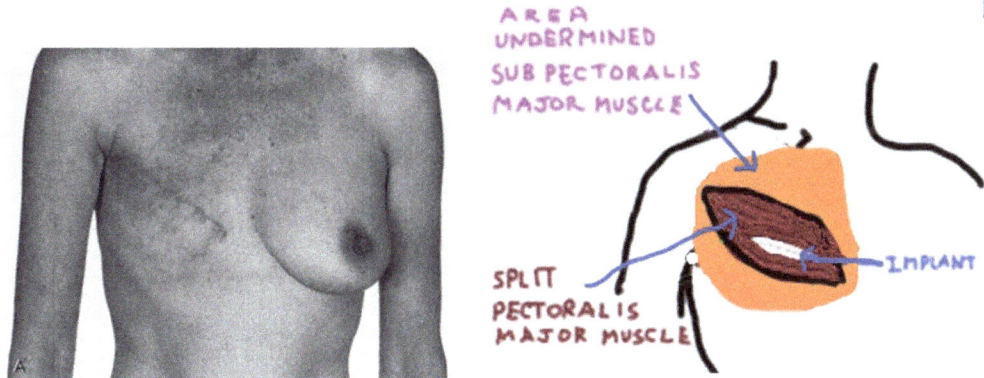

We sutured the split pectoralis muscle to close the implant pocket. We then placed a split-thickness skin graft on the exposed pectoral muscle to obtain a relaxed closure rather than making a tight skin closure by pulling the existing chest skin together.

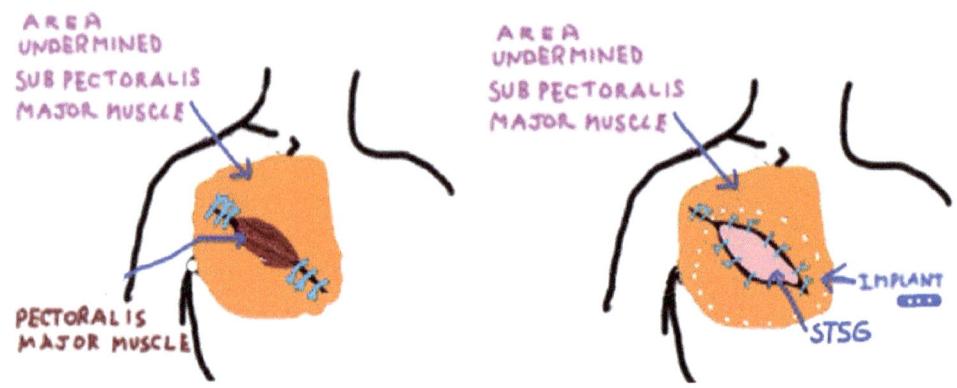

On the left breast, we did a prophylactic subcutaneous mastectomy with a mastopexy (breast lift). We also placed a sub pectoralis muscle silicone gel implant for symmetry. This type of reconstruction, after subcutaneous Mastectomy, is explained in more detail in chapter 9.

Her postoperative photo below is one example of a satisfactory reconstruction we accomplished for "Lynn" with relatively unsophisticated techniques. It would have been impossible without the development of the silicone gel implant by Dr. Thomas Cronin.

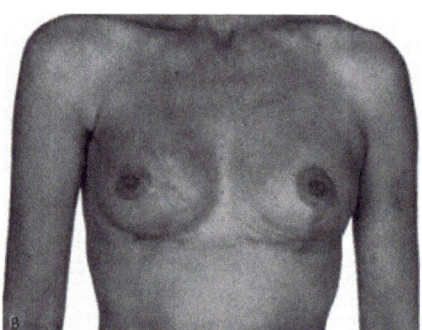

Thoraco-epigastric Flap

Dr. Thomas Cronin and I also reported on breast reconstruction using the thoraco- epigastric flap to add additional skin coverage for an implant. This technique was advantageous when the chest wall skin was too tight to place a silicone gel implant beneath it.

The drawings below illustrate the thoracoepigastric flap used in a secondary reconstruction after a traditional radical mastectomy, which removed the pectoralis major muscle. The thoroco-epigastric flap gets its blood supply from perforating vessels of the superior epigastric artery medially. The flap contains fascia, subcutaneous fatty tissue, and skin. It can be rotated as much as 90° after opening the old scar to relieve the tight skin of the chest. A silicone gel implant was placed immediately beneath the thoracoepigastric flap, which produced coverage for the implant. We closed the flap donor site directly.

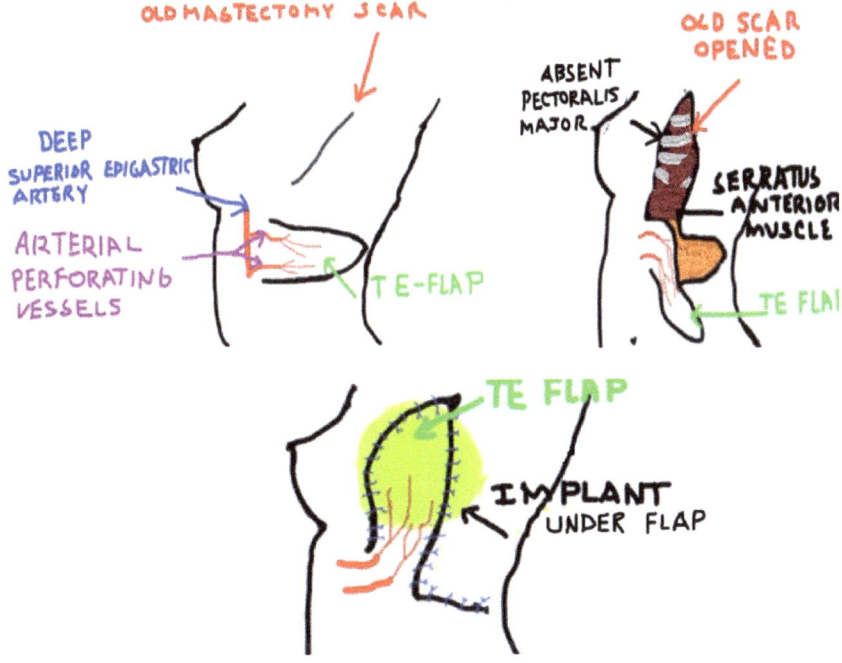

Dr. Thomas Cronin used a thorocoepigastric flap to reconstruct the patient below after her traditional radical Mastectomy. She also had significant radiation therapy with concomitant skin changes.

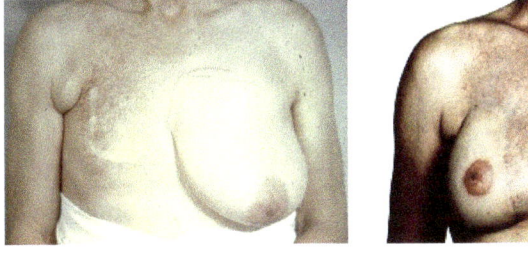

The pictures below are those of a 60-year-old woman, "Gloria," who waited 20 years after a left simple mastectomy (muscles intact) to have her breast reconstructed. We used a thoraco-epigastric flap with a silicone gel implant placed in a sub pectoralis major and serratus anterior muscular pocket as the drawings of this technique below demonstrate.

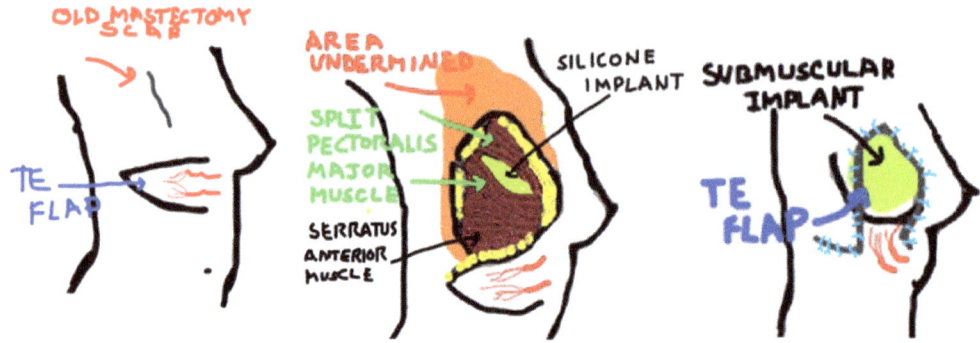

We reconstructed the nipple-areola using labium minus for the nipple and labium magnus for the areola. We augmented the right breast with a small silicone gel implant

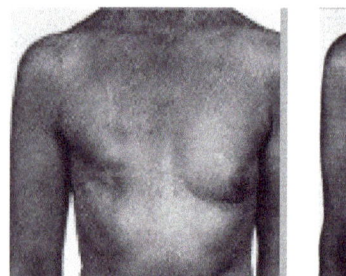 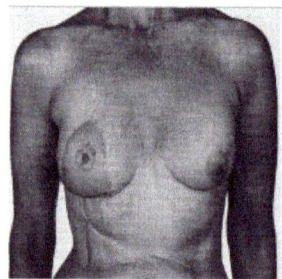 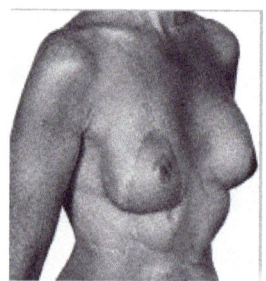

Latissimus Dorsi myo-cutaneous Flap

The routine utilization of the thoraco-epigastric flap technique soon became obsolete as it was superseded by the latissimus dorsi myo-cutaneous flap technique. The latissimus dorsi myo-cutaneous flap included an island of skin and subcutaneous fat on top of the latissimus muscle. The latissimus muscle is a large flat muscle that inserts on the humerus in the axillary area. Its blood supply from the thoracodorsal artery also comes from the underarm area. This flap can swing from the back, through the underarm area, to the anterior chest while maintaining its blood supply.

In most cases, a silicone gel breast implant is placed beneath the flap as needed for volume and protection. The diagrams below show the outline and movement of this flap for breast reconstruction. The first drawing shows the skin island oriented on the back. The numbers indicate the muscle's orientation before and after its utilization. Usually, the skin island is placed obliquely on the anterior chest, not necessarily at the location of the old scar.

This practice came about somewhat serendipitously when a patient of Dr. Tom Biggs had a modified radical mastectomy with a long, laterally positioned oblique incision. Dr. Biggs placed the latissimus skin island in the mastectomy incision, as was the routine. The island, therefore, had a curvilinear inferior and lateral position, which helped to produce an exceptionally lovely curvaceous breast. Making a note of that, we began to ignore the mastectomy scar, which was ofter horizontal, and place the island inferior and laterally. Dr. Thomas Biggs and I published a paper on the latissimus flap for breast reconstruction recommending this modified technique.

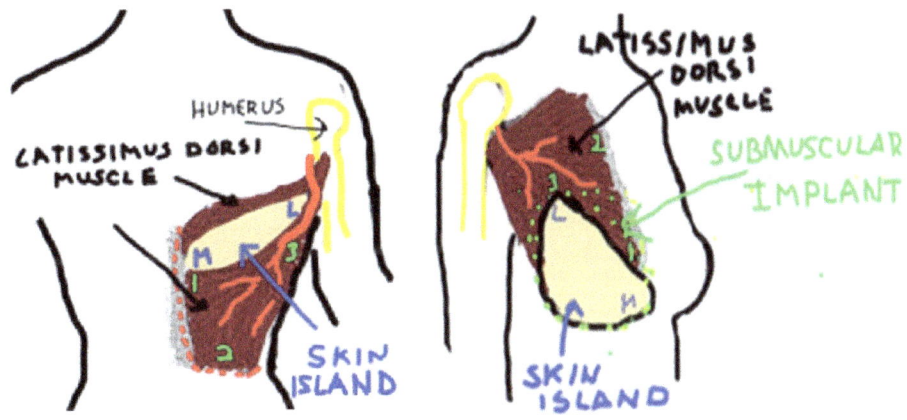

After that, Dr. Cohen and I analyzed the mastectomy scar and position for the latissimus flap. We described the mature breast as having an upper portion consisting of a long gradual slope leading to the point of maximum protection of the nipple and a shorter inferior curve joining the chest wall at approximately a 90° angle. The shape is similar to a right - angle triangle, as in the drawing below.

The Healing Mission of Plastic Surgery

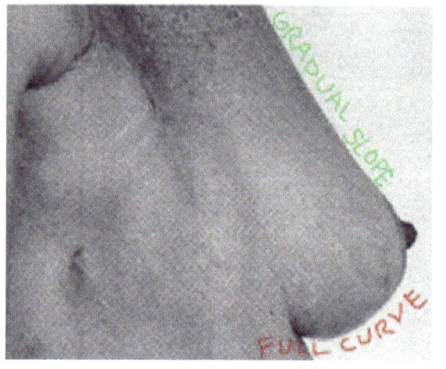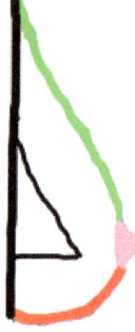

We were looking for the best orientation for placement of the skin island latissimus dorsi flap in secondary (delayed) modified radical mastectomy cases. It seems intuitive that in a secondary modified radical mastectomy, one would open the old scar and re-create the defect made by the Mastectomy and then replace there to replace that tissue excised at the time of the Mastectomy. That concept is standard procedure in many plastic surgery reconstructive scenarios. Therefore, when we first began using the latissimus flap, we would incise the old scar allowing that to open up and then placed the skin island into the re-created defect as the case below demonstrates. The photograph and diagrammatic representation show some limitations in this traditional intuitive placement of the skin island at the site of the existing mastectomy scar. The inferior aspect of the breast is not released satisfactorily.

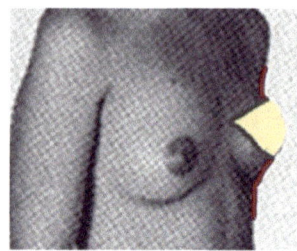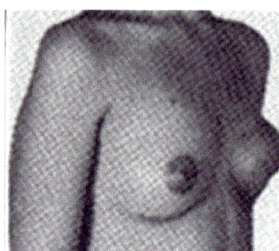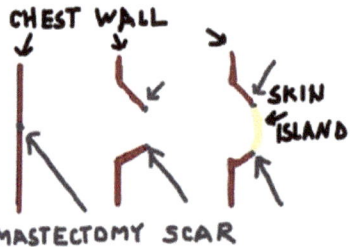

Conversely, in the photograph below, the existing horizontal scar from the Mastectomy was ignored, and curvilinear placement of the skin island inferiorly and laterally allowed the silicone gel implant to produce proper forward protection of the breast as one could envision from the drawing below. Therefore a more natural breast shape was attained in this patient shown below.

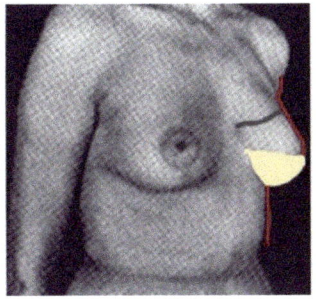 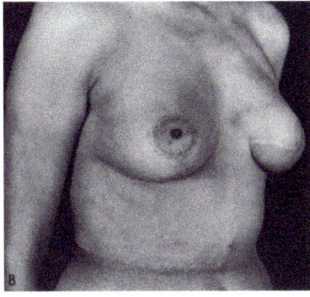 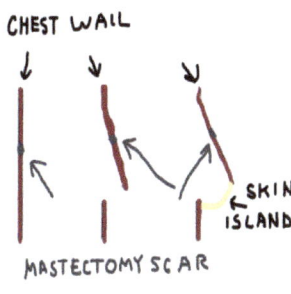

It would seem the "gradual slope" of the breast can be maintained by just elevating the existing chest wall skin and placement of an implant. However, the lower" full curve" portion of the profile needs the added tissue of the latissimus skin island to provide coverage for the projection the implant produces. To re-create the entire curve portion of the reconstruction, it became evident that an inferior and lateral release was best. We found that often the old scar could be ignored, and the flap skin island placed inferior laterally, offering the best breast shape. We recommended ignoring the most common horizontal mastectomy scar and placing the island in a new incision inferiorly and laterally shown in the drawings below. Our analysis reaffirmed the findings of the previous paper I published with Dr. Biggs.

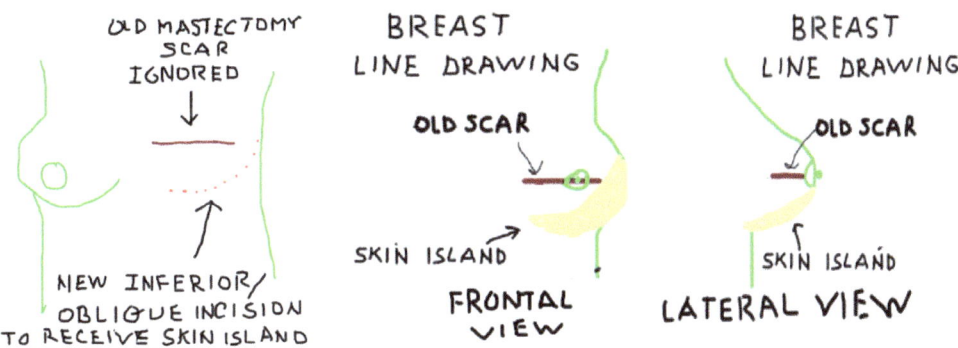

Chapter 9 contains a more thorough presentation of the latissimus flap for breast reconstruction

Primary nasal repair

I devised a variation on primary nasal repair in cleft lip patients. Patients who have complete clefts of the lip also have a significant deformity of the nose. The floor of the nose is absent, and repairing the lip reconstructs the anterior floor of the nose. A substantial part of the nasal deformity with complete clefts of the lip involves the tip cartilages of the nose. The cartilage on the cleft side will be splayed out laterally, and the dome of the cartilage, which should be in the nasal tip, will be lower and forward compared to the non-cleft nasal tip dome cartilage. The photo below shows a typical deformity with a complete cleft of the lip. The drawing shows the distorted tip cartilage on the right side and how this cartilage must be elevated and brought at least to the prominence on the better side. Because there may be some postoperative regression, we often try to make the tip even more prominent than the opposite side.

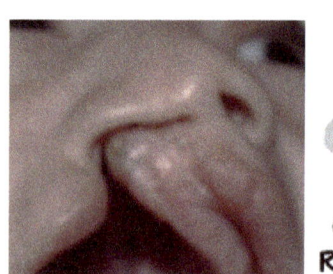 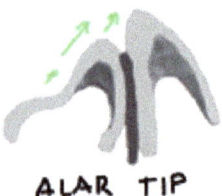 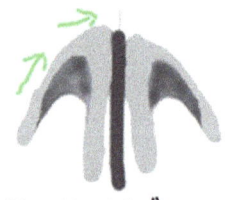 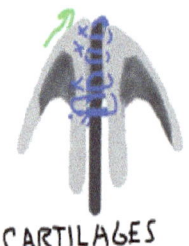

ALAR TIP CARTILAGES RIGHT CLEFT LIP   RIGHT ALA MOVED UP AND MEDIALLY   CARTILAGES SUTURED

When I started in plastic surgery practice, the routine was to repair cleft lips when the patient was three months of age. The nasal repair followed years later. Soon this practice changed, and many surgeons began to do primary work on the nose. Usually, significant improvement occurred with nasal surgery done concurrently with the original lip repair. However, because of modulation with growth, additional secondary surgery has always been beneficial in the teen years, in severe cases.

Below is depicted a technical variation of primary cleft lip nasal deformity repair, which I devised. I first made incisions to free the lateral portion and dome of the tip cartilage on the affected cleft side. I left a mucosal tab attached to the lateral end of this cartilage. I then elevated the cartilage superiorly and immediately so that the dome was at least as high as the opposite dome. To help stabilize the new position of the cartilage, I sutured the domes together. The mucosal tab aids in the closure of the donor wound from where the cartilage was advanced, thus. Preventing scar contracture with the closure of the intranasal wound.

The Healing Mission of Plastic Surgery

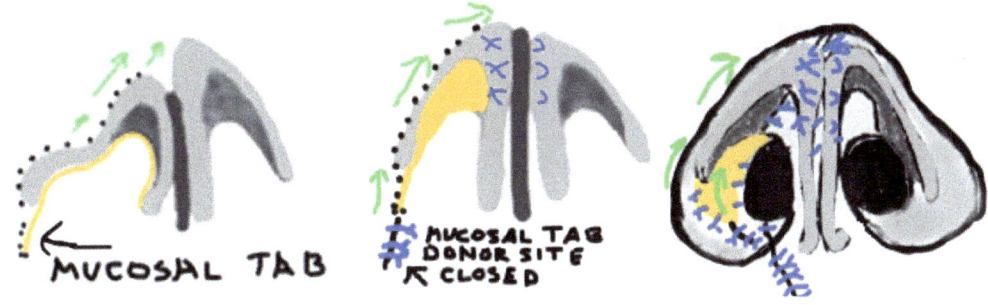

"Susy," below, had a complete cleft of the lip on the right side. I performed the above-described procedure at the time of the lip repair. Postoperative photographs are shown after several weeks and at one year. As you can see, compared to the preoperative condition of the nose, the postoperative nasal symmetry is good.

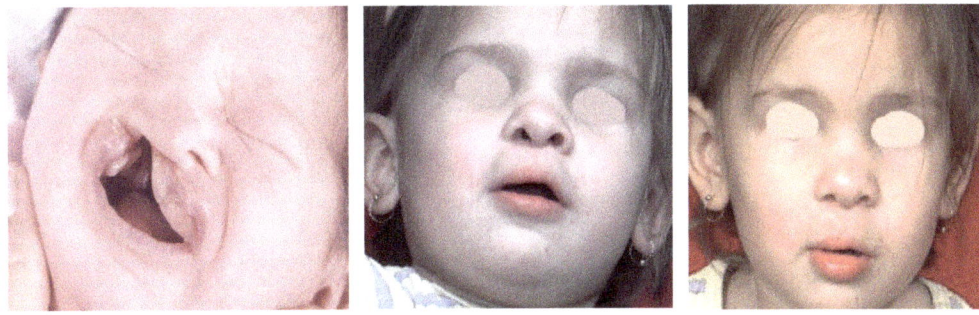

The patient below "Jesus" had an incomplete cleft of the lip on the left side. I did the cartilage advancement with the mucosal tab procedure for him simultaneous with the lip repair. His preoperative and two-year postoperative photos are below.

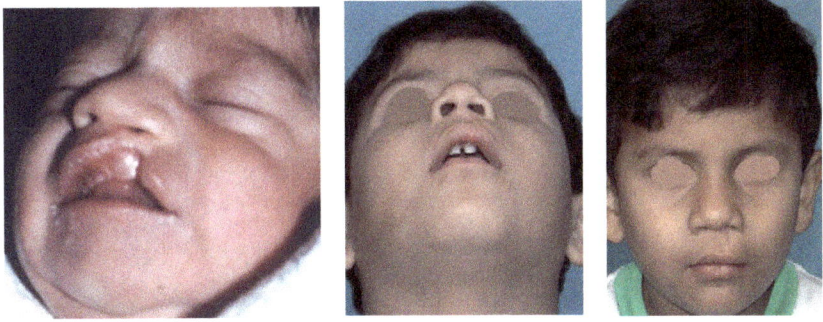

Innervated Cross Finger Flap

My partner Benjamin Cohen and I produced a novel improvement to a traditional procedure known as a cross finger flap. The original description of the cross-finger flap was made by Thomas Cronin in the 1950s. This procedure transfers tissue from the backside of the finger to the palm side of an adjacent finger for reconstructive purposes. We leave the base of the flap attached to the donor's finger while transferring dorsal finger skin to the palm side defect of the adjacent finger. We cut the bridge after two weeks when the new blood supply from the recipient's finger is sufficient for flap survival.

Our innovation takes advantage of the innervation of the tissue on the back of the fingers. That innervation comes from a small branch coming from the palm side digital nerve. In selected cases, we can include this dorsal branch with the flap so that it can supply sensation to the injured finger. It does not provide immediate sensation but relies on the healing of the repaired nerve to slowly regenerate. The first drawing shows the donor areas on the back of the fingers that the cross-finger flap uses. The second drawing shows the dorsal branch transgressing from the palm side digital nerve to the flap area on the dorsal side of the finger.

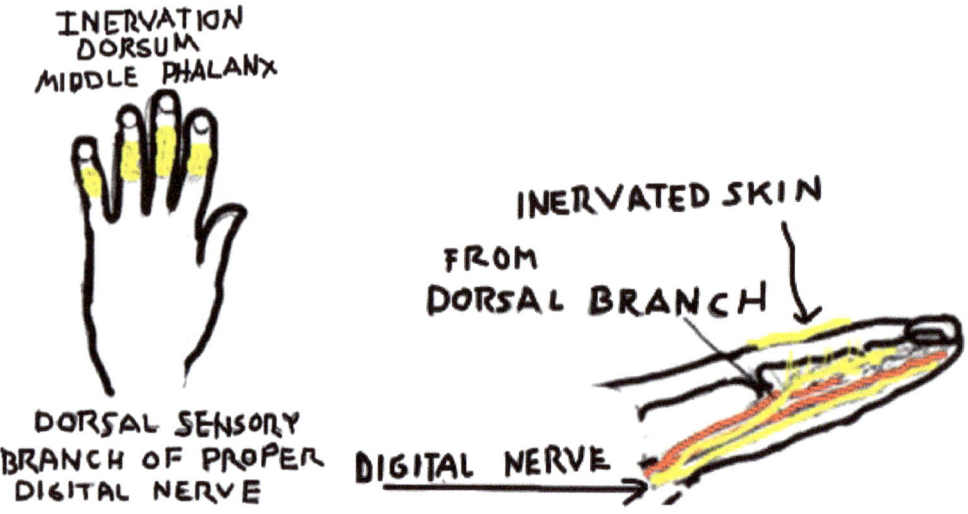

This worker below, "Robert," caught his fingers in a machine resulting in the injuries to his index and long finger shown below. The second photo shows the tissue on the backside of the ring and long finger, which I will transfer to the middle and index finger defects, respectively.

The Healing Mission of Plastic Surgery

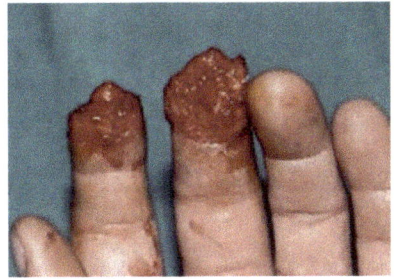
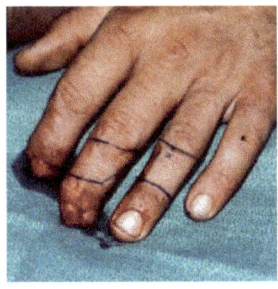

The first drawing shows the dorsal sensory branch in the donor finger. The second drawing shows the flap, elevated with the cut dorsal sensory nerve still attached. I will suture this nerve to the cut digital nerve in the injured finger.

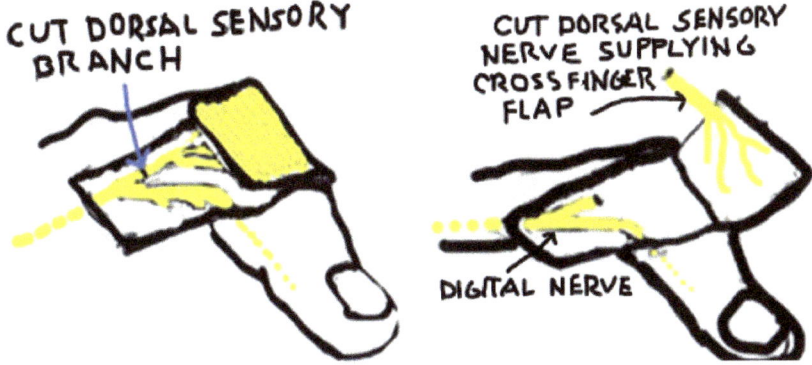

The following picture shows the flaps sutured to the injured index and long finger while the base of each flap remains connected to the donor finger. I separated the fingers at two weeks postoperatively. The last picture shows the final result several weeks later.

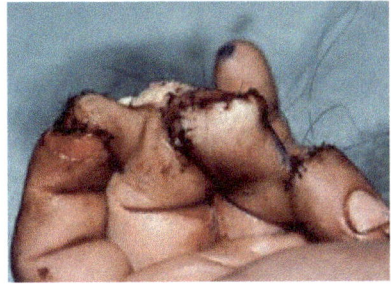
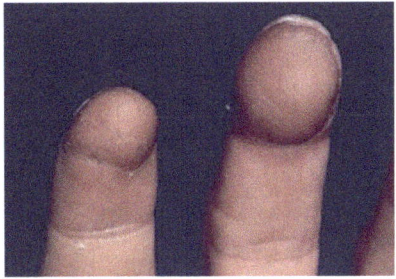

The additional case below shows "Jackson's" avulsion injury of the volar surface of the left little finger. The first drawing shows a skin graft on the donor area and the cross-finger flap with its attached dorsal digital nerve.

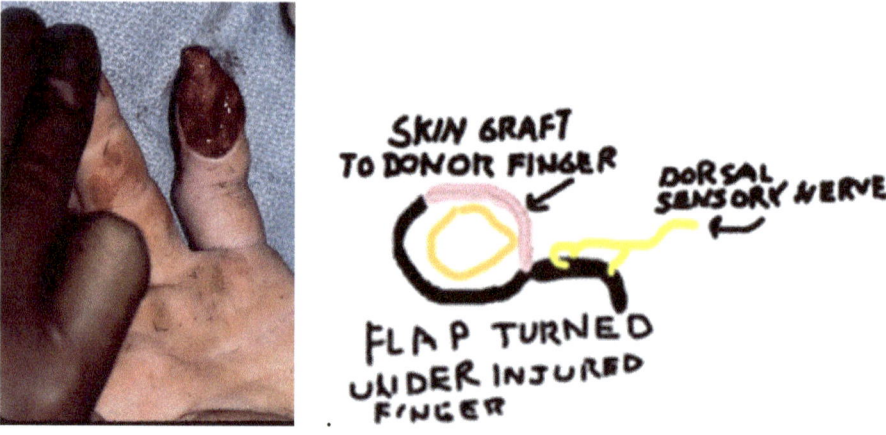

The following drawing shows the flap donor site repaired with a skin graft and the flap partially sewn to the adjacent injured finger. The dorsal sensory branch transferred with the flap is sutured to the digital nerve of the injured finger. The photo on the left below demonstrates this anastomosis in a patient during the operation.

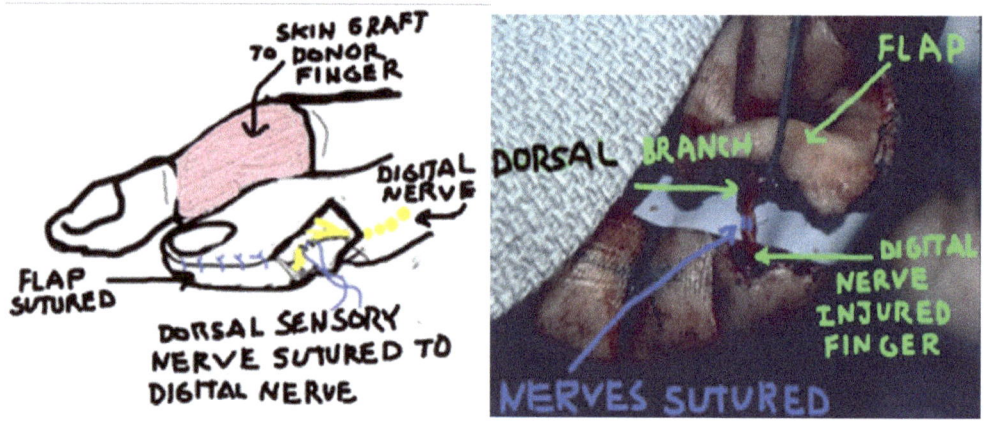

The last picture below shows the final result for "Jackson's." injured finger and the donor finger.

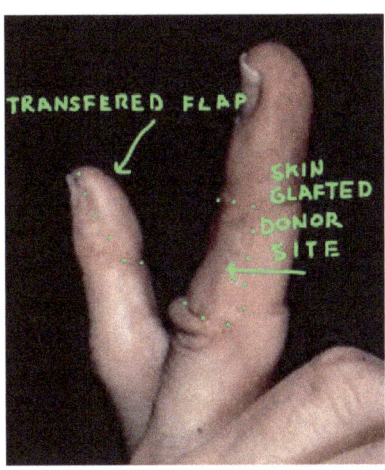

Over the years, teaching in such a program has been a two-way street. I have certainly learned many things from our residents, as well as hopefully imparting some knowledge to them as well. Because our residents had, on average, five years of training before they come to us, they often had a lot to offer. Many of them had five years of general surgery. But because they come from all over the country, from Boston to San Diego and from San Francisco to Miami, each one's experience was different. Also, some of our residents had ENT training for four or five years or general surgery experience plus some additional specialty fellowship such as hand surgery, burn surgery, or microsurgery.

It's been wonderful to see the residents mature and leave the program to become successful on their own. It makes us proud. As I have gotten older, it seems the residents keep getting younger. In some ways, they're like one's professional children. I always want to see them do well. I always anxiously await the results of their written and oral plastic surgery board examinations. I am rarely disappointed.

Besides teaching them various techniques of plastic surgery, I have tried to instill in them good habits such as preparing well for cases. I stress always keeping primary the best interest of the patient. Because I was in an academically oriented practice with plastic surgery residents, I received some fascinating cases that I might otherwise not have seen in private practice.

Cleft Palate with Lateral Synechia Syndrome

Cleft palate lateral synechia syndrome is quite rare. The following patient report by myself and Dr. M. Jabor and Dr. P Shayani represented the third case of cleft palate isolated bilateral alveolar synechia in the United States and the fifth worldwide at the time.

At birth, the infant's physical exam revealed fibrous bands connecting the upper and lower jaws bilaterally with severe trismus limiting the mouth opening to approximately 5 mm. The fibrous bands spanned from the posterior alveolar ridge of the maxilla to the poster alveolar ridge of the mandible bilaterally, as demonstrated by the drawing and photographs below.

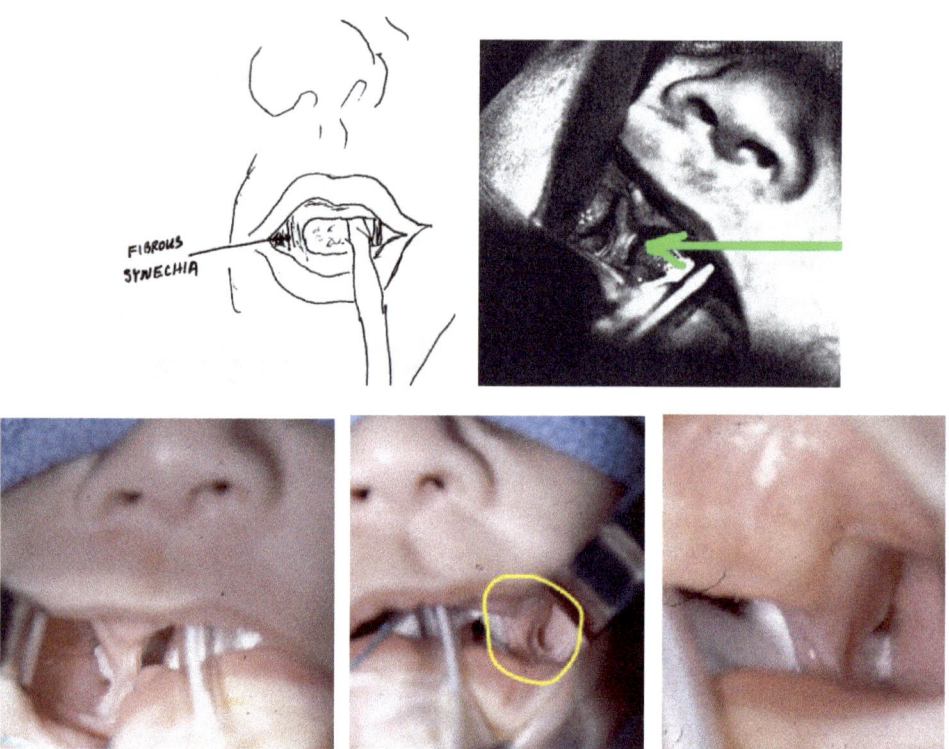

I also noted a U-shaped posterior cleft palate. I decided against immediate surgical intervention because there were no breathing or severe feeding difficulties. The infant was allowed time to grow while being closely followed. I instructed the mother to manually manipulate the jaws of the child while at home by placing a fingertip between the jaws. She was able to slowly stretch the opening 1st to 10 mm then to as much as 14 mm, which made feeding easier. When the baby was four months of age, I took the child to surgery.

An experienced pediatric anesthesiologist successfully performed oral tracheal intubation of the patient. On close inspection, I observed that the fibrous bands extended from the poster maxilla in an area corresponding to the third molar down to the area of the mandibular trigonal. I made a sagittal incision along the length of the fibrous band and on the buccal and lingual side of the fibrous bands. The incised fibrous bands were then used as individual flaps and were folded over and sutured so that no two opposing raw edges were present, which might have allowed for scarring to re-create the problem. The blue and green dots help to understand the repositioning of the tissue after the incision severing the fibrous band. I did each side in this same manner.

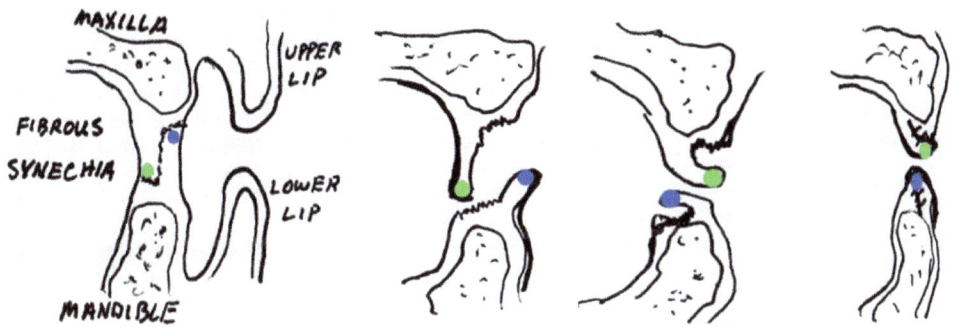

However, some trismus was still persistent after the operation. I encouraged the very cooperative mother to continue manually stretch the jaw, which resolved the trismus within a couple of months. On the left below is the early post-op result. At one year of age, when the mouth would open fully, I repaired the palate; the post-op picture after palate repair is on the right. The patient continued to mature and grow normally.

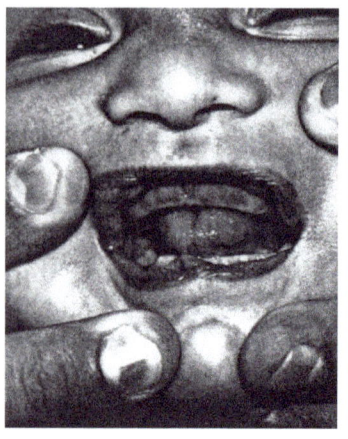 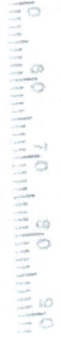 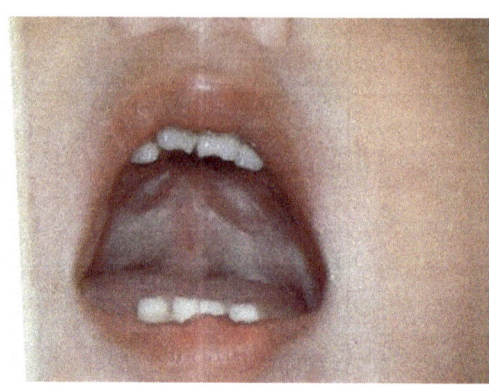

Novel Dermabrasion

I did another project with doctors Jabor and Shayani, that described an innovative approach to traumatic tattoos. Traumatic tattoos result from the accidental deposition of pigmented particles within the dermis. Dirt, carbon, asphalt, and other substances can traumatically stain the dermis and result in black or blue pigmentation of the skin depending upon the depth of embedment. The mechanism of injury for these foreign particles is abrasive or explosive trauma. The abrasive tattoos are more common and occur secondary to friction with a road surface such as a fall from a motorcycle or bicycle. The explosive type of traumatic tattoos involves blast injury with firecrackers, firearms, dynamite, or bombs as the source. Regardless of the mode injury, the best cosmetic result is obtained by the early treatment before the wounds heal and epithelialize over the foreign particles. Complete spontaneous closure of the facial wounds may occur within 72 hours, making treatment more difficult.

Part of the initial management includes cleaning the pigmented areas with saline and soap, followed by the application of petroleum-based antibiotic ointment to improve the miscibility of the pigment. Following this conventional dermabrasion with a diamond burr may be successful and sufficient for many traumatic tattoo injuries. For a patient presenting after epithelization of the wound, the treatment may include excision of the largest carbon deposits with a number 11 scalpel followed by primary closure with small monofilament nylon sutures.

However, profoundly stained tissue that contains small concentrated areas of pigmented debris is exceptionally problematic. I published a new technique for the removal of these tiny, deeply stained traumatic tattoos. Refractory pigments deposited into the deepest layer of the dermis can be successfully removed by an innovative technique that utilizes a 1 mm otologic cutting burr and a striker drill shown below. I use the tip of the burr to drill down perpendicular to the small pigmented areas, and the abrasion removes the deep pigment. Often the burr penetrates deeply, resulting in a tiny full-thickness defect. This process is repeated as many times as necessary until all the resistant pigment is gone. The small imperfections produced are left open to heal by secondary intention and generally lead to minimal or no scar.

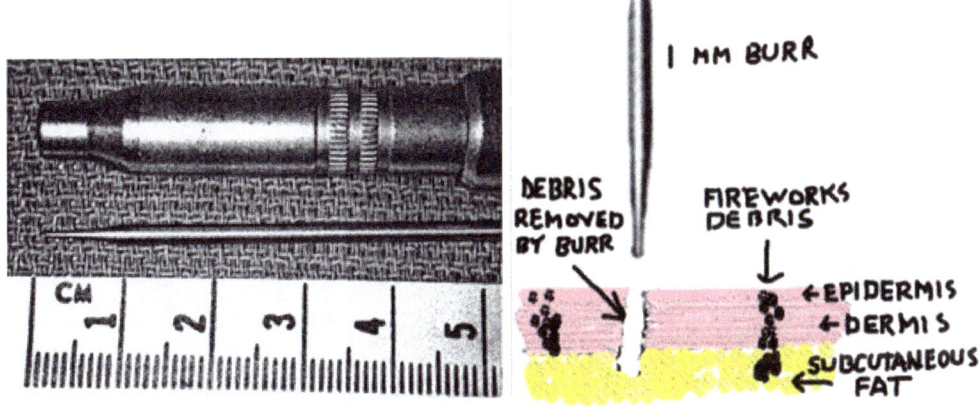

Fireworks exploded in the face of the boy whose photographs are below. As the pre-op picture demonstrates, he had reasonably discrete small deposits of fireworks debris that were too deep to remove with standard dermabrasion techniques safely. I used the above-described novel method to treat him. I was thrilled that this technique worked so well for him. He and his mother were delighted that I was able to help him with this new technique.

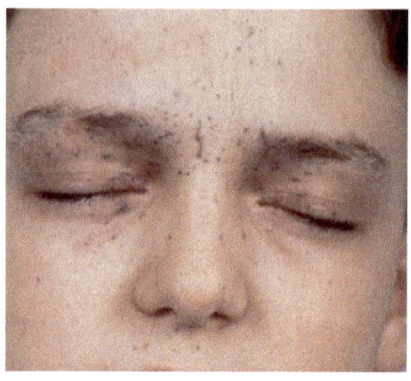
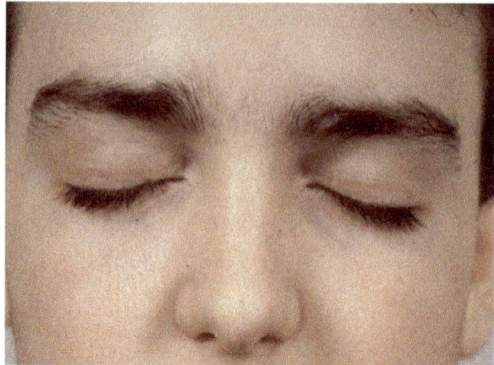

The S flap nipple reconstruction

The S flap nipple reconstruction was a method I devised for nipple reconstruction. I found this technique especially beneficial when there was a horizontal scar running through the area where the nipple needed to be. I discuss nipple-areola reconstruction techniques in chapter 9, Breast reconstruction, after Mastectomy.

TRAM flap after abdominoplasty

The pedicle TRAM flap for breast surgery utilizes tissue from the lower abdomen. A pedicle of rectus muscle brings skin and subcutaneous fat to the chest. The superior epigastric vessels supply blood flow to the pedicled rectus muscle flap. Perforating vessels from the muscle traverse the subcutaneous fat to sustain the viability of the overlying skin. Performing a "tummy tuck" or abdominoplasty obliterates these perforating vessels. However, some experimental studies show that some revascularization takes place between the muscle and the newly adjusted overlying skin after such a procedure.

Dr. Tom Biggs and I wrote a paper on the use of the TRAM flap after abdominoplasty. We do not recommend this is a routine procedure, but only in particular circumstances. For example, if the patient wants and could benefit from a repeat abdominoplasty, this procedure might be considered. Also, alternative reconstructive measures must be available in reserve in case the abdominal tissue has an insufficient blood supply to survive. The patient shown below "Carol" had a previous abdominoplasty. I performed a bilateral subcutaneous mastectomy and successful bilateral reconstruction with pedicle TRAM flaps. Her preoperative, intraoperative, and postoperative photographs are below. My plan, if the abdominal tissue was unusable, was to utilize silicone gel implants.

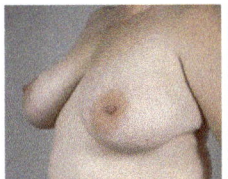 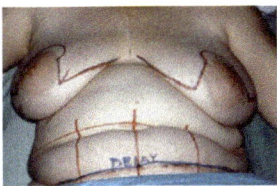 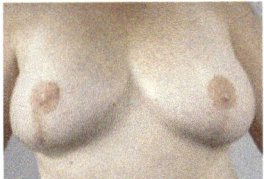 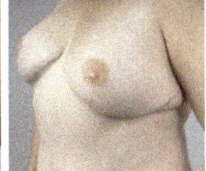

Breast Reconstruction

I wrote several other papers on breast reconstruction co-authored with Thomas Cronin and one with Dr. Robert Wright. Some of that information will be in Chapter 9, Breast Reconstruction, after Mastectomy.

Augmentation

I wrote a paper on augmentation mammaplasty with Thomas Cronin. Some information on that will be in Chapter 8, Thomas Cronin, and the Silicone Gel Breast Implant.

Endoscopy

I wrote an early article on the endoscopic approach for the resection of forehead masses, together with doctors Amado Ruiz-Razura, Christopher Livingston, and J.Timothy Katzen. The technique used one or two small incisions within the hairline and endoscopic equipment to develop a plain beneath the periosteum and frontal bone, as indicated in the drawing below. I removed osteomas easily with a chisel. The usually "mint patty" shaped lipomas are situated between the periosteum and the frontalis muscle, which is the muscle that raises the brow. I removed lipomas by cutting through the periosteum from the space dissected endoscopically.

The picture below is an impressive view through an endoscope of an osteoid osteoma, a benign bony lesion that caused a bump on the forehead. These lesions usually separate quite readily with a chisel, making the endoscopic approach quite practical for them. Here the osteoma has been cleanly separated from the frontal bone and is ready to be grabbed with small forceps and removed through the small scalp incisions as shown in the drawing and intraoperative photo

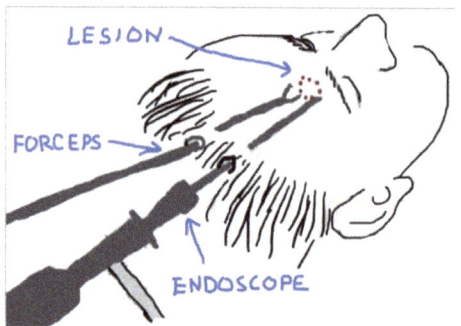 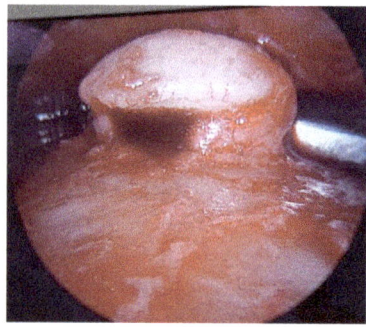

The patient below "Gregory" had a lipoma of the forehead demonstrated in the first photo, which indicates the incision placement. I removed the lipoma endoscopically through a small incision in the scalp rather than a direct skin incision on the forehead. The removed lipoma is shown in the middle photo looking from above the head. The immediate post-op result is on the right.

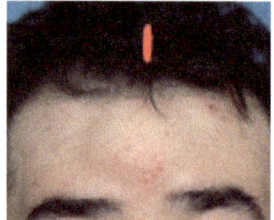 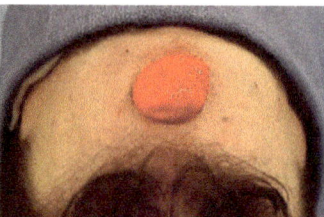 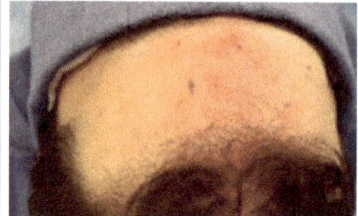

Chapter 6

The Emergency Room and Trauma

Traumatic injuries all over the body are in the purview of plastic surgery, particularly the face and hands. The emergency room has played an essential part in every plastic surgeon's life. Young surgeons in training learn how to evaluate and treat traumatic injuries in the emergency room. Throughout my training in medical school, general surgery, ENT surgery, and plastic surgery, the emergency room played a significant role in my exposure to complicated traumatic injuries. Often injuries are treated in the department. Other times the initial treatment is followed by procedures in the operating room, either immediately or later. The emergency room has a unique environment. As a medical student from 1967 to 1971, I had a relatively small amount of exposure to the emergency room. I saw a variety of ailments and sutured several minor lacerations.

Internship

My real baptism in the emergency room came as an intern at the Kansas City General Hospital. The interns were on 12- hour shifts in the emergency room, which could be quite demanding. Fortunately, when a significant trauma came in, I had excellent backup from the general surgery residents, who would arrive within two to three minutes after being called. I also have fond memories of some of the nurses who helped me in the emergency room.

On one of the first shifts I had in the emergency room, a patient was wheeled in on a stretcher by an ambulance crew. The patient was yelling and flailing about, making no sense. Before I had much of a chance to examine the patient, the nurse working with me had gone and got a large syringe of injectable glucose and said: "she needs this." The nurse knew this patient from numerous previous visits to the emergency room with diabetic problems. The patient was having erratic behavior because of low blood sugar. After briefly assessing her, I took the large syringe and gave her an intravenous injection of glucose. In an almost miraculous way within one minute or so, she began to calm down and became oriented.

I was then able to call the internal medicine resident house officer to come to the emergency room to admit and take over the care of the patient. If that nurse had not been there, I might have eventually figured out what the problem was, but it would have taken more time and certainly would have been a more trying ordeal. I sincerely appreciated her help. On one of the first nights in the ER, I had three gunshot victims. I was sure relieved the general surgery residents responded so promptly to help me care for these patients.

That internship year was a crazy mixture of nerve-racking experiences and exhilarating ones as well. Trauma was a significant part of the emergency department experience. Every shift, there would be patients with minor lacerations to repair or perhaps a nasal fracture to straighten with manual manipulation.

A memorable case involved a young man who was in an automobile accident and came in at the end of my shift. He was terrified by the blood everywhere at the accident site and the reactions of the people around him. He had blood all over his scalp and on his shirt. It appeared that his ear had been totally avulsed. As my relief intern came in, I told him I would finish taking care of this patient so he would not fall behind as the ER was already busy. On further inspection, although severely lacerated and mangled, his ear was hanging on the side of the head connected only by a small bridge of tissue. After anesthetizing the area with a local anesthetic, cleaning everything up, and accessing the available tissue, I realized his ear was like a puzzle cut into many still interconnected parts. As I slowly and carefully re-approximated the cartilage and then the skin, it seemed that a new ear, of standard shape, emerge from the mangled tissue and blood that I had first observed.

The young man was lucky that the blood supply through the small residual connection of the ear to the side of the head was robust enough that the entire ear lived. The patient was thrilled. He thought he had lost his whole ear. I was impressed at what I had accomplished as a lowly intern. It did not take extraordinary skill but only careful patience and visual perception to be able to put the parts back into place again.

When completed, the ear looked very good. This case did have a significant impact on me. It caused me to think much more about plastic surgery as a possible career goal, partly because I immediately saw the results of my efforts. I remember going home to my wife after that shift in the emergency room and telling her about this great case I had. Later she told me she knew then I would eventually end up practicing plastic surgery.

On another occasion, in the Kansas City General Hospital ER, I saw a patient who had broken a light bulb in his hand. The x-rays, which were not very good, only showed a little bit of swelling in the palm. All the bleeding had stopped. It looked unlikely that any glass remained in the palm. I asked him if he thought any glass was still in his palm. He said the bulb shattered in his hand, and there was a lot of blood, but he didn't know whether any of the glass might remain in his hand. He had a 2 1/2 cm cut in the middle of the palm of his right hand. Strangely, he did not complain of any numbness of the fingers, and he was able to bend all the fingers. I cleaned the surface of his hand with antiseptic. Then I anesthetized the wound with local infiltration of anesthetic.

Before suturing the laceration, I carefully lifted some of his skin to look into the wound. As I explored the injury, I immediately came upon some glass, which did not surprise me. However, the further I looked, the larger the piece of glass seemed to get. It was such a large piece of glass; I could not pull it back through the existing wound. Finally, after carefully orienting it, I was able to maneuver the glass out of the palm gingerly. It seemed that the size of the glass fragment was much larger than the 2 1/2 cm length of the cut. I don't quite know how such a large piece became hidden in the wound.

He was astounded when I showed him the large lightbulb fragment. I removed several smaller pieces of glass carefully with forceps. It was incredible to pull such a large chunk of glass from the palm, but even more surprising that no significant nerves, tendons, or blood vessels were severed. After thoroughly cleaning the wound and assuring myself that I had removed all the glass, I sutured the laceration and sent the man on his way.

General surgery

After my internship, I decided to do a year of general surgery at St. Joseph Hospital in Houston as a prerequisite to beginning the ENT residency program in Galveston. During my general surgery residency year at St Joseph Hospital, we had a rotation at Breckenridge Hospital in Austin. One night there, I had three patients brought in by ambulance. They had been in an automobile that had inadvertently entered an industrial area where there was a natural gas pipeline leak. Their car exploded in flames, severely burning all three occupants of the vehicle. I helped stabilize them in the emergency room with the help of senior surgery residents I called down to the ER.

We admitted them to the ICU, but their injuries were more complicated than what we could handle at Breckenridge at that time. Therefore, we called the burn center at Brooke Army Medical Center. The next morning, a few hours later, a team arrived. It was almost like a SWAT team. One particular patient with third-degree burns of the entire chest was having some difficulty breathing because of the tight and stiff nature of the chest eschar. The full-thickness burned skin had no sensation. The burn surgeon immediately prepped the patient in the ICU bed and, without using any local anesthesia, took a large knife and made incisions through the eschar around the entire chest.

This splendid bold action allowed the chest to expand more fully. The patient's breathing immediately improved. The eschar had acted as a restrictive breastplate. We transferred these three burn patients that day. I was extremely grateful for the expert help we received from the Brooke Army Medical Center burn unit team.

Also, at Breckenridge Hospital in Austin, a trauma patient came into the emergency department with injury to his chest with difficulty breathing. X rays showed a collapsed lung on one side. With the help of a more senior resident, I placed a chest tube between ribs into the space created by the collapsed lung, a rather daunting task that first time. Placing a chest tube can be a life-saving maneuver in many traumatic circumstances. Gentle suction on the tube allowed the lung to re-inflate and fill the chest cavity again. After several days of healing, I removed the tube, and the patient did well.

During that year of general surgery at St Joseph, I had many other experiences with trauma. I remember seeing a man in the ER who had been in an automobile accident, sustaining an abdominal injury. To help diagnose his condition, I placed a big needle in the abdomen and got back blood. I notified my supervising staff surgeon, and we took the patient to the operating room to explore his injury. Upon opening the abdomen, there was blood everywhere. The mood became a little hectic as we looked for the source of the bleeding.

We discovered he had a ruptured spleen, which we needed to remove to control the bleeding. Once we excised the spleen, everything calmed down. We cleaned up the belly, washed it out, and looked for other injuries. Exploration of the rest of the abdomen revealed no other issues. We closed his incision, and he did well post-operatively.

ENT

During the three years of ENT residency in Galveston, which followed the general surgery year at St. Joseph Hospital in Houston, I took care of numerous ER patients. Many had severe facial lacerations and facial bone fractures that needed to go to the OR for treatment. I took care of many nasal fractures in the ER.

During my ENT residency, I had a particularly significant and suspenseful encounter in the emergency room. The emergency physician called me in to see a patient involved in a motor vehicle accident. The patient had tremendous swelling in the neck with difficulty breathing. On palpating the neck, there was crepitation, which is a crackling or popping sound and sensation caused by the air in the subcutaneous tissue.

This man had severed his trachea, although there was no laceration in the anterior neck. He was fortunate to have made it to the emergency room alive. I needed to do an emergency tracheostomy. We quickly prepped the patient in his trauma bed. With the help of a medical student, I was able to accomplish this unusually difficult tracheostomy and place a breathing tube into the severed trachea to secure his airway. The severe swelling of the tissues from the subcutaneous air, which had spread throughout the neck, made the task dangerously tricky.

Quickly locating the severed trachea was necessary to avoid a catastrophe. If this had not gone well, the patient could have expired, right before my eyes. The first of two drawings below represent the condition of this patient with a severed trachea and swelling from subcutaneous air in the neck. I needed to transect this swollen tissue to find the end of the trachea nearest the lungs to place the tube. The second shows a tracheostomy tube (dark blue) in place which secured his airway.

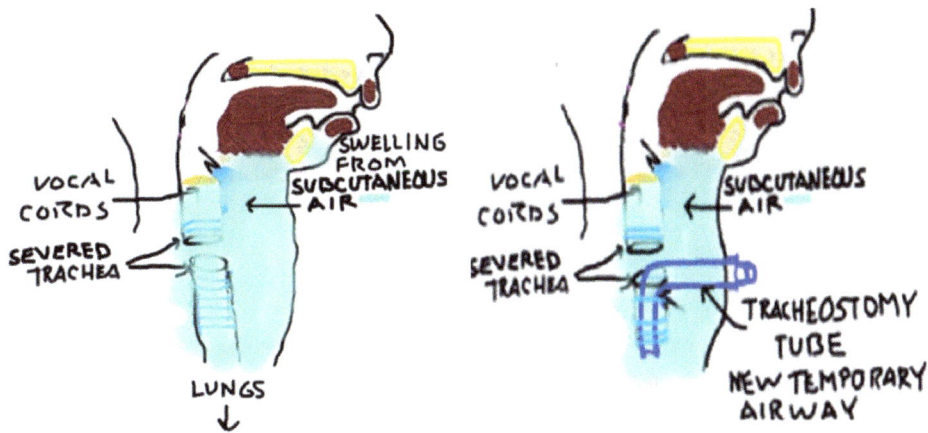

The patient was asleep under anesthesia with an anesthetic tube already in place, securing the airway for most of the many tracheostomies I did during my ENT residency. In that circumstance, the procedure is usually routine, safe, and not particularly stressful. The only exception was in already intubated premature infants, where the tiny nature of the structures made the procedure delicate, precarious, and stressful.

Plastic surgery residency

One night early in my career, I was called to an emergency room to see a patient who had an accident with a chainsaw. This man lived on a farm and frequently used a chainsaw. When I first saw him, he was lying on a stretcher in the emergency room. It was apparent he had a significant facial injury with blood covering his face. I was surprised and happy to find him alert and coherent. He said he had been cutting wood on his farm with a chainsaw when suddenly the chain caught on something, kicked up and back to hit him square in the face.

On the first inspection, it seemed he should have lost his right eye. This injury started at the right brow, went straight down through the upper and lower eyelids through the cheek into the maxillary sinus, and caught the corner of the mouth lacerating both the upper and lower lip. Finally, it went through the lateral chin and ending high in the neck.

To my surprise, I was able to retract the eyelids and saw no injury to the globe, and his visual acuity was normal. I, therefore, proceeded to anesthetize the areas by injection with xylocaine. I then washed out the wounds. On closer examination, there still didn't seem to be any way that this injury would have spared his eyeball. Both the upper and lower eyelid lacerations were full-thickness. Beneath the cheek laceration, there was even a minimal fracture of the lower rim of the bony orbit. The wound also extended into the maxillary sinus.

As I began to repair the injury, I was pleased with how little tissue was lost. Everything came together exceptionally well. This man refused hospital admission. I only saw him back once to remove the sutures several days later. When I called him later to come in for further follow-up evaluation, he said he was doing fine and didn't like to come into the city, so I obtained no further follow up.

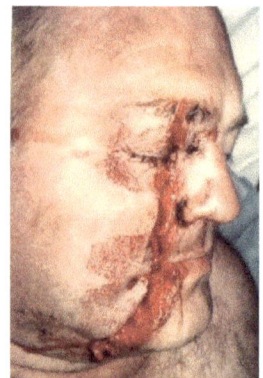 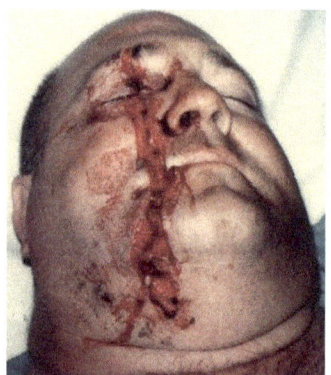 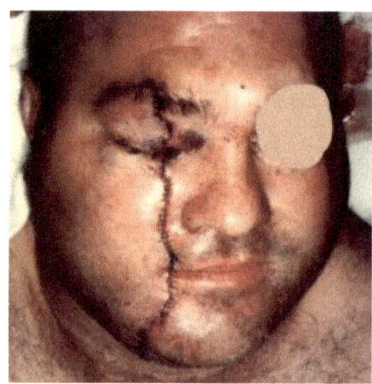

This case was impressive to me on two accounts. First, it gave me a healthy fear of chainsaws. Secondly, it reiterated that it is hard to figure everything out as I still do not know why the chainsaw did not damage this patient's globe. A miracle? I surmise that the chainsaw could have barely touched the upper and lower eyelid but still pulled the lids away from the eyeball, tearing them, but thereby sparing the eye itself.

After I began my private practice, I was frequently called to the emergency room to take care of traumatic injuries. In this chapter, I will share some exciting experiences I had from the emergency room.

Plastic surgery practice

One traumatic experience I had about 1978 occurred when I was on my way home from the hospital one evening. I told my wife I would stop and get some Mexican food at Felix Mexican Restaurant on Westheimer rd. They had delicious chili con queso. I parked on the side street right by the restaurant and went in to get our food. They had it ready, so it took only a couple of minutes. As I came out of the restaurant, I heard a loud yell from a woman running toward me from the small house behind the restaurant. She had a baby in her arms and was screaming that the baby was not breathing.

I dropped my package and took the baby from her. She seemed to be about three months old and was not breathing. I could not feel a pulse, so I began resuscitating her there next to the sidewalk in the dim light from the restaurant windows. A couple of other people came out of the restaurant, and I told them to call an ambulance. The 911 service did not start in Houston until 1983. An ambulance arrived after what seemed like an eternity. I carried the baby into the ambulance with the mother and continued to give CPR until we arrived at St Joseph Hospital emergency room, which only took 8or 9 minutes. I turned everything over to the ER. My resuscitation had failed, and shortly after our arrival, the emergency department physician pronounced the baby dead. The mother was distraught. I assume in retrospect that this was a case of sudden death infant syndrome

Nasal Trauma

A prevalent traumatic injury seen in the emergency room is a nasal fracture. Sometimes this is taken care of in the ER under local anesthesia, especially if the patient presents only a short time after the injury. Depending on the severity, it is common to wait about a week for swelling to subside. A nasal reduction means returning the parts to their pre-injury position. A closed nasal reduction resets the components without an incision and needs to be done within three weeks so that the parts have not healed too much for manipulation. Reduction requires open surgery if the nasal fractures have solidified.

Below "Jason" is shown before and after a closed reduction of a recent traumatic nasal fracture. I tried to restore the nose to its pre-injury contour. I achieved this with a combination of manual pressure and manipulation with surgical instruments but with no incision either externally or inside the nose.

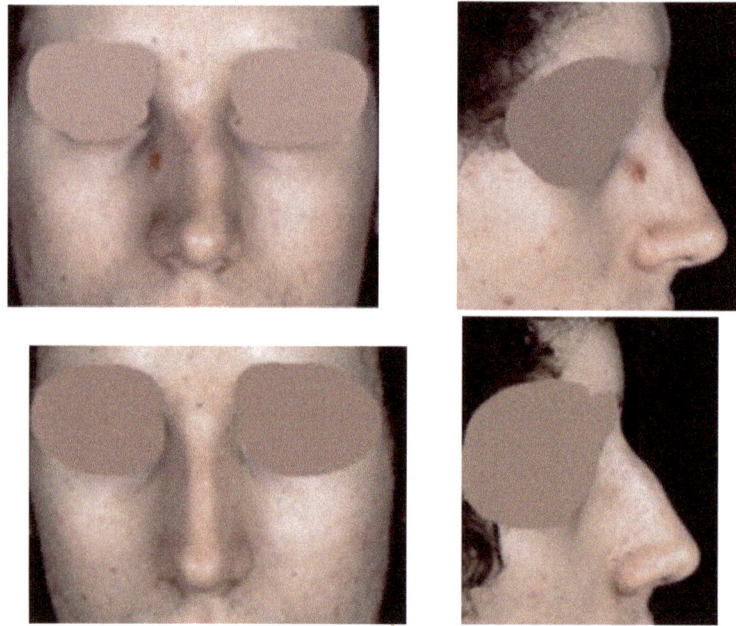

"Suzie," below, had old nasal fractures purportedly related to various sports. She was unsuitable for a closed reduction. Therefore, I elected to recommend an open reduction of her fractures with a septorhinoplasty at the same time to improve her nasal breathing. She had a crooked nose with a bump on the bridge and left side of the nose. She had difficulty breathing through her nose. I performed an open reduction but also straightened her nasal septum to help her breathe. I also, at her request, refined the nasal tip and lifted it to give slightly more projection. Chapter 16 contains a detailed discussion of rhinoplasty.

The Healing Mission of Plastic Surgery

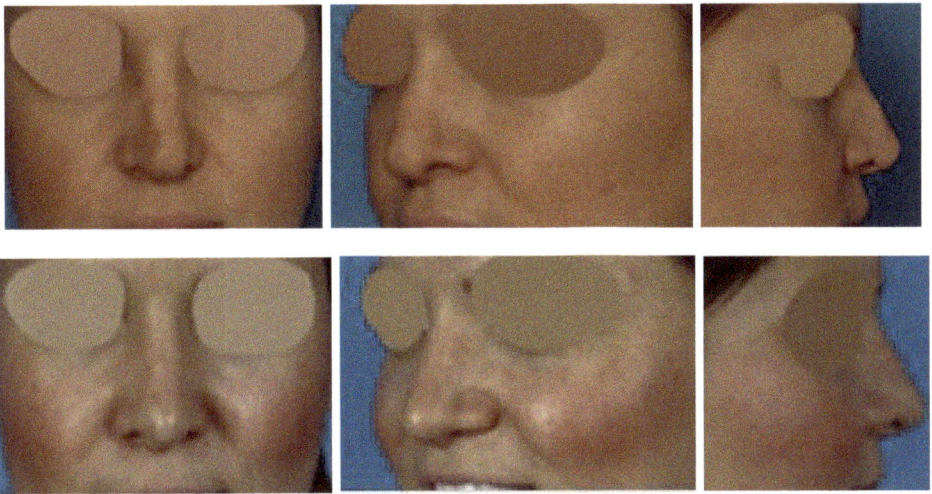

Facial Trauma

Orbital Trauma

"Hank," shown below, suffered an orbital floor "blow out" fracture in an altercation. I treated him with a thin Teflon® sheet placed on the bottom of the orbit after lifting the eye slightly for access. This implant wafer replaced the bony floor, which had been pushed downward into the maxillary sinus, which is immediately below. This maneuver restored the proper position of the orbital contents and gave him a functional and symmetrical post-op result.

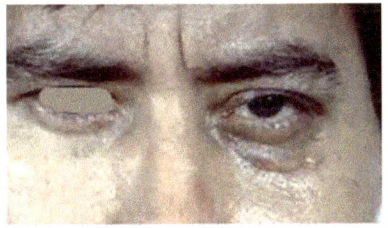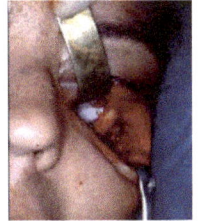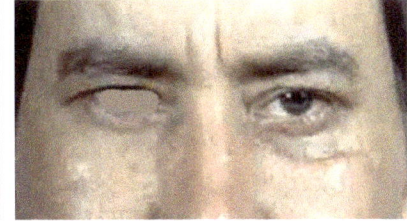

Two assailants accosted and bludgeoned "Jesus," shown below. He sustained a "blowout" fracture of the left orbital floor. The picture on the left only shows soft tissue swelling and bruising. In the second photo, he is trying to look up, but his left eye is stuck because soft tissue has descended into the left maxillary sinus under the eye through a defect in the floor. This inability to look up with the left eye indicates entrapment of the extraocular muscles of the left eye.

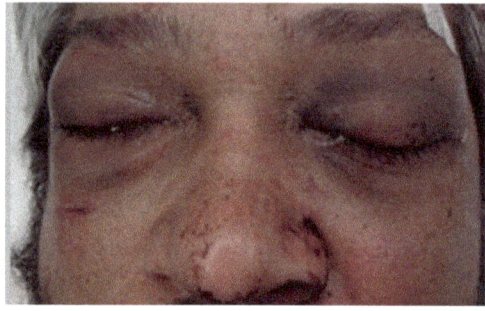 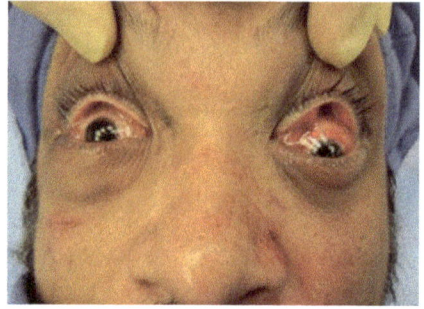

The orbital defect, simulated in the model shown below, can ensnare periorbital fat and periocular muscles, causing limitation of eye movement. Fisticuffs with a blow to the orbit can create pressure which "blows out" this thinnest most fragile orbital bone.

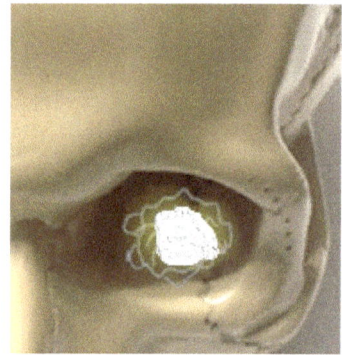 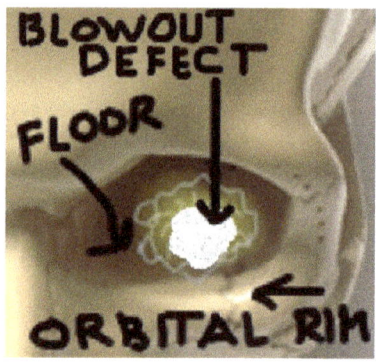

I explored the orbit through a lower eyelid incision and teased the fat and muscle tissue trapped in the maxillary sinus back up into the eye socket.

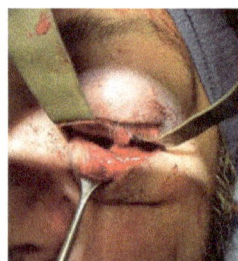 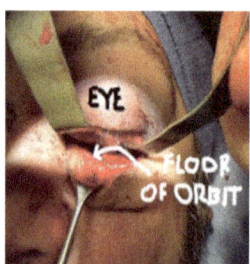 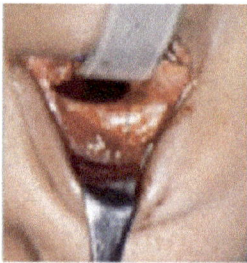 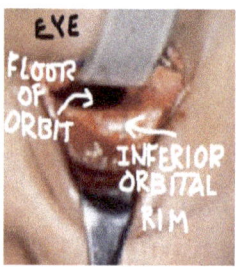

I placed a polyethylene-coated titanium implant on the floor of the orbit trimmed to cover the defect. I secured it at the inferior orbital rim with screws. This implant restored the orbital floor and kept the orbital contents in place. The model below left diagrammatically shows the placement of the synthetic implant on the floor. The post-op photo shows "Jesus" can now look upward with the formerly entrapped left eye.

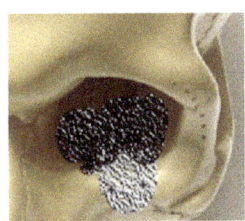 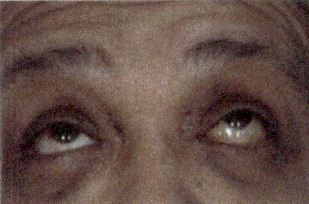 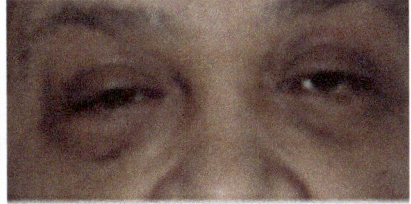

Orbital Rim fracture

Another patient with a similar orbital floor fracture is "Ronald" below.

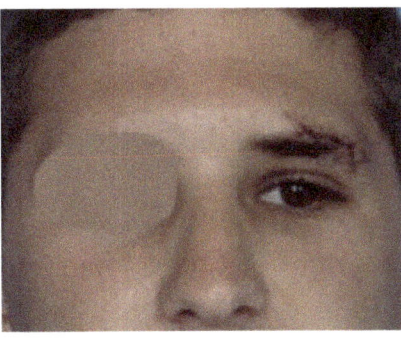 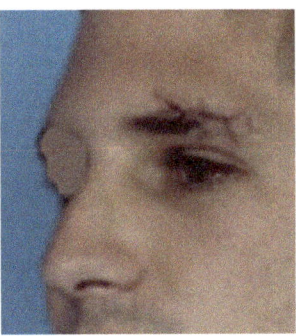

The intraoperative photos below show an orbital floor implant secured to the inferior orbital rim.

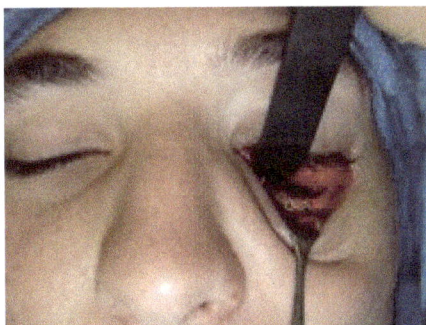 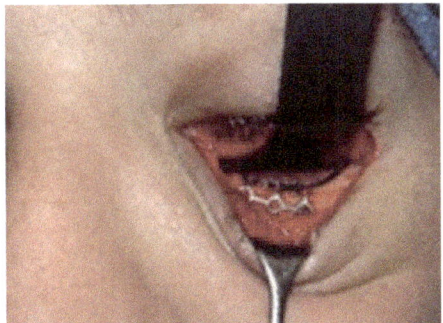

His postoperative photos demonstrate the free upward movement of the globe.

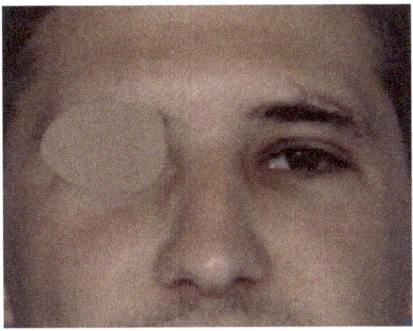 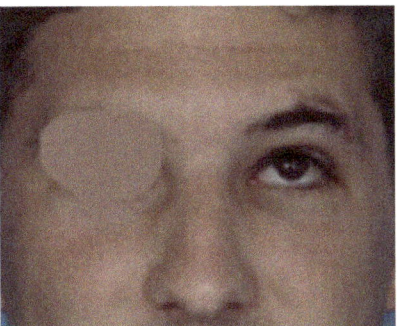

A long bicycle ride

In 1977 while I was a plastic surgery resident, I was called to the emergency room to see the grandson of the Chief of radiology at our hospital.

The young boy had fallen and hit his nose on a table. He had a large laceration that created a flap on the bridge of the nose. I cleaned and repaired this injury very meticulously under the watchful eye of the child's mother and grandmother. This injury healed well with minimal scar. Unfortunately, this was not the last time this young man would need my services.

A few years later, after I was in practice, I again was called to the emergency room to see "John." Little did "John" know what was in store for him when he began his bike ride on a crisp winter afternoon. As 15-year-old boys will do, "John" was out for a bicycle ride near his home. Suddenly, tragedy struck as "John" was riding on the street; he and a motor vehicle came just a little too close together. The rigid side mirror of a passing truck struck "John" in the face as he rode in the opposite direction.

Luckily the impact did not kill him or render him quadriplegic. As it was, he had severe facial soft tissue and bony injuries. An ambulance scene and he was brought him from the scene to the emergency room at St Joseph Hospital. I saw him there, and he was alert and oriented and in no severe distress as he was breathing comfortably. I ordered X-rays and prepared him for the operating room.

I explored his wounds under general anesthesia. There was a markedly displaced broken nose and comminuted (split into multiple fragments) fractured bones between the eyes. A deep laceration ran across the face and the bridge of the nose nearly avulsing it. The injury exposed the nasal septum and other internal aspects of the nose. A laceration along the orbital rim revealed orbital contents and a fracture of its medial wall and roof extended to the right forehead frontal bone. Additionally, he suffered a comminuted fracture of the maxilla (upper jaw).

The various displaced bones were put back into their best position and wired into place. A spacer was placed into the orbit to cover a defect in the orbital wall. The trauma displaced the tendons that ordinarily hold the medial eyelids to the nasal bones. So, the eyes seem to be too far apart. I secured these tendons with wire brought through the nose from side to side to restore the eyelids to a normal position and mold the nasal bones into place. Next, I repaired the many soft tissue lacerations and applied a nasal splint externally. "John" did well after the extensive surgery, and I discharged him from the hospital a few days later, knowing, however, he would undoubtedly need additional future surgery to finish his reconstruction. The pictures below show "John's" his appearance after his first major operation

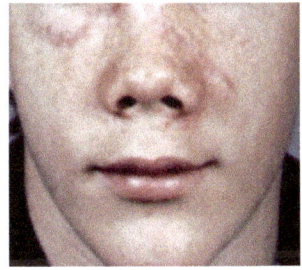
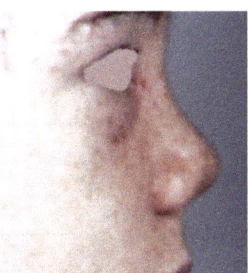
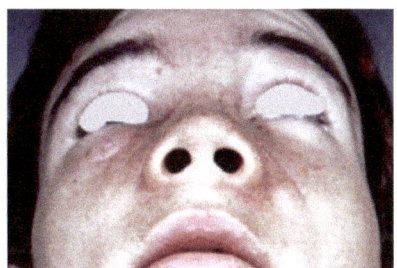

About eight months later, he was ready for another surgery. Some residual problems were difficulty breathing through the nose, a shortened and wide nose with too little projection, and a right eyeball that was retracted inward and was too low compared to the left eye. Fortunately, the movement of the eyes was normal. He needed bone grafting to the floor of the orbit to reposition the globe. Therefore, we again took him to the operating room to undergo surgery.

This time I took cranial bone from the skull to build up the orbital floor to raise the eyeball. Also, I performed a revision of the nasal reconstruction with a strip of cranial bone to the bridge of the nose and increased the nasal airway. Also, I did dermabrasion (sanding) of facial scars to help improve his appearance. His intended short bike ride led to two major surgeries and a long recovery. The pictures below pictures show his result about ten years after his last surgery.

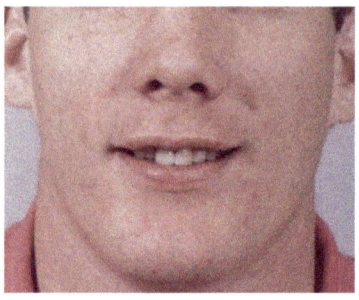 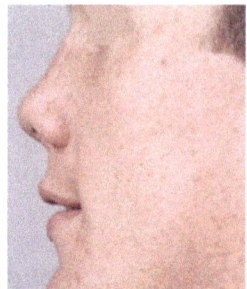 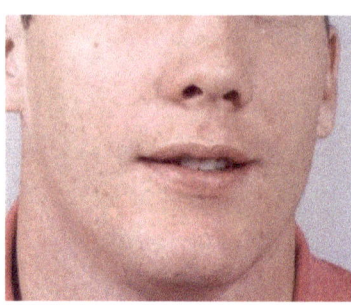

The ER is the scene of ubiquitous facial lacerations from multitudinous causes. Most are handled well by the emergency room physician. When they are troublesome in some way, he may call in a plastic surgeon. For example, "Henry" below suffered some traumatic loss of skin. Although not necessarily intuitive, I elected the convert the wound into a vertical closure with a good result.

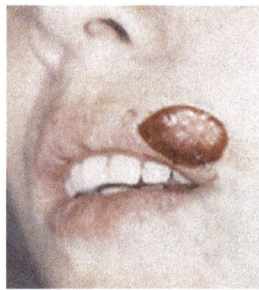 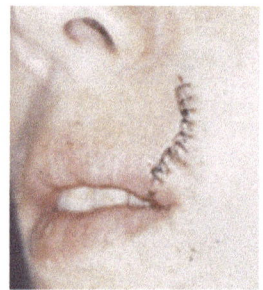

The young man below "Noah" suffered a severe laceration extending from the left lower eyelid to the lower cheek at the level of the oral commissure. The gash went into the maxillary sinus; however, the facial bones were stable. Straightforward repair of the lacerations produced the results shown.

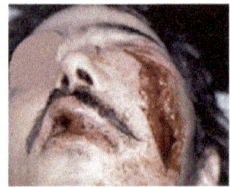 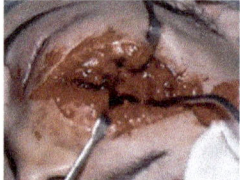 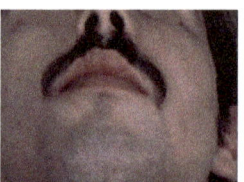 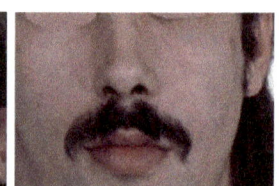

MVA

The lady pictured below "Donna" suffered trauma in a motor vehicle accident. The preoperative photo and the x-ray showed a fracture just to the left of the midline of the jaw. I reduced the fragments into their proper position manually. I then stabilized the mandible with the combination of an arch bar on the teeth and stainless-steel wire ligatures across the fracture, as shown in the first drawing below. A few years later, I would have used titanium plate and screw fixation, a more efficient repair, as illustrated in the last picture.

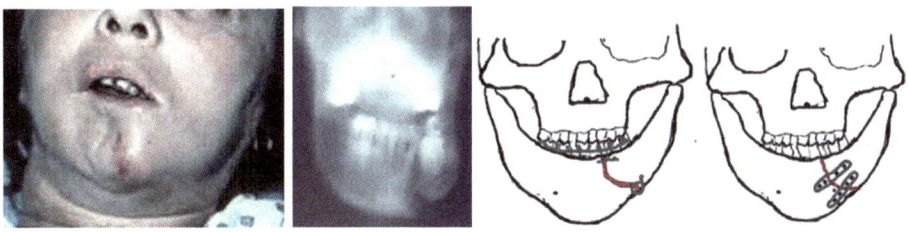

The following three photos are early postoperative results that show the jaw realigned.

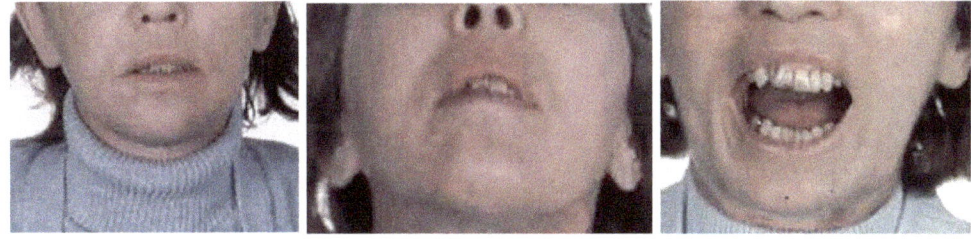

Three-wheeler accident

A young teenage boy "Greg" was having fun driving a three-wheeler on the beach. However, something went wrong. He flipped over and crushed his face. He was brought to the hospital by ambulance. The initial examination in the emergency department revealed multiple midfacial fractures, and a nose smashed flat. Regrettably, he also ruptured the right eye.

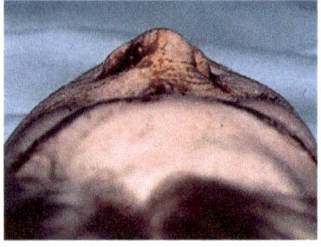 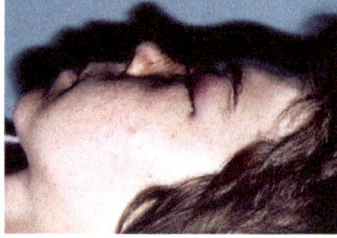 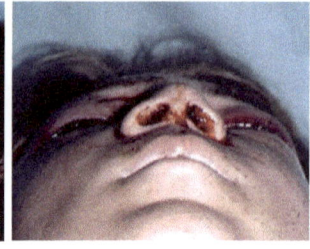

After stabilizing his condition in the emergency department and confirming he had no neck or brain injury, I took him to the operating room for exploration and repair of his injuries. Providentially, they were no injuries other than the facial ones. I consulted an ophthalmologist who came to surgery with me to repair the ruptured globe. However, he lost eyesight entirely in the right eye. His facial lacerations provided us some access to the bony defects. I made additional incisions in the mouth under the upper lip and in the scalp to obtain further access to the fractures. I found a lot of midface destruction, and the frontal sinus behind the forehead was marred and needed exploration.

I employed bone grafts to help repair the damage and elected to take them from the skull. I harvested bone grafts from the outermost of the three layers of the cranium. I took rectangular strips as in the first two photos below with chisels and an electric bur. (I also used this technique on a case presented in chapter 1). I repeatedly lifted the nasal structures from the face, but they invariably fell back down. Therefore, I secured one of the grafts at the glabella as a cantilever upon which that I could "hang" or suspend the remaining nasal bones and cartilage. The cantilever nasal graft from the skull extended from the forehead to the nasal tip.

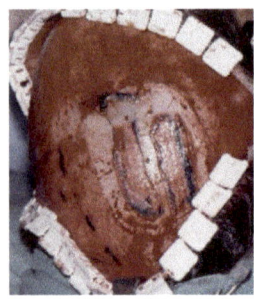 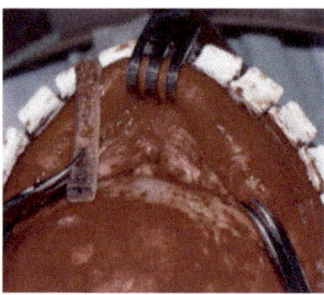 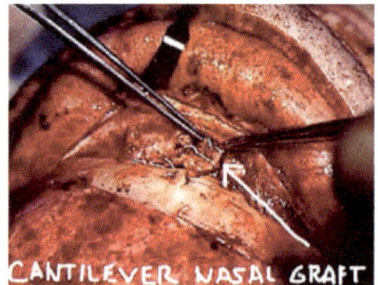

The first photo below demonstrates the cantilever support of the nasal tip. The drawings show my utilization of bone grafts to buttress the comminuted midface fractures. I fixed them with wire ligatures.

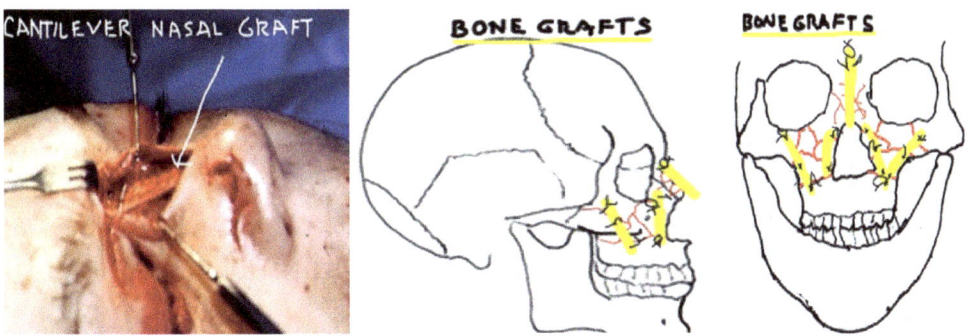

Although "Greg" lost sight in the right eye because of the ruptured globe, the remainder of the surgery was quite successful, and I was quite pleased with the repair of the midface and nose. I have followed him for many years, during which he continued to do well.

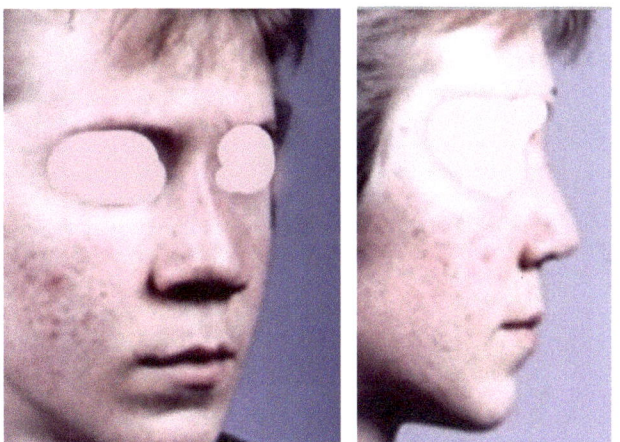

You're Fired

Long before "going postal" became a commonplace designation for workplace violence, I had a challenging case along those lines.

One Friday afternoon, while I was operating, a call came in from the Emergency Department. It was from a trauma surgeon who said he had a patient with a gunshot to the face. He said it was a severe injury, and I needed to get down there as soon as possible. I finished the part of the case I was doing expeditiously and proceeded down to the emergency room.

The patient "Mark" was alert and stable, but his lower face was torn apart and bleeding. He had severe damage to the soft tissues of the upper and lower lip. It was evident the jawbone was severely fractured and unstable. I packed the wounds and prepared him for surgery. I returned to the operating room and finished my case, which my resident had been tending in my absence. While my elective case went to the recovery room, we "turned over" the operating room for the trauma case. The timing and logistics were a little hectic. We brought him to the operating room, and the anesthesiologist intubated him without difficulty.

The intraoperative photos below show the injury to the upper and lower lip. The plastic suction catheter in the last photo demonstrates the opening from the mouth through the shattered jaw and out the left cheek.

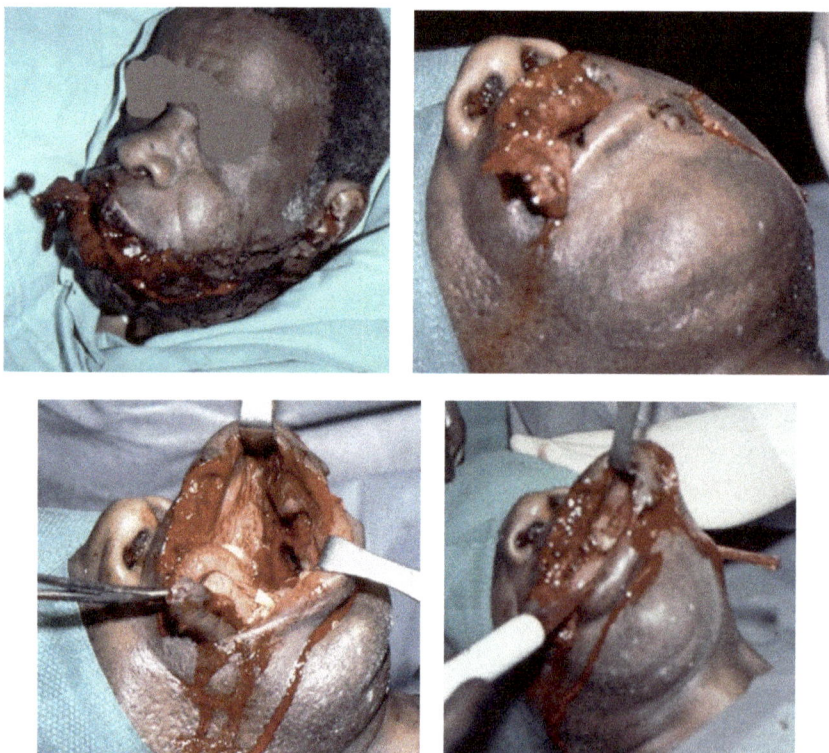

His wounds were extensive. Because most of his teeth were missing, he could not have his teeth wired together. I first aligned the multiple fractures of his jaw as well as possible. I stabilized them with screws and an external acrylic device, shown below, which I customized during the operation. Now there are sophisticated external fixation devices available, which preclude the need for such customization.

This device stabilized the bone after I placed large pins into the major bone segments and then connected the pins externally with the acrylic bar made right then and there in the operating room. Next, I repaired the intraoral soft tissues which closed over the fracture fragments of the jawbone. Finally, I sutured the damaged deep soft tissues and skin. Below is an early postoperative photo with the external fixation device in place.

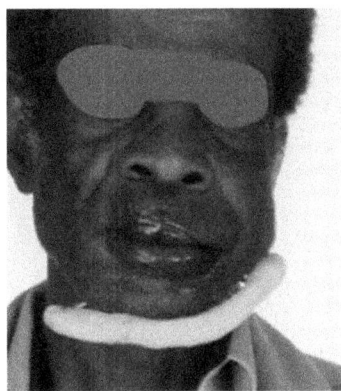 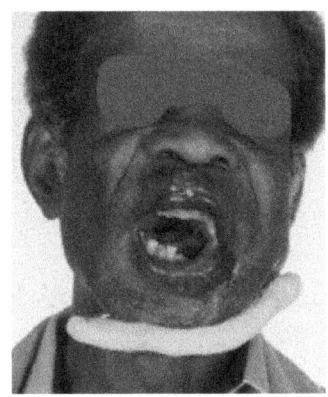

Later I found out that my patient worked for the local bus company and had fired an employee earlier that day. The employee returned to the workplace and shot my patient, who was lucky to be alive. The recovery phase was quite extensive. First off, the pins and acrylic bar needed to remain in place for seven or eight weeks. He then needed to go through a minor procedure for removal of the bar and the pins. Because of the loss of alveolar (gum) soft tissue, I had to perform a skin graft so that he would be able to wear a denture. Eventually, he was fitted with dentures, obtained a functional recovery, and returned to work. The last two photos are his final postoperative results with dentures in place.

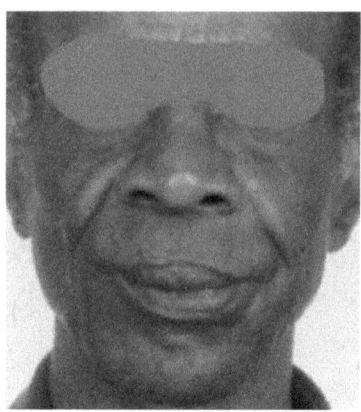
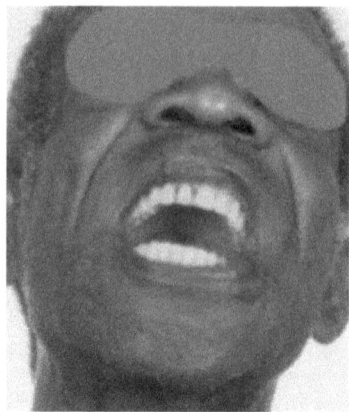

Hand Trauma

Trauma to the hand is one of the most common reasons for emergency room visits seen by plastic surgeons. The subject of hand surgery is too extensive to cover comprehensively, but I will show several examples of cases that I have treated during my career.

Thumb Replantation

"Angie" severed her right thumb at the level of the mid proximal phalanx in an industrial accident. The severed part was saved and brought to the emergency room with the patient. In triage, I decided that she was an appropriate candidate for replantation for several reasons. First, the thumb effectuates 40% of the hand's function. So, it is the most significant digit. Secondly, the severed thumb resulted from a fairly sharp, non - crushing amputation. Thirdly she arrived in the emergency room only about an hour after the injury with the severed part. I took her expeditiously to the operating room. I first identified the vessels, nerves, and tendons both in the stump and the amputated part. My amateur drawing below illustrates the pertinent anatomy.

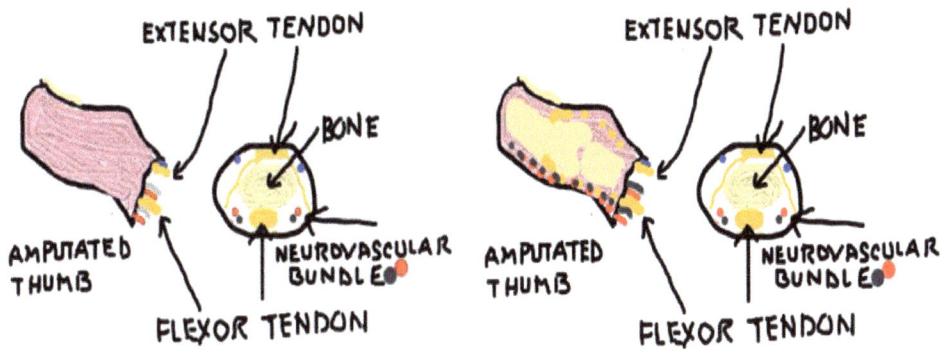

I commenced the replant procedure by stabilizing the proximal phalanx by pining the amputated part to the stump. I anastomosed the digital arteries and a small dorsal vein to re-establish blood supply to the amputated thumb. I repaired the flexor and extensor tendons, as shown in the drawing below.

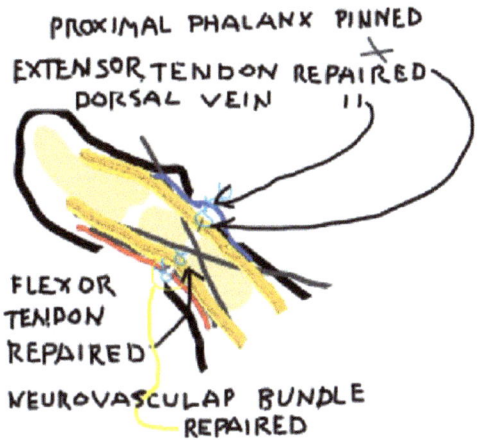

Everything went smoothly with the replantation; however, the venous drainage was suboptimal. Therefore, I elected to utilize leeches post-operatively to improve the survival chances of the replanted thumb. These parasites were known to be used in medicine more than 3000 years ago in Egypt and India. The first description of their use in replantation by Foucher et al. in 1981 showed them to improve survival of re-planted fingers with good arterial supply but inadequate venous drainage- precisely the problem I had with this case. That report was only a short time before my case. I urgently sent for medical leeches, and I use them to good effect in Angie's case. That is a picture of a "medical" leech below.

The Healing Mission of Plastic Surgery

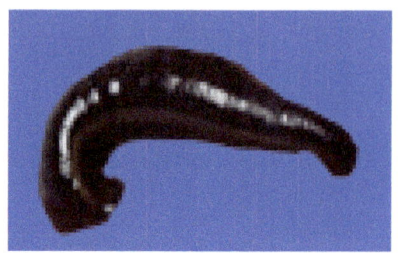

Leeches both ingest blood and produce an anticoagulant, hirudin, whose effects last several hours. I used several of these parasites for a few days. It was a little tricky using them as they did not instinctively go for the congested part where I wanted them to attach. Therefore, I constructed a small tent out of a paper cup to try to contain and direct them to the congested replanted thumb, which I wanted them to affect. They successfully decongested the replanted thumb. Although the replant ended up slightly smaller than the unaffected thumb, the operation was successful, with full function, as seen in the photos below.

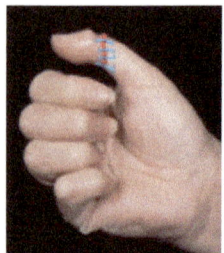 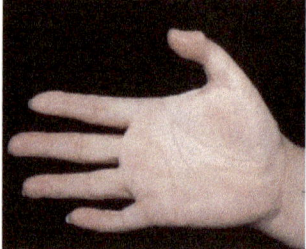 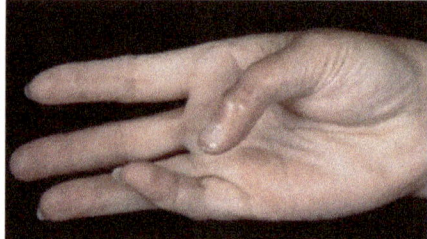

All digit amputations are not candidates for replantation. Sometimes the amputated finger may have been crushed and, therefore, may be unsuitable. Distal amputated fingers are more favorable than proximal. Some digits, such as the thumb, are better candidates. Complete single-digit amputations may be better treated by merely tidying up the stump and discarding the part. This passivity may seem counterintuitive in this age of microsurgery. However, a stiff non- functioning finger can result after replantation, which would be detrimental to hand function.

For example, as a surgeon, if I had a total amputation of my index finger, I would not have it replanted. The rehabilitation would take a long time, and I might end up with a poorly functioning finger, which was just in the way. Without a replant, the stump would heal rapidly, and my long finger would readily substitute for the index finger. I would be able to resume work as a surgeon in just a few weeks. Apropos, a fascinating article by Dr. P.W. Brown discussed survey results of one hundred eighty-three surgeons with missing digits, mostly from trauma. The amputations comprised fingertips, multiple fingers, variable thumb loss, and even a full hand. All but three began or resumed the practice of surgery after their injury. It seemed that adaptation, incentive, and motivation were more critical for hand function than the number of digits.

Finger Tip Trauma

Fingertip trauma is one of the most prevalent injuries seen by plastic surgeons in many emergency rooms. The treatment for simple lacerations without loss of tissue is suturing. If the area of tissue loss is small, it may be left to heal secondarily with only dressing changes. If the wound is superficial with skin loss, a split-thickness skin graft might suffice for repair, as in Roberto's case below. The donor graft was taken from the wrist because it is in the field and will heal with a favorable scar. Some surgeons do not like this donor site, thinking it might conjure the notion of a previous suicide attempt.

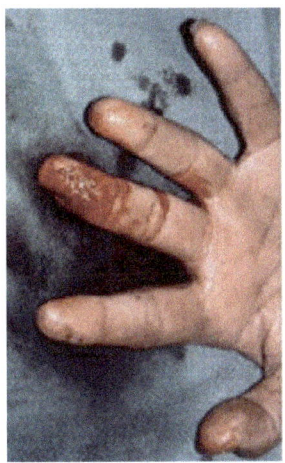
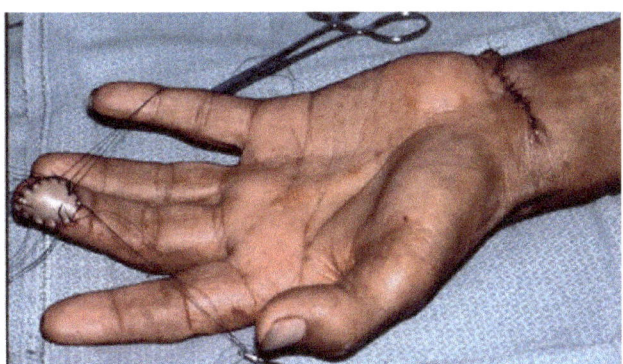

An exceptional circumstance exists in young children. Some times a very distal amputation even including bone can be sutured back in place and will sometimes be successful. If it fails, removal of the part allows various other methods of repair. Below is an example of a near-complete distal amputation of a finger in a small child, which was treated successfully by suturing the piece back into place.

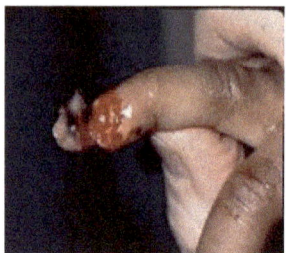 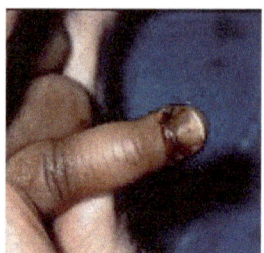

The case below of "Timothy" exemplifies still another fingertip repair method. He experienced a loss of skin and soft tissue bulk of his right long finger. The intraoperative photos below are of the defect and the proposed flap at the base of the thumb outlined in blue ink.

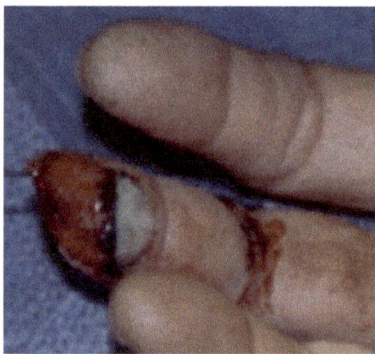 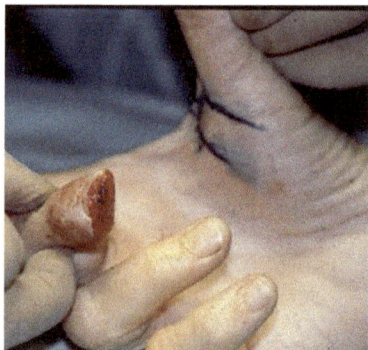

The thenar area at the base of the thumb is a donor area accessed by bending the injured long finger. I sutured the end of the flap over the fingertip wound. I waited two weeks before separating the finger from the thenar area. New blood supply to the transferred business end of the flap from the recipient finger made the separation possible after two weeks.

The Healing Mission of Plastic Surgery

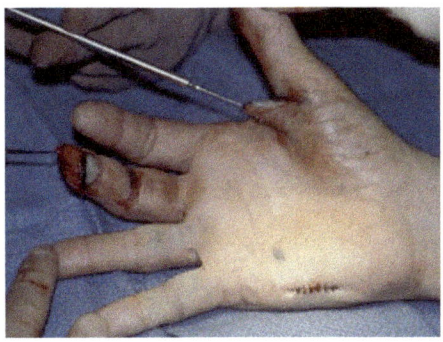
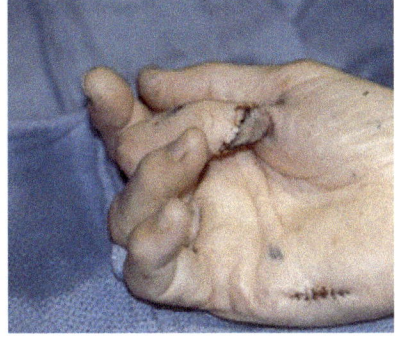

The case illustrated below of "Martin" shows a distal loss of fingertip tissue. The second photo shows the volar surface of the finger. I made a V incision that preserves some soft tissue connections to maintain blood supply. It is advanced to cover the defect with excellent thick tissue, as shown in the third photo below. A skin graft would have left thin coverage over the distal bone and likely would have been hypersensitive or painful.

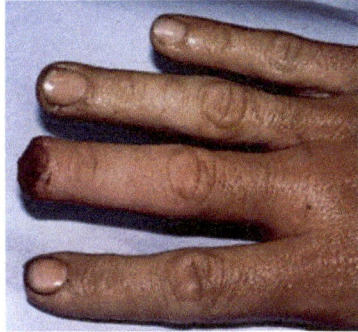
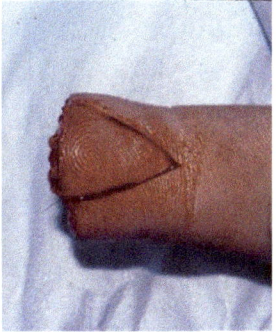
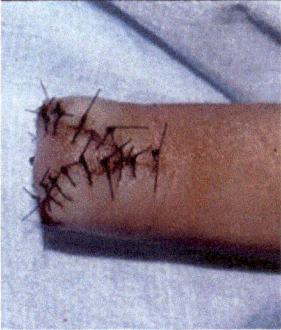

Another method to obtain full, soft tissue coverage for fingertip injuries is a cross finger flap. I described in detail the innervated cross finger flap in chapter 5. Here in "Kevin's" cases, I utilized this same technique for an extensive soft tissue loss in his little finger. The first intraoperative photo below shows the depth and broad nature of the injury. There is an exposed tendon and absence of distal neurovascular bundles. I have outlined in blue the flap from the dorsum of the adjacent ring finger. The second photo again demonstrates the injury and the flap. I will elevate the skin and turn it toward the little finger. The dots show how the flap will be oriented as it is unrolled and sutured to the little finger.

The Healing Mission of Plastic Surgery

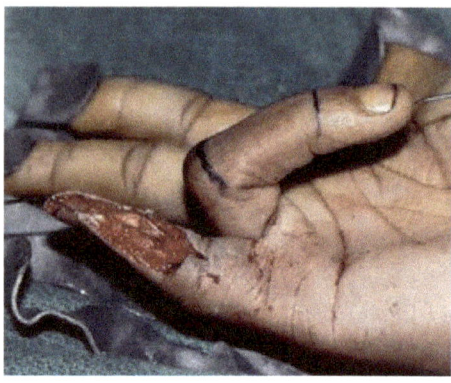
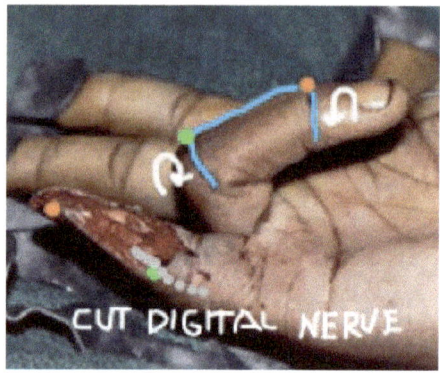

The turning of the flap and connection of the nerves is challenging to understand. I have altered the same photo, so you may have to go back and forth to comprehend the procedure. I have turned the flap toward the little finger. I then sutured the cut end of the digital nerve from the little finger to the nerve branch, coming with the flap from the ring finger. The anastomosis is superficial to the small grey rectangular plastic sheet. This nerve repair provides sensation to the skin that will "read" little finger. I outlined the cross-finger flap cut edge in light blue. Dots in the above photo drawing, when compared to the middle picture below, help orient the movement of the flap onto the little finger. The nerves are grey, and the nerve repair location is in dark blue.

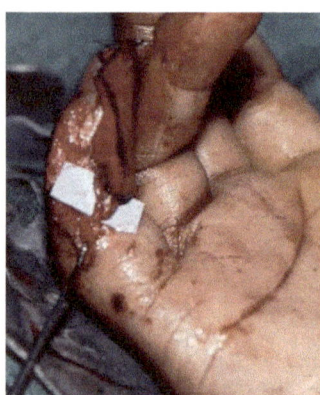
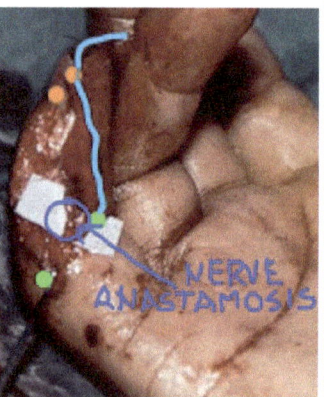
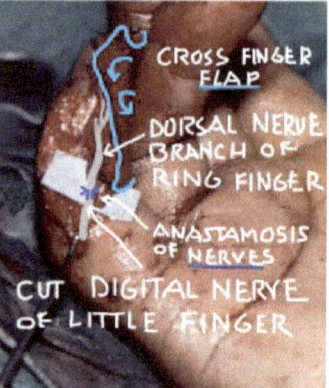

The intraoperative photo below shows I have sutured the cross-finger flap in place. The photo drawing outlines the flap from the ring finger in light blue. The dots orient proximal and distal aspects. The grey illustrates the nerves and dark blue, the nerve repair. After two weeks I separated the flap from the ring finger

The Healing Mission of Plastic Surgery

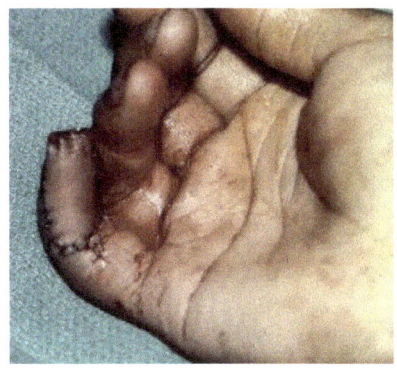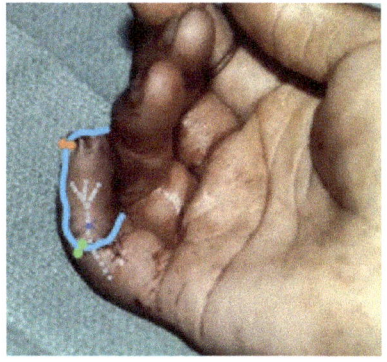

The flap has provided good thick, soft tissue coverage with sensation. The most significant drawback is the color mismatch. I have treated smaller superficial fingertip defects with a graft from the side of the palm or the instep of the foot for a better color match. "Kevin" regained capable sensation and range of motion with full extension and full flexion after several weeks. Sometimes the donor finger will have some restriction of movement, necessitating physical therapy.

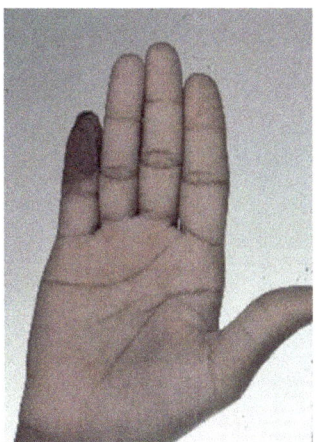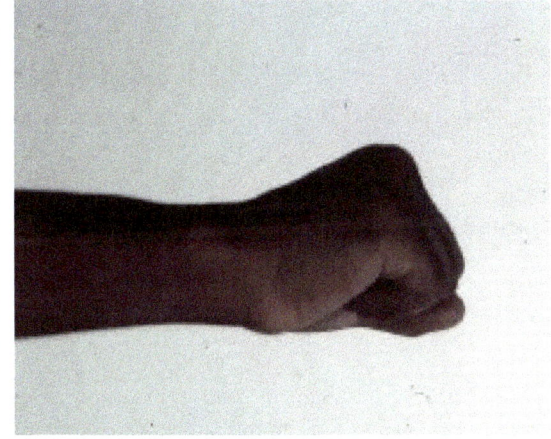

Gunshot wounds of the hand

A particularly exciting story involves one of my former residents, Dr. Charles Stuart. He helped me with this very noteworthy, traumatic injury to the hand. While "minding his own business," the patient had been shot in the proximal phalanx of the right index finger. That's the bone between the knuckle and the middle joint of the finger. The injury had destroyed some bone and also obliterated a portion of the two tendons that extend the index finger. The x-ray below shows a void in the proximal phalanx of the index finger where the bone was blown away and then that the fracture stabilized with stainless steel pins. The index finger has two tendons for its extension, whereas the other fingers only have one. The intraoperative photo below shows the soft-tissue defect where the two index finger extensor tendons had been.

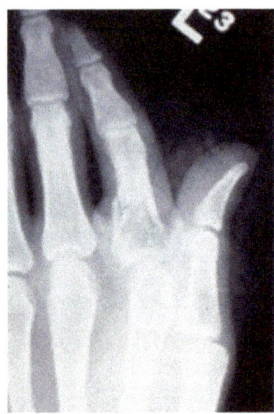
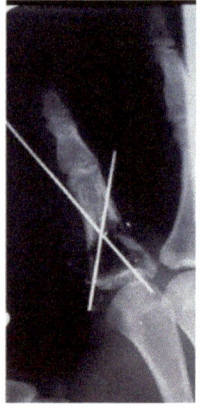
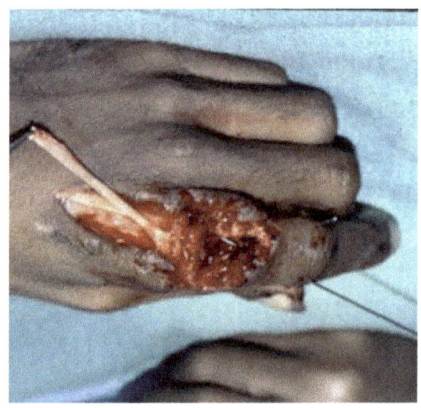

I decided to take one of the tendons which had been severed by the bullet and use it as a tendon graft. Together with the remaining tendon, I reconstructed one extensor mechanism for the finger with parts from each of the two tendons. I harvested a bone graft from the man's foot, as shown in the middle photo below. I used this bone graft to replace the lost bone at the base of the proximal phalanx of the index finger. The last intraoperative photo shows the donor tendon graft, which I used to cross the defect and reconnect to the distal severed portion of the other index finger tendon. Also, the bone graft is ready for placement into the bony defect.

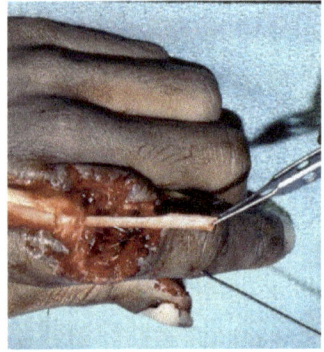
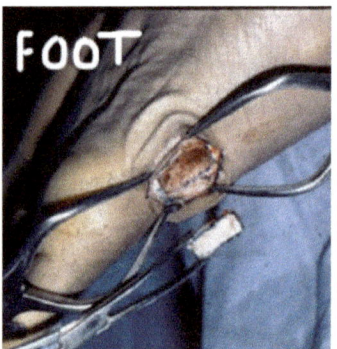
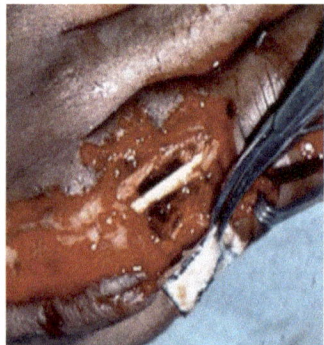

The final pictures, taken postoperatively, show the man able to bend his index finger to make a full fist as well as fully extend the digit after only his primary operation.

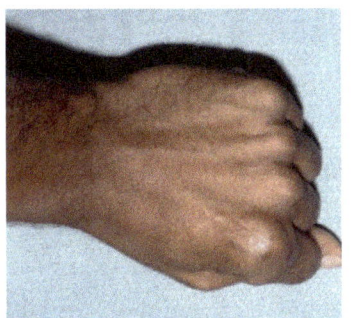 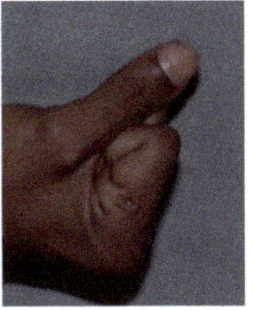 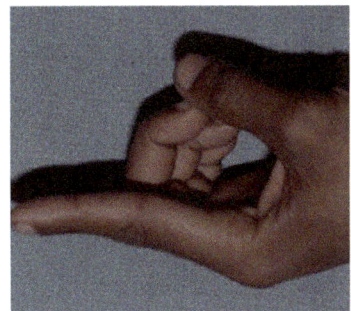

Three things are extraordinary about this case. I performed extensive reconstruction primarily at the time of his injury, which saved the man significant extra surgery and time. More often, a situation like this would require multiple separate procedures. The second thing is that he received such an excellent functional result without the need for therapy or revisional procedures. The third extraordinary thing about this case was the lengths to which Dr. Stewart went to get follow up on this patient.

Dr. Stewart wanted to present this case at a conference at the end of his residency. He needed some postoperative follow-up photos to document the excellent function the patient had regained in the finger and hand. The resident was having trouble locating the man to get him to come into the office. The phone number was no longer working. He went to the address the patient had listed in his hospital records, which was in a dilapidated and rough part of town. He went up and knocked on the door but got no response.

Then in desperation, he walked around the side of the house and called into an open window the patient's name. After Dr. Stewart waited a while, the patient finally came to the window, recognize the doctor, and agreed to have his hand examined and photographed. So that is how Dr. Stewart got the documentation he needed to present this case at the upcoming conference. I was impressed with Dr. Stewart going beyond the call of duty to follow up on our patient.

"Dwane" also received ballistic trauma to his right hand while he was proverbially "minding his own business." An assailant shot him with a handgun. He had quite a bit of soft tissue injury as the projectile went through and through the hand. He also had a bony loss at the head of the thumb metacarpal as seen in the X rays

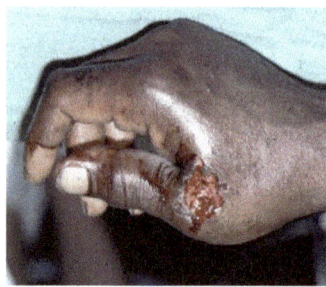 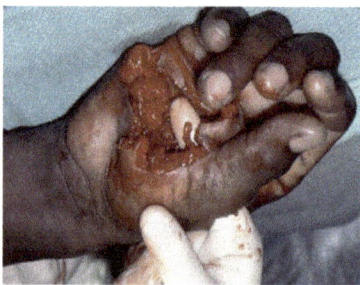 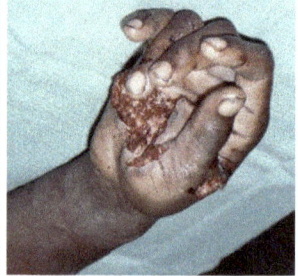

I used pins with a custom made acrylic external fixator to stabilize the thumb and placed a bone graft to the metacarpal defect. I also apportioned a skin graft to the palm to replace lost skin.

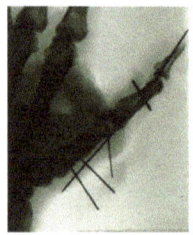 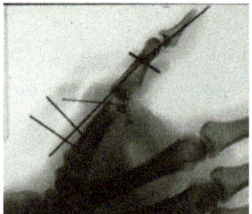 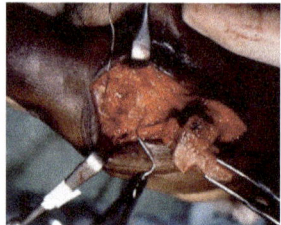 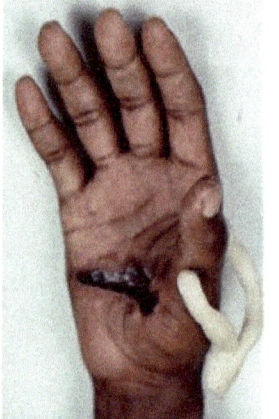

I left the pins and external fixator in place for several weeks. Below are pictures of the post-operative results after a few months.

The Healing Mission of Plastic Surgery

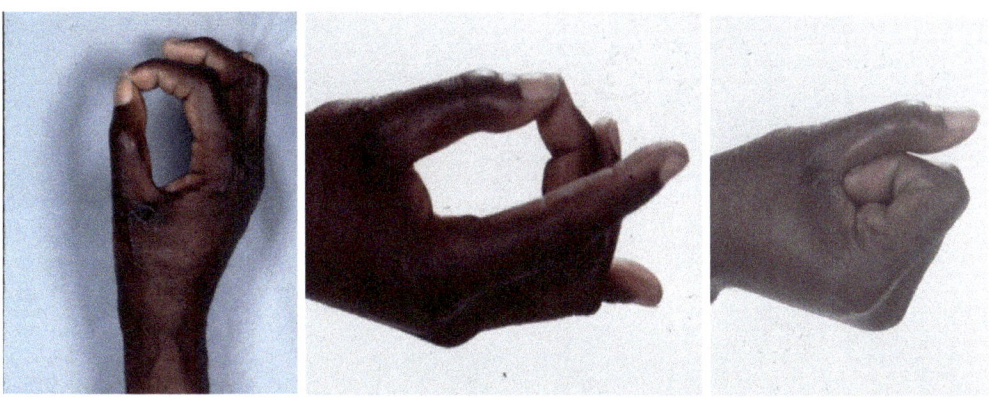

The patient below suffered an injury to his right ring finger with a loss of full-thickness skin. In his case, I raised a small flap from his trunk to replace the missing tissue. I sutured his finger to the small flap and left it attached to the abdomen for two weeks before separation.

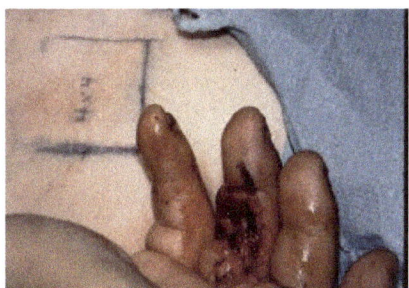 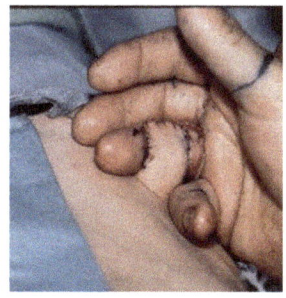

Nail gun

One day I was called to the emergency room to see a patient attached to a 2X4. He was a construction laborer who had been working on a new house. He came in with his hand nailed to a 2x4. Although this looked quite serious, it was a relatively straightforward matter of numbing the wound with a local anesthetic, cleaning the area, and removing the metal with a pair of pliers. Luckily, the man and had hit no critical structures. The first two pictures show the man's hand attached to the board. The third photo is after I sawed through the metal to separate it from the board. The fourth photo is an x-ray showing the position of the nail. The final picture shows the nail removed with a pair of sterile pliers.

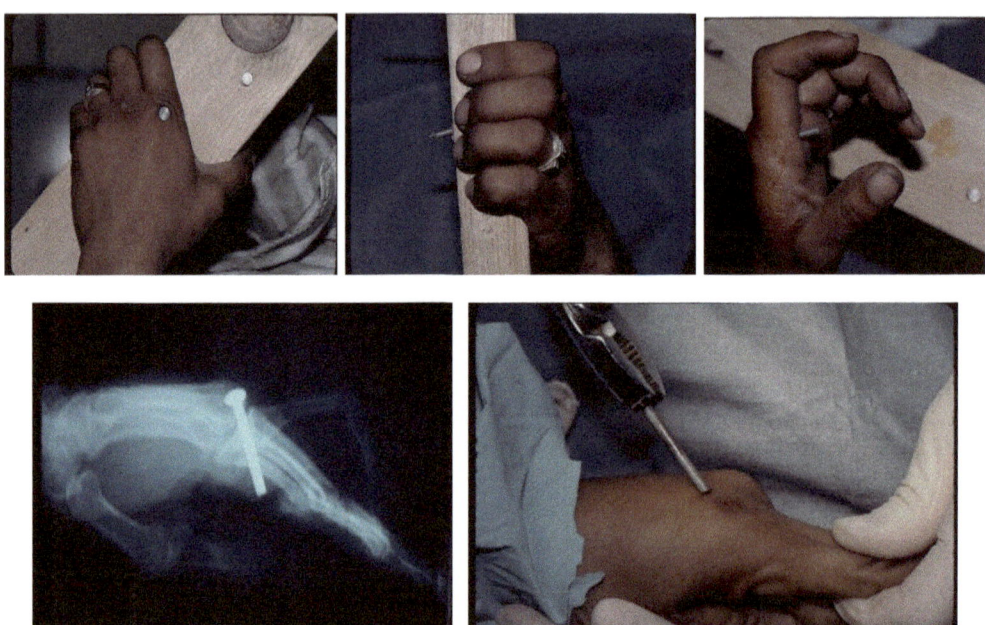

Tendon lacerations come in many variations from single, one finger injuries to the proverbial spaghetti volar wrist laceration, which injures many structures. The photo below illustrates how one must identify and label the proximal and distal ends of the severed structures so that they can be appropriately matched and repaired. The drawing shows most of the structures potentially damaged in such an injury, namely the flexor tendons, the ulnar and radial arteries, the ulnar, and median nerves, etc. I repaired the nerves and arteries with the aid of the operating microscope. This kind of extensive injury will likely leave the patient with significant functional deficits, which will probably require additional surgery and comprehensive physical therapy.

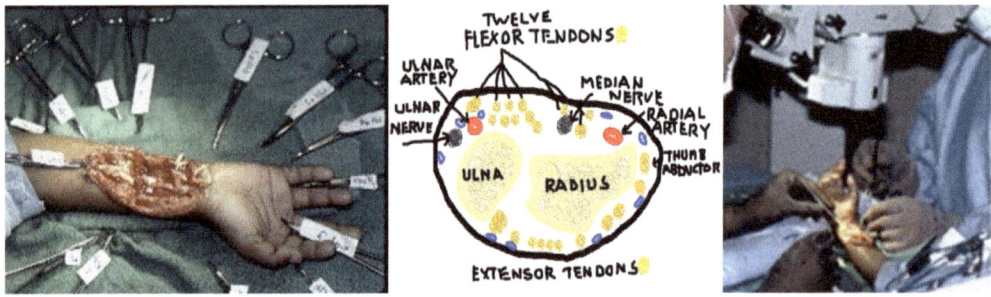

Tendon lacerations of the hand or fingers may be treated differently depending on the exact location of the cut. "Bobby" suffered an injury of the left thumb and was unable to flex the thumb. I took him to the operating room and explored the thumb. I found a severed tendon, as shown below. (flexor pollicis longus). I repaired the flexor pollicis longus with a routinely used suturing technique (blue sutures). His functional prognosis was excellent.

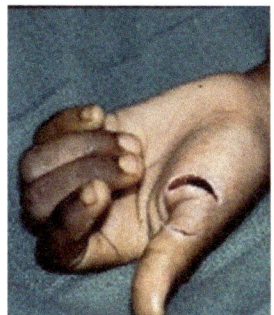
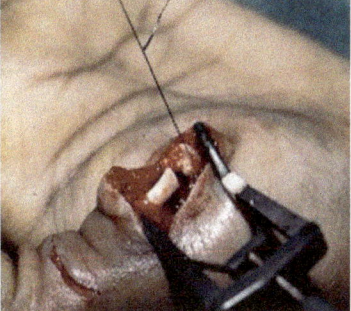
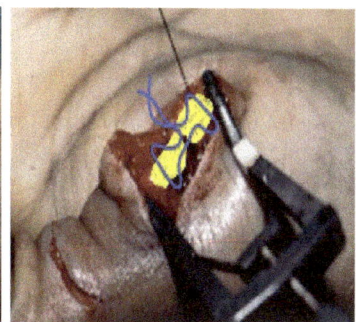

"Jerome" below suffered a single tendon laceration in a favorable location near the distal tip of the volar surface of the finger. In this case, I drilled a hole through the bone from the dorsal side to the volar side of the distal phalanx. I inserted wire suture (dark grey) through this opening and secured it to the proximal tendon. The tendon was advanced distally to underlap the small stub of distal tendon and even slightly into the bone. I tied the wire, securing a button to the dorsal aspect of the fingertip, and left it in place for a couple of weeks to allow for healing of the tendon. I placed additional sutures between the overlapped tendon segments (blue).

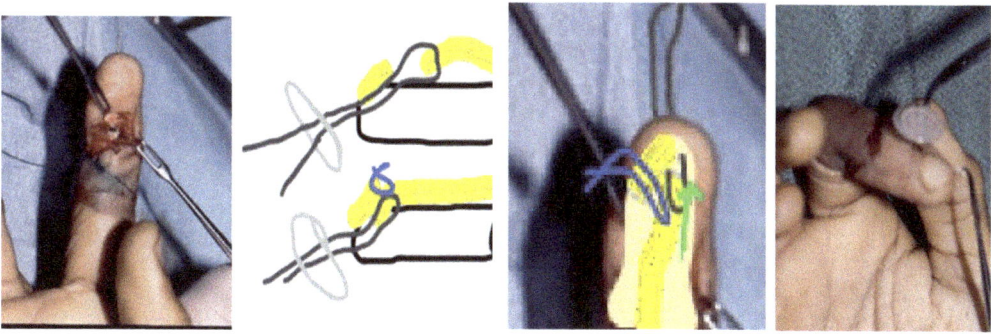

Below are his functional postoperative results.

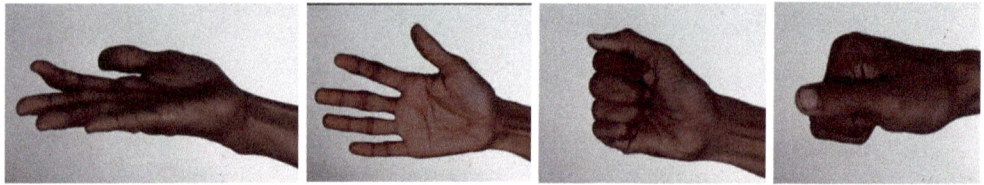

"Oscar" injured a single finger, but the tendon laceration was in an area prone to scar tissue formation, potentially limiting the postoperative results. The photo below shows the hand in a relaxed position. The ring finger has an abnormal extended orientation while the other digits show their typical flexed configuration. The straight ring finger indicates a complete laceration of its two flexor tendons. The first drawing shows the relationship between the flexor tendons. The profundus tendon starts in a deep position and comes through a split in the superficialis tendon to end up at the distal phalanx (D) while the superficialis tendon stops at the middle phalanx(M). The second drawing shows the severed tendons, with the proximal ends temporarily being held in position with needles (light blue) during the tendon repair.

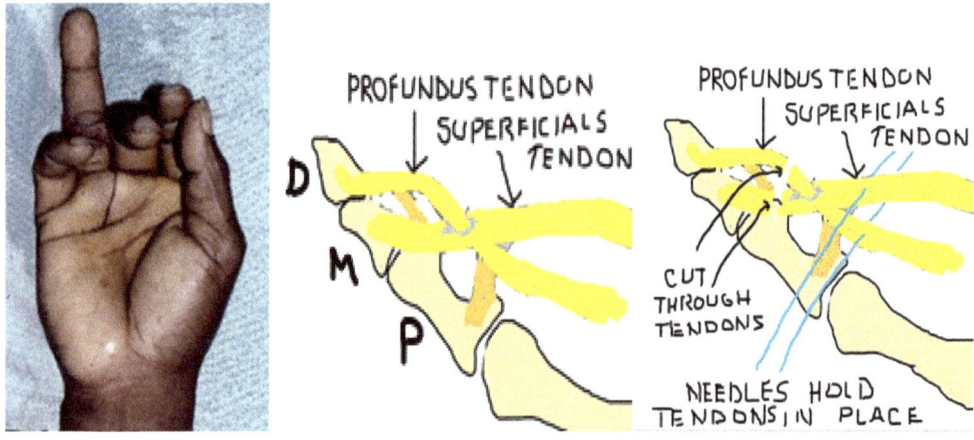

Both tendons are repaired with a dark blue suture deep and with a superficial suture layer in light blue.

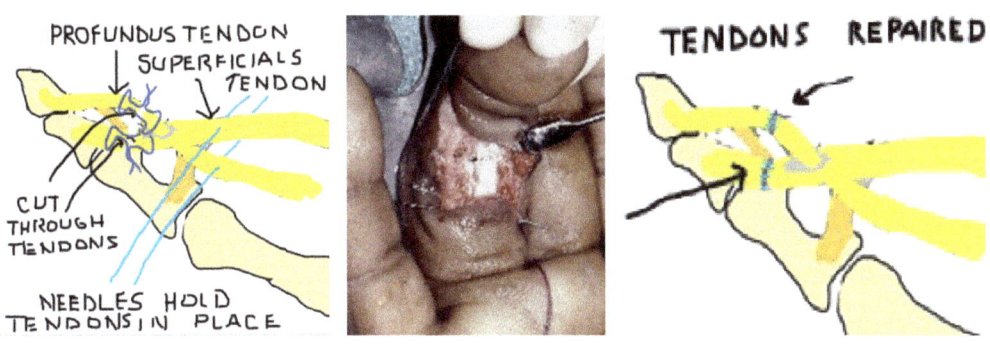

This type of injury will require specialized hand physical therapy for an optimum result.

Carpenter stories

During my almost 30 years in practice, I have seen hundreds of hand injuries. Many of these relate to carpentry. A few times, it seems that the victim of the accident was a young man just beginning to learn how to use power tools. These injuries varied from minor lacerations, which I repaired without resulting in any permanent deficit, to significant injuries that left permanent impairment from loss of digits or significant nerve injuries that never recovered full function. Another category was the experienced carpenter, who had been using power equipment for 20 years or more, who slips one time and loses a finger or thumb. Because of this observation, I am quite cautious about the use of power saw equipment

Dog bite

Over the years, I have treated many patients with dog bite wounds. In adults, the most common areas are the hands and arms. I remember one elderly lady who had two dogs, which would periodically fuss with one another. She commonly broke up their feuding. I met her one night in the emergency room because of multiple lacerations to both hands. I had to clean these wounds and irrigate them with antibiotic solution copiously and then suture them. These went on to heal uneventfully. However, several months later, I was called to the emergency room to see the same lady. This time her injuries were much more significant. She had fractures of the metacarpal bones in her right hand from the severe dog bite. This time we had to take her to the operating room, where we cleaned the wounds, pinned the fractures, repaired the lacerations, and put her hand in a splint. This injury took her many weeks to heal. Because of her age, she had some residual stiffness in her knuckle joints, even after physical therapy.

One of my cousin's daughters called me because her child of about five years old had been bitten in the cheek by the family dog. I met the family in the emergency room and decided that I could handle the lacerations in the emergency room. I repaired the injury after locally anesthetizing the cheek. I let the mom and dad stay and help keep the child calm while I sutured the cheek.

Incidents like this caused me to be a little suspicious of dogs around my children, and now, my grandchildren.

"Bobby" was bitten by his family dog losing most of the ear helix. The photos below show the result of the primary repair. The second photo is after healing when he is ready for reconstruction.

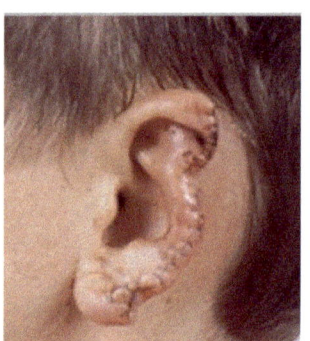 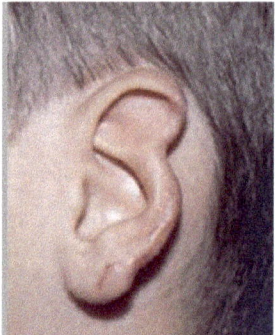

Below I planned to reconstruct him with a flap of skin from behind his ear.

In the first photo, I made a red mark on the scar edge of the healed ear wound. Also, the second red line behind the ear indicates an incision I will make to suture the cut edge of the ear down. The area enclosed in blue will be the actual flap skin, which I will transfer to reconstitute the ear helix. The diagram is from a different viewpoint, with the incisions still indicated in red. Dots of different colors indicate the edges of the incisions. I have marked the flap surface in blue.

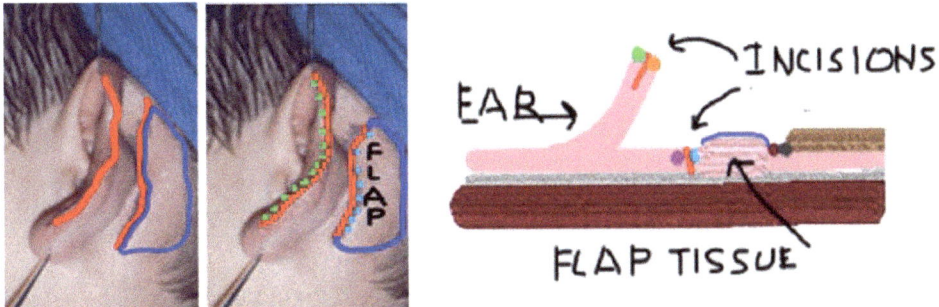

By carefully following the colored dots in the two drawings below, you can see how I brought the ear close to the side of the head. I split the healed injured edge of the ear open so that I can temporarily suture one side to the side of the head (orange and purple dots). I will suture the other side of the split to the proximal portion of the dark blue flap tissue (green and light blue dots).

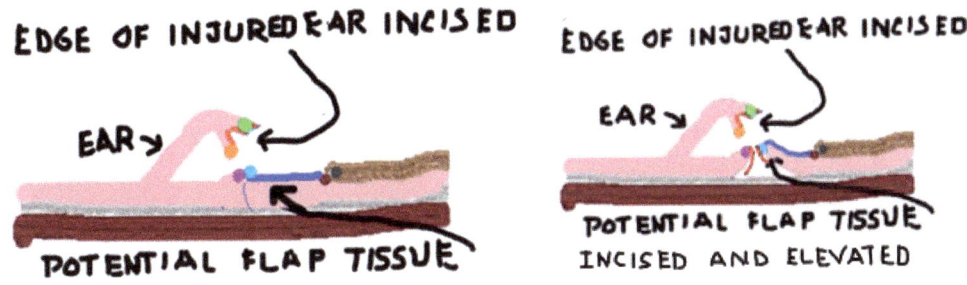

In the photo below, I have sutured the ear to the side of the head. I illustrate this first stage in the drawing on the left, where I have approximated the gold and purple dots and the green and light blue dots. So, in this first stage, I connected the ear (green dot) to the proximal edge of the flap (light blue dot). The distal part of the flap (red dot) is still attached to the side of the head. I left the ear sutured to the side of the head for two weeks so that small blood vessels would grow into the flap from the ear.

The Healing Mission of Plastic Surgery

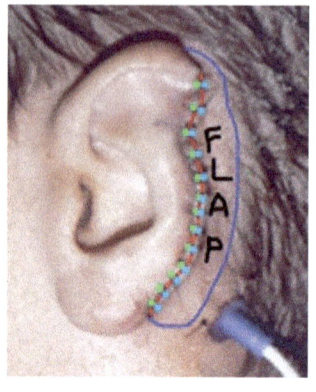
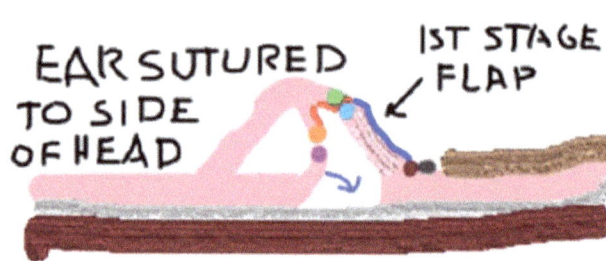

Below, I have released the distal side of the flap (red dot) from the side of the head (after two weeks). It now had enough blood supply from the ear side of the flap to survive. The lower drawing shows the flap folded on itself and sutured in place as the new helix. The flap donor site is cover with a split-thickness skin graft. The postop photos are from a few months later.

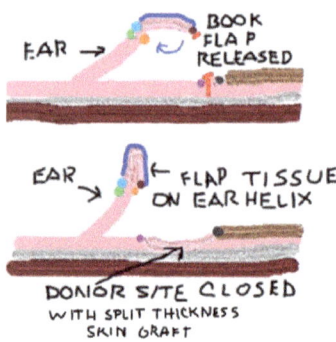
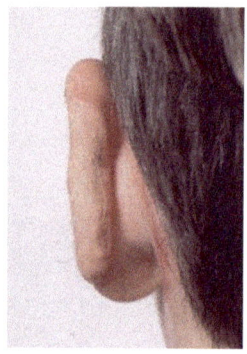
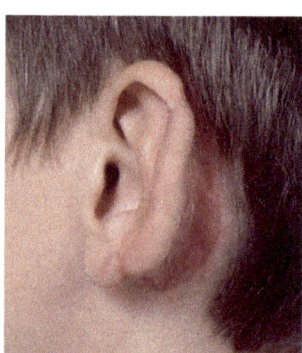

"Anastasia" presented with a dog bite injury to the nose, as shown below.

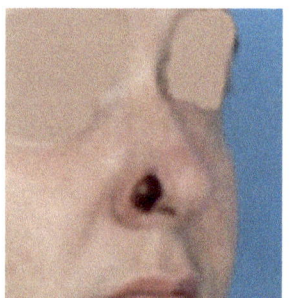
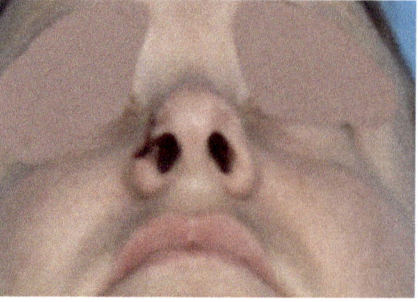
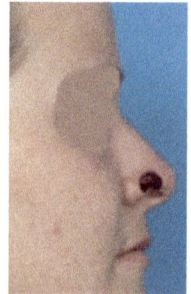

I reconstructed her with a nasolabial flap, as outlined in blue below.

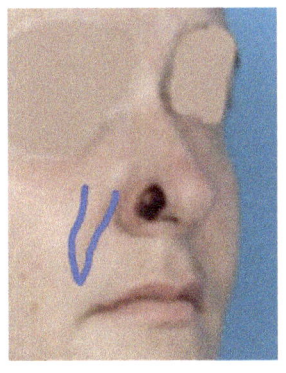
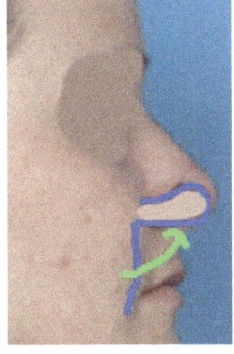

After the initial flap movement, I needed to perform two more small revisions to obtain the final result.

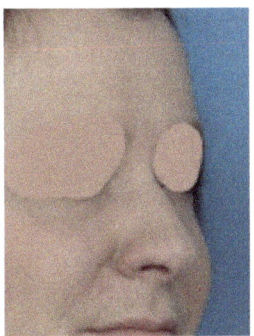
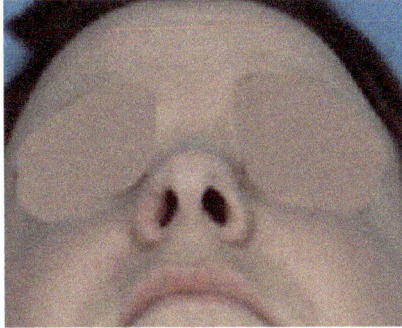
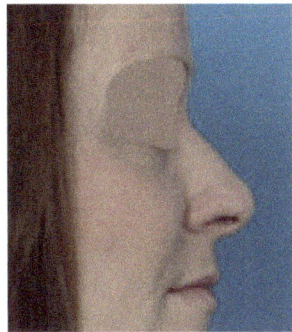

Human bite

"Charles's" human bite of his nose was not from a truculent act, but rather reportedly from a passionate amorous encounter. The original wound was allowed to heal secondarily as the amputated part was not available. Below are multiple views of the preoperative defect.

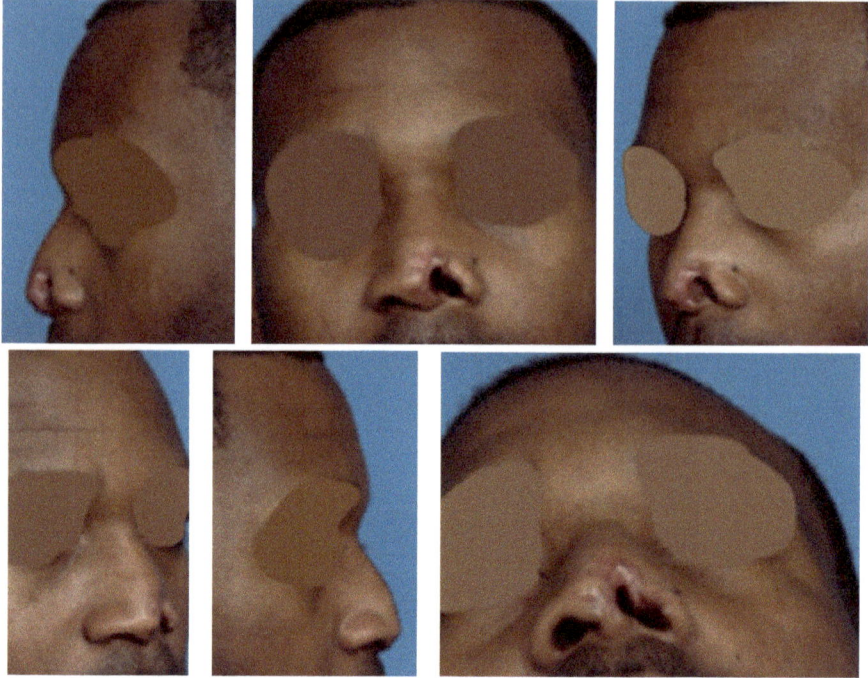

Analysis of the defect below indicates the loss of most of the left ala, including cartilage support. There is also a loss of a significant amount of internal nasal lining with dense scar tissue present at the edge of the wound. I have drawn anatomic subunits of the nose in blue ink.

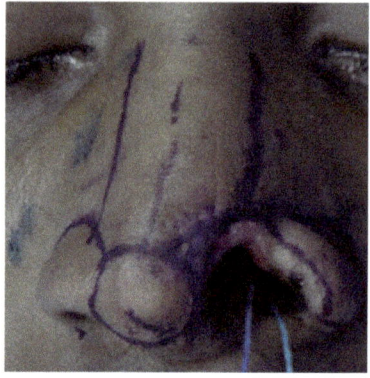

Because of the size and nature of the defect, I planned to perform a paramedian forehead flap on "Charles." I have drawn the flap outlines on his forehead in the first photo below. I planned to introduce new cartilage in the nasal tip at the second stage. Below I measure the size of the cartilage I will need to utilize. The distal part of the flap needs to be the right size to cover the cartilage later when I place it in the nasal tip (right photo).

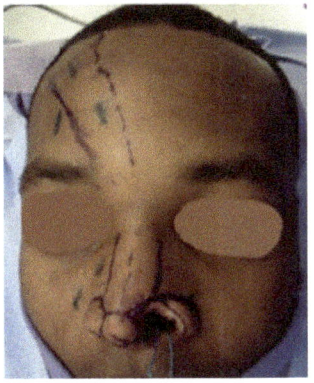 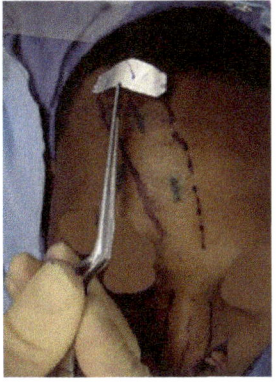 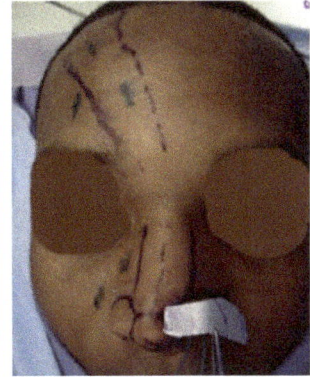

Rather than excise and discard the indurated scar tissue around the defect, I lifted and turned it over to produce nasal lining, as shown in the photos below, providing a more accurate picture of the size of the defect the forehead flap needs to cover.

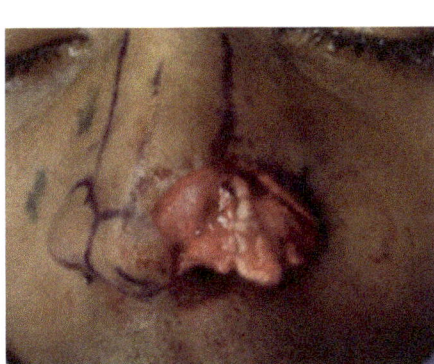 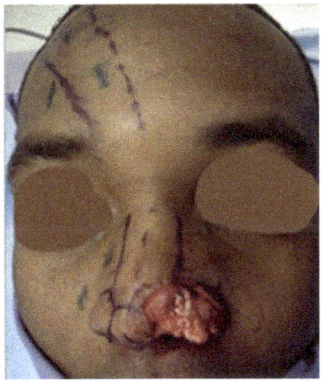

In the first stage, I turned down the forehead flap to bring full-thickness tissue to the nasal tip defect. The intermediate result after the first stage is pictured below.

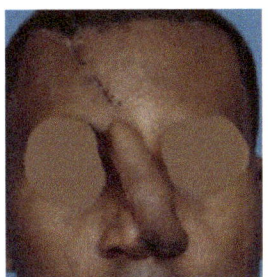 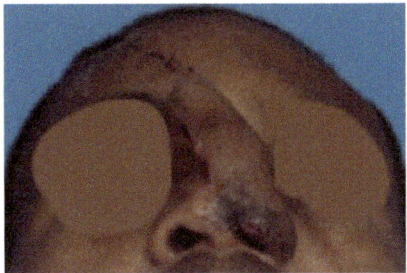 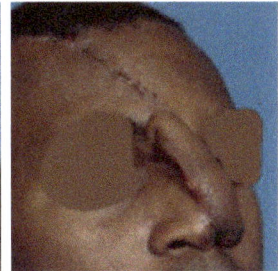

At the second stage, I dissected the flap free from the nasal tip and lifted it to reexpose the surface defect, as in the first photo below. Next, I sutured in place the cartilage I harvested from the nasal septum and fashioned for support of the nasal ala, as shown in the second photo. I then replaced the flap on the nasal tip, covering the cartilage graft. I used the white nasal splint is used for nostril sizing and stenting.

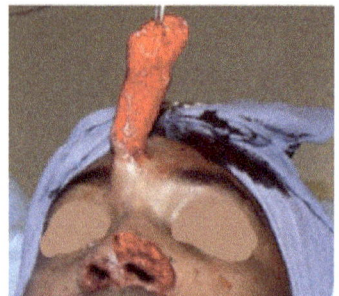 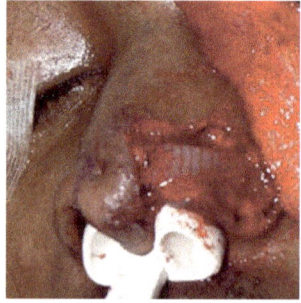 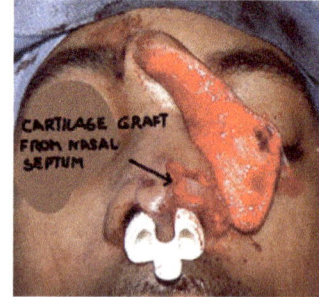

I used the small cotton bolsters below to help shape and define the nasal tip.

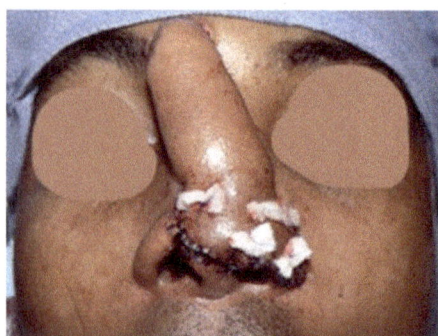 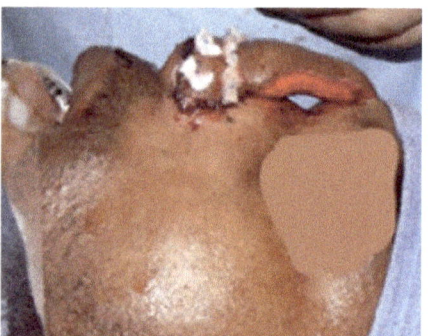

In the final stage, I returned the unused portion of the forehead flap to the forehead. The postoperative pictures below are a few months later. The contour of the nose is good, but the color match is not. At this point, I began treating "Charles" with topical bleaching agents to the flap to improve the color match. His early postoperative photos are below.

The Healing Mission of Plastic Surgery

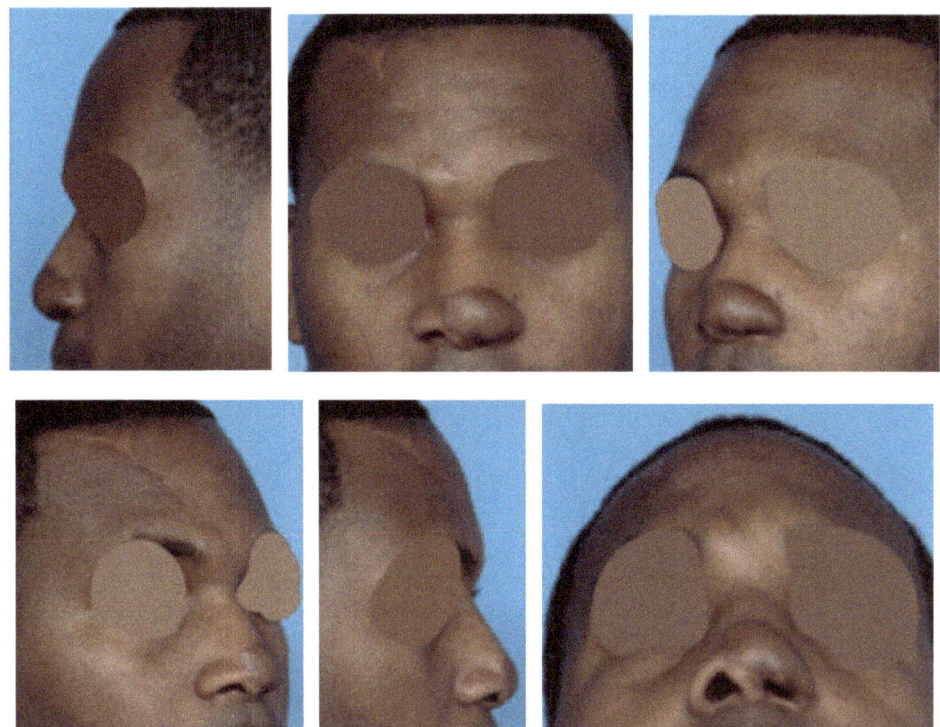

Chapter 7

The Cleft Palate Clinic

I found it immensely gratifying to take care of patients with cleft lip and or palate. A significant portion of my career was devoted to these patients. I became interested because of the work of my mentors and partners Dr. Thomas Cronin and Dr. Raymond Brauer. From the beginning of their careers, they took care of patients with cleft problems. In the late 1940s, they met when they were still in the army. They worked at Wakeman General, an army hospital under a prominent plastic surgeon named Truman Blocker, who later became the head of the University of Texas Medical Branch in Galveston.

They told me stories about the plastic surgeons meeting to discuss cleft lip and palate care calling it "the children's hour." I believe they took care of local children and dependent children of army personnel with cleft problems. Later I will explain how this connection will come full circle again.

Cleft lip and or palate are some of the most common congenital anomalies, affecting about one out of every 700 newborn babies. Clefts are splits in the lip, gum line, or palate. They can be on one side or both sides. They occur when something goes awry with embryological development. Functional and other problems such as difficulty feeding, airway or breathing problems, ear infections with hearing loss, speech impediments, psychosocial dysfunction, and facial disfigurement are common.

Proper care and treatment can substantially improve this potentially devastating problem. Achieving such is usually very satisfying work for the plastic surgeon. The etiology is primarily genetic and is inherited.

There may be some environmental factors such as drugs like steroids, Dilantin, or Valium or even infections such as rubella or toxoplasmosis.

My following amateur drawings summarize the very intricate embryologic development of the labium and palate. In these drawings, I depict the head and face of the embryo during its formation. They show various components of facial development from 5 to 10 weeks post conception. The upper lip and nose form from a compilation of three parts, which grow and develop, as shown in the diagrams. These components are the maxillary prominence and the medial and lateral nasal prominences. At five weeks, they are just mounds on the developing face of the embryo. At six weeks, the components are coming closer together towards the midline.

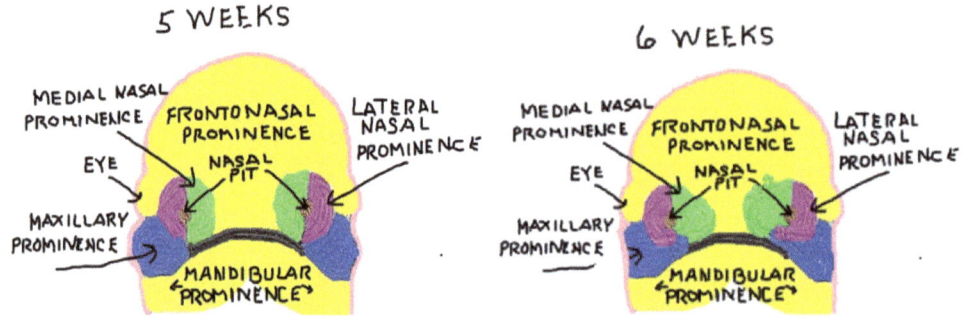

By seven weeks, the medial and lateral nasal prominences and the maxillary prominence moving towards the midline have formed the rudimentary nose. Rapidly the medial nasal prominences and the maxillary prominences morph into the upper lip (labium), which is fully assembled by ten weeks after conception. By comparison, the developing child already has a heartbeat, which typically can be seen on an ultrasound at six weeks after conception.

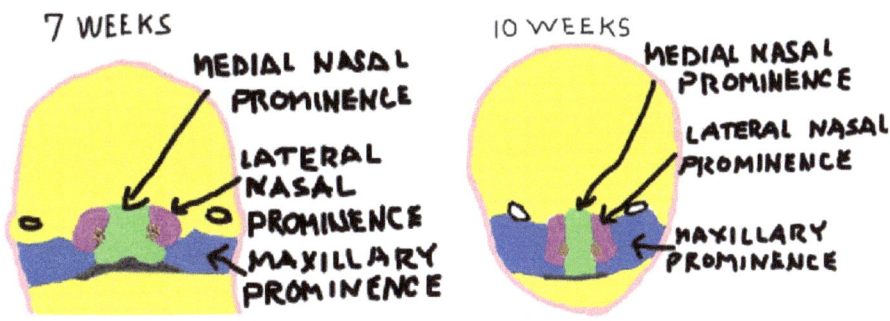

The drawing below shows bilateral clefts of the lip, which result from the failure of the prominences to fuse.

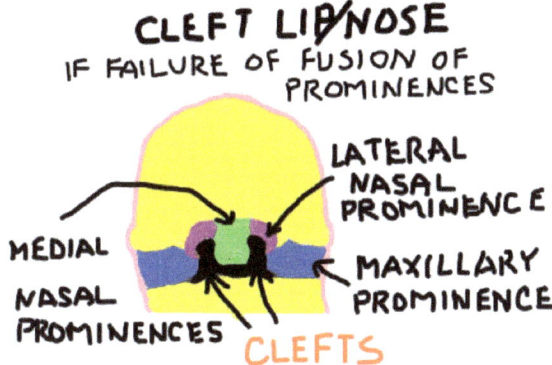

Additional drawings below represent the embryologic formation of the palate. The illustration on the left below is of a view looking to the roof of the mouth. The palatal shelves develop on either side, and the premaxilla forms anteriorly. The drawing on the right is a coronal plane cross-section of the mouth and nose. The palatal shelves grow toward the midline, as shown in the second drawing.

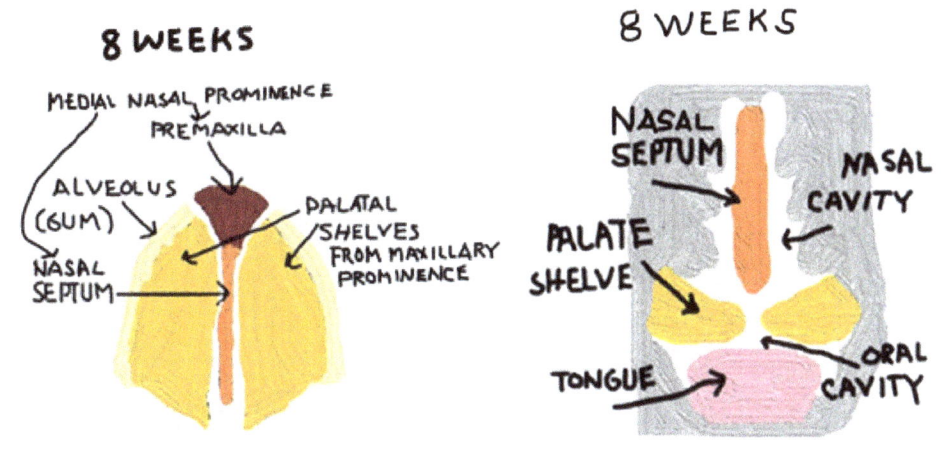

By the 10th week, the palatal shelves fuse in the midline and anteriorly with the pre-maxillary segment. The premaxilla constitutes part of the anterior palate and the central gum, which is also called the primary palate.

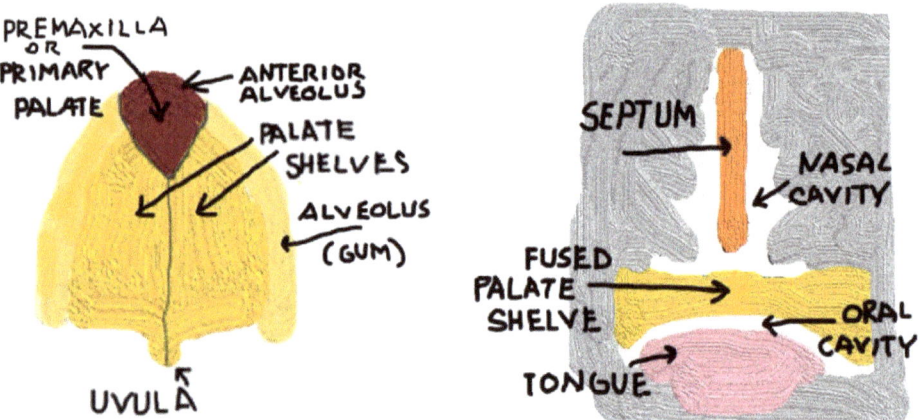

If fusion does not occur, clefts of the palate may result. Almost any area of fusion can fail. Some diagrammatic representations of the resultant clefts are below.

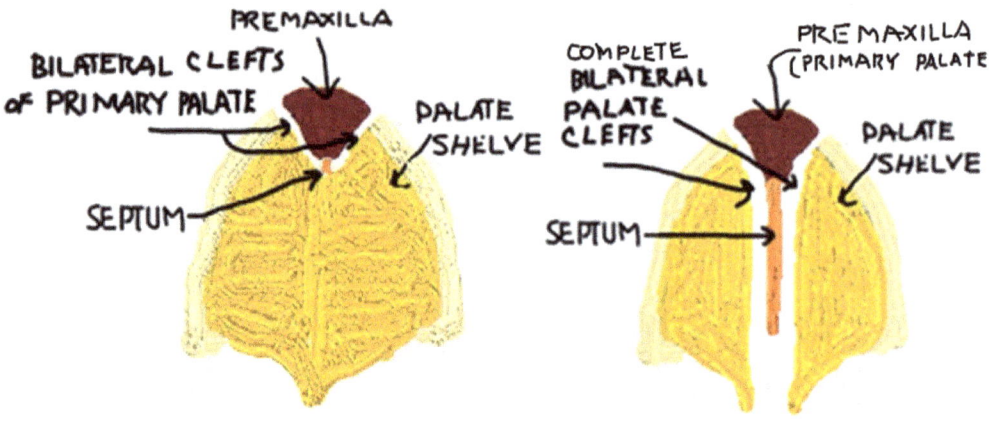

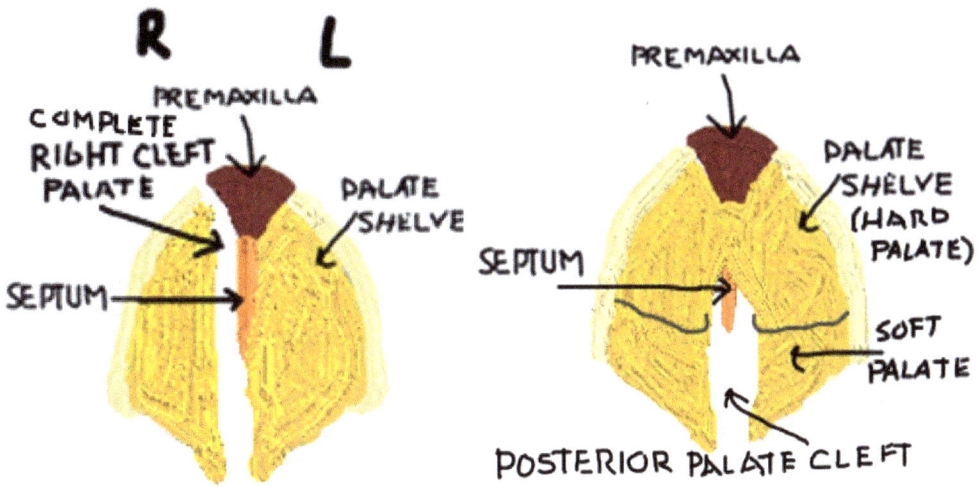

Embryology is a fascinating science that one would think would very much engage the general public because of the contentious issue of abortion. However, I remember that when I started medical school in 1968, abortion was something about which I hardly knew anything. It was a mysterious taboo subject. I knew it was "wrong," but not much else. How times have changed. A myriad of scientific facts is now available to any interested person. Still, some of our politicized media disingenuously characterize such a fetus or developing baby as merely a "glob" of tissue.

Having studied embryology, it is still astounding to me that so much development takes place so soon after conception. By ten weeks after fertilization, the nose, lips, and palate have formed, and the heart has been beating for two weeks.

On a very personal note, many years ago, my wife was 16 weeks pregnant when she had a miscarriage at home. Fortunately, I was home at the time to help her. I held our premature baby in one hand and baptized him. We contacted a friend, Don Earthman, who was associated with a local funeral home, which had a particular area in one of their cemeteries to bury the remains of babies who died from early miscarriages. Taking advantage of their service was consoling to us because often such very premature babies are just discarded as medical waste.

Cleft lip and palate variations

Examples of children below, all patients of mine patients demonstrate the diverse nature of this affliction. The first picture below shows a microform cleft of the baby's right lip. The embryologic fusion was almost but not quite complete. The second picture is of an incomplete cleft of the next baby's left lip.

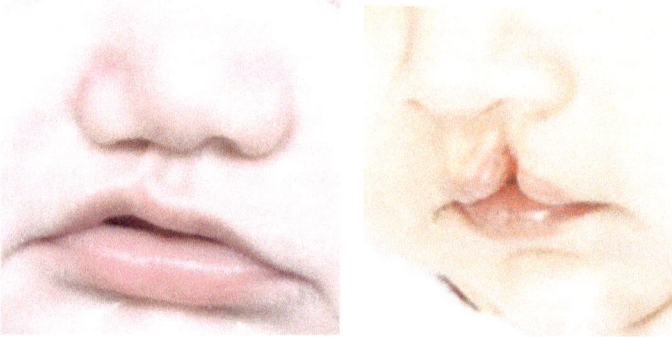

Below is another baby with a complete cleft of the left lip. The second picture below is of a baby with a full wide cleft lip and palate on the right side.

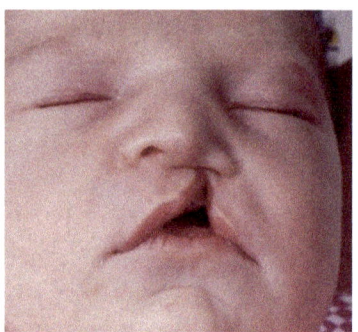
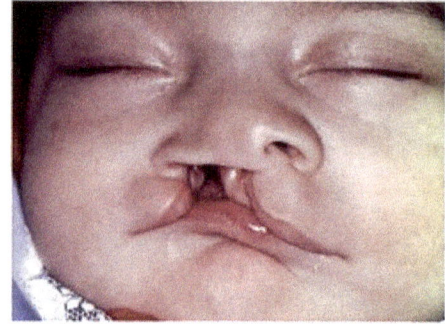

The next group of patients below begins with a baby with a bilateral incomplete cleft lip. Note there is only a small amount of distortion of the left nasal ala while the right nostril is normal. The second young boy has complete bilateral clefts of his upper labium. The nasal alae are splade out laterally but are symmetric. There are two teeth in the pre-maxilla twisted 90 degrees.

The Healing Mission of Plastic Surgery

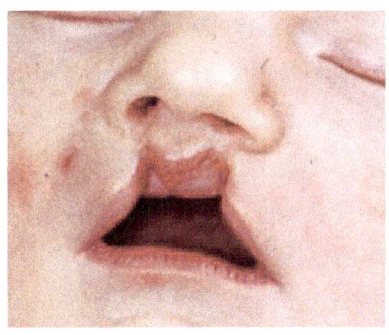
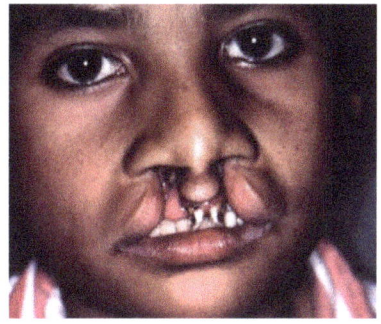

The first photo below shows an extremely wide bilateral cleft lip and palate with extreme distortion of the nose. The picture on the right below shows a baby with bilateral clefts of the labium and the roof of the mouth but also lower lip "pits." Such deep dimples are an expression of the autosomal dominant Van der Woude syndrome, which is a relatively common cause of cleft lip and palate.

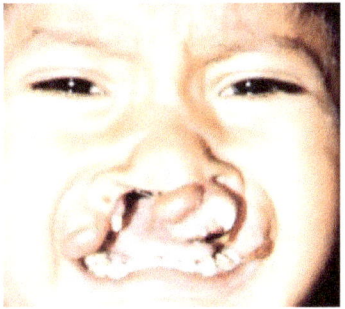
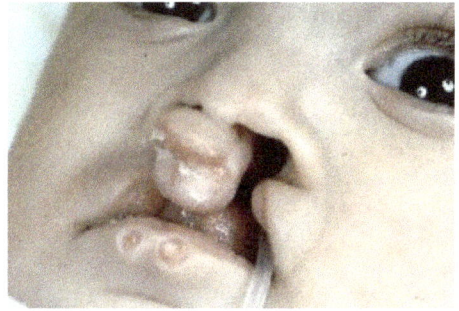

The first picture below shows a rare, very partial midline cleft palate; this could be confused with a previous failed attempt at a palate repair. The second photo shows a somewhat typical incomplete cleft palate, as well as a partial cleft lip and a partial cleft of the alveolus.

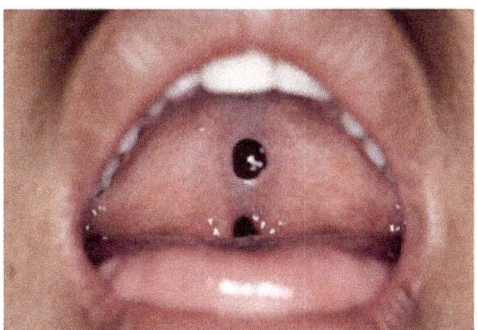
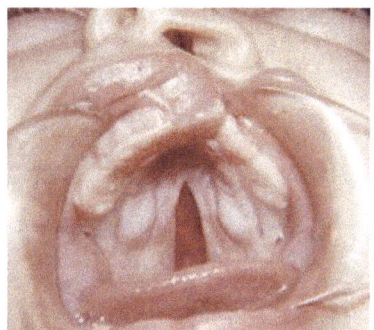

The two patients shown below have complete bilateral clefts of the labium (lip) and palate. I have labeled some of the structures to clarify abnormal anatomy. The premaxilla is the central part of the gum (alveolus), which has been separated from the lateral gum segments by the bilateral clefts. One can see the vomer, the lower bony part of the nasal septum, because of the wide-open palate.

The lateral view shows the premaxilla disconnected from the lateral alveolar segments and also protruding abnormally even in front of the lateral lip segments. This anterior protrusion can be addressed preoperatively with maxillary orthopedic maneuvers such as elastic pressure or taping to reposition this segment. Also, sometimes I will perform preliminary lip adhesion surgery to reposition the premaxilla. I will show examples later.

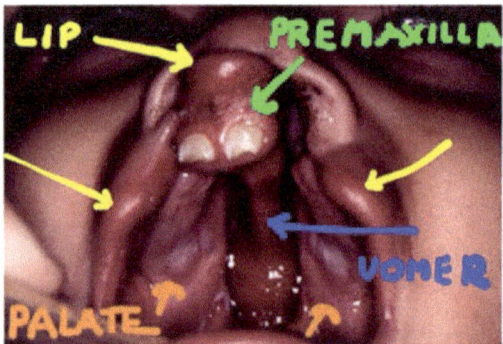
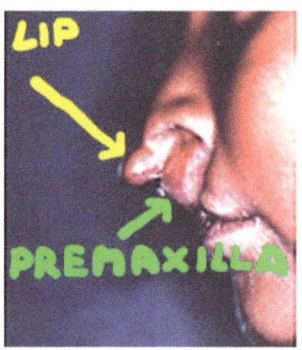

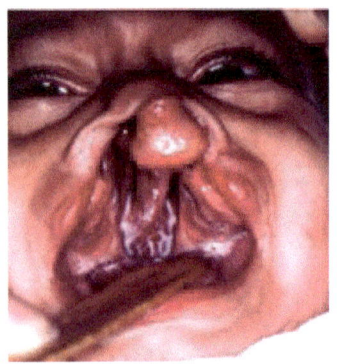
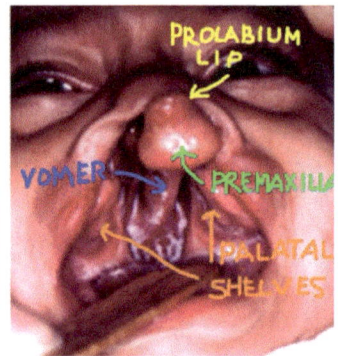
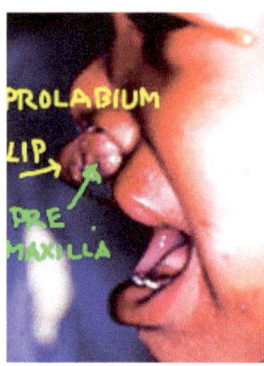

The photograph below shows a complete cleft of the lip and palate on the baby's right side. The palate cleft is extensive, and the nasal distortion is severe. The second photo shows a child who has a cleft running through alveolar ridge and gumline on both the right and left, which then extends the full length of the palate. Note the extreme flaring of the nasal alae in this child with complete bilateral clefts of the lip and palate.

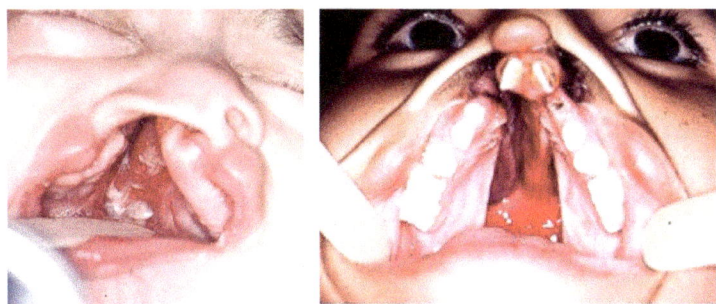

Treatment goals

The treatment goals include normal speech and hearing, minimization of growth disturbances, functional dentition, good aesthetic results, psychological well-being, as well as patient and parent education. It takes very specialized care to obtain optimal results for the patient with such very complex deformities. Treatment not only involves surgery by the plastic surgeon but may require extensive orthodontic treatment, management of the middle ear disease by the otologist, and perhaps comprehensive speech therapy.

I enjoyed seeing many of my patients go from infancy to young adulthood. I became very proud of many of my patients because they were able to overcome with aplomb the limitations nature imposed. I would often ask my young patients what they wanted to be when they grew up. I would encourage them to find something in which they were very interested. I discussed the field of medicine with some, pointing out the great variety available within it like surgery, internal medicine, pediatrics, etc. Also, when some children expressed interest in mathematics, I tried to inspire them to look at engineering, because like medicine, it has myriad variations from which to choose, such as mechanical, civil, electrical, chemical, etc. I tried to emphasize, to the vast majority of my older cleft patients, that their attitude and belief that they could achieve a worthwhile life goal was the first and most crucial aspect in accomplishing it.

I strived to give my cleft patients function and appearance as close to normal as possible. Only by enlisting the help of my cleft palate team colleagues, especially in the fields of speech pathology, orthodontia, otology, and oral surgery were my efforts ever realized

Over the years, neonatal nurseries, pediatricians, and families of other cleft patients, etc. referred many newborn cleft patients to me. One thing that changed in the middle of my career was that, because of improved ultrasound examinations, I began seeing expectant mothers who were already informed their child had a cleft of some sort. I was able to tell them about what to expect and especially reassure them that their unborn child's cleft lip and palate problems were correctable. I believe this has been very helpful to the families of these children.

Cleft lip and palate patients may have their essential functional surgeries completed in childhood; however, they may still request secondary surgery because of residual abnormal structures or function related to the cleft lip or palate. They sometimes also seek aesthetic improvements in areas unaffected directly by the cleft lip and palate. They may pursue additional surgery for residual deformities, including short tight or scarred upper lips, nasal asymmetry, midface under development, relative overgrowth of the lower jaw, and occlusal or bite problems.

The psychological discomfort the patients suffer does not necessarily parallel the severity of the residual deformity. Neither does improvement necessarily correlate to the real success of their surgery. In these patients, functional success includes normal speech, mastication, respiration, as well as normal hearing. Aesthetic success is much more arbitrary and depends on the patient's acceptance of the "final" result.

When I evaluated secondary cases, it was vital that I understand the patient's goals and assessed whether their objectives were obtainable. I was gratified in many instances by intervention in such cases, where I was able to achieve enhancement of the residual deformities through additional surgery. Patients must have a realistic attitude and want surgery. Some of the standard operations involved the movement of the upper jaw forward for an underdeveloped midface. Such orthognathic procedures could also remedy some bite problems.

I frequently performed nasal surgery to improve nasal contour or asymmetries. Perhaps one of the most frequent interventions I executed in my practice was a revision of the scar of the upper lip. Occasionally I took skin and muscle from the lower lip and brought it to the upper lip to improve contour and function in a two-stage procedure. Examples will follow.

In the early 1950s, my mentors, Dr. Thomas Cronin and Dr. Raymond Brauer, involved other practitioners, such as an orthodontist and a speech pathologist, to help obtain the optimum result for their patients. In the early 1980s, there was a push to have teams certified by the American Cleft Palate Association to care for the cleft patient.

Although Drs. Cronin and Brauer used the team concept de facto since the 1950s; I initiated a formal team in 1987 at St. Joseph Hospital with their cooperation and support. Dr. Paul Tessier, the world-famous father of craniofacial surgery, was the inaugural speaker for the opening of the clinic. The Clinic was supported by the Thomas Cronin endowment of the St Joseph Foundation (now the Christus Foundation for Healthcare), which was set up by the Dunn Research Foundation and matched by the Sisters of Charity of the Incarnate Word.

Cleft palate team

The cleft clinic team consultation is an excellent convenience for the patient and the patient's families. The American Cleft Palate-Craniofacial Association recommends a multidisciplinary team be involved in all cleft patient care. As coverage becomes more restricted with the domination of managed-care, it has become more difficult for most patients to obtain multi-disciplinary team care. We were constantly battling with insurance companies, especially for the orthodontic work that a majority of the cleft palate patients need. I have to say my general impression is that care for cleft lip and palate patients has deteriorated somewhat in the past few years because of difficulties with insurance issues. Hopefully, this will improve with time.

The cleft palate clinic followed hundreds of patients and saw a few dozen new patients every year. The clinic offered an excellent opportunity for residents in training to see many patients with cleft lip and palate conditions in a concentrated manner. It is preferable to see cleft palate and cleft lip patients as newborns to initiate a comprehensive treatment plan. Sometimes the first crack at a particular surgical procedure has the best opportunity for the optimum result. I frequently saw cleft lip and palate patients for consultation who had had surgery elsewhere.

When I saw such secondary cases, I never knew whether my result might have been better for the patient. I frequently saw patients with suboptimal results for consultation. However, I know that a portion of my cases have turned out to have suboptimal outcomes, and perhaps they will see other cleft palate surgeons before I have a chance to improve on the results. So, I always give the benefit of the doubt to the previous surgeon in such cases. Often, after consulting with a family and giving them recommendations for future surgery, I would have them return to their original doctor to consider proceeding with that care.

This type of clinic offers an excellent opportunity for plastic surgery residents to see many patients with cleft lip and palate conditions in a concentrated manner. Cleft lip and palate surgery, is taught to plastic surgery residents through multiple modalities, including personal contact in the cleft palate clinic and hands-on instruction in the operating room. Didactic teaching through conferences and reading of the medical literature is also relevant. Analyzing, drawings of cleft lip, and palate procedures such as those which I will describe below is also helpful in learning how to treat patients with this common congenital problem.

This clinic offered free consultations for patients with cleft lip and palate problems as well as other facial reconstruction problems. All of the patients saw the core team members, including the speech pathologist Dr. Donna Fox, the orthodontist Dr. Dan Louie, the otologist Dr. Paul Gidley (and for a time Dr. Al Maillard) and myself as the plastic surgeon. All the team members saw all of the patients. We developed a plan of care for the patients after everyone had seen them. The coordinator saw that the patients followed through with various lab tests, consultations, studies, or exams at that they might need. These free consultations were supported by the Thomas Cronin Endowment Fund in the St. Joseph Foundation (later the Christus Foundation for Health Care). The above consultants were paid a small stipend. I never took a stipend or a salary as Medical Director although the Foundation would have allowed that.

I was the Medical Director from 1987 until I arranged for the Clinic to move from St Joseph Hospital and to merge with the Shriners cleft palate program in 2014. I did this after the Sisters of Charity of the Incarnate Word sold St Joseph Hospital. The clinic became the Cronin and Brauer Cleft Lip and Palate Clinic at Shriners Hospital for Children Houston under the directorship of Dr. Steve Blackwell. Dr. Blackwell had been director of the cleft palate program at the University of Texas Medical Branch in Galveston, where Dr. Truman Blocker had become chancellor after WWII. The destruction caused by Hurricane Ike in 2008 led Dr. Blackwell to move the program from UTMB to Shriners Hospital in Houston.

The 2014 merger brought full circle a generation of plastic surgeons succeeding Dr. Truman Blocker, Dr. Thomas Cronin, and Dr. Raymond Brauer, who were now treating cleft lip and palate patients together at Shriners Hospital. So, beginning in 2014, a new type of "Children's Hour" continued as I worked with Dr. Steve Blackwell.

Most importantly, this merger created a more comprehensive cleft lip and palate team, which can offer treatment to all children with cleft lip and palate problems regardless of their financial statuses. Medical specialties, including plastic surgery, pediatrics, anesthesiology, otolaryngology, radiology, psychiatry, genetics, are now represented. The dental specialties of orthodontics, oral surgery, and pediatric dentistry are integral participants. The team also includes essential allied health professions such as speech pathology, audiology, social work, psychology, child life, and of course, nursing.

I continued to participate in the care of clinic patients until my 2016 retirement. The Christus Foundation continues to support the clinic, now titled Cronin and Brauer Cleft Lip and Palate Clinic at Shriners Hospital Houston.

In the photo on the left below are Drs. Tom Cronin and Ray Brauer with one of their happy cleft patients at the former Cronin Brauer Cleft Palate Clinic at St. Joseph Hospital. The picture on the right below is the ribbon-cutting ceremony for the merger of the cleft palate program at Shriners with the Cronin & Brauer Cleft Palate Clinic in May of 2014, with representatives from the Shriners and the Christus Foundation. Dr. Blackwell, the medical director, is second from the left.

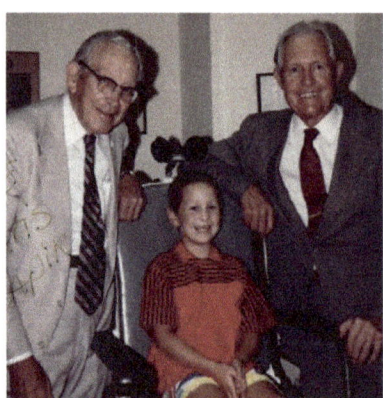 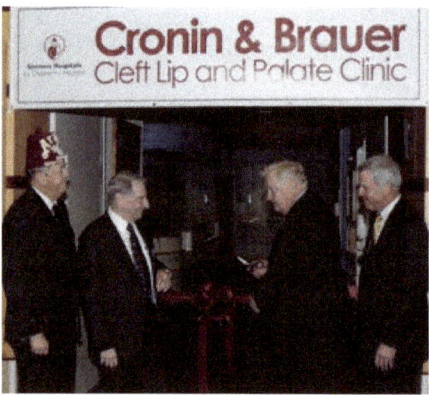

Unilateral cleft lip repair

Repair of cleft lips not only improves the patient's aesthetics but also aids in speech articulation and social interaction. As discussed in Chapter 2, such repairs address issues of the body- image and self- image and can be very important for the patient's self- esteem.

The pictures below illustrate some principles involved in the repair of clefts of the lip. The goals are to produce a normally functioning, symmetrical, intact lip of appropriate length with an aesthetic cupid's bow and inconspicuous scars. It is not merely a matter of cutting the two sides and sewing them together. Older cleft lip repairs did not appreciate that the cupid's bow was present in the lip but "hidden in plain sight." In the first picture below, there are four blue dots, three on the non - cleft side (left) of the lip and one on the cleft side (right). They represent the two peaks, and the valley of the cupids bow medially and the position of the peek on the cleft side (right). The first principle is the cupids bow peak medially next to the cleft (large dot) needs to rotate downward to be level with its counterpart on the non-cleft side.

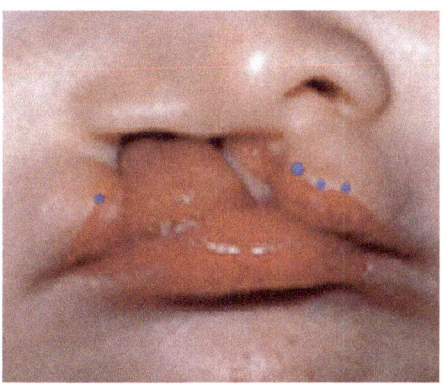 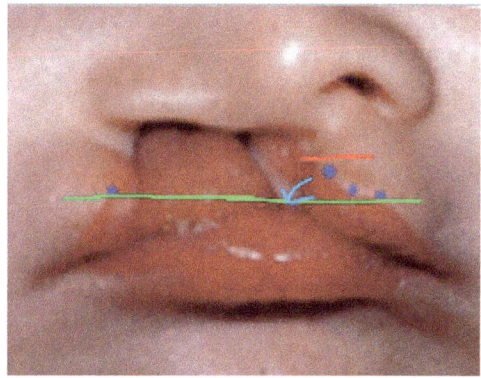

In the diagrams below, a "back cut" (red line) is made somewhere above that cupid's bow peak so it can rotate down

(gold arrow) to match the opposite cupids bow peak. Tissue from the lateral lip (green arrow) fills the gap created by the back cut, which lengthens the lip and maintains the new position of the peak. I will show how this is done with different techniques later.

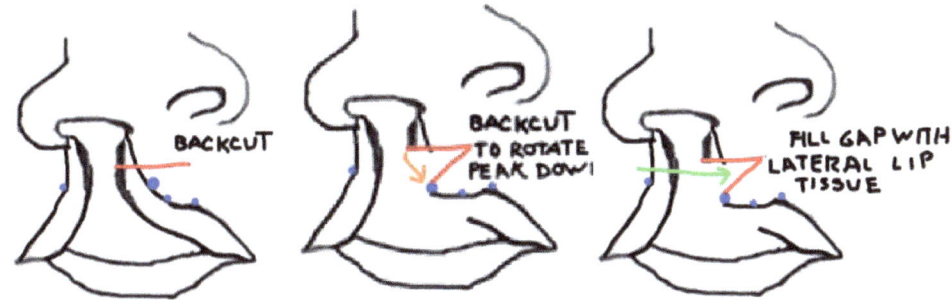

Another fundamental concept in cleft lip repair is re-orientation and restoration of the orbicularis oris muscle, as indicated by the drawings below. The surgeon frees the muscle on either side of the lip, reorients the direction of the muscle fibers into a more horizontal position, and sews them together, thereby reconstituting the oral sphincter and establishing normal lip function.

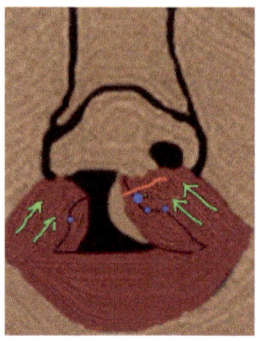 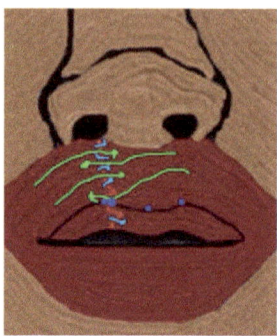

The most common cleft lip repairs today place the" back cut" either just above the peak or high just below the columella of the nose. Charles Tennison, a San Antonio plastic surgeon, described the first technique shown below. He made a "back cut" close above the peak and used a triangular flap from the lateral labium to fill the gap created after the rotation of that point downward.

The drawings below represent the Cronin (Thomas) modification of the Tennison repair. Further changes of this technique by a Canadian plastic surgeon, Dr. D.M. Fisher, using a smaller triangular flap than the original Tennison repair, have led to improved results. In the drawings below, the portion of the incision in purple constitutes the "back cut," which allows the large blue dot cupid's bow peak to rotate downward, which levels the cupids bow. The triangular flap from the lateral lip fills the gap created by the rotation of the labium downward. This technique is useful in narrow or wide unilateral clefts.

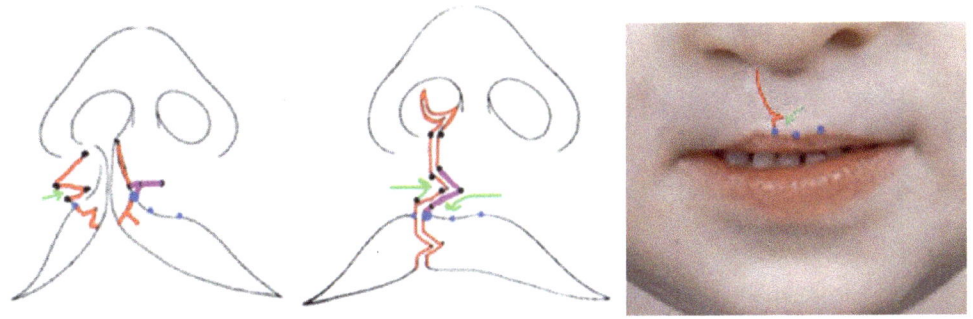

Ralph Mallard originally described the other most common technique with a "high" back cut to allow the peak to rotate down. Incidentally, he was Thomas Cronin's first plastic surgery resident at Jefferson Davis Hospital in Houston in the 1950s. His "rotation advancement technique" makes the "back cut"(purple) at the junction of the lip and nasal columella. Advancing lateral lip tissue fills the gap. Various modifications of this technique, not described here, are also utilized today.

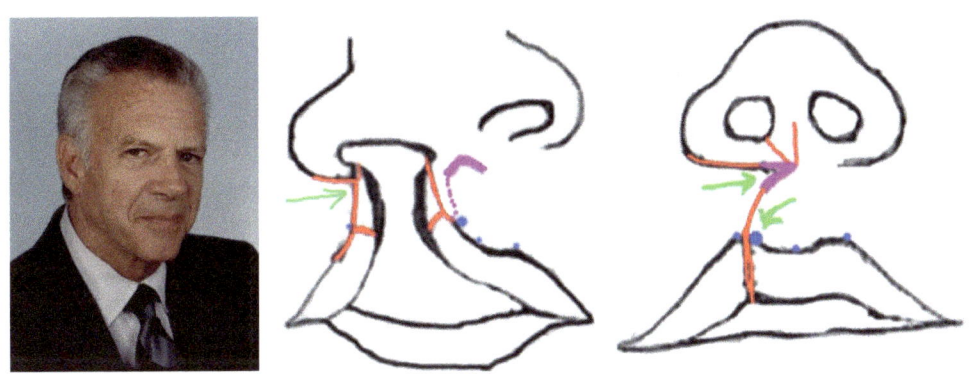

Preoperative maneuvers

By far, most unilateral cleft lips are done in one procedure, although occasionally, a partial repair known as a lip adhesion precedes by a few months the definitive surgery. I sometimes do various preoperative maneuvers when the patient presents with an exceptionally wide unilateral cleft. External taping, as shown in the baby below, sometimes together with an acrylic palate splint, can help to stretch the tissues and even mold a protruding gum (alveolus), making the lip repair easier.

The Healing Mission of Plastic Surgery

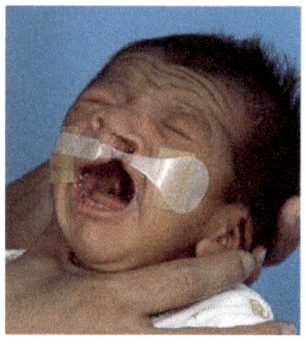 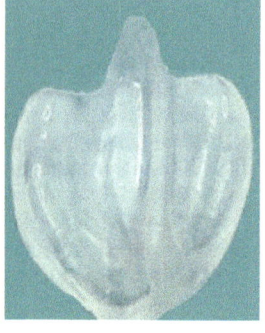 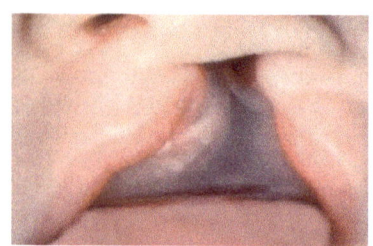

The device below is an acrylic palatal plate with an expansion screw. Because the external taping tends to collapse the cleft, an expansion device is sometimes used to prevent this and to align the palate and alveolar segments better. These maneuvers can take the place of doing lip adhesion surgery before the definitive lip repair in very wide clefts. However, it takes a lot of time, patience, and effort from the parents. It is not unusual or surprising that the parents sometimes abandon these maneuvers along the way.

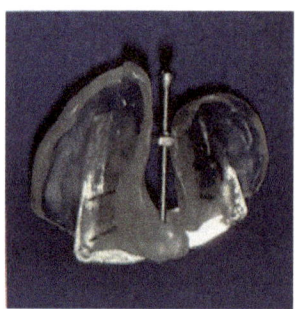

An extension of these preoperative "orthopedic" maneuvers is naso-alveolar molding (NAM), which can sometimes make not only the lip repair easier but also the concurrent nasal tip repair easier. The pediatric orthodontist usually orchestrates (NAM). Below on the left is an example of a palatal plate with a nasal extension. The photo drawing on the right shows its placement in an infant. Over several weeks, gradually adding to the splint extension, together with external taping, the nose, as well as the alveolar portion of the palate, can be molded and made more favorable for surgical repair.

The Healing Mission of Plastic Surgery

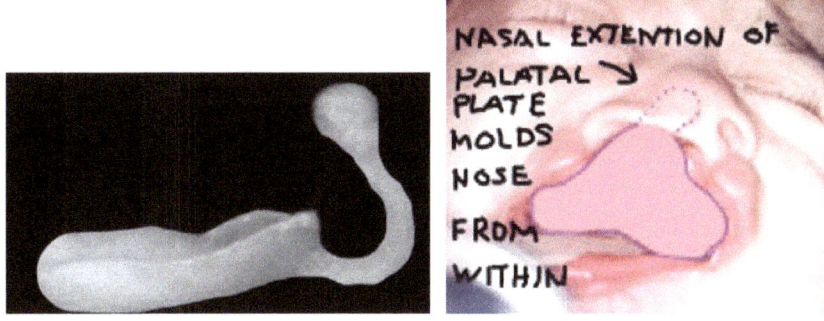

Below are pictures of "Pete," the first patient with a cleft lip that I repaired after I completed my residency and was in private practice. I was able to approach this patient confidently because of the expert training Dr. Tom Cronin and Dr. Raymond Brauer gave me. The first picture shows "Pete,s" incomplete cleft of the lip. The second picture is my plan of a Cronin modification of the Tennyson triangular flap repair outlined in blue ink on the patient's labium. I made incisions on the blue lines, rotated the peak down, and advanced the lateral lip triangle into the gap created by the back cut. I thereby equalized the cupids' bow peaks. Internally I repaired the orbicularis muscles.

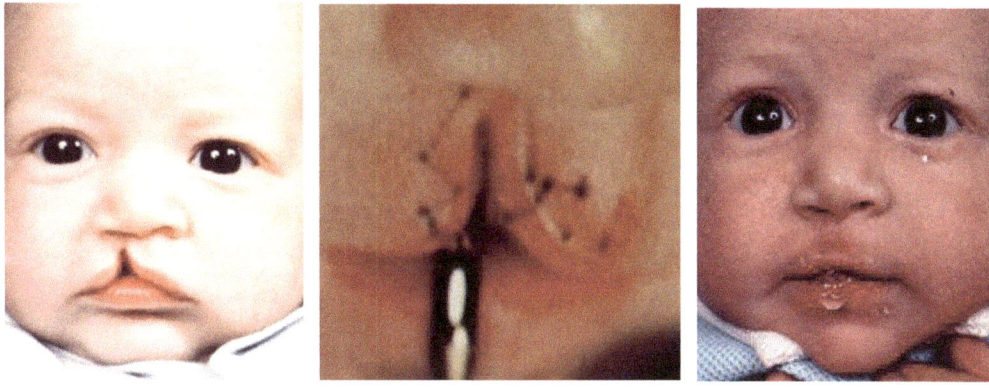

The photos below show the postoperative result. Notice that the cupid's bow that was " hidden in plain sight" has been "revealed" to produce a pleasing contour.

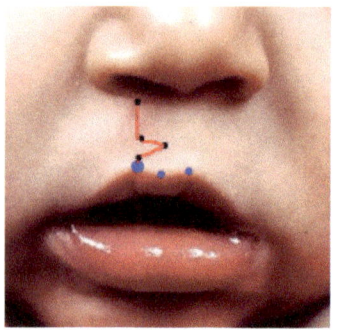 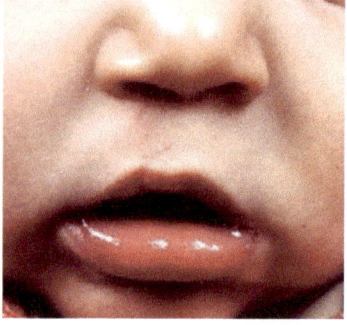 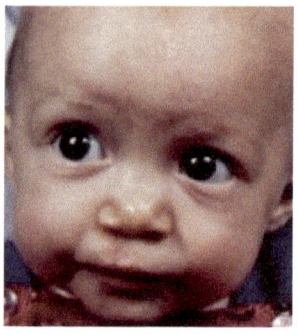

"Bobby," below, had an incomplete cleft lip, which I repaired in one procedure. Although the cleft was incomplete, there was a fair amount of distortion on the left side of the nose. The postoperative photo shows not only lip repair but improvement in the symmetry of the nose.

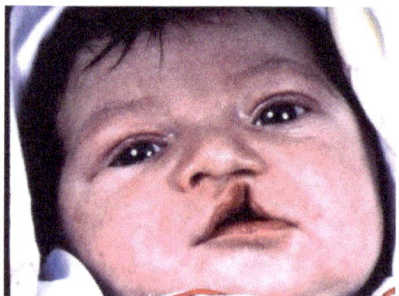 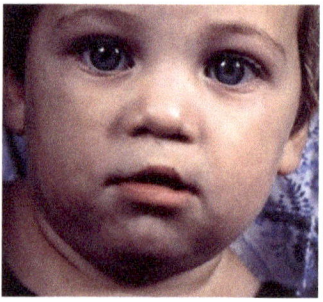

"Freddy" below had a very wide cleft on the right side. I did a preliminary lip adhesion, shown in the central picture below. In this operation, the edges of the upper part of the cleft were partially incised and sutured together, thus changing a wide cleft into a more manageable incomplete labial lip. A few months later, after the tissues had softened and stretched, I performed a second operation with a low triangular flap for a definitive lip repair with a more predictable result. His postop result a couple of years later is on the right below.

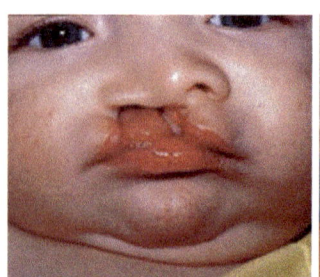 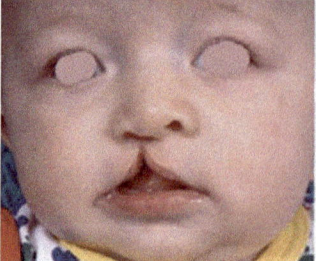 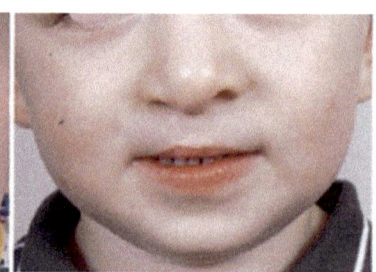

"Pascal" below also had a wide cleft with extreme distortion of the nose. He also had a lip adhesion procedure preliminarily. The definitive repair (modified Tennison) involved both the lip and the nose. His postoperative result below after those two procedures is two years later.

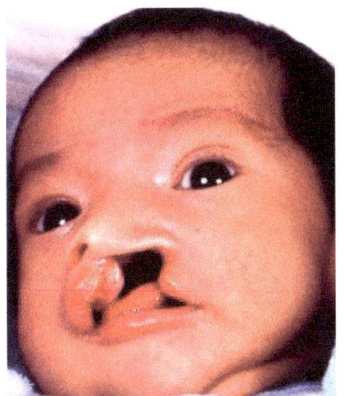 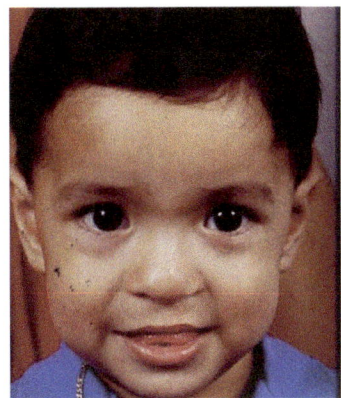

"Gregory," below, had a complete left-sided unilateral cleft lip and palate. The middle picture shows the extensive cleft palate. This view also demonstrates the significant distortion of the nasal ala on the left side. The final image shows the result after one procedure (modified Tennison) to repair the cleft lip and nose.

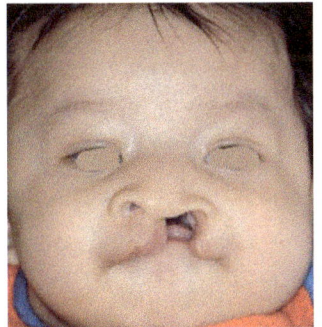 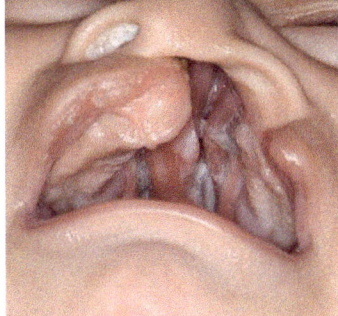 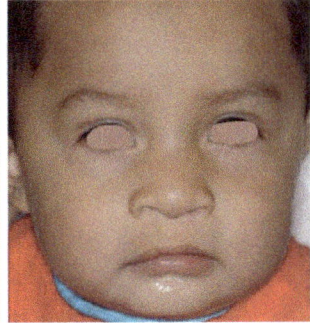

"Stanley, below" presents with an incomplete cleft lip as it does not extend into the nasal cavity. Nevertheless, the cleft is extensive along the alveolar ridge or gum line, and although the cleft does not extend into the left nostril, there is significant nasal distortion. Below are his preoperative picture and six-year postoperative result following a modified Tennison repair.

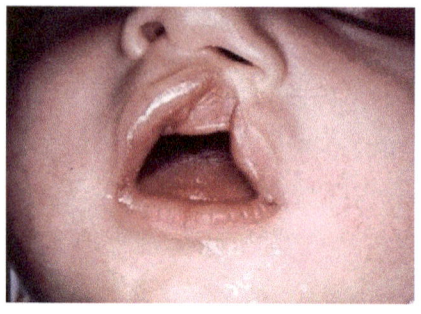 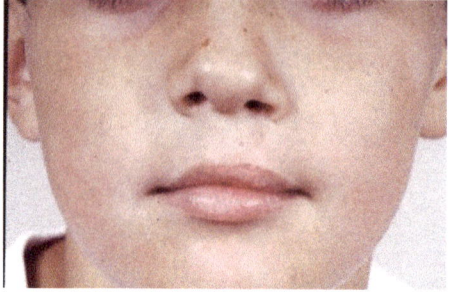

"Felicity" shown below has a minor incomplete cleft lip and no palate involvement. Her postoperative photo after a Millard rotation advancement procedure (high back cut) is about a year later. This patient may never need any further surgery, unlike many patients who have more involved clefts.

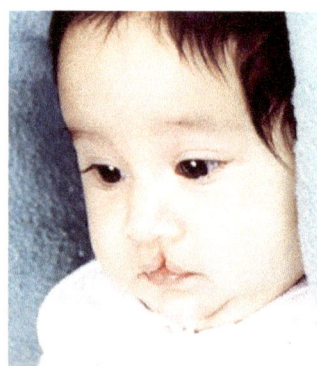 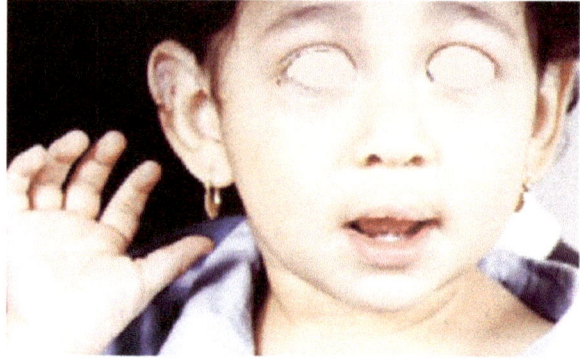

The baby below "Francis" had a wide cleft of the lip and palate. I performed three operations on him; one was a modified Tennison repair of the labium at about three months, the second was a palate repair at about one year, and a third operation on the nasal tip just before he was to start regular school. The post-operative photo is at about ten years of age.

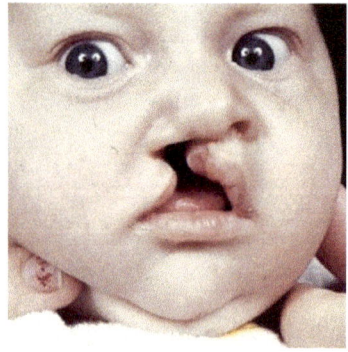 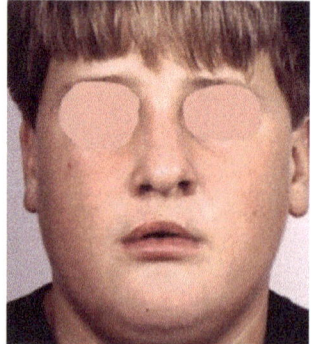

"Blaise" shown below has an extensive cleft of the lip and palate. I repaired the cleft lip at approximately three months of age (modified Tennison) and the cleft in the roof of his mouth at about ten months of age. His postoperative result is a few years later.

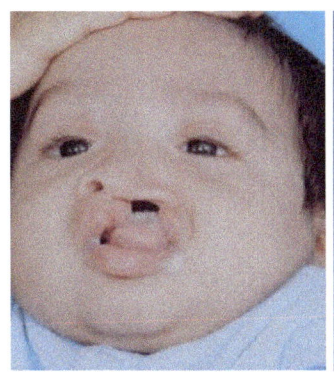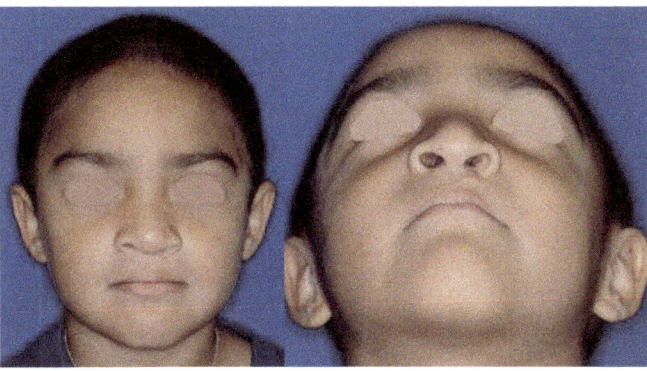

Bilateral clefts of the lip and palate

Preoperative maneuvers for bilateral cleft lips

Bilateral clefts of the lip and palate are less common than unilateral clefts. However, various preoperative orthopedic maneuvers are used even more frequently in these bilateral cases. I often used external pressure with elastic bands or with taping I conjunction with palatal plates. Sometimes, these are sophisticated dynamic splints with elastic or spring dynamics.

The picture below on the left is of a model of a bilateral cleft palate made from an impression taken of a child's palate. The green arrow points out the central gum line or premaxilla. The nasal septum or vomer is labeled in blue while the lateral segments, including the gum line, are shown in orange. The palatal device in the second photo can pull the premaxilla posteriorly by the action of the rubber bands on a pin placed through the premaxilla. This pressure pulls the premaxilla back and encourages the lateral palatal segments to grow anteriorly. This maneuver repositions the premaxilla and aids in the repair of the wide bilateral cleft lip.

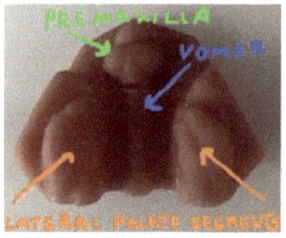
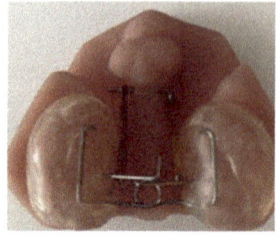

The maxillary orthopedic appliances below are additional examples of the ingenious devices orthodontists design to help the plastic surgeon care for bilateral cleft lip and palate children. The one on the left below is to move the premaxillary gum posterior, thus making the lip repair easier. The one on the right differentially expands the palate segments.

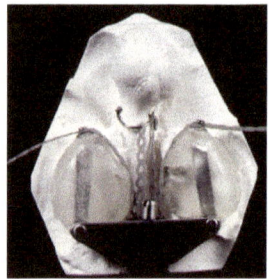
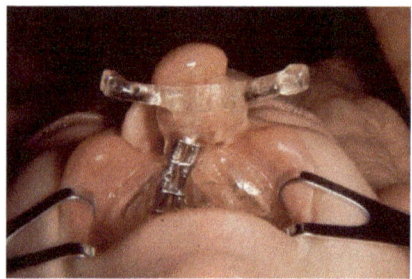

As in unilateral lip repair occasionally, lip adhesion surgery is done in bilateral cleft lips before the definitive lip repair to make the lip repair easier. The main objective is to move the premaxilla backward, so the lip repair is not so tight. The first photo below shows a baby with a bilateral cleft of the lip and primary palate. The premaxilla is protruding forward, and the prolabium is way ahead of the lateral lip segments. The second and third photos are after a temporary lip adhesion. Partially sewing the lip together like this will apply pressure to the protruding premaxilla and over several weeks cause it to move back closer to the palate and thereby make the repair of the lip easier.

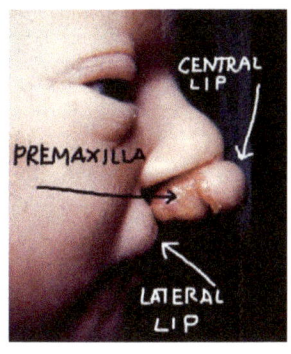 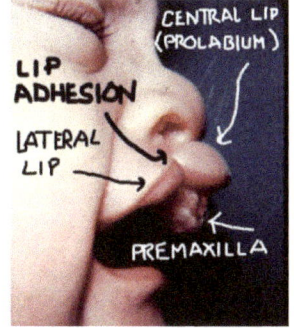 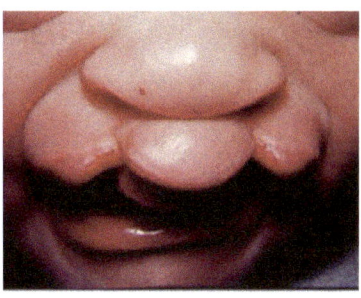

The two photos below before the adhesion show the premaxilla is positioned forward on a "stalk" of vomer anterior to the intact hard palate. One can visualize the vomer portion of the nasal septum from the palate side.

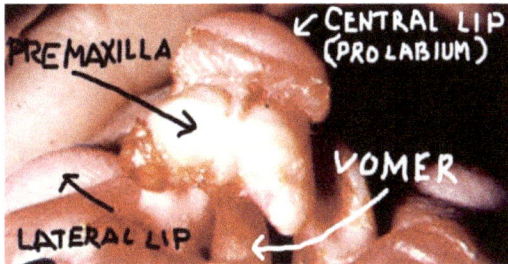 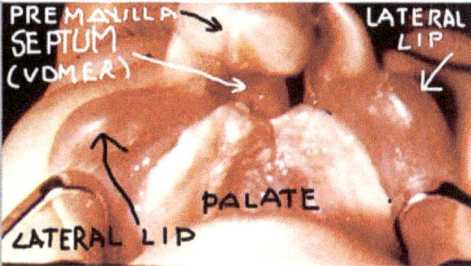

The photo below is after the adhesion has been working for several weeks. One can see that the premaxillary alveolus is now immediately adjacent to the hard palate. The lip is, therefore, less tight, making the definitive repair of the labium without undue tension possible. If I had initially attempted a complete lip repair, it might have pulled apart because of too much stress on the closure.

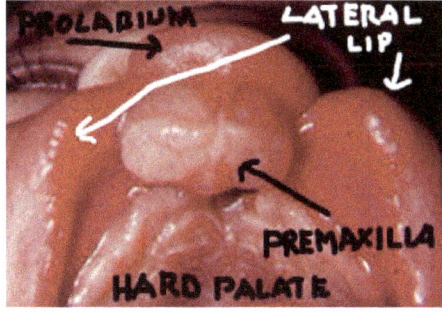

Repair of bilateral cleft lip

I usually repair bilateral cleft lips with straight-line incisions on both sides of the philtrum. In this baby below with an incomplete double cleft lip, the prolabial mucosa (Z) is too thin, so muscle and mucosal flaps (X) are brought below the prolabial segment to augment the central vermillion to produce the result shown in the third photo.

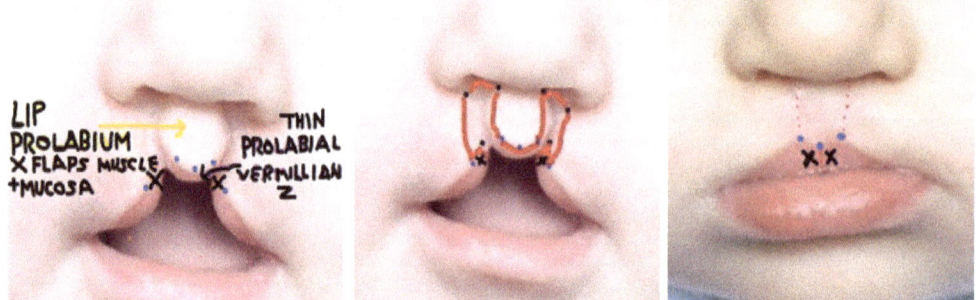

Again, in the two drawings below, I make straight-line incisions, remove excess skin, identify, and free the muscle. I then turn down the lateral X flaps, containing muscle and mucosa, and bring them under the prolabium to the midline to augment the prolabial vermillion. In the second drawing, I flipped the thin Z mucosa under the lip for the lining. The blue stitches show the closure of the inside mucosa (yellow).

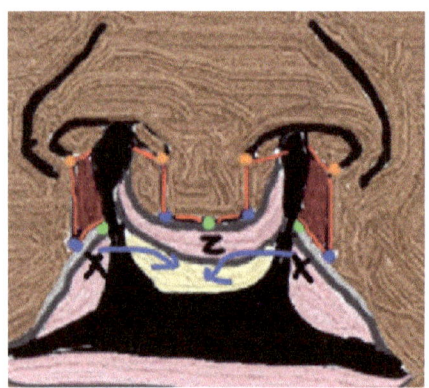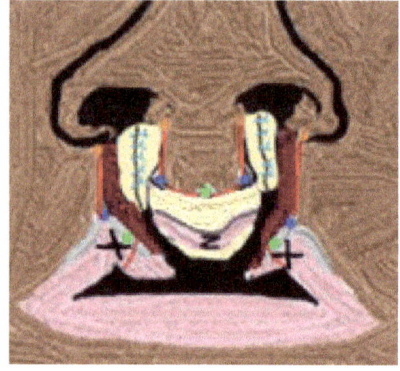

In the drawings below, I free the muscle from either lateral lip segment, reorient them from vertical to horizontal, and stretch them under the prolabium, to be sutured together in the midline. Usually, there is no muscle in the central labial segment of complete bilateral cleft lips. In the second drawing, I have sutured the muscle in the X flaps to build up the central lip vermillion. Repair of the orbicularis oris muscle reconstructs the oral sphincter. In those cases where the premaxilla is still too far forward, the lip repair exerts elastic tension, which will tend to push the premaxilla backward just as it does in cases of a lip adhesion. The last diagram shows the final straight line, closure.

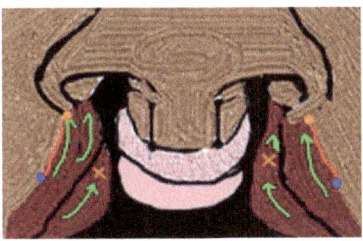 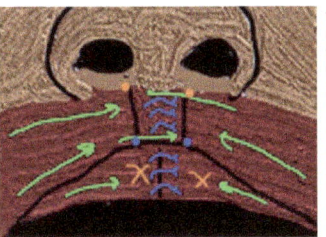 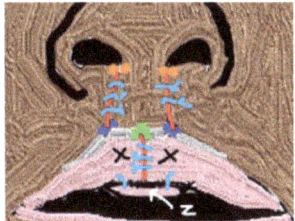

The baby below "Matthias" has bilateral incomplete clefts of the lip with a short prolabial lip segment centrally. There is only mild asymmetry and distortion of the nose. The second photo shows his post-operative result after one procedure. Also, note the improved nasal symmetry.

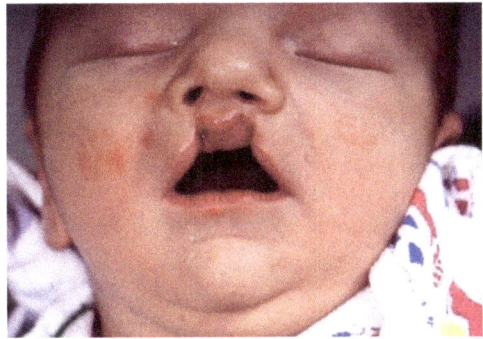 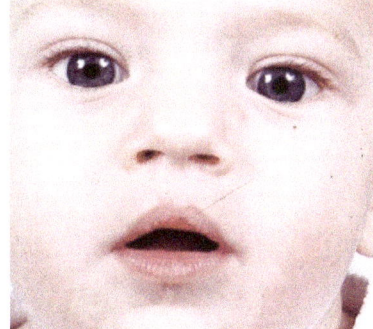

Although "Margarete," pictured below, had complete bilateral clefts of the lip and alveolus, she was fortunate to have an otherwise intact hard and soft palate, which was very favorable for the future growth of the face. I performed a single-stage cleft lip repair.

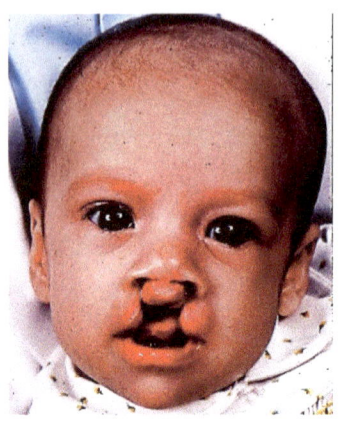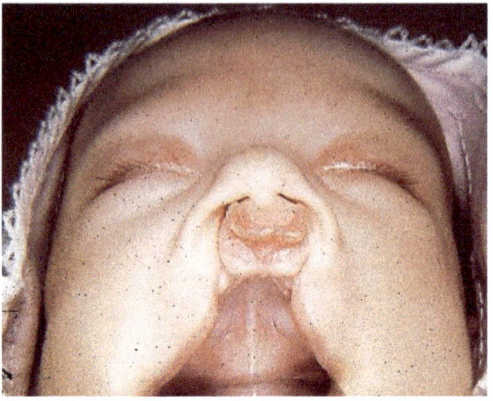

Below are her postoperative photos a few years later.

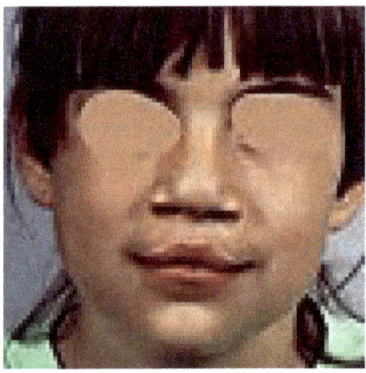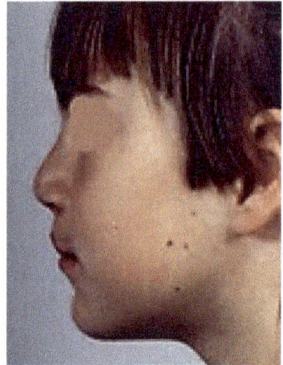

The patient below, "Marylin," had complete bilateral clefts of the lip. The central prolabial portion between the clefts is relatively large and overlaps the lateral lip segments on both sides. So, this is a narrow cleft, although it is complete on both sides.

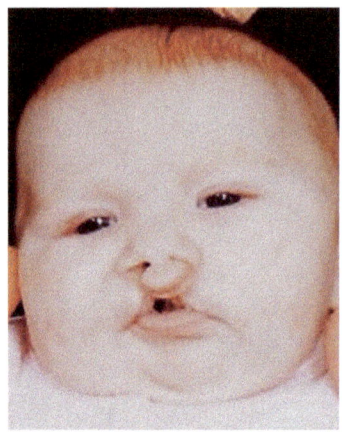

Her postoperative pictures from a few years later are below.

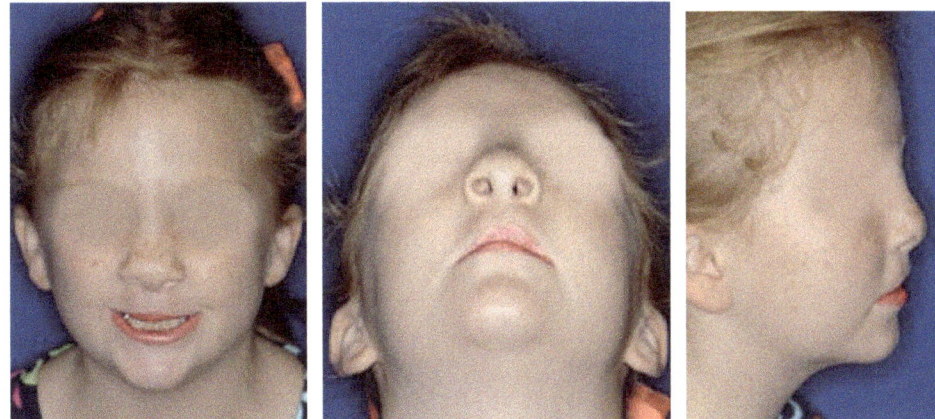

The baby boy below "Juan" has bilateral wide complete clefts of the lip and palate. The second photo is a few years after the repair of both sides of the labium in one operation.

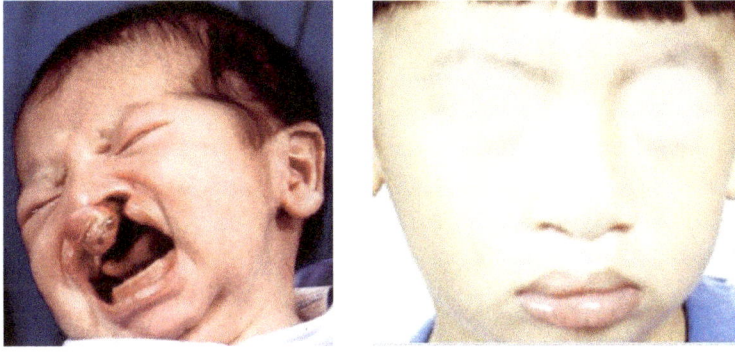

The baby below, "Jerome," had a complete bilateral cleft of the lip. I treated him with external elastic taping, which created backward pressure to recess the protruding premaxillary segment. I then performed tensionless straight-line lip closures.

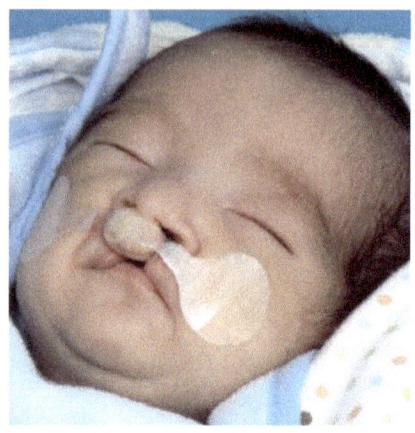 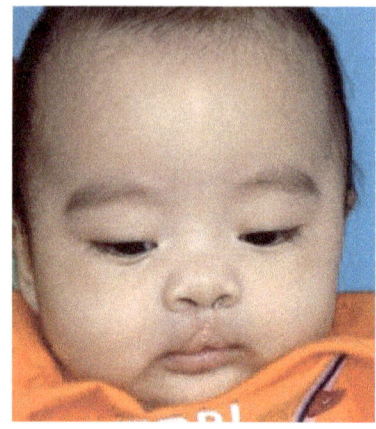

"Ophelia" shown below had complete bilateral clefts of the lip and palate. The prolabial portion of the upper lip is quite small. The premaxilla or central part of the gum is also tiny and twisted to the left side. I did a preliminary bilateral lip adhesion, picture in the second photograph later.

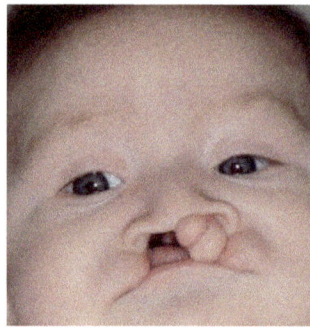 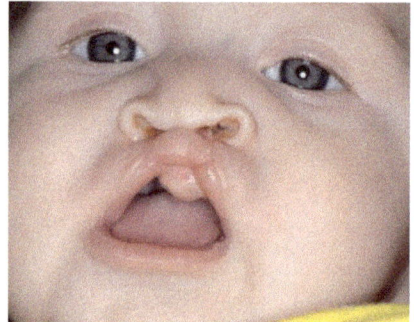

A few months later, I did the definitive lip repair. Below you see "Ophelia's" postoperative result a couple of years later.

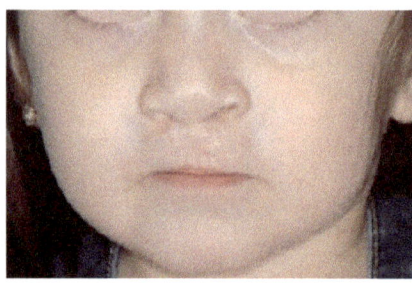 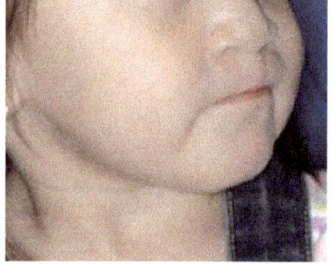

"Oscar'," below, had a complete bilateral cleft of the lip and palate. His premaxilla and prolabium protruded anteriorly. I treated him preoperatively with elastic straps for several weeks to push the premaxilla back to make the lip closure easier. His pre-op and seven years post-operative photos are below.

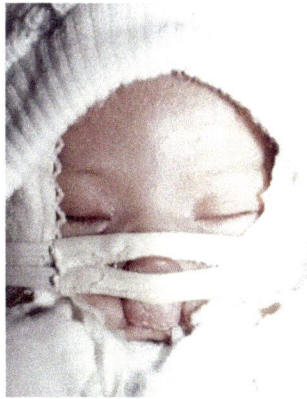 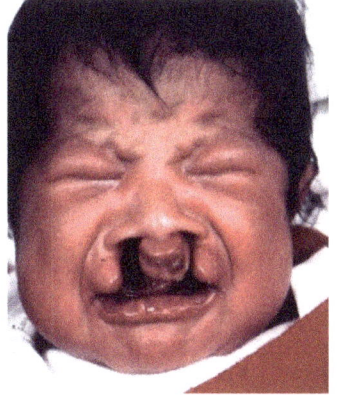 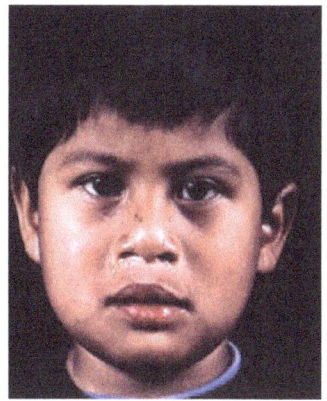

"Martin" was my last cleft lip patient before my unexpected early retirement. His before photo below demonstrates a wide cleft with severe nasal distortion. I did a small triangular flap technique for lip closure and also worked the nose at this first operation. His early after picture is below.

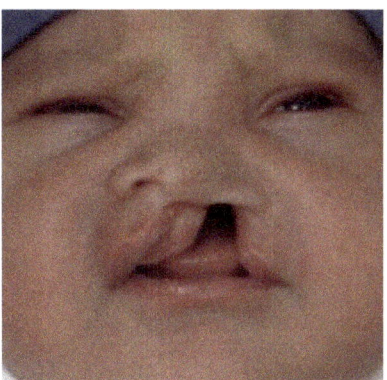 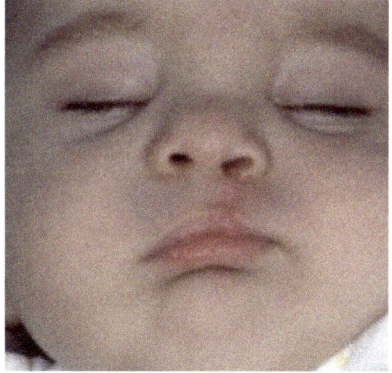

Cleft palate repair

Vomer flap

The two drawings below illustrate what is known as a vomer flap closure of the anterior palate. A vomer flap was once commonly used as the first stage in a two-stage palate repair. Now, most palate repairs are one stage, but the vomer flap may be the first part of that one-stage operation. The vomer is the bony part of the nasal septum immediately above the palate. In the first drawing below, the vomer is pointed out by the purple arrow.

It extends from the hard palate vertically upward into the nose as the nasal septum. In this vomer flap technique, the surgeon makes an incision along the blue line. He/she then undermines the mucosa and periosteum of the vomer and turns the vomer flap laterally towards the right side across the opening between the palate and the nose.

In the second drawing, the yellow represents bone exposed after the elevation of the vomer flap. The orange represents the underside of the mucosal and periosteal vomer flap, now sutured to the patient's right palate segment. This flap now separates the oral cavity from the nasal cavity for the anterior palate.

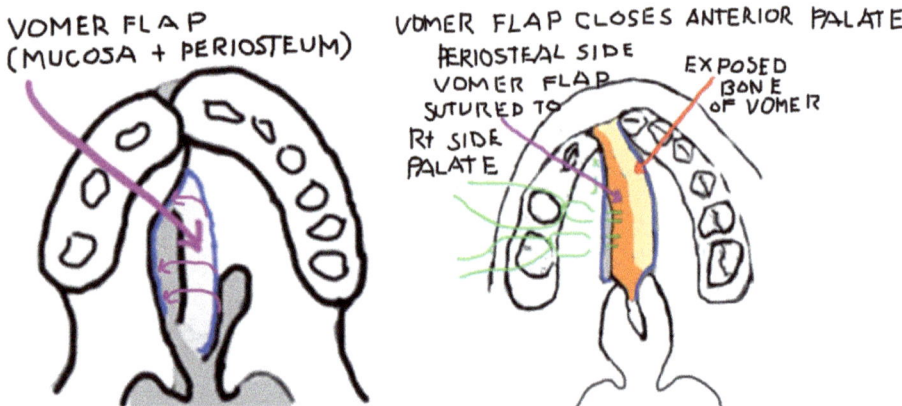

The two drawings below illustrate one of the two most common methods of palate closure. This one is known as a push back palatoplasty procedure. Often the first part of this two- flap operation is to complete a vomer flap as shown in the previous drawings above. The maroon color represents the levator veli palatini muscle, which is critical for normal speech but is abnormally split by the palate cleft. The red lines represent the greater palatine vessels, which are the blood supply for the flaps. The blue lines indicate incisions made to elevate the flaps. The green arrows indicate the proposed movement of the flaps posteriorly and medially.

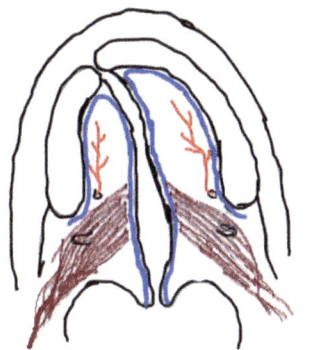 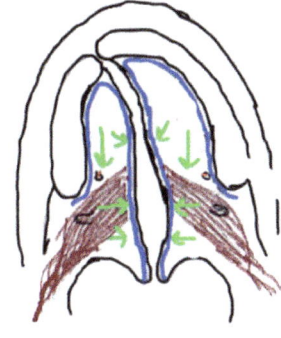

In the two drawings below, yellow represents bone of the hard palate exposed by the backward and medial displacement of the flaps. The main objective of palate surgery is to close the abnormal openings between the oral cavity and the nasal cavity and reconstruct the levator veli palatini muscle, which is critical for speech. Pushing the muscle back and sewing it together across the midline reconstitutes the levator portion of the velopharyngeal sphincter needed for normal speech.

The palate can now move upward and back to touch the posterior pharynx, preventing abnormal nasal air escape. Specific speech sounds require this sphincter action. The yellow area represents bone, which sometimes is left exposed as I show in this drawing. Otherwise, it may be covered by stretching and suturing the flaps back after the muscle repositioning.

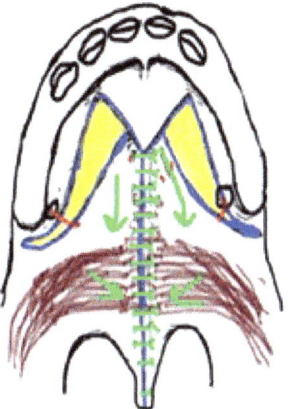 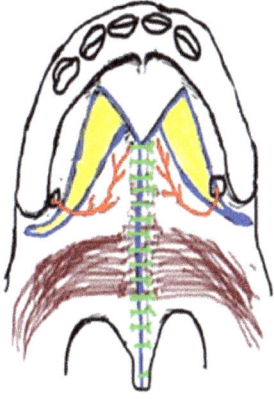

A second standard method of repairing the palate is known as the Furlow or double reverse Z-plasty technique. In the first drawing below, the surgeon first does a vomer flap. Then, as outlined in blue, he/she cuts the edges of the palate and creates four flaps from the soft palate tissues. One flap from each side contains mucosa and muscle, while two flaps contain only mucosa. The purpose of the Z-plasties is to lengthen the soft palate by borrowing lateral tissue.

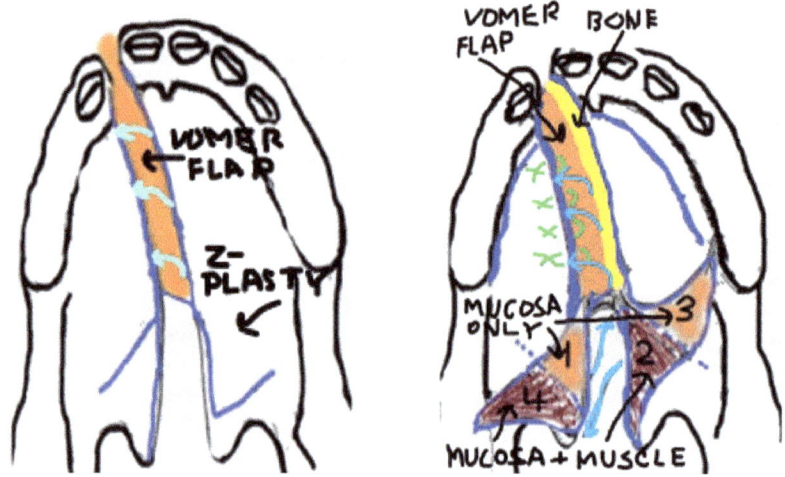

As shown below, rearranging these four flaps both completes the muscle sling and lengthens the soft palate. Also, the now intact palate separates the oral cavity from the nasal cavity anatomically and physiologically. Again in the drawings, the blue is for incisions. The surgeon closes the anterior part of the palate after making relaxing incisions laterally in the anterior palate on either side, which may expose some palate bone. The green color represents sutures.

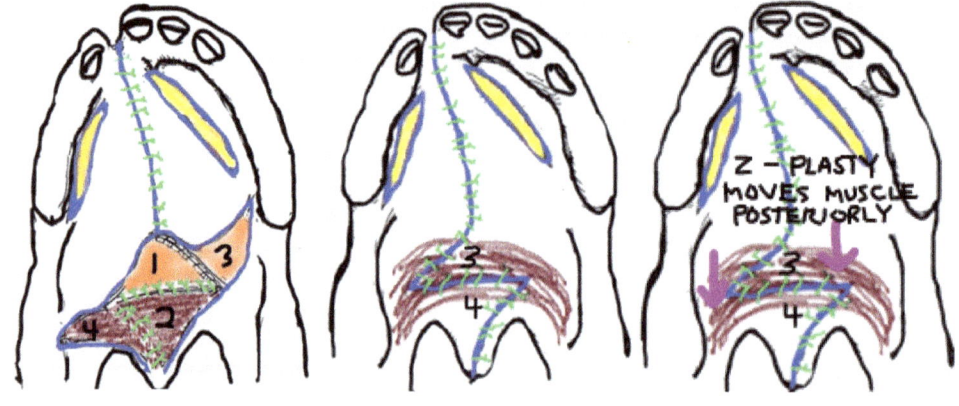

I produced the larger than life model shown below as a teaching device for plastic surgery residents. It can demonstrate various flaps and layers of tissue so that the three-dimensional anatomy of palate repair is better understood. The middle picture shows a small flap in the sulcus between the gum and the lip designed to close that portion of a congenital cleft, which sometimes is most difficult. The last photo on the right demonstrates a vomer flap being elevated and moved from the model's left palate to the right side to close the anterior palate.

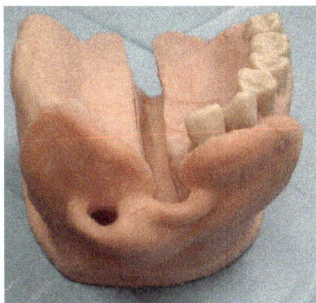 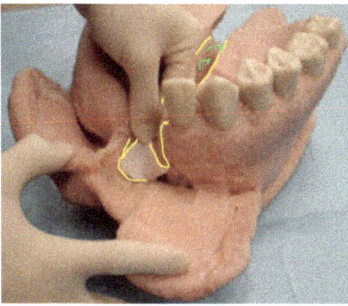 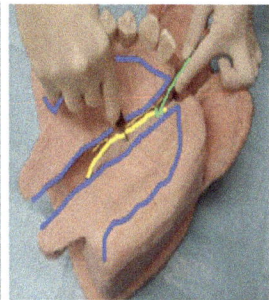

On the left below, an intraoperative photo shows a cleft palate opening in the roof of the mouth pointed out with the green arrow. Planned incisions for the two-flap technique are outlined in blue. The second picture shows the palatal flap on the patient's left side elevated.

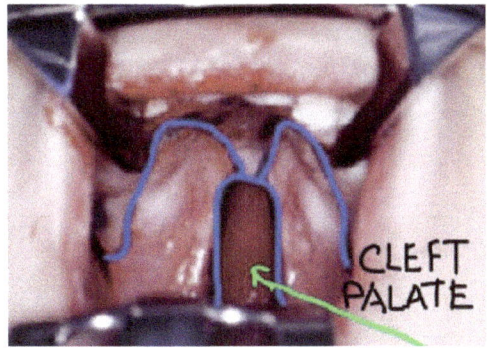 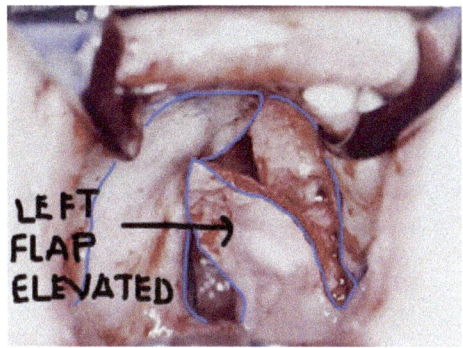

The next picture below shows both flaps have been pushed backward and sutured together in the midline to repair the opening in the palate and to allow the muscle repair to be posterior enough. The final picture shows the result of the palate surgery a few years later.

The Healing Mission of Plastic Surgery

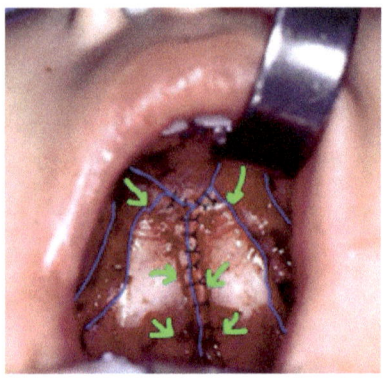 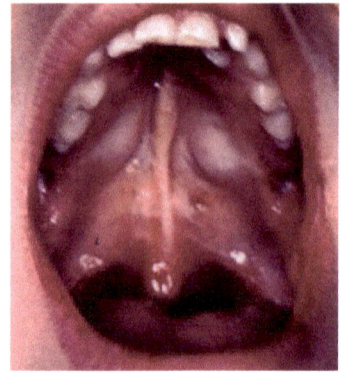

Below left, I show a before picture, and on the right, I show a photo after palate repair. In the first picture, you can see the reddish mucosa in the nasal cavity because of the wide cleft in the palate itself. In the second photo, one sees the intact roof of the mouth after the repair has fully healed.

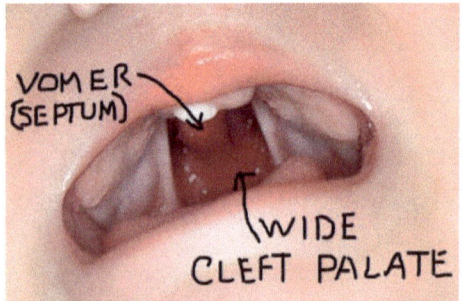 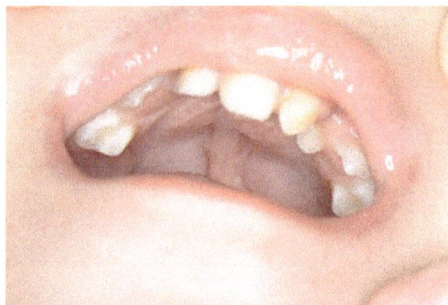

Again the primary purpose of repairing the palate is to allow for normal speech. Other benefits include better oral hygiene, better chewing, and less likelihood of ear infections, etc.

Velopharyngeal insufficiency (VPI)

A patient with an unrepaired cleft palate has very nasal speech, probably unintelligible, because of extreme nasal air escape (hypernasality). The most crucial reason for repairing the cleft in the roof of the mouth is to give the patient an opportunity for normal speech. However, initial palate repair does not always result in the physical structure capable of normal speech. Perhaps as many as 25% of patients who have a cleft palate repair have less than normal speech usually because of some level of continued hypernasality.

Of course, other speech issues are sometimes present, such as articulation errors. Sometimes these issues may be resolved with speech therapy. Otherwise, additional surgical intervention may be necessary to give the patient the structure needed for the development of normal speech. The first drawing below shows normal velopharyngeal closure, which prevents nasal air escape. When the soft palate moves upward and backward, and the pharyngeal wall constrictor muscles move slightly forward, the sphincter separates the oral from the nasal cavity. With most speech sounds, there is only air escaping through the mouth.

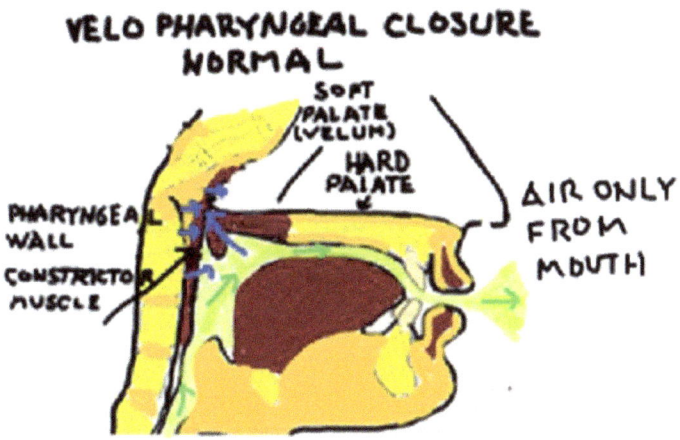

In contrast, the drawing below shows insufficient velopharyngeal sphincter action. In this case, air also escapes through the nose creating abnormal speech resonance.

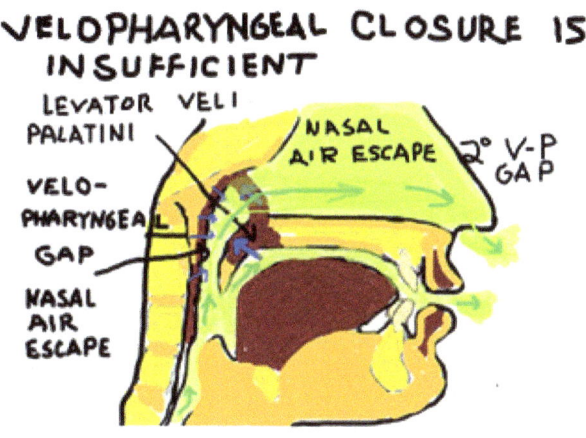

Because normal speech is so vital for human communication and interpersonal relationships, it is crucial to correct this problem. Sometimes revision surgery or even multiple revision surgeries are needed, but the vast majority of cleft palate patients can obtain normal speech. Several ingenious procedures developed by various plastic surgeons are available to help these patients achieve normal speech. I will briefly describe the most common ones.

Pushback palatoplasty

A palatal lengthening procedure (or pushback palatoplasty) performed on a previously repaired cleft palate may correct the problem. Probably the most common operation for velopharyngeal incompetence after palate repair is such a revision surgery on the palate. In that procedure, the surgeon elevates flaps from the hard palate and frees the levator veli palatini muscles and moves them back closer to the posterior pharyngeal wall. This procedure is similar to primary palate repair but adds to the posterior repositioning of the muscle sling. The first drawing below represents the situation of velopharyngeal insufficiency (VPI) with nasal air escape. The second drawing shows the palatal flaps outlined in red, which, when elevated, provide access to the levator muscles.

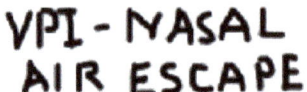

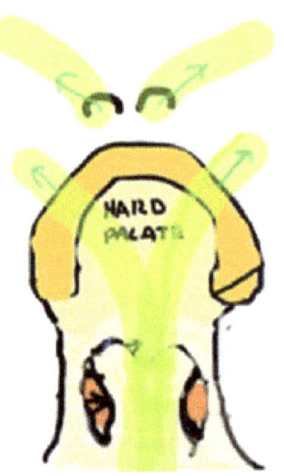 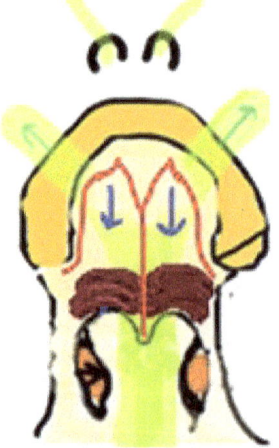

The next drawing below indicates the surgeon has pushed backward the levator veli palitini muscle so that it is nearer to the posterior pharyngeal wall preventing abnormal nasal air escape with speech. The surgeon has pushed back the palatal flaps from the hard palate leaving the raw pink area of exposed bone. Sometimes the surgeon frees and pushes the muscle back separately from these flaps and returns them to their original position. In that case, there is no exposed bone.

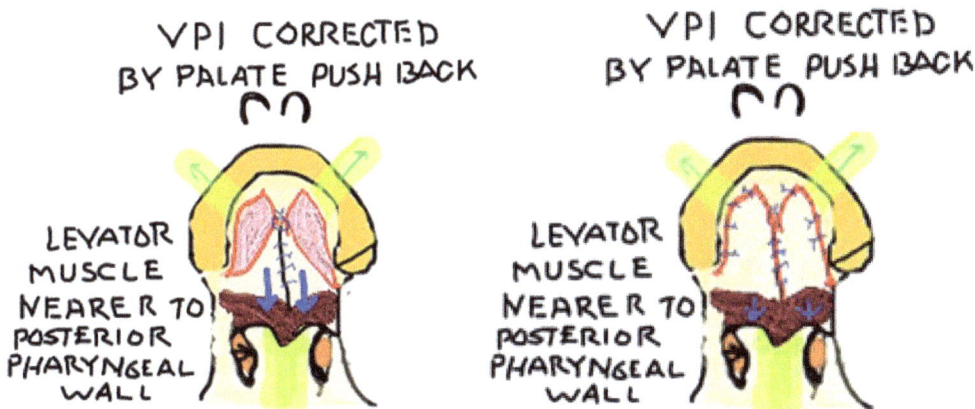

The drawing below is a sagittal view representing this same pushback palate procedure. Because of the repositioning of the levator veli palatini muscle posteriorly, it's action now is sufficient to complete the sphincter action together with the posterior pharyngeal constrictor muscles. Therefore, the VPI is corrected, and there will be no abnormal nasal air escape with speech.

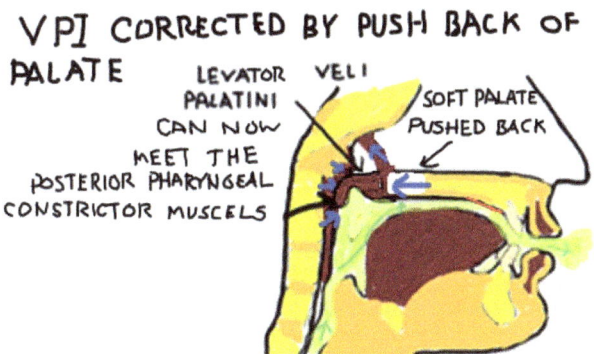

The first drawing below represents a view at the level of the wide-open velopharyngeal sphincter with a palate that is not posterior enough for sphincter closure. The second drawing represents active closure of the sphincter after correction with a pushback palatoplasty. The soft palate moves up and back through the action of the levator veli palitini muscles. In contrast, the pharyngeal constrictor muscles move the posterior and lateral pharyngeal walls anteriorly and medially, thus together closing the sphincter.

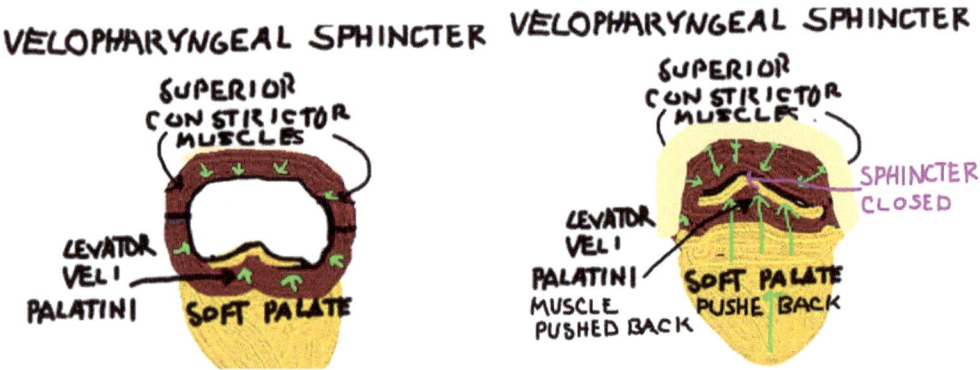

Another palate operation used to correct hypernasal speech caused by velopharyngeal insufficiency is the double reverse Z plasty described earlier. If that was not the original palate repair method, it could be used as a revision procedure to good effect to correct VPI by moving the levator veli palitini muscles more posteriorly so that closure can take place.

Pharyngeal flap

Alternatively, a pharyngeal flap procedure in which a flap of tissue from the posterior pharyngeal wall is connected to the posterior palate to prevent nasal air escape may be corrective. The pharyngeal flap is usually reserved for more severe cases or for cases that have failed to obtain natural resonance even after a secondary palatoplasty. The flap acts as an obturator by partially obstructing the velopharyngeal area.

This procedure changes the anatomy and is not physiologic. For that reason, I reserved this procedure more or less as a last resort for the correction of VPI. However, experience has shown this to be a very worthwhile procedure in many instances, and it has corrected cleft palate nasal speech in countless patients. In this procedure, the surgeon elevates a superiorly based flap of tissue containing mucosa and pharyngeal constrictor muscle from the posterior pharynx. The surgeon then turns the flap forward to meet an incision made in the posterior soft palate and sews them together.

The first sagittal plane drawing below illustrates a patient with velopharyngeal incompetence. There is nasal air escape with speech. The red lines indicate incisions in the posterior pharyngeal wall and the posterior aspect of the soft palate. The second drawing shows the superiorly based pharyngeal flap elevated from its inferior edge and turned forward and sutured into the receiving incision made in the soft palate. This superiorly based pharyngeal flap is an effective method that usually corrects the velopharyngeal insufficiency, as demonstrated in the drawing.

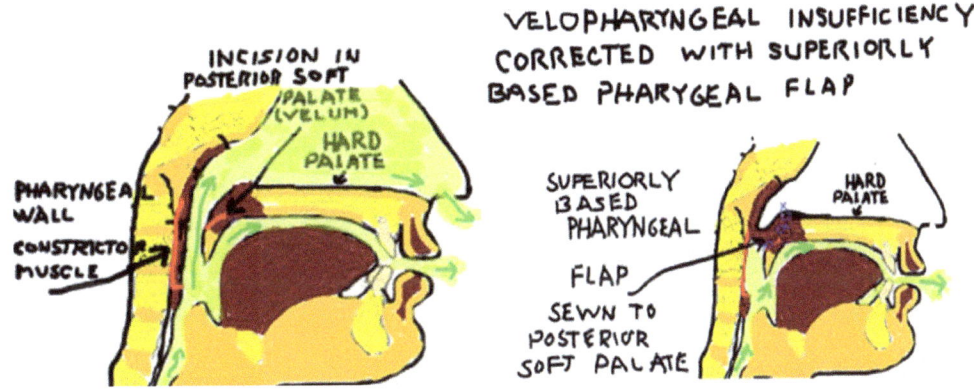

The two drawings below represent the views from inside the mouth. The first shows the pharyngeal flap outlined in red on the posterior pharyngeal wall. The dotted red line indicates an incision in the posterior edge of the soft palate for the insertion of the pharyngeal flap. There are a few somewhat different technical methods of making this connection. The second drawing shows the donor site sewn, and the flap turned upward and forward and sutured to the posterior soft palate. As noted before, this procedure usually corrects the velopharyngeal incompetence and prevents abnormal nasal air escape.

The Healing Mission of Plastic Surgery

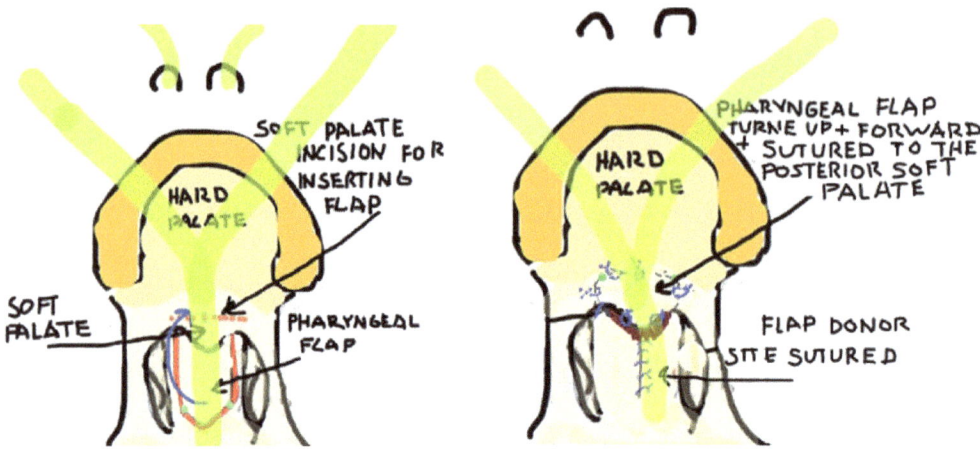

The drawings below represent the pharyngeal flap procedure at the level of the sphincter. A small port remains open on either side of the flap so that the patient can still breathe through the nose as in the first drawing. The patient retains mobility of the soft palate and now will be able to actively close off the oral from the nasal cavity to prevent nasal air escape with speech, as illustrated in the second drawing.

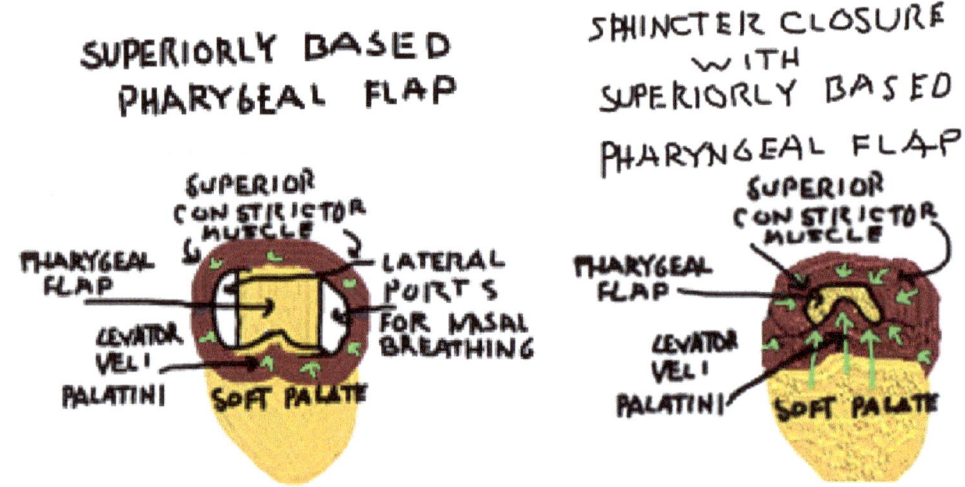

Sphincter Pharyngoplasty

Sphincter pharyngoplasty is another standard and useful procedure for the correction of velopharyngeal incompetence. There are several variations in this procedure. A typical example uses the palatopharyngeal muscles from the posterior tonsillar pillar. The surgeon develops superiorly based flaps of mucosa and muscle and turns them 90° upward and towards the midline of the posterior pharynx. The surgeon then overlaps them to create a muscle mound in the posterior pharynx opposite the soft palate. They act in two ways, both as a dynamic action to aid in the closure of the velopharyngeal sphincter and as a muscle mass for the levator veli palatini to abut.

The first draw shows the palatopharyngeus muscles constituting the posterior tonsillar pillar on either side. This muscle connects the palate to the pharynx inferiorly. The surgeon elevates the superiorly based flap, including the mucosa and muscle. The second drawing shows the flaps after the surgeon rotates them 90° towards the midline. The surgeon makes an incision in the posterior pharyngeal wall opposite the velum and sutures the overlapping flaps to the posterior pharyngeal wall.

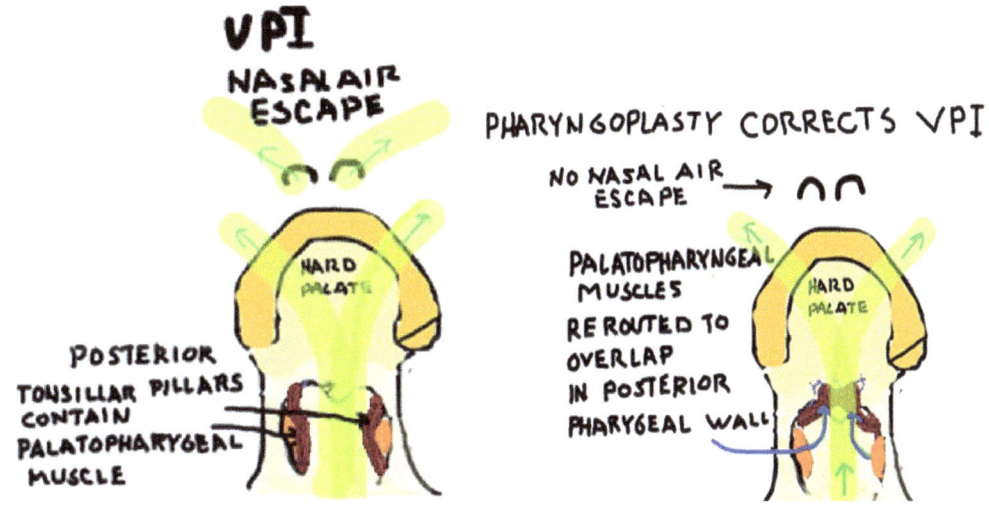

Below, the sagittal view of the sphincter pharyngoplasty operation shows the palatopharyngeal muscle overlapped from either side, creating a fuller posterior pharyngeal wall for the velum (soft palate) to oppose.

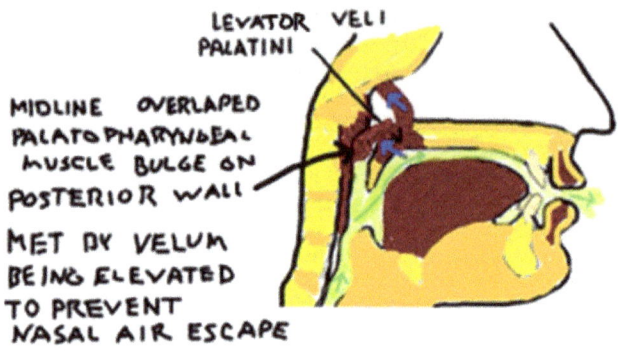

The first drawing below shows that the sphincter pharyngoplasty leaves a smaller central opening for breathing through the nose rather than a small opening on either side as with the posterior pharyngeal flap. The second illustration shows a closed sphincter with the action of the palate moving back and up and the posterior pharyngeal wall moving forward and medially with the aid of the palatopharyngeus muscles

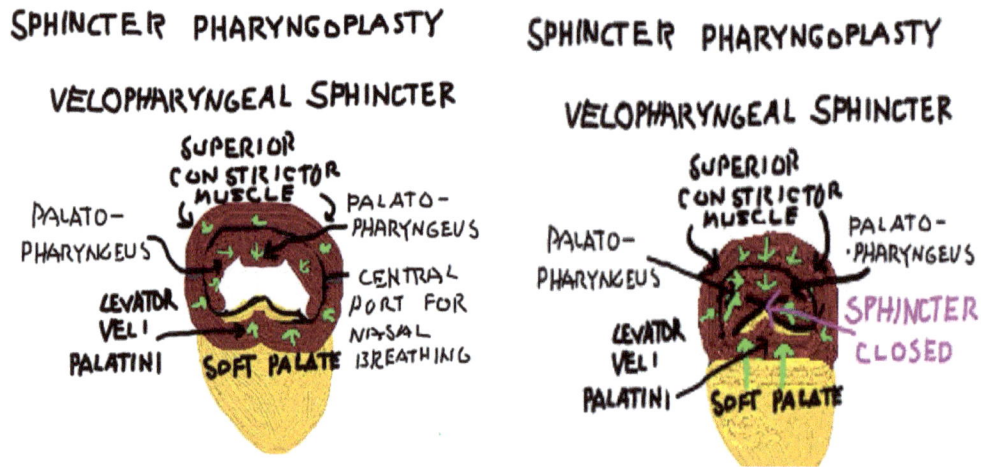

Augmentation posterior pharyngeal wall

A less standard procedure is to augment the posterior pharyngeal wall so that a previously repaired palate has less distance to go before it can fulfill its function as part of the velopharyngeal sphincter. I have used various synthetic materials with success for augmentation of the posterior pharyngeal wall to correct velopharyngeal incompetence. Other substances used for this purpose are cartilage and, more recently, fat grafts. In the drawing below, the purple represents an implant placed beneath the constrictor muscles of the posterior pharyngeal wall opposite the soft palate. The surgeon places the implant as high as possible in the posterior pharynx beneath the constrictor muscles. The surgeon makes the vertical incision well below the site of the implant, so they do not overlap. As demonstrated in the second drawing, the soft palate has less distance to go to reach the posterior pharyngeal wall because of the implant.

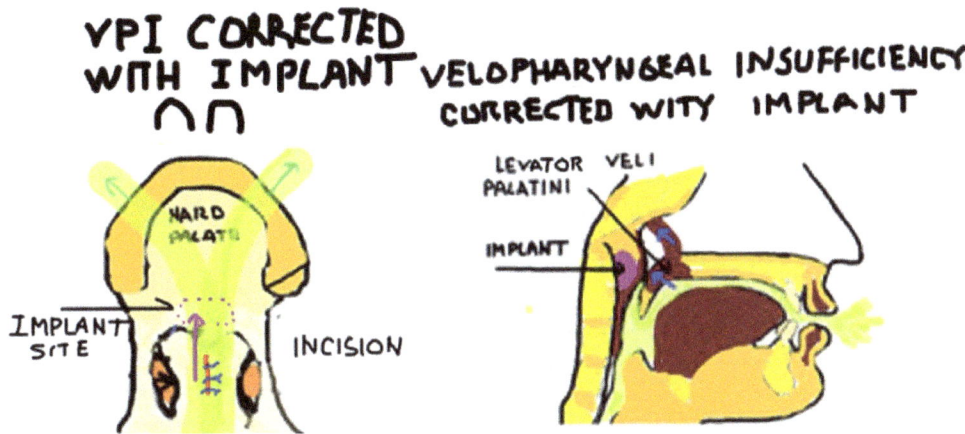

The sphincter level views below show the position of the implant and the physiological action of obtaining sphincter closure

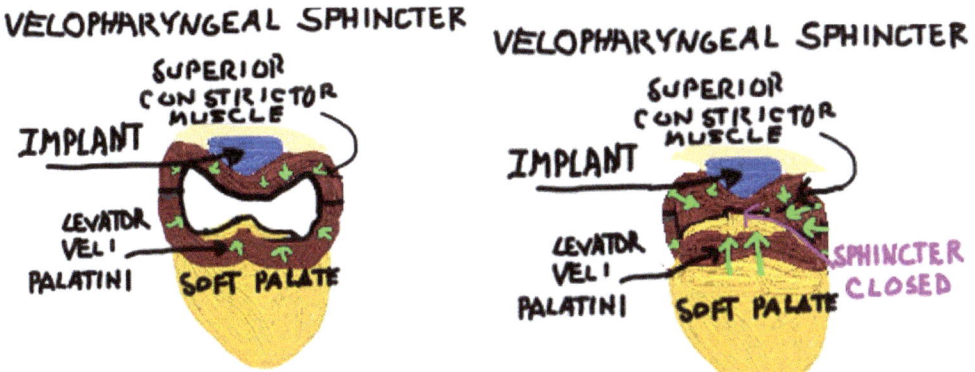

Most patients will be able to obtain natural resonance with good speech after a primary cleft palate repair. Appropriate utilization of the above techniques will correct the minority who have residual VPI after palate closure.

Bone grafting

Most patients with complete clefts of the labium and palate will require bone grafting into the alveolar cleft area, usually between the ages of six and 12 years of age. There are three reasons for bone grafting. The first reason is to buttress the teeth adjacent to the cleft; the second is to improve the contour of the upper lip and finally to support the nasal ala.

The most common source for bone is the iliac crest in the hip area. Other possible sources of bone are the skull, the tibia, and the chin. There are also bone substitutes that are sometimes employed. One option for bone grafting is a bone morphogenetic protein (BMP), which is a protein that stimulates the formation of new bone.

I have used BMP in a unique way that I believe has not been described. I have utilized BMP together with bone harvested from the nasal turbinate and the bony nasal septum, which does not seem to add to the discomfort the patient already has from the alveolar dissection. It is much less involved than iliac or cranial bone graft harvesting.

The first photo below shows exposure in the alveolar cleft area. The middle photograph shows the bone, harvested from the turbinate and nasal septum, being wrapped up like small tacos with the carrier sponge. I place these "tacos" in the alveolar cleft as a bone graft with BMP stimulation, as shown in the third photo.

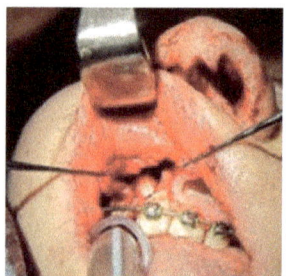 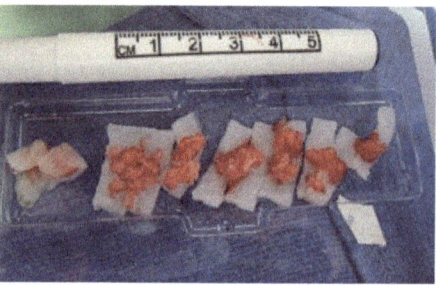 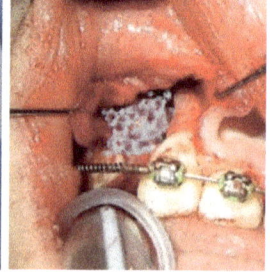

The first picture below is preoperative. The second photo shows where I placed the graft under the ala base in the alveolus. The third picture is the postoperative result.

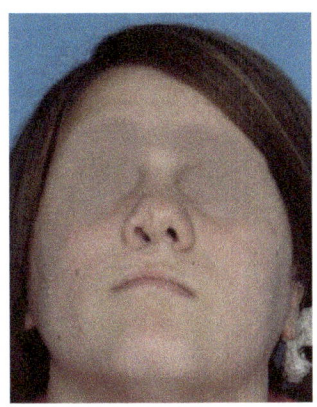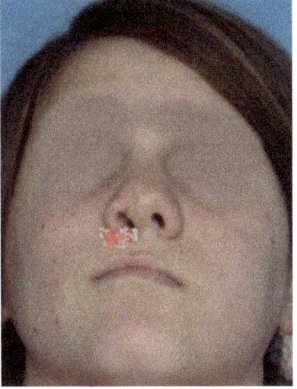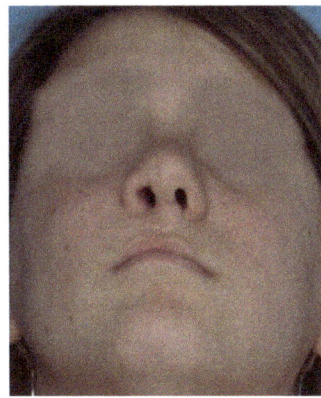

A patient like this might now be able to receive osseointegrated dental implants. Cleft lip and palate patients need a sophisticated multispecialty team for optimum care.

Secondary cleft lip and palate surgery

When we see secondary cases, we never know whether our result might have been better for the patient than what the patient received. We frequently see examples of suboptimal secondary cases in consultation. However, we know that a portion of our cases have also turned out to have suboptimal results, and perhaps they are seeing other cleft palate surgeons. So, we always give the benefit of the doubt to the previous surgeons in such cases.

Patients go to doctors seeking relief of discomfort. Patients see plastic surgeons because they want correction of imperfections, which may be functional, reconstructive, or aesthetic. They do this to improve body image, self-image, and self-esteem. Mainly, they want to feel better about themselves. Cleft lip and palate patients may have their essential, functional surgeries completed in childhood. However, they may still seek secondary surgery because of residual abnormal structures related to the cleft lip or palate.

They sometimes also desire aesthetic improvements in areas unaffected directly by the cleft lip and palate. Patients often want additional surgery because of such problems as tight or scarred upper lips, nasal asymmetry, midface under development, relative overdevelopment of the lower jaw, and occlusal or bite problems.

The psychological discomfort the patients suffer does not necessarily relate to the severity of the residual deformity. Neither is improvement necessarily proportional to the measurable success of the surgery. In these patients, functional success includes normal speech, mastication, and respiration, as well as normal hearing.

Aesthetic success is much more arbitrary and depends on the patient's acceptance of the "final" result. When I evaluate secondary cases, I need to understand the patient's goals and assess whether the goals are obtainable. I have been gratified in many instances by intervention in such cases, where improvement through surgery is possible for the residual deformities. The patients must have the right attitude and want surgery. I saw patients with similar remaining problems. One might wish nothing while the other is ready to try anything to gain improvement. Standard operations may include the movement of the upper jaw forward for an underdeveloped midface. Such a procedure can also correct some bite problems. Another typical intervention is nasal surgery to improve the contour of the nose, including asymmetries.

Furthermore, revision of the scar of the upper lip is frequent. Occasionally an operation is done in which we take tissue from the lower lip and bring it to the upper lip to improve contour and function. It requires two stages to complete the transfer of this flap. Several examples of these different secondary procedures will follow.

The first example is a simple revision of a bilateral cleft lip. "George" illustrates a short upper lip that also has a "whistle" deformity. I excised the two old vertical scars. I then brought tissue from the lateral mucosa to the midline. I then re-sutured the lip lengthening the philtrum. He started with two vertical scars and ended up with a goalpost shaped scar.

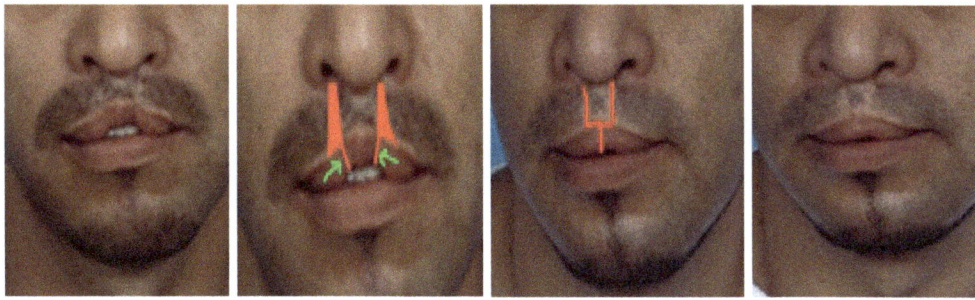

The patient below, "Martin," had some residual problems after bilateral cleft lip procedures. He especially wanted his stubbed nose released. He also had a wide philtrum of his lip.

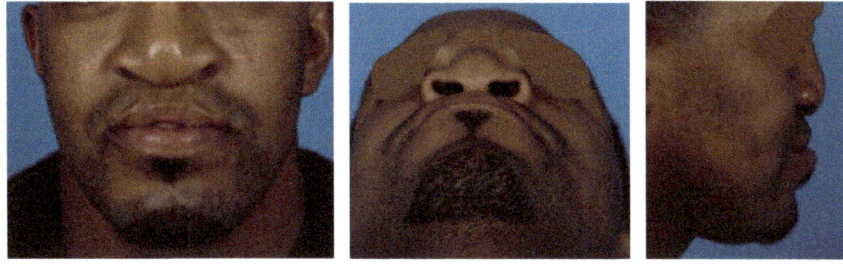

I performed a lip revision to narrow the philtrum and improve the lip scars. At the same time, I did a rhinoplasty. I released the nasal tip and elongated the columella; which allowed for much better nasal tip projection

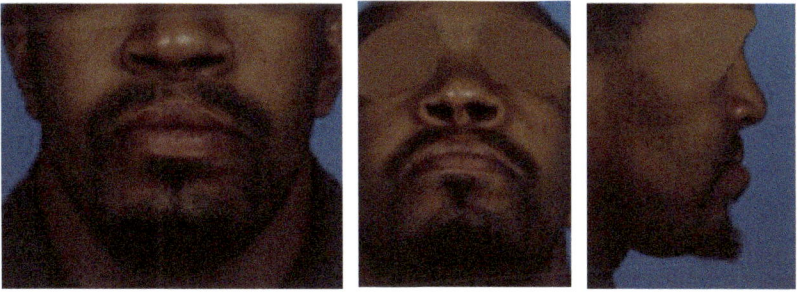

The next example is more complex.

Up from the valley

One afternoon I received a call from a plastic surgeon in the Texas Rio Grande valley. He had just seen a 15-year-old boy with significant residual deformities from a congenital cleft of the lip and palate that he thought was quite challenging. Because he was not doing this type of

The Healing Mission of Plastic Surgery

surgery, he wanted to refer him to me for workup and treatment. (Probable 10% or fewer plastic surgeons do 90% or more of the lip and palate work.) A week or so later, the 15-year-old boy "John" and his mother came to the office for a consultation.

This boy "John" had already had approximately eight surgical procedures. The first lip repair surgery was at three months of age in Germany at an army hospital. The last surgery was about five years previous. He had several residual problems, including the distortion of the nose, difficulty breathing through both sides of the nose. He had a prominent lip scar with a deficiency of tissue near the midline of the lip. Also, he had some teeth that were erupting in a disorganized manner. There was also a hole in the palate, which led from the oral cavity to the nasal cavity. Two additional problems were the most significant. One problem was that the midface and upper jaw area were deficient, giving him a malocclusion. The other was a retruded chin, which was too long vertically. "

John" is shown below as he first presented to me at 15 years of age.

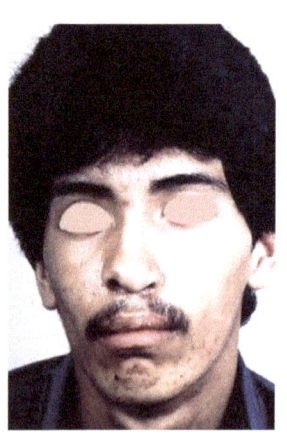 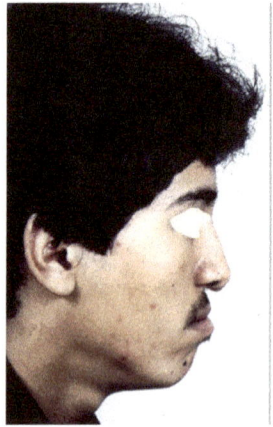

His was quite a complicated case, so I arranged for him to come to our cleft palate and facial reconstruction clinic, where he could get consultations by doctors in other disciplines as well as plastic surgery. We made a surgical plan, including an orthodontic workup, which would need to be carried out locally in the Rio Grande valley. So, we had the cleft clinic orthodontist correspond with the patient's orthodontist in the valley.

The first surgery involved a revision of the cleft lip, extraction of two mal-positioned teeth, and closure of fistulae openings between the palate and the nose. "John" now had better oral hygiene and improved dentition. About eight months later, after the orthodontic work had progressed, I performed a major surgery in which I moved the upper jaw (midface) forward and secured the new position with titanium plates and screws, as shown in the photo below. Planning for the maxillary advancement included impressions of the bite and plaster dental models. I then used an articulator like the one shown below to align the predicted postoperative bite through pre-operative "surgery "on the plaster models.

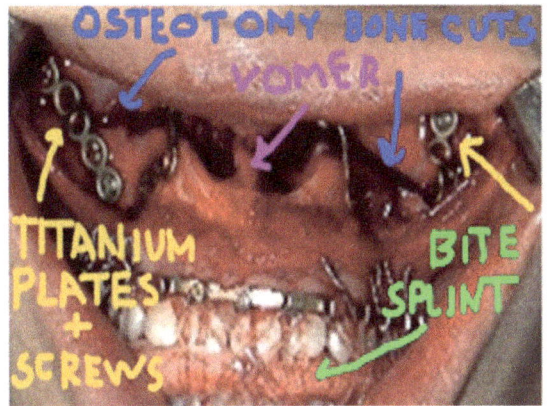 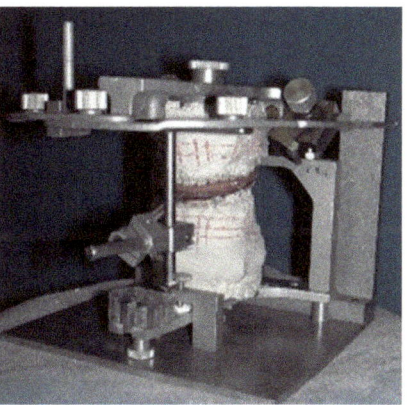

This patient's upper jaw was too far back, and his top teeth were behind his lower teeth. I brought the jaw forward so that post-op his face was more balanced, and he now had a normal occlusion. At that time, I also augmented the midface with synthetic material.

During the early postoperative time, he had his teeth locked together, and he was on a liquid diet for a couple of weeks. I then took off the rubber bands between the upper and lower jaw. This procedure was quite successful and gave him a sound bite. I performed the third stage a few months later. I then operated on his nose, straightening the nasal septum

The Healing Mission of Plastic Surgery

to help correct the breathing problem, and adjusted the external shape of the nose to give it a more pleasing and symmetrical appearance. At that time, I also worked on the chin bone, cutting it and moving the chin bone forward and upward to improve his general profile and to help him obtain better lip competence.

Comparing his preoperative pictures with the below postoperative photos demonstrate a vast improvement after this series of significant surgeries. A lot of credit needs to go to the orthodontist as well for helping to line up "John's" teeth in preparation for the operation and to fine-tune their position postoperatively. The last two photos are his final result after the three procedures.

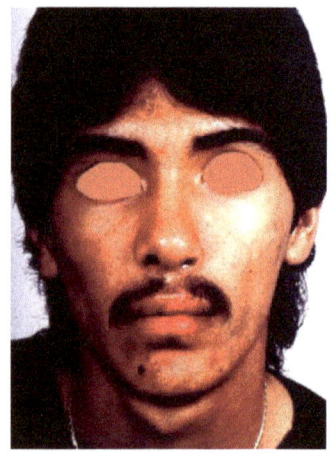
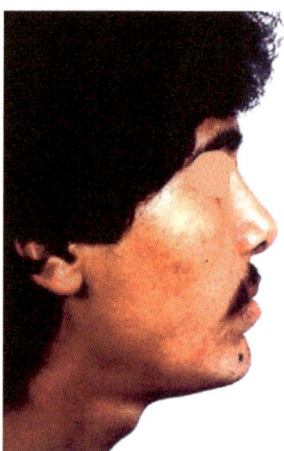

I first saw the patient below, "Franklin," as a 19-year-old who came to me to see if I could do anything for him. He had had a unilateral cleft lip and palate repaired in childhood. However, he still had openings in the roof of the mouth into the nasal cavity. He was also interested in any cosmetic improvement possible. His preoperative photos are below.

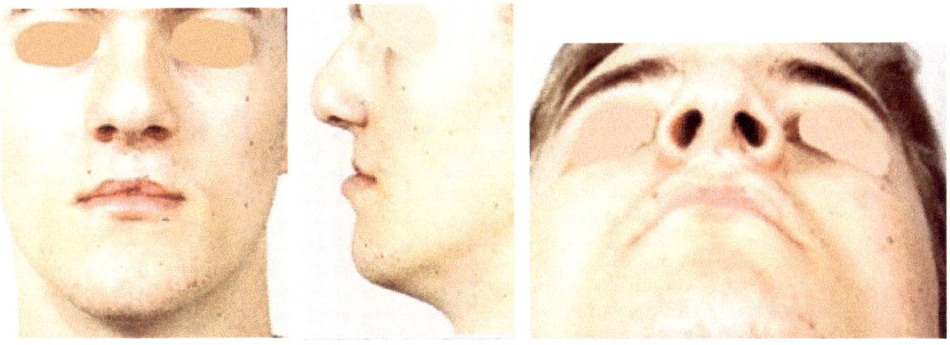

I did three operations on him. The first was the repair of the residual abnormal openings (fistulae) between the mouth and the nose through the palate. The second operation was a Le Fort I for maxillary advancement. I brought the midface forward after having made osteotomy cuts through the facial bones. The third procedure was a rhinoplasty with cartilage grafts to the tip of the nose. His post-operative photos are below.

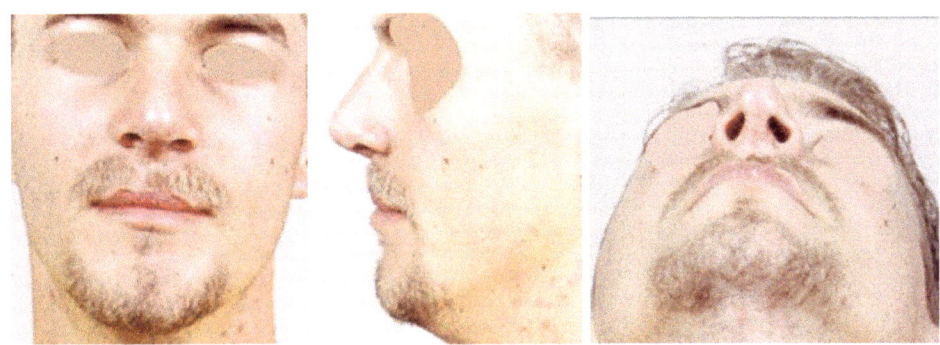

"Major" presented for secondary revision surgery. I performed a rhinoplasty, a genioplasty (moved the chin forward and upward and slightly to the left), and lip revision. His pre- op and post-op photos are below. Several years later, he and his wife brought their newborn child to me to repair his cleft lip.

The Healing Mission of Plastic Surgery

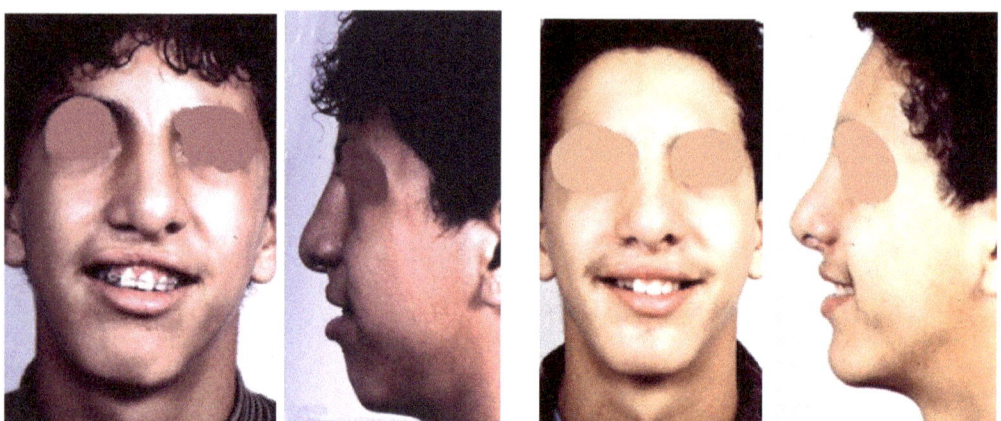

"Angelica" shown below had a tip rhinoplasty and also had a Le Fort I operation, in which I advanced the upper jaw or maxilla forward. The Le Fort I operation was to correct her malocclusion as well as improve her profile. Pre-operative photos are below. In the preoperative occlusion below, her upper central incisors are posterior to the lower front teeth.

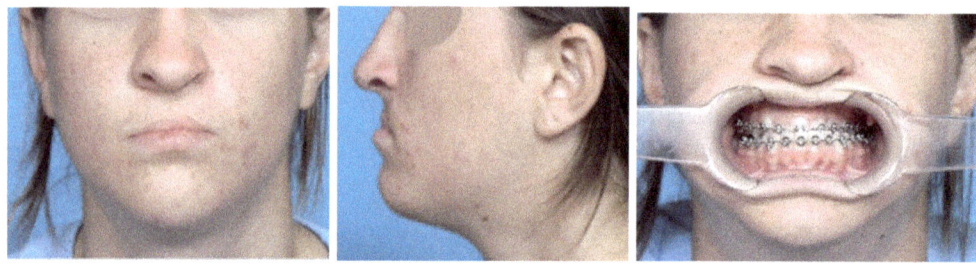

In the intra-operative photo on the left below, the green arrows point out the osteotomy cuts. The yellow arrow shows a lack of bone in the pre-maxillary area on the patient's left. The second photo shows I have pushed down the Le Fort I lower jaw fragment to mobilize it fully. The purple arrow points out the vomer (or nasal septum). The blue arrow shows a tear in the floor of the nose, which I must repair before completing the surgery. The green arrow points to the left maxillary sinus, which I transected as part of the operation.

The Healing Mission of Plastic Surgery

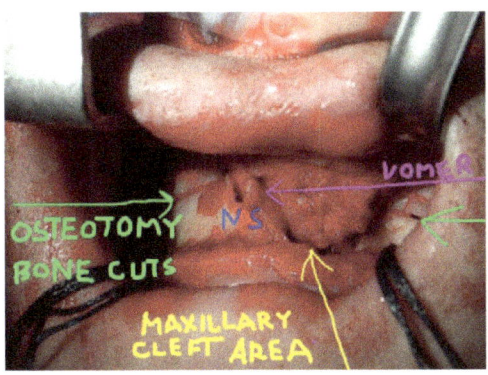 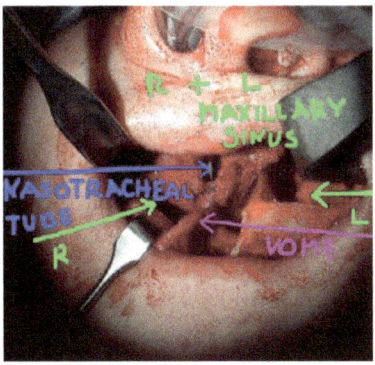

When a Le Fort I is done on a patient with cleft palate often, there is significant scar tissue, which makes mobilization of the Le Fort I fragment difficult. That was the situation in this case, so I utilized these large disimpaction forceps to help mobilize the maxilla so it could be reposition anteriorly.

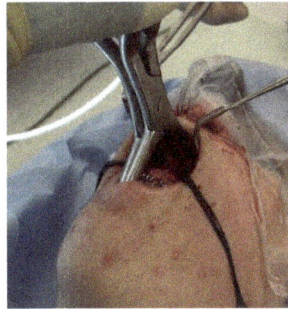 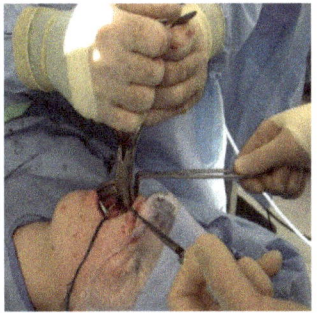

Below are "Angelica's" postoperative photos. In the postoperative occlusion below, her upper central incisors are slightly anterior to the lower front teeth, and she has an improved occlusion compared to her pre-operative situation

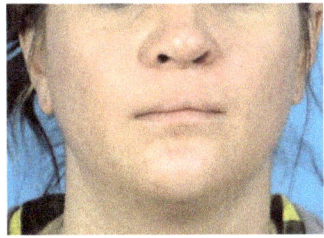 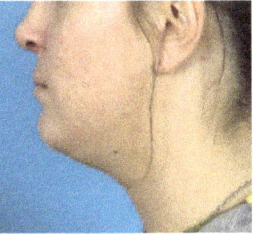 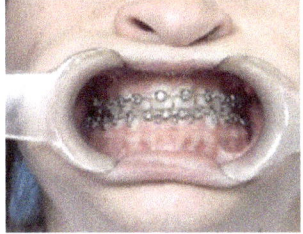

This teenager "Joseph had received proper medical care for his cleft lip and palate but had a retruded midface. I performed a Le Fort I advancement of the midface and a rhinoplasty, thereby correcting the

profile imbalance, improving his occlusion, and giving him more nasal symmetry.

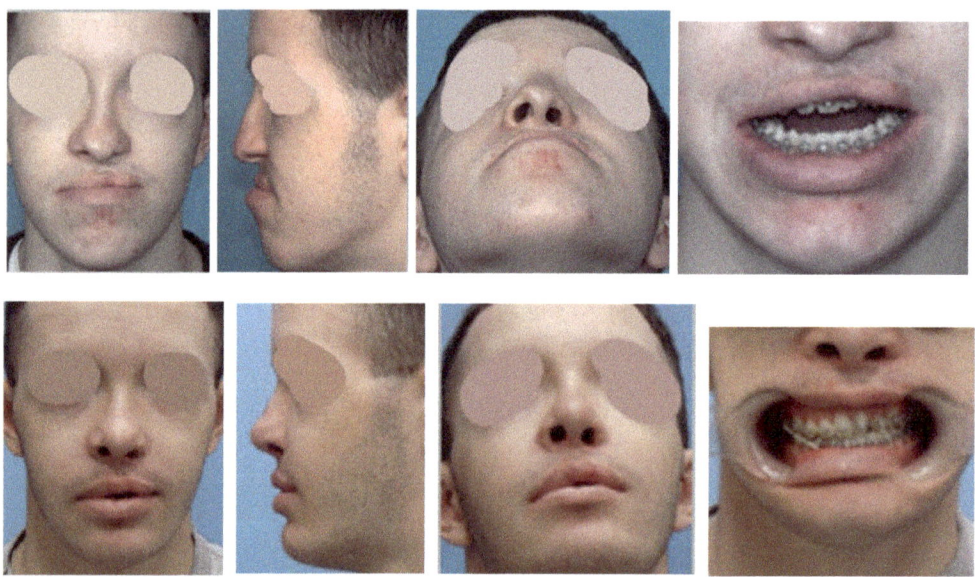

The patient below was a patient of Thomas Cronin. He wanted to perform a rhinoplasty on this patient, but because of her midface retrusion, he first arranged for me to do a Le Fort I advancement of the midface. Her preoperative and postoperative photos are below.

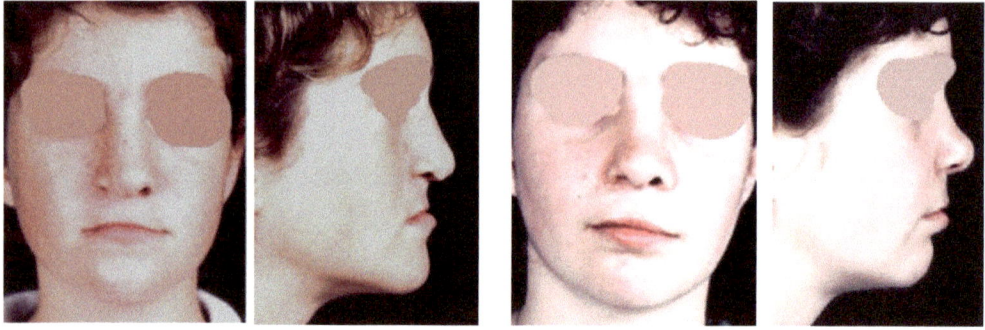

"Roberto" had a maxillary retrusion with a class IIII malocclusion. A Le Fort I advancement improved his profile as well as his occlusion. His pre and postoperative photos are below.

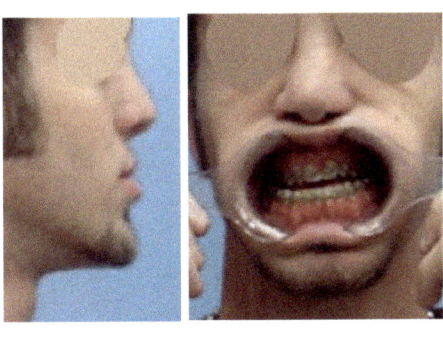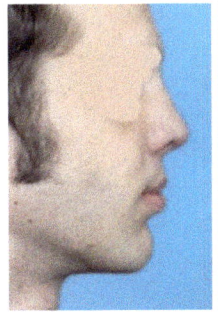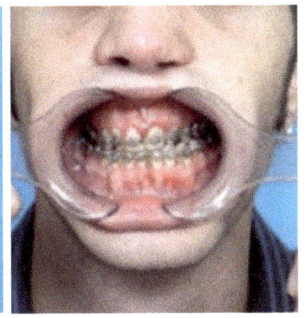

The patient below "Donna" is like many other patients who were born with complete bilateral clefts of the lip and palate. She had already undergone standard procedures on the labium and palate and several revision surgeries. I believed she could benefit from additional surgery. After discussing this with the patient and her mother, we decided that a cross lip Abbe flap would be beneficial. So, the last of her operations was an Abbe flap, which brought tissue from the lower lip into the upper lip in a two-stage procedure like the previous patient shown near the end of chapter 1. Her upper lip was too short and was a little flat on profile.

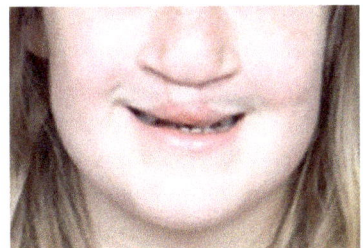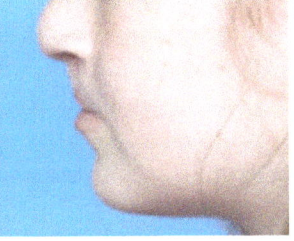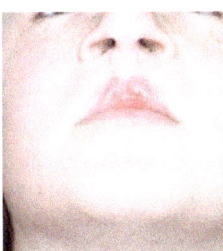

I first worked to free the tethered nose by freeing the philtrum portion of the upper labial tissue. I allowed it to slide upward, thereby lengthening the short nasal columella.

Next, I brought tissue from the lower lip into the upper lip. The first interoperative picture below shows a wedge of lower lip tissue, still connected by a small bridge, turned into the upper lip. You can see I have already sutured the lower lip flap donor site. One can appreciate the release of the tip and lengthening of the columella in the second photo below.

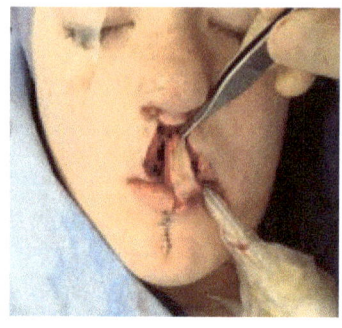 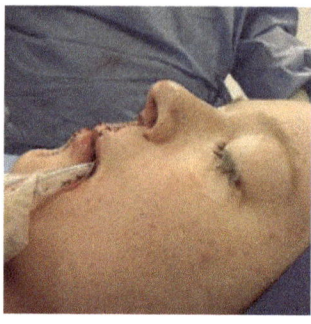

The three post-Abbe flap pictures below demonstrate that the lip has been lengthened and made fuller, giving a better profile. Also, I have increased the nasal columella, thereby allowing the proper projection of the nasal tip. This procedure significantly improved the patient's facial aesthetics, thus improving her body image and giving a boost to her self-esteem.

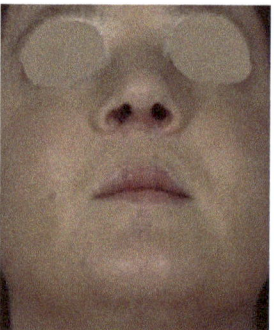 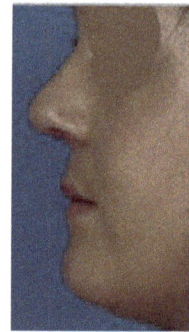 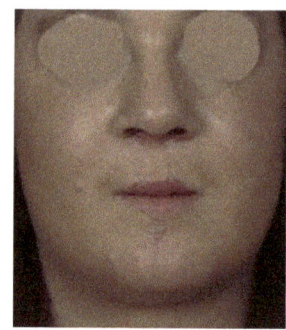

One of the ancillary activities undertaken by the Cronin and Brauer Cleft Clinic was an annual Christmas party for the patients and their families, which we conducted for about 20 years. Pictured below are my wife and me together with other volunteer hosts for the party.

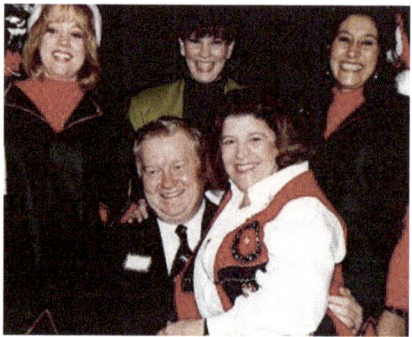

This Christmas party was fun and quite therapeutic for many of the patients and their families. We ordinarily had many arts and crafts activities, music, Santa Claus, and sometimes a magician, as well as food and drink. Many parents said that their children began to talk about this party when Thanksgiving came around. Other activities replaced this party when the cleft clinic merged and moved to the Shriners Hospital.

We tried to get some of our adult or older teenage patients to come to the party to be good role models for the younger cleft patients. Among those, we could always count on was Steven Decker, a former bilateral cleft lip and palate patient. He is pictured below with me for a Christus Foundation for Health Care brochure. Steven demonstrated his poise and friendly presence when he made a brief presentation (with totally normal speech) for the ribbon-cutting ceremony at the Cronin and Brauer Cleft Palate Clinic at Shriners Hospital for Children. The interim photos on the right below demonstrate some of Steven's previous issues and his progress through the cleft clinic.

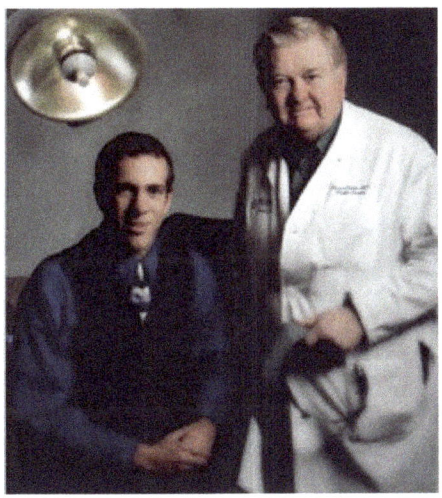 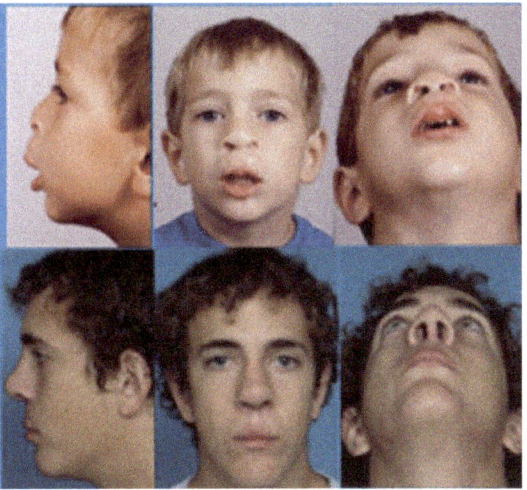

In the montage below are aggregated just a few of the patients I was privileged to be able to treat at the Cronin Brauer cleft palate clinic during my plastic surgery career.

The Healing Mission of Plastic Surgery

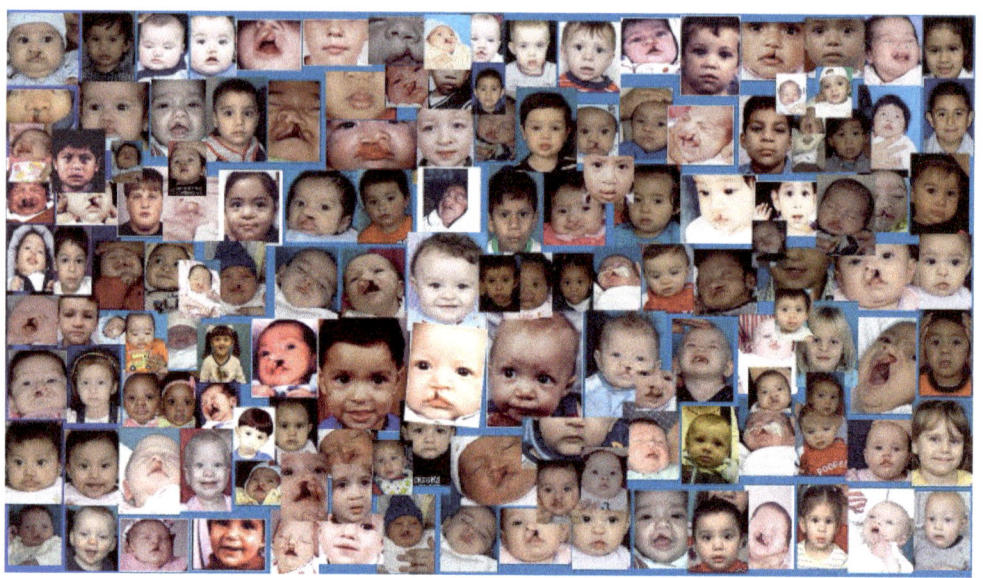

Chapter 8

Thomas Cronin and the Silicone Gel Breast Implant

History

As far back as the 19th century, there are reports of breast augmentation with various materials such as ivory, bone, glass, metal, and paraffin. We can only imagine how those results looked and felt. Before the development of modern breast implants, augmentation by injection of silicone liquid or other substances was reasonably common, especially in Japan and other far eastern countries. I saw eight or ten patients with problems because of these injections. Most had indurated lumps in the breasts, which were often painful. Some patients, in which the silicone or other substance had migrated very superficially into the skin, developed nonhealing sores that were uncomfortable and continuously inflamed.

Some of these patients needed mastectomies to rid themselves of these hygiene and pain problems. When possible, I did a subcutaneous mastectomy; that is, I removed the breast tissue from beneath the skin if the skin was not involved. I then place a modern breast implant beneath the skin flap or deeper beneath a layer of muscle. These patients were quite appreciative of getting out of their pain yet still being able to have the appearance and feel of breasts. I present a particularly tragic example of one of these injection cases in chapter 12 under the subtitle Leather Chest.

In the 1950s, surgeons occasionally used various synthetic sponge implants such as Ivalon for breast augmentation. Below on the left is a diagrammatic representation of a breast sponge specimen cut in half. Before implantation, it is very porous and pliable, similar to a kitchen sponge. After implantation, there is fibrous ingrowth for a few millimeters into the sponge. Still, there is also gradual shrinkage of the implant and collapse of the interstices causing these breast implants to become extremely firm inevitably. Because of this complication, few surgeons performed this procedure. The drawing on the right below represents a firm, shrunken implant with fibrous ingrowth on the periphery, as it might look after removal from a patient and cut in half.

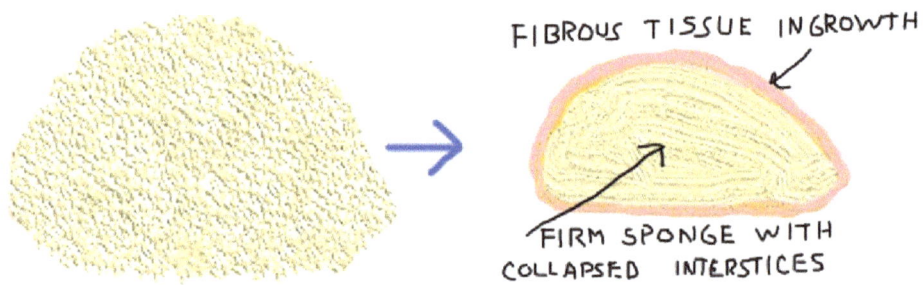

As the 1960s began, all this was about to change radically because of Drs. Thomas Cronin and Frank Gerow

Dr. Frank Gerow (below on the left) was a plastic surgery resident working with Dr. Thomas Cronin (below middle) in the early 1960s. He squeezed one of the new plastic bags filled with blood and told Dr. Cronin that he thought it felt soft like a woman's breast. Below right is pictured an old glass bottle for blood transfusion next to the plastic bag container for blood.

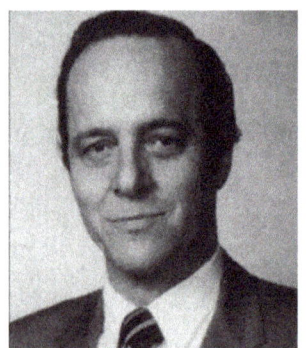 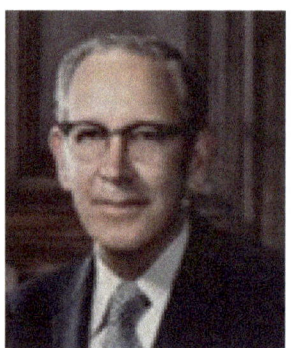 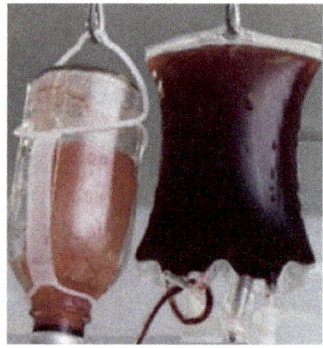

After hearing Dr. Gerow's analogy, prescient Dr. Cronin recognized the potential for a new breast implant and immediately got to work on this new idea. He had recently heard about silicone gel at a medical conference in New Orleans from a young doctor from Midland Michigan, home of Dow Corning. He learned that Dow Corning had developed an inorganic polymer silicone gel that was tissue nonreactive and variably flexible, depending on polymerization. Little did Dr. Cronin know at the time of that conference that this serendipitous information would become so relevant so soon. With the idea of a new breast implant in mind, he contacted Dow Corning and arranged for a visit to their Midland Michigan facility to find out more about this new silicone polymer

Dr. Cronin worked with researchers, including Silas Braley, at Dow Corning's Center for Aid to Medical Research. They studied the tensile strength of various silicone elastomer membranes. Dow Corning's silicone was named Silastic in honor of Silas Braley. They implanted twelve dogs with four to six Silastic balloons, each filled with Dextran, electrolyte solution, or silicone gel. These sacs remained in place from a few days to 18 months. The cavities all showed a low -grade fibrous response.

They decided that the choice of the filler for the Silastic elastomer would be silicone gel, partly because they believed the cohesive gel stuck to itself to such a degree that it was almost leak proof. If a tear developed and gel extruded from the bag, the gel would remain contained within the pseudo-membrane, which formed around the implant. Also, they observed the gel to be very non-tissue reactive. They next produced prototypes of breast implants such as those shown below. These consisted of a thick silicone gel encased in a thick and sturdy silicone teardrop sack with Dacron patches on the back. They thought that the Dacron patches assured the stabilization of the implant position.

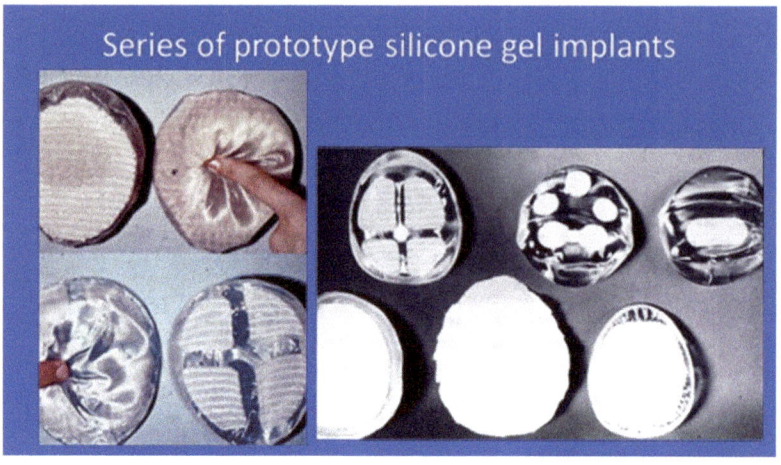

Finally, as related by Dr. Tom Biggs (pictured below), the prototype breast implant was a biscuit sized one placed in a dog named Esmeralda in Houston. As a resident, doctor Tom Biggs had the task of looking after this dog with the first implant. The implant remained in place a few months and seemed not to harm the dog. Esmeralda eventually chewed out the implant.

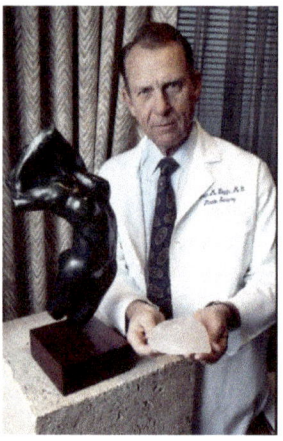

The first human breast implant patient was a 30-year-old divorced mother of six who wanted to have rose tattoos removed from her breasts. She saw Dr. Gerow in the resident clinic. He removed the tattoos. He then offered her the chance to become the first breast augmentation patient with a new "natural feel" silicone gel implant. She agreed as long as he also pinned back her prominent ears. This initial augmentation took place at Jefferson Davis Hospital in Houston in 1962. She did well after surgery and later that year remarried. Fifty years later, with her original implants in place, she was still happy with her decision to be the first breast implant patient.

"Augmentation mammaplasty: a new 'natural feel' prosthesis" was presented at the Third International Congress of plastic surgery in Washington DC in 1963 and published the following year, creating tremendous excitement among plastic surgeons who were looking for a practical method for breast augmentation.

Dow Corning began marketing these "natural feel" silicone gel breast implants in 1964. They were teardrop shaped, had a thick cohesive gel, a thick shell, and Dacron backing. The thinking was, fibrous ingrowth into the Dacron would prevent unwanted movement of the implant. The photo on the right is a box of different size samples of Dow Corning breast implants that Dr. Thomas Cronin had in his office to show to patients considering breast augmentation.

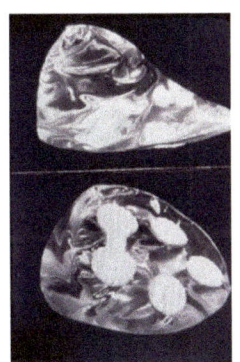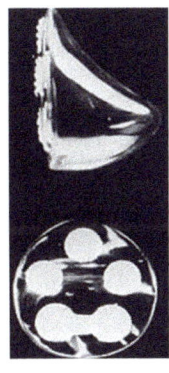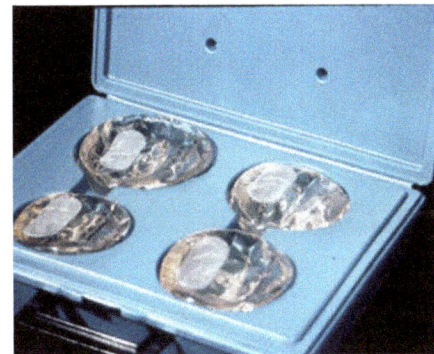

These implants were a quantum leap better than available sponges. Augmentation mammaplasty became one of the most popular plastic surgery operations. The manufacturers initially surmised that these implants would last the patient's lifetime. At first, the silicone gel breast implant was used exclusively for augmentation mammaplasty. However, very soon, it was recognized that it offered potential help for patients needing breast reconstruction. Reports soon followed of its use by itself or with various tissue flaps for the restoration of the breast after mastectomy for cancer. I devote chapter 9 to breast reconstruction after mastectomy breast reconstruction.

Dr. Cronin used a small durometer like the one shown below to document the postoperative softness of the augmented breasts. He would record this data in the patient's medical record.

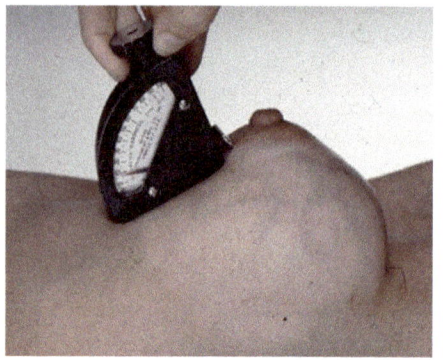
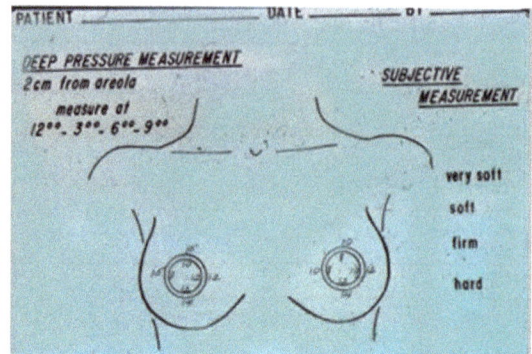

These new implants worked well and so pleased the majority of augmentation patients. Although highly successful, these implants were sometimes plagued by scar formation, which resulted in hard and occasionally painful breasts, necessitating scar removal and replacement with new implants. Below are pictured the scar capsules removed from breasts, which became too firm. Scar encapsulates the right implant below. I have removed the implant on the left, so only the scar capsule is present.

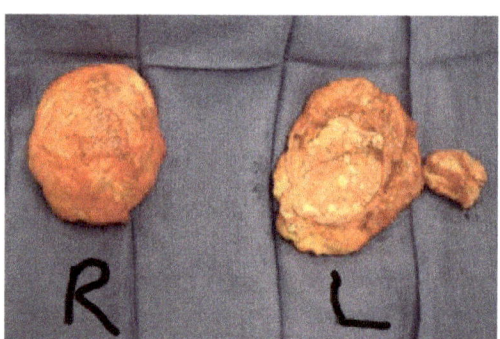

Thinking that the Dacron patches might be causing the excess scar, they were made smaller and finally done away with altogether. During the 1970s, the implant manufacturers produced implants with thinner shells and less viscous gel, which led to unforeseen complications of increased leakage and rupture of the implants; and did not solve the problem of spherical capsular scar contracture. The gel consisted of a mixture of gel with polymerized chains of various lengths. The shorter chain silicone gel polymers tended to leach or "bleed" through the silicone shell. If an implant had been in place for some time and then removed for some reason, the surface might feel slightly tacky because of the "bleed" of some of the shorter chain polymers through the silicone shell membrane.

The first picture below shows a second-generation thin shell, thin gel implant, prone to leakage and failure. This implant, removed from a patient, has both a tacky surface from gel "bleed" and a ruptured shell with thin gel extruding from the implant. The two xero-mammograms below demonstrate the complication of silicone leakage outside of the implant capsule into the upper breast tissue of two different patients. This finding might require not only removal of the implant but also silicone granulomas, which may have formed from scar tissue forming around the extruded gel.

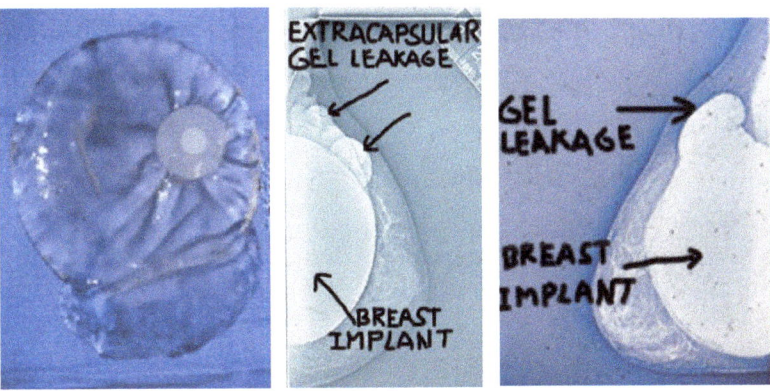

The photo on the left below shows a leaking implant and the capsule which had contained it before removal. On the right below are capsules from the right and left breasts. The right-sided implant was intact, and on the left side in the metal bowl, I placed the "ruptured" implant with the shell hardly recognizable in a pool of relatively liquid silicone gel.

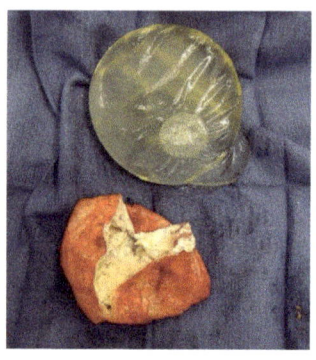 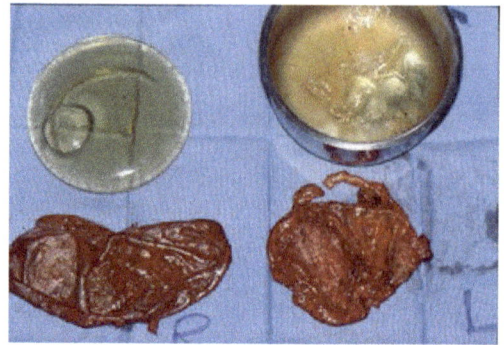

Several manufacturers introduced new silicone implants, such as the polyurethane-covered implants, textured implants, and double lumen implants with an outer lumen filled with saline and saline-filled implants.

Beginning with the December 1990 Connie Chung face-to-face TV program, which featured women who blamed implants for autoimmune diseases, an "implant crisis" was born. A new industry developed by plaintiff attorneys suing implant manufacturers and, in many states, the plastic surgeons as well. These autoimmune diseases could be quite debilitating and painful. Rheumatoid arthritis and lupus erythematosus are examples of autoimmune diseases. There was no cause and effect proof of this, as the allegations were mostly anecdotal. A problem for the manufacturers became proving the negative that implants do not cause various autoimmune diseases, which was the main thrust behind large implant suit settlements.

Nevertheless, the FDA placed a moratorium on the use of silicone gel implants in 1992, resulting in multiple lawsuits and a massive class-action lawsuit. The class-action lawsuit involved more than $3 billion. Of course, the lawyers probably got most of the money. As a result of talented personal injury lawyers, the implant manufacturing companies and insurers paid billions of dollars to the attorneys and plaintiffs. Therefore, the most notable and largest implant manufacturer, Dow Corning, filed for bankruptcy in 1995.

These suits were handled differently in different states. In Texas, all the individual lawsuits included the plastic surgeon along with the various manufacturers of the implants. I received about 50 malpractice lawsuits. Eventually, over several years, I was dismissed from all of these lawsuits. Nevertheless, as you might imagine, this entire episode was extremely stressful.

This implant crisis caused unwarranted fear for many patients; some of them had their implants removed or exchange for saline implants unnecessarily. Dozens of subsequent studies did not show an increase in autoimmune diseases in women with breast implants or significant problems with cancer detection with implants in place.

Between 1992 and 2006, the FDA restricted silicone gel implants to reconstructive and replacement applications. Although there have been many studies, everything seems to point to the fact that autoimmune diseases occur in approximating the same rate in people without implants as in people with implants. Many of the original allegations regarding disease associations remain unproven. In 2006, silicone gel implants were allowed back on the general plastic surgery market, although there remained some restrictions on the use of silicone gel implants. The newest implants are improved because the shell allows for less seeping or "bleeding" of gel through the sack to the outside, and the gel is more cohesive and less runny.

Now about 70% of the market is silicone gel-filled and 30% saline-filled implants. All the implants bags are made of silicone, whether they are saline or gel-filled. There are now fourth-generation implants filled with a very cohesive gel, which tends to maintain its integrity and shape without relying upon the implant sack. These "gummy bear" implants are especially useful in reconstruction and refractory cases of fibrous contracture. Although much improved, these are very much like the original implants devised by Thomas Cronin.

A unique form of cancer, anaplastic large cell lymphoma, has recently been associated with silicone implants. In 2011 the FDA identified a possible association between breast implants and the development of anaplastic large cell lymphoma. In March 2017, the US FDA updated its warning about a link between breast implants and this very rare type of cancer. Breast implant-associated anaplastic large cell lymphoma (BIA – ALCL) is a unique and highly treatable type of lymphoma that can develop around breast implants, especially textured ones. Complete capsulectomy is curative in most cases.

It is not a type of breast cancer. The lifetime risk for this disease appears to be about one case for every 30,000 textured implants and less for smooth surface implants. In contrast, the lifetime risk for breast cancer in women with or without implants is one out of every nine women!

Today we have improved implants with sturdier shells and more viscous cohesive gel again. These newer implants have gel with more uniform polymerization with little "gel bleed," thereby minimizing problems of contracture and implant failure. The drawing below represents a modern implant sliced in half through the thick shell with the cohesive gel staying put and not flowing out of the silicone sack.

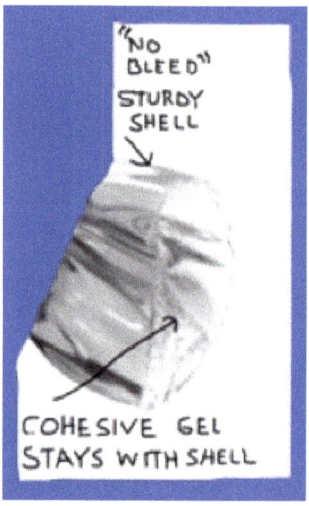

Dr. Frank Gerow's Eureka moment and Dr. Thomas Cronin's insight, perseverance, and boldness to take this idea from a mere concept to a practical product revolutionized breast surgery. It turned augmentation mammaplasty from a rare procedure to one of the most common plastic surgery procedures today. Together with its use in breast reconstruction, it has benefited hundreds of thousands of patients. Breast augmentation with silicone implants remains one of the most popular plastic surgery operations in the United States and the world.

Breast augmentation my personal experience

My personal experience with breast augmentation has been extensive, beginning with being taught this procedure by Drs. Thomas Cronin, Ray Brauer, and Tom Biggs during my plastic surgery residency. After I started my practice, the typical patient who came to see me for breast augmentation was a 30-year-old mother of two or three children, who said: "I use to be a C cup, but I nursed my three children and look at me now- deflated."

This typical patient wants only a moderate implant to replace what she lost or maybe just a little bit more. She wants to be proportional; she wants her clothes to fit better and to look beautiful in her clothes. The other somewhat typical patient is a young, petite breasted woman who has never been pregnant. She is the more complicated case because there is very little soft tissue coverage for an implant, which makes it harder to end up with a natural result. Initially, all of the breast augmentations placed the implant in a sub breast tissue parenchymal pocket. Later the submuscular technique also became quite common. If patients were a little ptotic (saggy), I would usually place the implant in a sub-glandular pocket above the muscle layer. If the patients tended to exercise and use their pectoral muscles a lot, I might also put the implant in a sub-glandular pocket. Otherwise, I more commonly used the submuscular implantation technique.

Although most patients are quite happy with augmentation mammaplasty, it is a challenging operation. An ongoing issue has been maintaining a natural feel despite the fact the body produces a scar tissue capsule around the implant. If that scar capsule becomes tight thickens, it will make the breast fill too hard. If that occurs, additional surgery to restore softness is required or recommended. An additional procedure to release or remove that scar tissue is often quite successful. Other possibly complicating issues are infection, bleeding, skin scar, and numbness, all of which occasionally occur. Rarely a patient has repeated severe scar contractures that are resistant to all treatment; such an exceptional patient may have to have her implants removed permanently.

Textured polyurethane-coated implants became available in about 1985. They seemed to elicit less scar tissue formation. Over time I also observed these implants to be quite sturdy and seldom failed. These implants were especially suitable for conditions in which a lot of scar tissue was likely such as in post-mastectomy cases or previous scar contracture cases. These implants were also taken off the market as a precaution in the early 1990s because of allegations that the polyurethane coating might break down and give off carcinogenic chemicals. I am not aware of any cases of cancer attributed to this process.

The good results obtained with the polyurethane-coated textured silicone implants caused the manufactures to produce textured surface implants made of only silicone. The textured surface was initially created for gel implants and later for saline implants. Although this textured silicone surface may offer some advantages, so far, it has not seemed as beneficial as the original polyurethane-coated textured implants in preventing scar formation.

Technique

I utilized a few special instruments in performing augmentation mammaplasty. I like the tissue retractor represented below on the left, designed by Dr. Tom Biggs. He liked to say that the assistant could hold this with one finger because of the counterbalanced handle and blade. Also, I used a headlight and an extended electric cautery wand with an insulated tip.

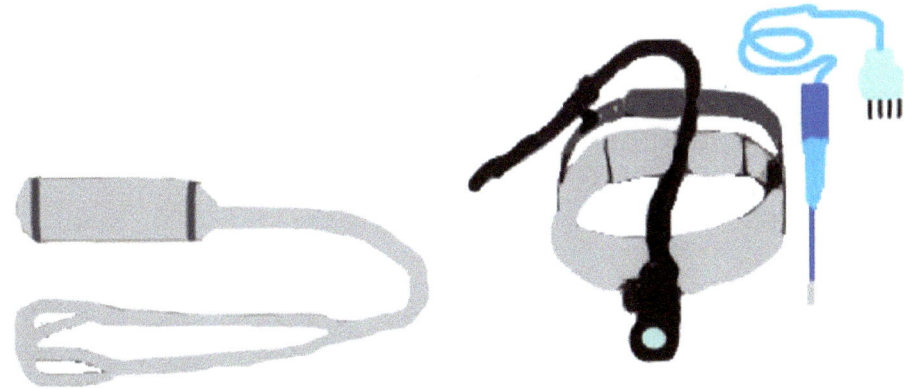

The surgical technique itself commences with making an incision. There are four possible sites for creating this cut. The most common placement is in the natural crease under the breast. Other potential incisions are around the nipple-areola, in the axilla, or near the bellybutton. I never did this last one. Next, the surgeon dissects a pocket either immediately beneath the breast parenchyma on top of the pectoralis major muscle or a layer deeper under the pectoralis major muscle. The first picture below shows a dissection of the breast parenchyma off the pectoralis major muscle with electrocautery to make a subglandular pocket. The second picture shows the electrocautery dissection below the pectoralis major muscle to make a submuscular pocket.

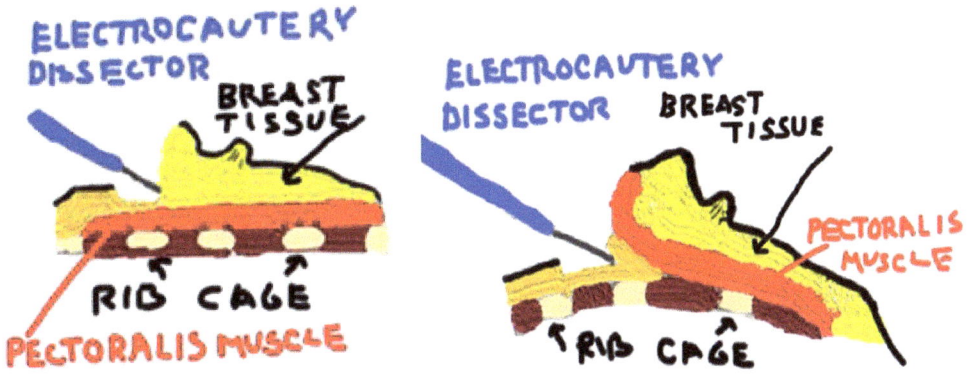

The surgeon then places the implant in the newly created space and closes the incision. The surgeon develops a pocket more extensive than the size of the implant. However, textured gummy bear implants require a pocket of the same size as the implant. The first view below represents the anatomic relationship between the chest wall, pectoralis major and serratus anterior muscles, and breast tissue. The second view shows a breast implant placed in a sub-glandular pocket beneath the breast parenchymal tissue but on top of the pectoral muscles. The third view shows a breast implant placed sub-muscularly, which is beneath both the breast parenchyma and the pectoralis muscle on top of the ribs.

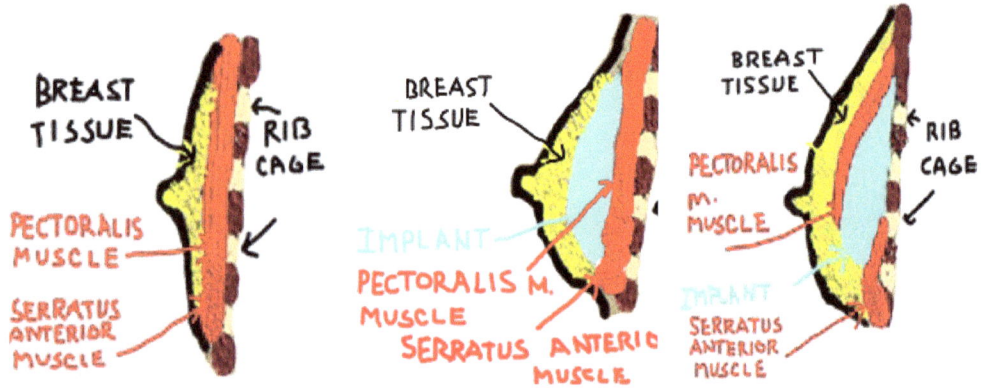

I performed the following examples of breast augmentation with an incision in the inframammary crease. I placed silicone gel implants either under the breast tissue (subglandular) or more buried under the pectoralis major muscle (submuscular). The first four examples below are patients in whom I performed augmentation with submuscular placed silicone gel implants. The first patient, "Dannie," is a 30 something lady who liked to sunbathe. She wanted to have fuller breasts to show off in her swimwear and to look more proportional in her clothes. She was happy with her moderate enlargement with the silicone gel implant placed sub-muscularly. Pre-op on the left and post-op on the right.

The Healing Mission of Plastic Surgery

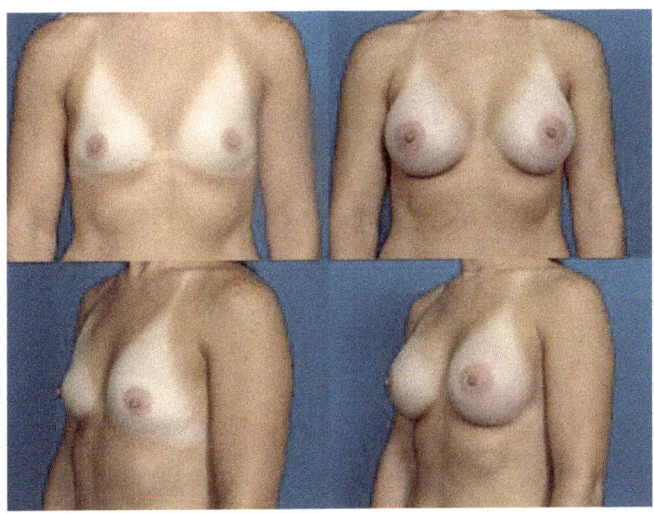

The second patient, "Barbara" had lost some weight and felt like her breasts were smaller than she would like. A small augmentation gave her back her desired breast size and made her breasts seem a little less saggy. Pre-op on the left and post-op on the right.

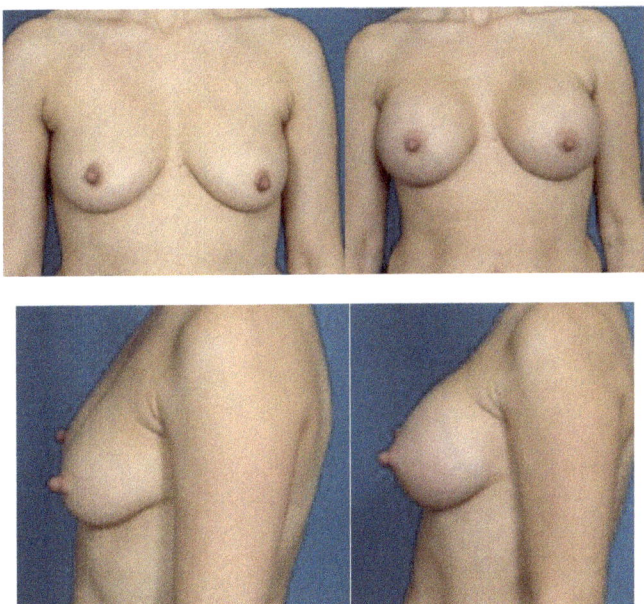

The next patient, "Mimi," shown below, was somewhat of a sun worshiper. She was looking to be more fulsome so that she could be "proud" of her chest. Pre-op on the left and post-op on the right.

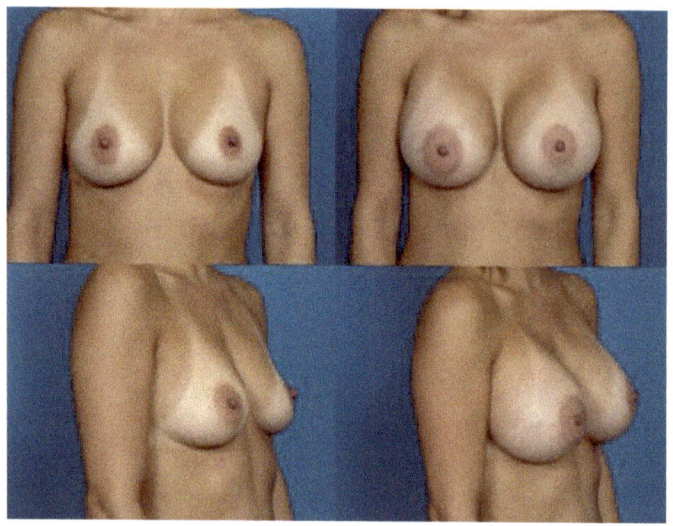

The patient below, "Diedra," was a twenty-something lady who was pleased to have a substantial augmentation. Pre-op on the left and post-op on the right.

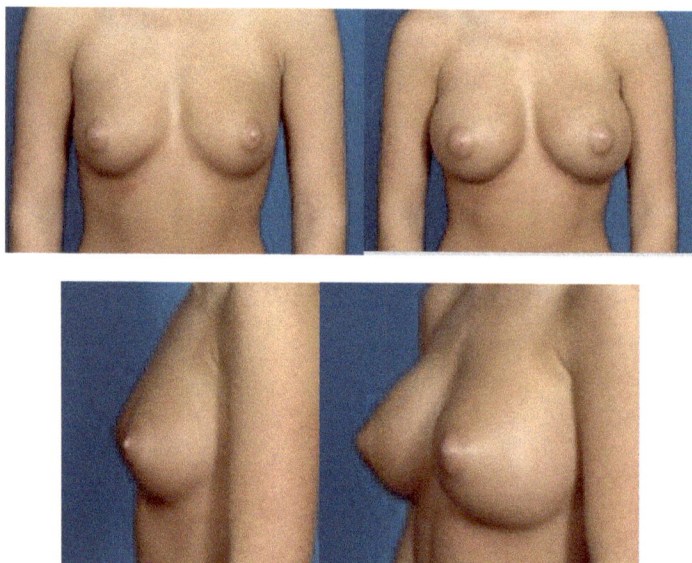

I treated the next group of patients with subglandular placement of silicone gel implants. This first patient shown below "Maggie" had been very disappointed her whole adult life that her nascent breasts never progressed. She was quite happy with the prospect of breast augmentation. Because she wanted a substantial increase in size, I selected a subglandular space that allowed the tissues to stretch more readily than they might in a submuscular plane. She was happy and satisfied with her augmentation. Pre-op on the left and post-op on the right.

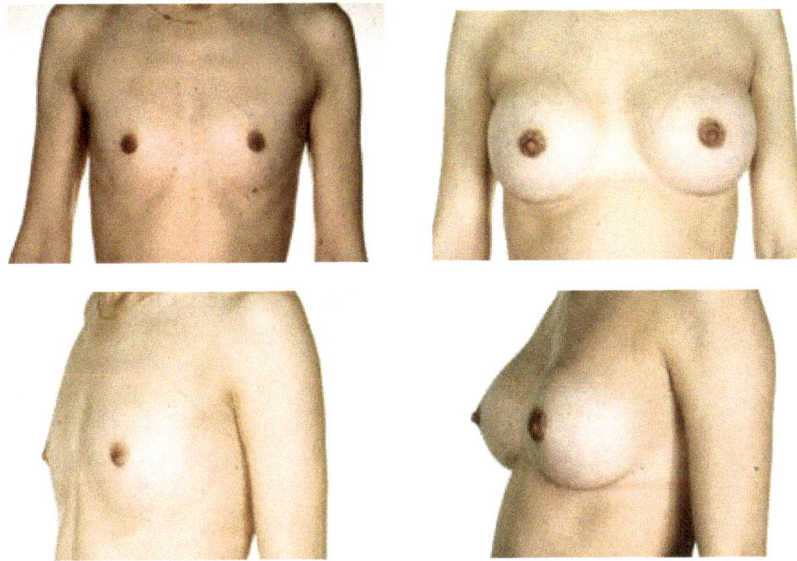

The patient with the pre -and postoperative views below was very athletic. She played a lot of sports, especially tennis. Together we chose a subglandular implant technique for her to avoid any potential muscle issues that could arise with a sub-pectoralis approach. Pre-op on the left and post-op on the right.

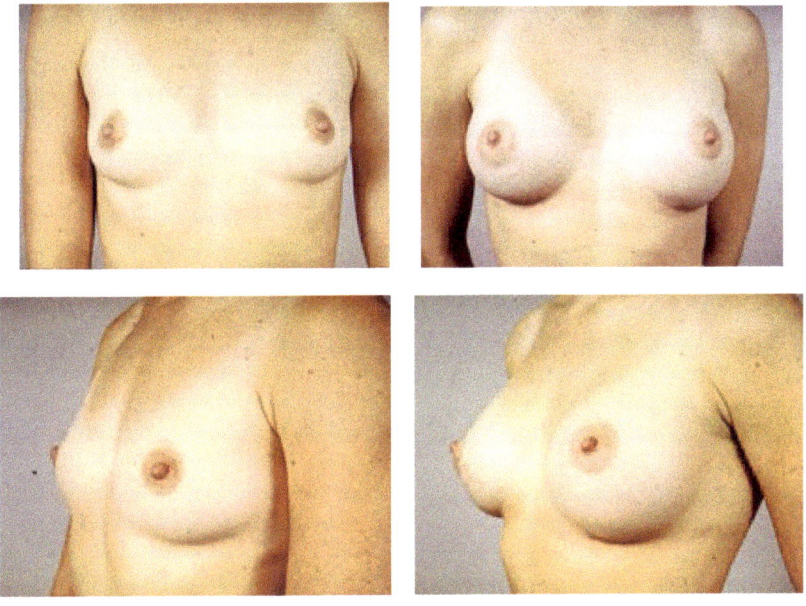

The Healing Mission of Plastic Surgery

The patient in the views below, "Sara," said she had been happy with her breast before she had three children. She felt like her breasts had become deflated after breast-feeding three infants. She just wanted to return the fullness she previously had. Because her breasts were a little bit saggy, I used a subglandular pocket to place the silicone gel implants. She was happy with her result done without a mastopexy (breast lift). Pre-op on the left and post-op on the right.

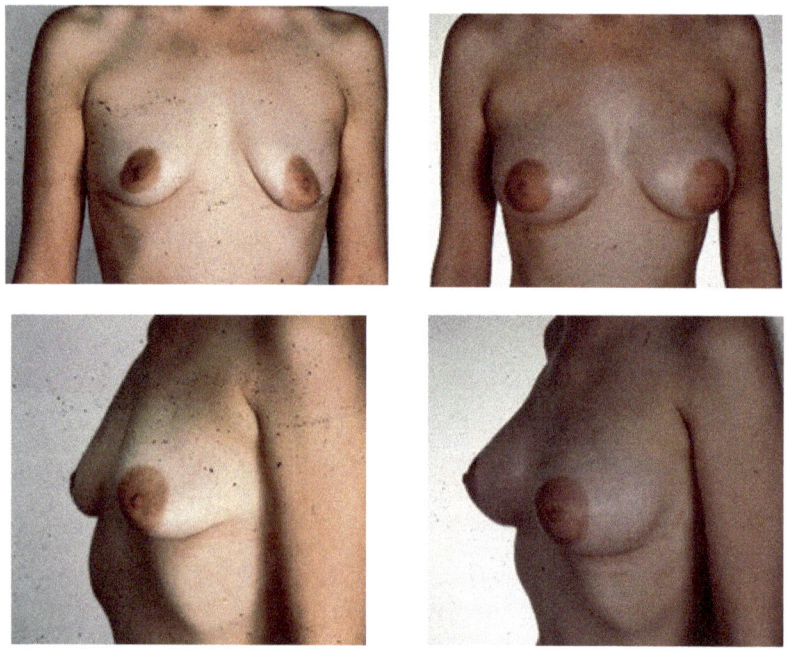

"Penny," whose pre and postoperative views are below, had well-shaped but small breasts.

She enjoyed poolside activities and wanted to look fuller and more attractive in a swimsuit. Pre-op on the left and post-op on the right.

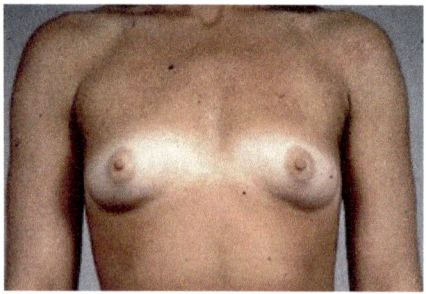
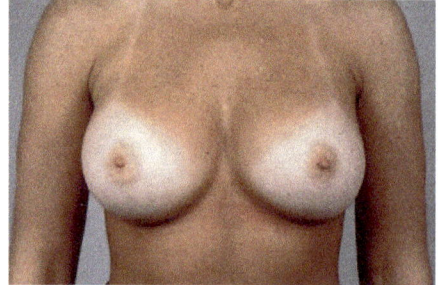

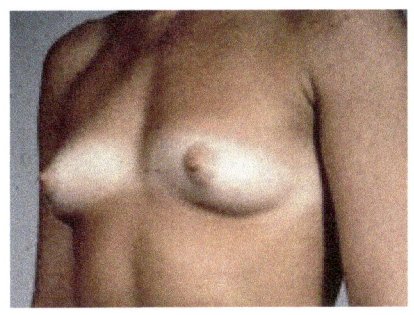 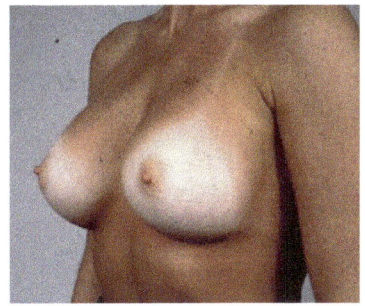

Augmentation of the breast with silicone implants remains one of the most successful and popular plastic surgery operations done today. As I mentioned before, most patients seek breast augmentation to look better in their clothes. However, many patients relate improved body image, self-image, and self- esteem, sometimes even enhanced sexual relationships after successful augmentation mammaplasty surgery. Production of newer implants with more durable shells that prevent leakage and "bleed" and better, more cohesive gel have ameliorated most of the drawbacks to the procedure that I discussed earlier.

Chapter 9

Breast Reconstruction after Mastectomy

Being diagnosed with cancer can be a frightening experience. For most women, this means their physician will likely advise some form of mastectomy. For a woman to also face the loss of the breast can be devastating. However, today the vast majority of women who need mastectomies can have reconstructions, allowing them to maintain or restore this badge of femininity. The results of reconstruction have improved in recent years because of less radical surgery and better reconstructive techniques.

Indications for breast the construction are the absence of the breast, lack of active chest wall cancer, and the patient's desire for reconstruction. Absolute contraindications include uncontrolled active local disease. A relative contraindication is metastatic breast cancer. In some instances, this is well controlled and may allow for breast construction.

Problems faced when undertaking a breast reconstruction are skin deficiency, lack of volume for a breast mound, absence of the nipple, and areola. Early in my career, I saw many cases post radical mastectomy in which the surgeon removed the pectoralis major muscle leaving only skin over the rib cage. Also, radical mastectomies wholly extirpated the axillary lymph nodes. These were the most challenging breast reconstruction cases. Two examples of patients post radical mastectomy are below.

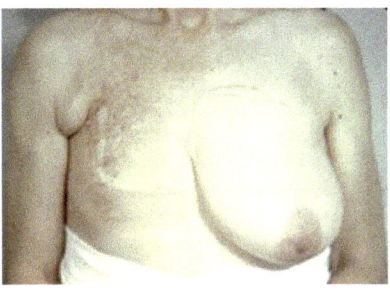 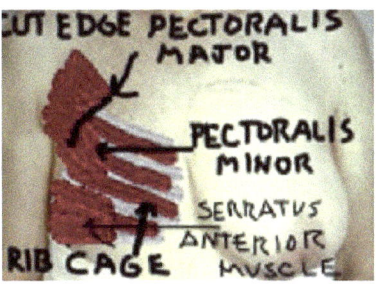

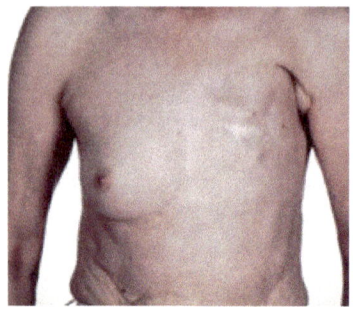 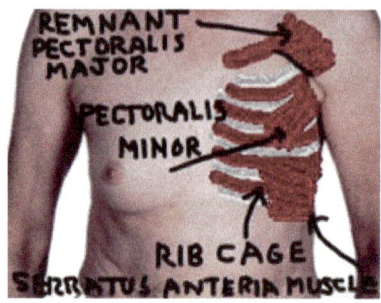

Over time the nature of mastectomy surgery for cancer changed. Modified radical mastectomy became routine during the majority of my practice years. In this surgery, although the surgeon removes the breast tissue, breast skin, and lymph nodes, the chest muscles are left intact as simulated below. These modified radical mastectomies were, therefore, less challenging to reconstruct than the previous radical mastectomies. Two examples of patients post modified radical mastectomies are below.

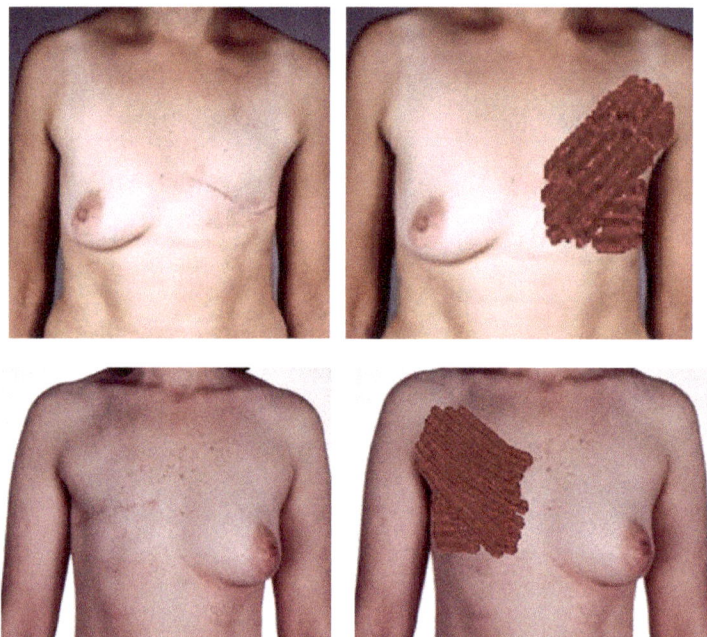

Later modifications were to remove the nipple-areola and breast tissue but spare the skin of the breast. Surgeons began doing less radical axillary lymph node dissections. With radioactive isotope and injectable dye for mapping purposes, often, only a single sentinel node was removed for diagnostic purposes. The first case shown below illustrates the transition between modified radical mastectomy and skin-sparing mastectomy. On the patient's left side, a modified radical mastectomy had been done similar to the previous two cases shown above. However, on the patient's right chest, the oncology surgeon will remove the breast tissue, but only the nipple and areola marked out in red, leaving the remaining breast skin of the right breast intact.

So, this first picture below shows what a significant difference in the starting point for breast reconstruction is for a skin-sparing (right side) versus a modified radical mastectomy (left side). Again, the chest muscles are left intact, as simulated in the second picture below.

The third and fourth pictures below represent two more cases of skin-sparing mastectomies. They illustrate the starting point for reconstruction with mostly intact breast skin and all the chest wall muscles remaining. I usually performed the repair at the same operation immediately after a skin-sparing mastectomy.

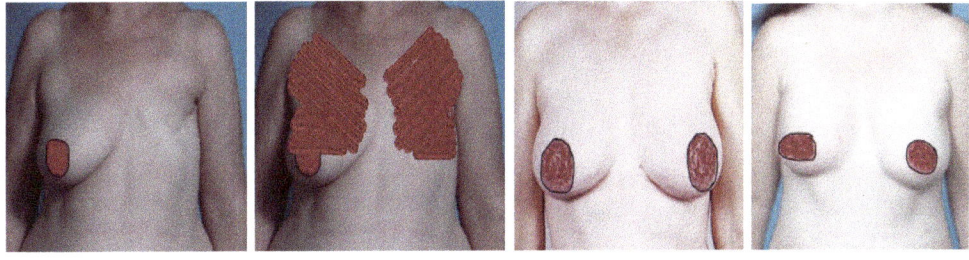

More recently, it has become common to do skin and nipple areolae sparing mastectomies (subcutaneous mastectomy) for smaller breast cancers that are not near the nipple.

That fact brings up another sidelight to the history of mastectomy surgery. At the Cronin Brauer and Biggs plastic surgery clinic in the late 70s and 1980s and 1990s, we performed many hundreds of prophylactic subcutaneous mastectomies, followed with immediate silicone gel implant reconstructions. (Remember approximately one out of every nine women will develop breast cancer in their lifetime.) These subcutaneous mastectomies excised the same tissue that skin and nipple-sparing mastectomies done for small cancer today remove.

However, in the past, the climate was very different. We did these prophylactic mastectomies obviously to prevent cancer. We performed them in patients who had strong family histories for breast cancer or had had multiple breast biopsies and seemed to be getting a piecemeal mastectomy over time. We also considered patients who had very dense breast tissue, which was very difficult to evaluate with the existing mammogram procedures. Although we were doing this in patients who did not have a diagnosis of breast cancer, the method was frowned upon and even criticized by the general surgery establishment as being not thorough enough?

I think it was unfortunate, but perhaps for that reason, we never gathered together and evaluated all of our patients to document the beneficial prophylactic effect of this surgery. I do remember there were numerous instances of finding a tiny previously undiagnosed cancer in the specimens, which of course, were carefully examined by the pathologist. In these cases, no further treatment was necessary as the subcutaneous mastectomy was curative.

On the other hand, I recall only one instance in which breast cancer developed right under the nipple in one of my post, prophylactic subcutaneous mastectomy patients. Local excision cured that patient. I will present some subcutaneous mastectomy with immediate reconstruction cases later in this chapter.

Goals

What are the goals of breast reconstruction? Excellent appearance in clothing is the primary goal. I aim for inconspicuous appearance without clothing. A soft natural feel is ideal. Also, underlying all the physical goals is the object of restoring a sense of wholeness to the patient. Many technologies are available. The most common ones are implant only, tissue expander followed by an implant, latissimus dorsi muscle and skin flap from the back usually combined with an implant, and the rectus abdominis flap of skin and fat from the abdomen, either as a pedicle flap or free flap often without an implant.

Another primary concern in breast reconstruction after a mastectomy is symmetry with the opposite breast. Psychologic, aesthetic, and oncologic (cancer) considerations are all germane in deciding what to do with the opposite breast. The options are nothing, breast lift (mastopexy), augmentation, reduction, or prophylactic mastectomy with reconstruction.

Consultation

When a new patient inquired about breast reconstruction, I obtained the how and why for the referral. I took a history, including existing treatments and previous history of surgery or illness. I made an assessment of the patient's general health, physical conditioning, expectations, and pain tolerance. Usually, the husband or another supportive person was present. At this time, I at least briefly discussed reconstruction options. Any plan for other treatments, such as chemotherapy or x-ray therapy, was noted. At first, consultation for reconstruction was always after the mastectomy.

Of course, now, most often, the patient sees the plastic surgeon before undergoing any ablative surgery. When I began my practice, most reconstructions were done years after the mastectomy surgery at the recommendation of the general surgeons. Now, of course, many restorations are done immediately following mastectomy surgery. My initial examination included an assessment of the patient's general physique, breast size and shape, and symmetry with the opposite breast. If the patient was already post-mastectomy, I noted existing scars, the quality, and looseness of the skin. I examined the possible donor sites, such as the abdomen and back.

Recommendation

To complete the consultation, after patient input, I gave my recommendations. If I favored a tissue flap, I expounded on the specifics of that surgery. If I recommended an implant, I explicated maintenance issues such as potential future replacement because of excess scar formation or leakage. I disclosed possible complications, risks, benefits, and alternatives. I tried to clarify postoperative care, such as wound drains, a urinary catheter, pain, dressings, diet, and activity. Finally, I may have shown the patient pictures of patients who had had a similar reconstruction. On occasion, I had the patient talk with a previously reconstructed patient. My guidance included advice about the opposite breast.

Reconstruction immediate versus delayed

The advantages of immediate reconstruction at the time of mastectomy are many. Breast restoration with good results seems to be somewhat more straightforward with the immediate repair because of the preservation of natural landmarks, as well as sparing more breast skin. Formal skin-sparing mastectomy has made immediate restorative surgery even more favorable. It is a single operation with a high degree of patient acceptance. The patient does not have to go through a period with no breast while she waits for reconstruction. The disadvantages of immediate repair include not knowing future treatments such as radiation therapy, which may affect the reconstructed breast. The operation may be more prolonged with more blood loss, and there may be a very slightly higher complication rate because of more surgery at one time.

Delayed reconstruction has some advantages. There is time for the patient to adjust to her disease and absent breast psychologically. She may better appreciate the imperfect results. Time is allowed to finalized ancillary treatment plans and for consideration of the opposite breast. However, there are disadvantages to delayed reconstruction. Another operation is required. Waiting for breast replacement can be a time of significant emotional/psychological trauma. On a practical note, there the loss of natural mammary landmarks. I usually recommended immediate reconstruction unless there were plans for post-mastectomy x-ray therapy.

Results I wanted include the return or maintenance of emotional well-being and self-esteem and a high level of patient satisfaction. Qualitative factors include the appearance in clothes, naturalness of shape, and feel as well as symmetry with the opposite breast. As with every surgery, complications sometimes occur. The rate of complications is low. The most common is an infection at approximately 2%, blood collection under the skin (hematoma), about 2%, an unfortunate aesthetic result of roughly 5%, scar tissue in excess around any implant approximately 20%.

Most of the time, revision surgery can salvage an initial unsatisfactory result. However, on very few occasions, my patient gave up on my ability to give her a satisfactory result, and either went elsewhere or resigned herself to not being able to get the results she wants. Revision surgery, for irregularity of breast shape or size, the position of the inframammary fold, the orientation of implants, or symmetry between the two breasts, is prevalent. Secondary surgery often dramatically improves the result.

In the past several years, I have seen improvement in the quality of breast reconstruction after mastectomy. Several reasons are evident. As demonstrated by the pictures above, general surgeons are doing less radical surgery, which spares the pectoral muscles, saves much of the breast skin, and preserves most underarm lymph nodes. Another improvement has been tissue - only reconstruction, which appropriates tissue from the lower abdomen or the back and occasionally from some other source such as the buttock. I believe that the higher the percentage of the patient's flesh versus implant the better the long- term results

Various techniques

There are several conventional techniques used today. Implant only reconstructions, usually in two stages with an interim tissue expander is the most common. Other methods use a flap of the patient's tissue, most commonly from the lower abdomen, as part of the reconstruction. A pedicle flap based on the rectus muscle or an abdominal free flap that includes blood vessels to the tissue is commonplace. Performing a free flap requires the anastomosis of the flap vessels to recipient blood vessels at the chest. The other standard tissue method is the latissimus dorsi myo-cutaneous flap technique previously mentioned in chapter 5.

Reconstruction with abdominal tissue

Most of the reconstructions in which I used the abdomen as a donor were pedicled transverse rectus abdominis myo-cutaneous (TRAM)technique. This technique uses skin, subcutaneous fat, and muscle from the stomach to reconstruct the breast, usually without an implant. I routinely left the tissue attached to a pedicle of muscle to maintain its blood supply. However, the flap can also be done a free TRAM flap by separating it from the body and reattaching its blood vessels at the chest wall. An advantage of the TRAM flap is no implant is usually required.

The abdomen is usually made smaller and tighter, a plus for many patients. However, some patients will have morbidity associated with the abdominal donor site, such as difficulty sitting directly up from a supine position. Excellent results aesthetically are possible, often with a very natural feel. The result with tissue only reconstructions tends to improve over time rather than deteriorate as with some implant techniques. Disadvantages include the possibility of the abdominal donor area developing a hernia, a lengthy operation, a painful early postoperative experience, and a significant recovery phase.

The photos below illustrate the pedicle TRAM flap technique. The first photo shows a sizeable radical defect after mastectomy of the right breast. I have incised the lower abdominal tissue, and it is ready for elevation. The drawing in the middle shows the rectus muscle pedicle, and the route the flap will be tunneled under the abdominal skin to the breast defect. In the third picture, I have lifted the TRAM flap, which still connected to the rectus abdominis muscle pedicle through which its blood supply flows. With bilateral reconstructions, the right rectus muscle remains connected to the right half of the abdominal tissue, and the left rectus muscle remains attached to the left half of the skin and subcutaneous tissue flap. In unilateral cases, usually, I used the contralateral muscle, as illustrated in the drawing.

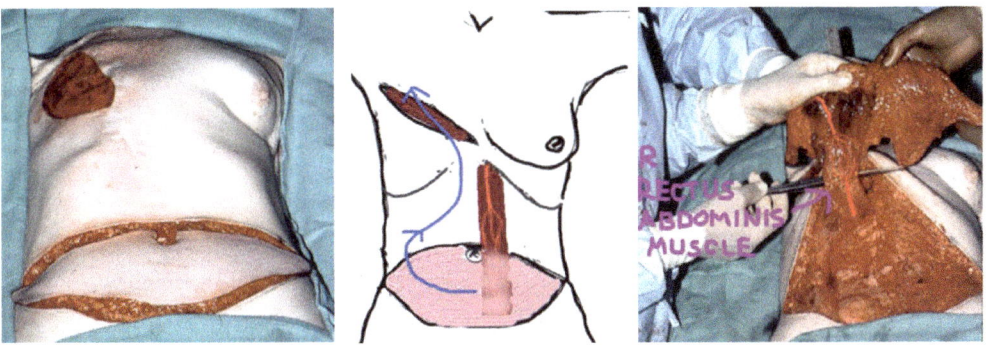

The pictures below show I tunneled the TRAM under the upper abdominal skin and brought it out onto the right anterior chest. I closed the abdomen with mesh reinforcement. I rearranged the tissue into the shape of a breast. Most of the time, no implant is needed. When the lady wants a fuller chest, I can place an implant either at the time of the TRAM flap or later.

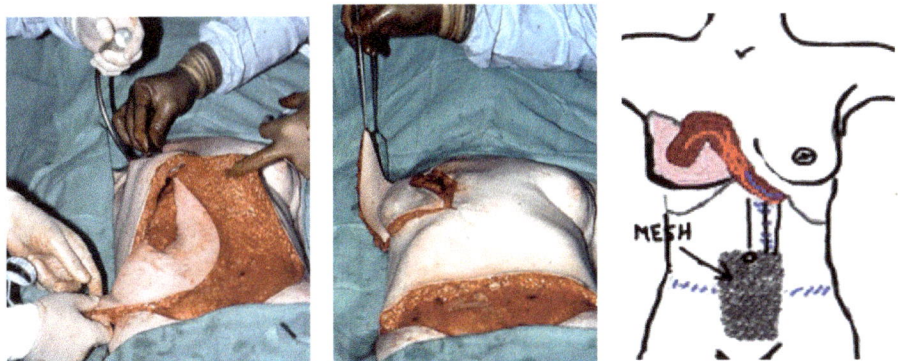

With free flaps, the surgeon completely separates the tissue from the body, transfers it to the chest, and reconnects the blood supply. An example of a free tissue myocutaneous(muscle and skin) flap, with connecting blood vessels ready for transfer to the chest, is shown below.

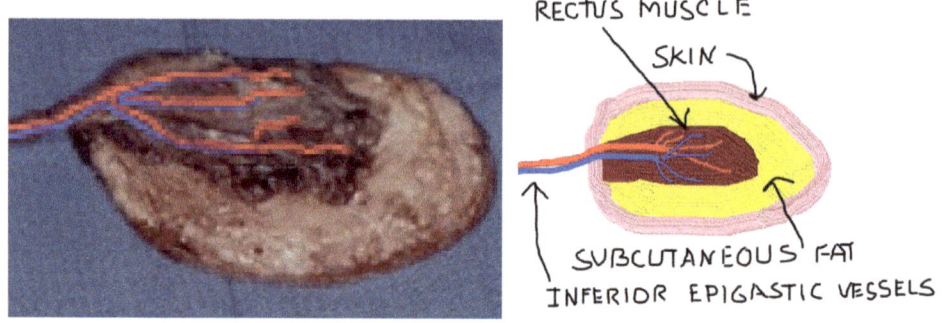

TRAM flap used in secondary breast reconstruction

The patient below "Adelaide" had a prior right mastectomy and recently completed radiation therapy. One can see skin discoloration as an effect of the radiation. I did a single pedicle tram flap on the right. The nipple was reconstructed by sharing from the left nipple and skin graft for the areola. I did nothing to the left breast.

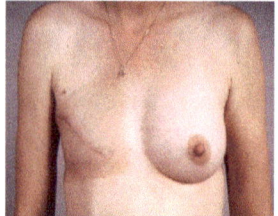 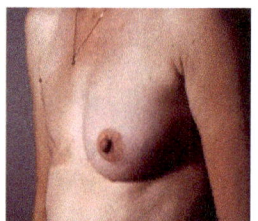 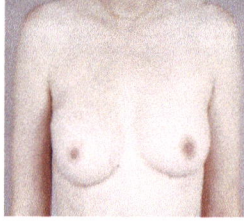 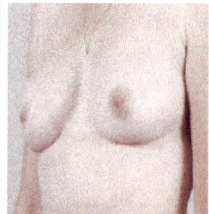

Annie,''' shown below, had a modified radical mastectomy with an oblique scar on the left. She wanted to have fuller breasts; therefore, I did a minimal mastopexy together with breast augmentation on the right side. I performed a large TRAM flap on the left and added a small implant to match the new right breast size. I reconstructed the nipple-areola with a small local flap and tattoo.

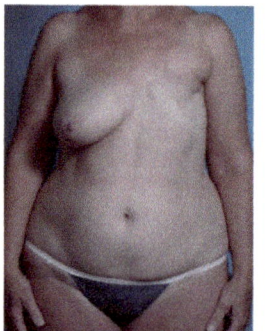 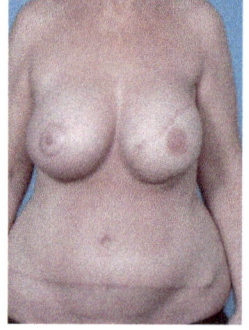

I recommended a delayed TRAM flap reconstruction for "Cloe" below. Although she had a lot of residual skin after a mastectomy and could have had an implant reconstruction, she did not want an implant. She had adequate abdominal skin and fatty tissue, which she wished to utilize.

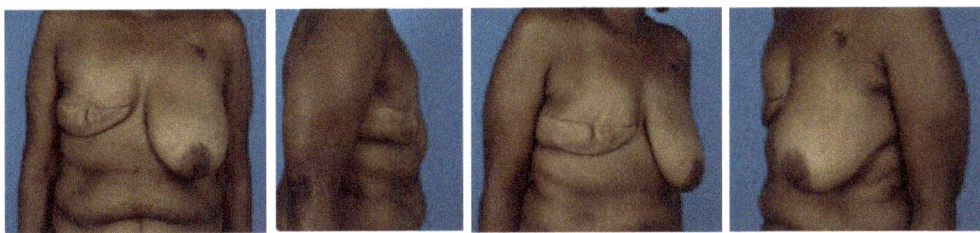

Therefore, I performed a pedicle TRAM reconstruction for her. At the same time, I did a mastopexy on the opposite breast. Below are her postoperative results after several months.

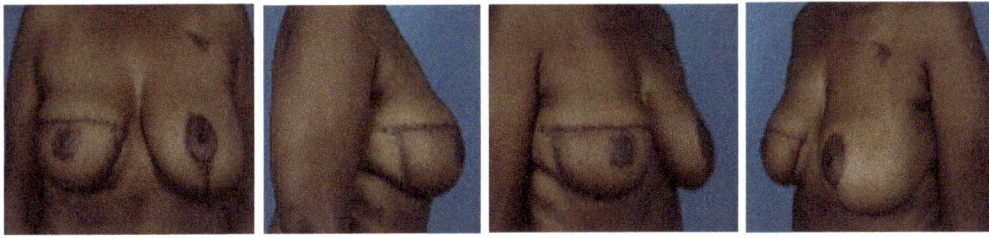

Zarita", shown below, had a modified radical mastectomy. Because I was able to obtain a sizeable cutaneous portion of the TRAM flap, I placed it horizontally at the level of the old scar. The intermediate picture shown is instructive in a few ways. It shows that the right breast is a little bit large and extends a little too far inferiorly. It also shows a fresh, red, somewhat hypertrophic abdominal scar. The final picture shows the result after a minimal mastopexy on the left and adjustment of the TRAM flap position on the right to create better symmetry. I reconstructed the nipple-areola with a keyhole flap and tattoo. You can see that the abdominal scar has faded quite a bit by that time.

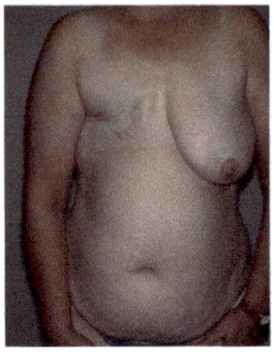 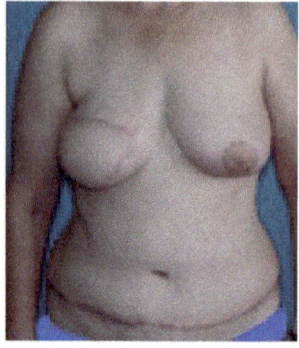 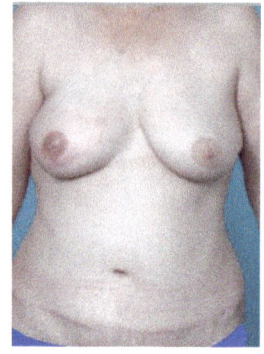

"Cheyenne" shown below was recently diagnosed with a second breast cancer. The first pictures below show her after a left modified radical mastectomy and before she had a right skin-sparing mastectomy.

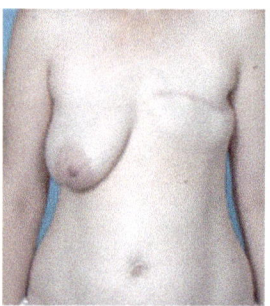 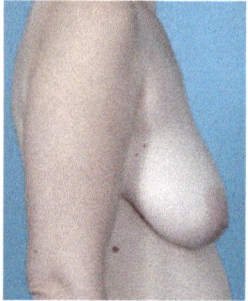 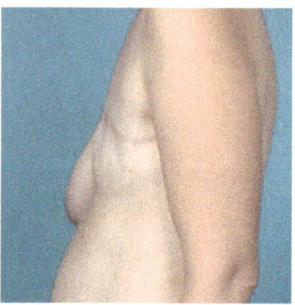

Her case illustrates the difference between an immediate skin-sparing mastectomy TRAM reconstruction on the right and a delayed post modified radical mastectomy TRAM reconstruction on the left. These breasts had a natural feel, and this patient looked very healthy in her clothes. She did not seek nipple reconstruction.

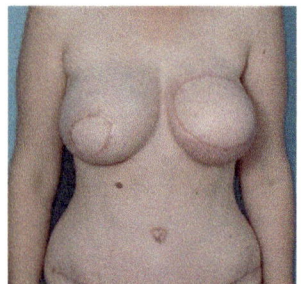 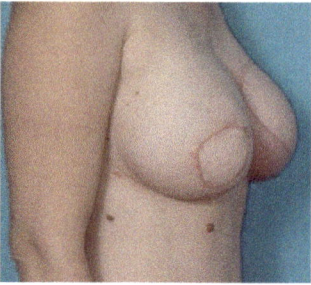 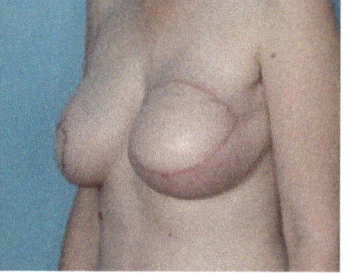

TRAM flap used in immediate reconstruction

The patient shown below "Georgianna" had a previous lumpectomy for breast cancer on the left and now has new breast cancer on the right. The general surgeon did bilateral mastectomies, removing the nipple-areola and breast tissue while sparing the remaining skin of each breast. I performed immediate bilateral pedicle TRAM flaps.

The initial postop result is in the middle photo below. Most of the pre-existing breast skin remains, but the central portion of the surface of each breast is part of the abdominal flap. Most of the flap tissue is beneath the pre-existing breast skin, giving the reconstructed breast its volume. I did nipple-areola reconstructions at a second operation. I utilized the excess skin island tissue to make the nipples with the keyhole technique described later. The final result is on the right below. Now the only scar left on the breast is that circle defining the areola.

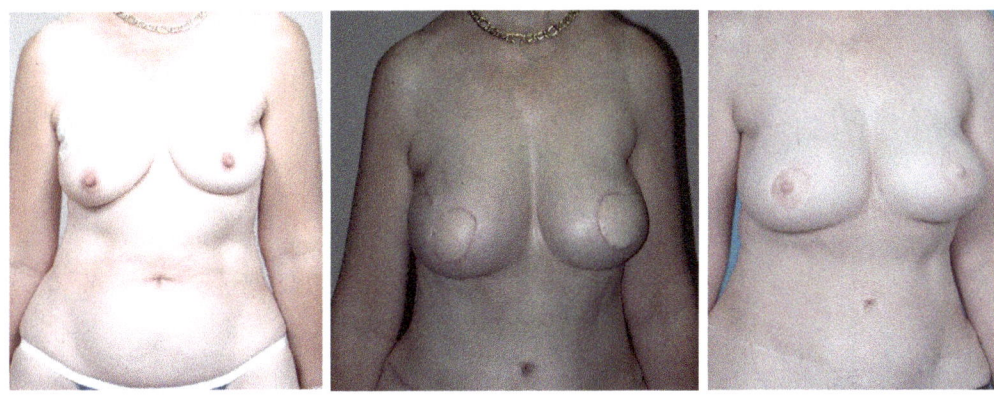

The lady shown below "Judy" came from Louisiana to have her breast cancer treated by a surgical oncologist friend of mine who referred her to me. I performed an immediate TRAM flap after the skin-sparing mastectomy on the left. I did a nipple-areola sharing from the right breast to the left one to reconstruct the left areola. The only thing I did on the right breast was to borrow some of the areola tissue for the left side, as mentioned above. This patient was unusual in that she rejected my first suggestion that she have a reduction mammaplasty on the right so that we would be able to match it with reconstruction on the left more readily. She had quite large breasts, which she adamantly wished to keep. I was delighted that I could give her the type of reconstructed breast she wanted. She returned every year for many years and did very well.

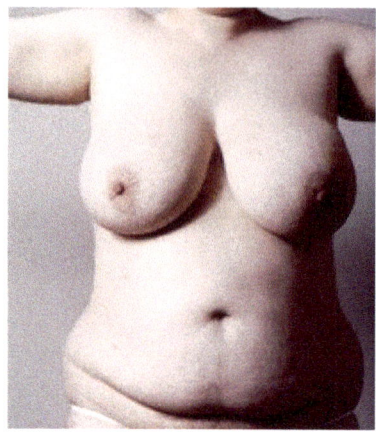
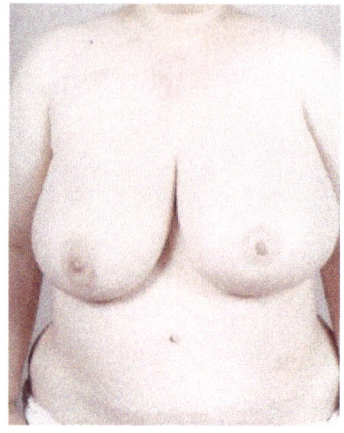

The patient below "Guinevere" had small bilateral cancers and underwent bilateral skin-sparing mastectomies by a general surgeon. I performed immediate reconstructions with bilateral pedicle TRAM flaps. The intermediate postoperative intermediate result is in the center photo below. At a second operation, I utilized small local skin flaps from the tram flaps to make the nipples together with the tattooing of the areola. The final result is on the right below.

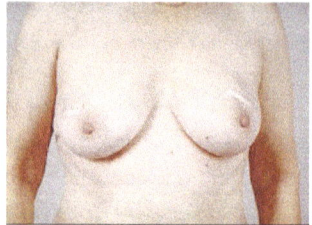
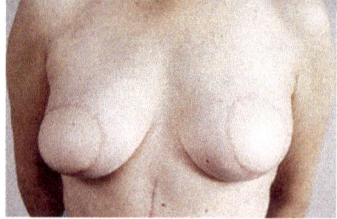
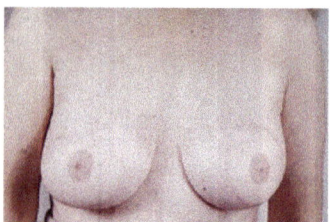

The patient below "Victoria" had bilateral mastectomies by her general surgeon. The pre-mastectomy picture is on the left below. I performed bilateral immediate pedicle TRAM reconstructions with no implant as she preferred. The intermediate result after the tram flap is in the middle below. In contrast, the final result after nipple-areolar reconstruction with the keyhole technique and tattooing is on the right.

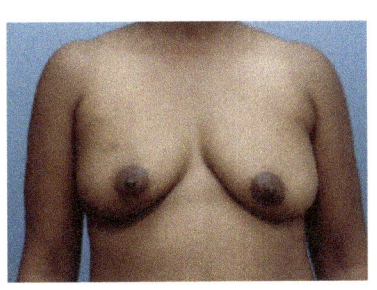 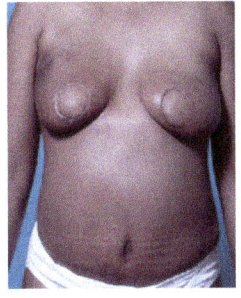 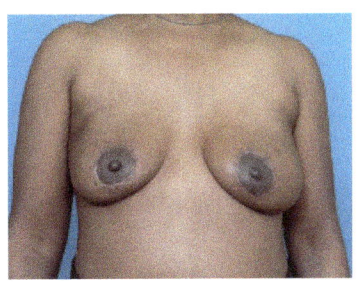

"Priscilla" is shown below preoperatively after her general surgeon did an open biopsy of the left breast. She developed a small hematoma hence the bruising. The general surgeon then did a left skin-sparing mastectomy, and I did an immediate reconstruction with a pedicle TRAM flap and a silicone implant on the left. I also did an augmentation mammaplasty on the right with a silicone gel implant; I made the nipple-areola with a keyhole flap and tattoo. Her postoperative result is on the right below

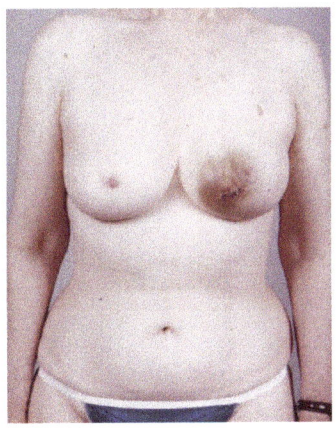 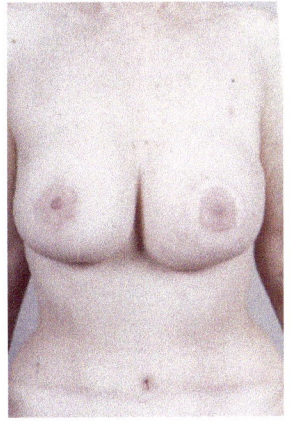

"Margaret" shown below previously had a left partial mastectomy and radiation. Because of recurrent disease, she underwent bilateral skin-sparing mastectomies. I performed immediate bilateral pedicle TRAM flaps, and her intermediate postoperative result is in the center below. A few months later, I did bilateral nipple-areolar reconstruction with the keyhole technique and tattooing of the areola. Her final result is on the right below

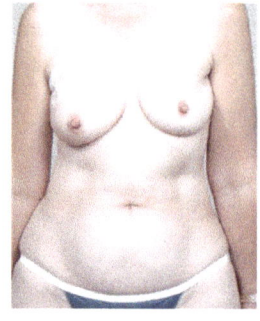 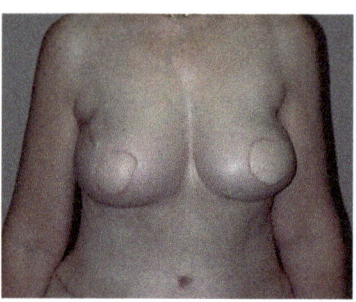 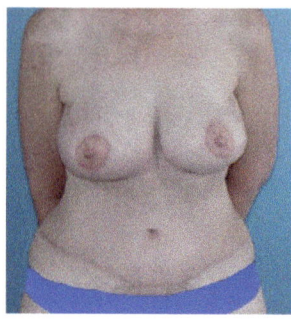

"Gertrude," shown below, developed cancer in her right breast. Her general surgeon recommended bilateral skin-sparing mastectomies. Because of the existing biopsy scar on the right, the general surgeon removed somewhat more breast skin on that side. I performed bilateral immediate TRAM flap breast reconstructions. On the left skin-sparing mastectomy side, she has the ideal situation of only a scar at the edge of the nipple-areola. These breasts feel quite natural. I did a keyhole flap and tattoo for the nipple-areolar complexes.

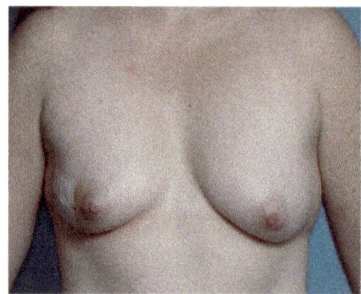 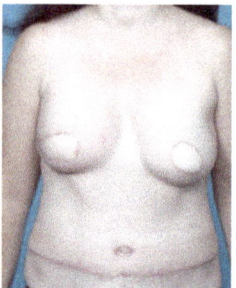 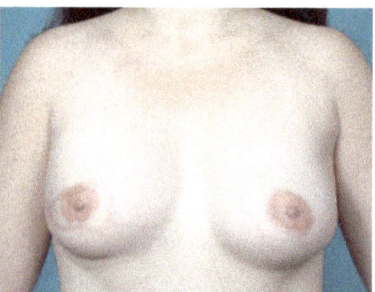

A lateral pre and final post-op view are below.

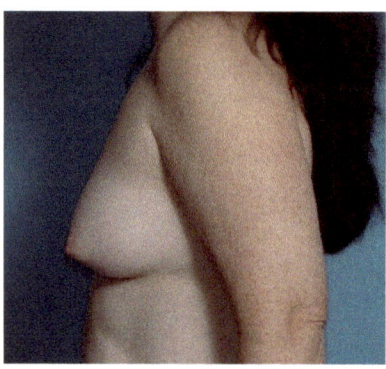 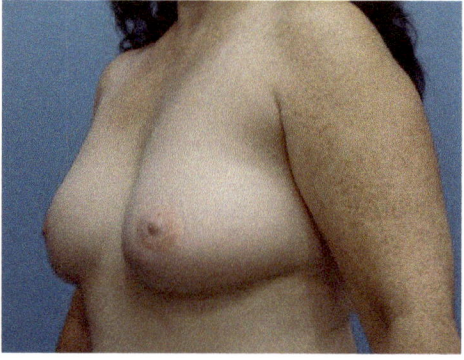

I did immediate bilateral TRAM reconstructions followed by keyhole nipple and tattoo for "Lolita, below. Because of the location of the biopsy scar on the right side, the general surgeon removed more skin on the right, and therefore a more significant skin island was needed for matching the breast size.

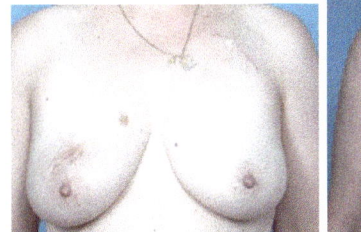 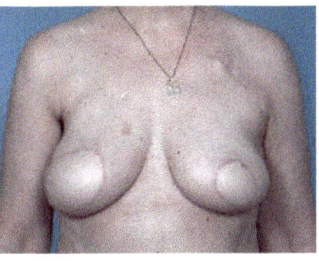 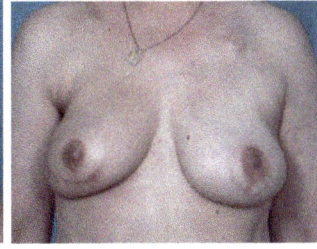

"Ramona," shown below, was diagnosed by her general surgeon with bilateral ductal carcinoma in situ. He recommended bilateral skin-sparing mastectomies and sent her to me for planning immediate breast reconstructions. During our consultation, she expressed the desire for fuller breasts.

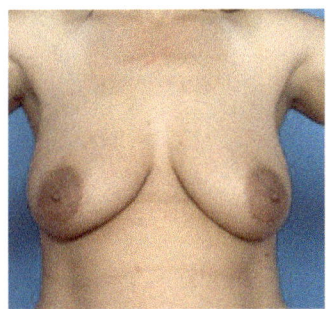 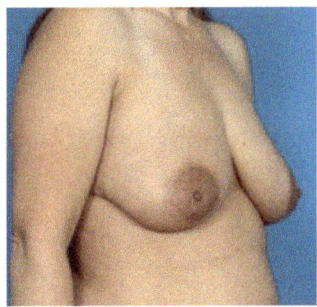 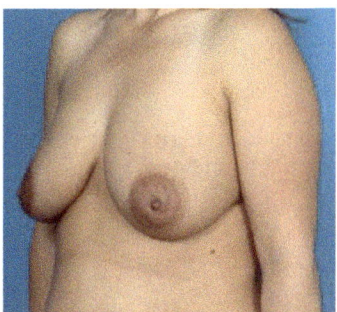

Together we decided to do bilateral pedicle TRAM flaps for restoration at the time of her mastectomies. Pictures of her intermediate result after that one operation are below.

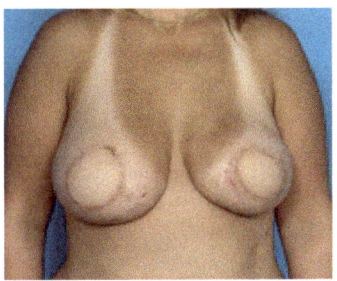 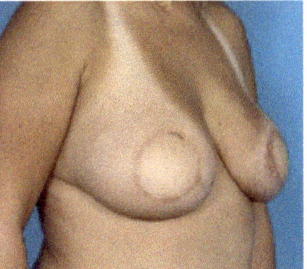 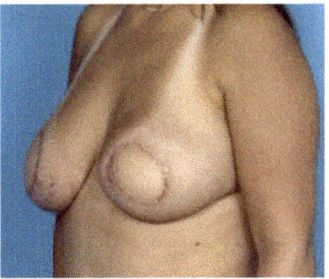

At a second operation, I performed a keyhole nipple reconstruction with a tattoo for the areola. I also placed a small silicone gel implant beneath the flap to add some additional volume. Her final result is shown below, together with the abdominal donor site pre and post-op.

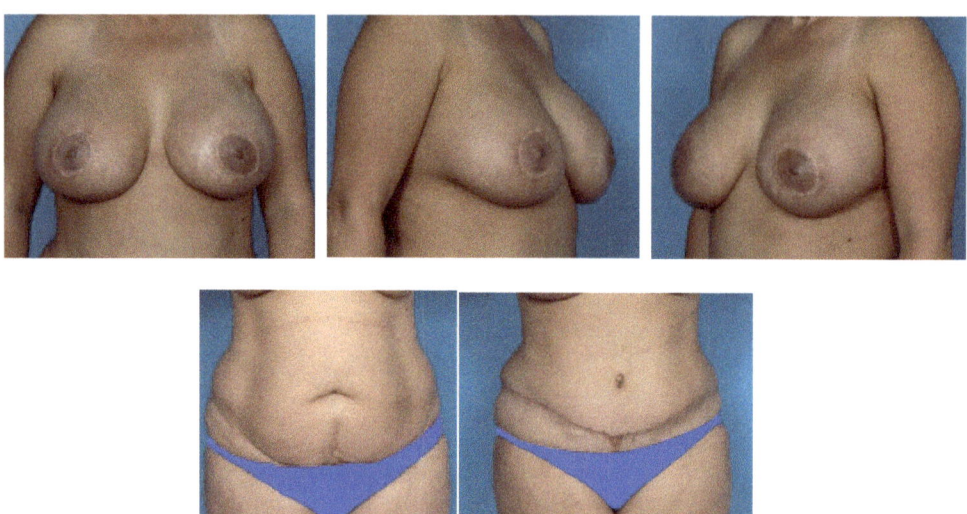

Latissimus dorsi myocutaneous flap technique in secondary breast reconstruction

The latissimus dorsi myo-cutaneous flap technique predated the TRAM flap technique and has been somewhat replaced by it. This technique uses skin, subcutaneous fat, and muscle from the back. The tissue is left attached to a pedicle of muscle containing its blood supply. The plastic surgeon passes the flap from the back through the underarm around to the anterior chest wall. This technique usually requires an implant, but not always. The latissimus procedure supplanted the thoraco-epigastric flap method described in chapter 5. In turn, the TRAM technique partially superseded the latissimus. An advantage is an outstanding blood supply, which means the latissimus flap rarely fails. It may also be easier on the patient from a pain and recovery standpoint compared to a pedicle TRAM flap.

The drawings below show this flap used in secondary breast reconstructions. The first drawing below shows an elliptical outline of skin and subcutaneous fat on top of the latissimus muscle of the right back. Through the elliptical skin incision, the latissimus muscle is dissected free except for its pedicle in the axilla containing innervating nerves and blood supply. The middle picture below shows the latissimus muscle elevated, except for its axillary connections to the humerus, and viewed from the patient's right back. The plastic surgeon must carefully preserve the blood supply (drawn in) from the axilla. The picture on the right shows the same muscle with the overlying skin and fat, which I have lifted from the back. The view is from the patient's right anterior chest. I have marked the medial and lateral aspects of the skin island in blue and the muscle orientation in green.

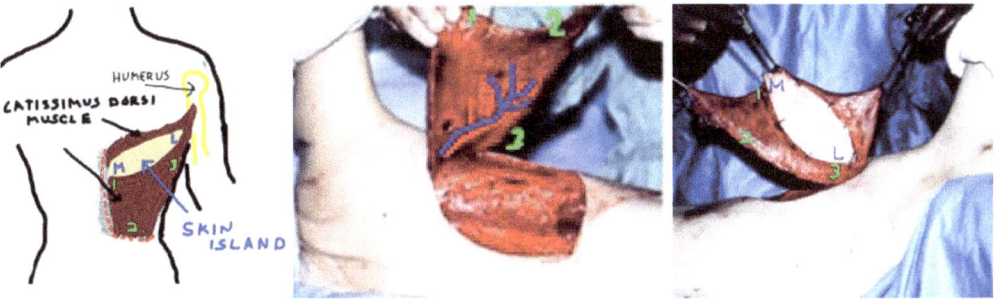

As shown below, I have tunneled the flap through the axilla to the mastectomy defect on the anterior chest. Although occasionally it can be used without an implant, it is routine to use a silicone implant beneath this myocutaneous tissue to obtain the necessary volume for the breast reconstruction, as illustrated below.

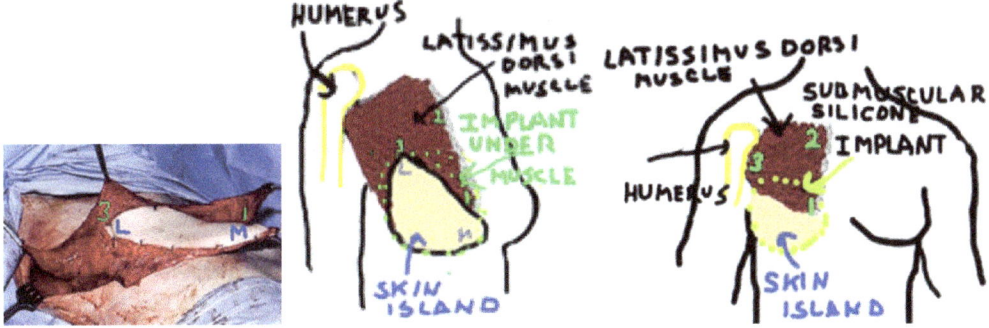

The latissimus dorsi myocutaneous flap breast reconstruction was a significant improvement over the thoracoepigastric flap described previously in Chapter 5. Initially, the majority of the patients done had had radical or modified radical mastectomies. It was intuitive that the plastic surgeon would open the old mastectomy scar, re-create the defect, which existed immediately after the mastectomy, and orient the skin island there.

Planning

The patient below "Jacqueline" had a radical mastectomy, which left her with thin skin flaps and an absent pectoralis major muscle. One can see the outline of ribs through the skin. I frequently saw such patients early in my career in the late 1970s and early 1980s. I planned a secondary reconstruction with a latissimus dorsi myocutaneous flap and silicone gel implant.

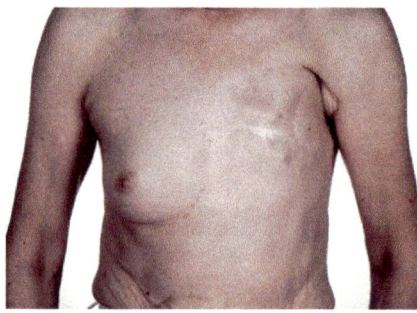
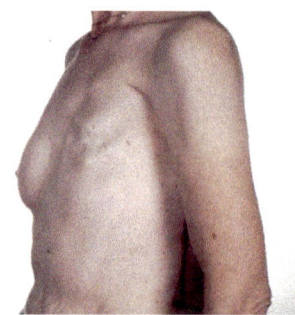

In many of the first latissimus dorsi reconstruction cases, I utilized a pattern such as the one shown below to plan the orientation of not only the skin island but the muscle coverage as well.

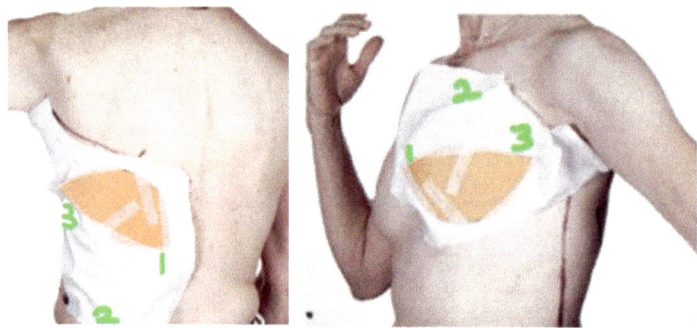

Even though she had had a radical mastectomy, "Jacqueline" obtained an agreeable result because we were able to utilize a considerable amount of muscle, to overlay the ribs in the upper chest, as well as a large skin flap. In this secondary case, I ignored the old mastectomy scar and placed the skin island inferiorly and laterally, as explained previously. She declined nipple-areola reconstruction.

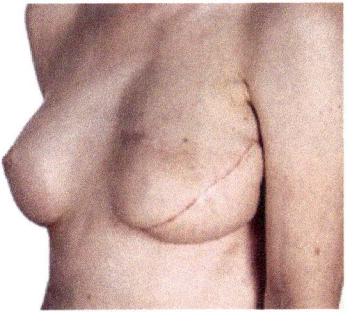 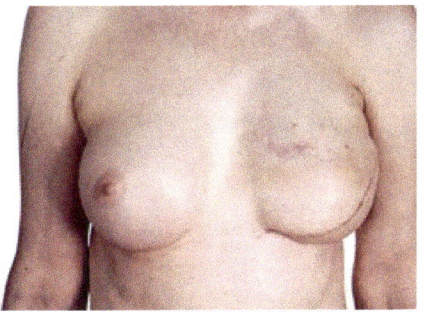

"Xena" shown below had had a modified radical mastectomy previously. I performed a latissimus flap breast reconstruction on the right. I brought tissue from the back, including skin, subcutaneous tissue, and muscle to the anterior chest. Despite the horizontal scar, I inserted the skin island low at the inframammary fold to create the full curve of the lower breast. I then placed a silicone gel implant beneath the flap. I also used a silicone gel implant for augmenting the left chest. I used a small local flap and skin graft for the nipple-areola. The last picture shows the donor site scar on the back.

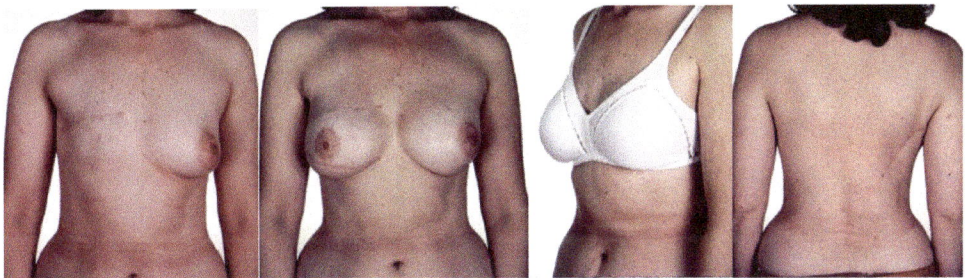

"Jane" below had had a modified radical mastectomy and postoperative radiation therapy. I reconstructed her with the latissimus flap and silicone gel implant. I placed the skin island low and lateral, ignoring as the horizontal mastectomy scar. She looks quite natural in her bra

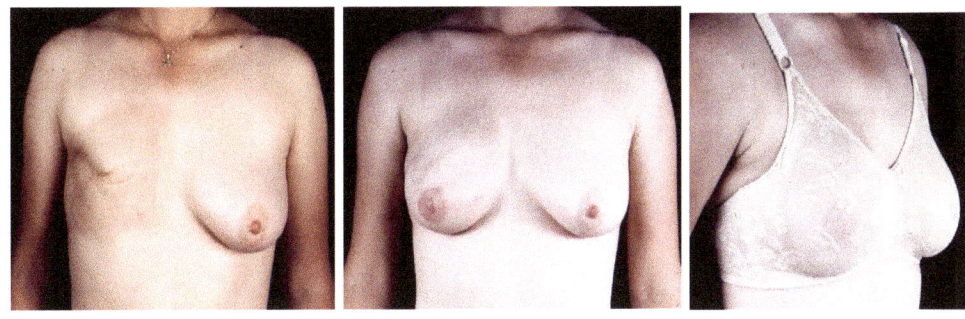

I performed bilateral latissimus dorsi myocutaneous flaps with silicone gel implants for "Francine" below. I avoided the horizontal mastectomy scars and positioned the skin islands inferiorly and laterally. I did the keyhole technique for the nipples and tattoo for the areola. Thus, this mature woman obtained the result shown,

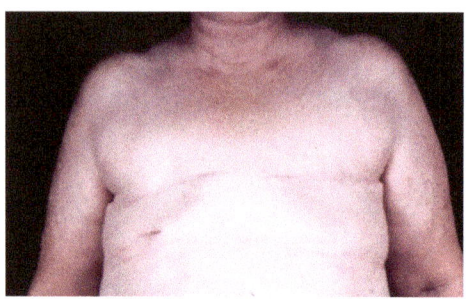
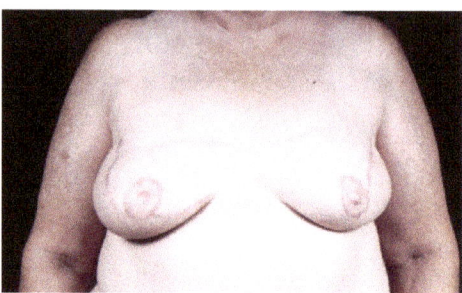

Marsha pictured below had an unusually long vertical scar after her mastectomy.

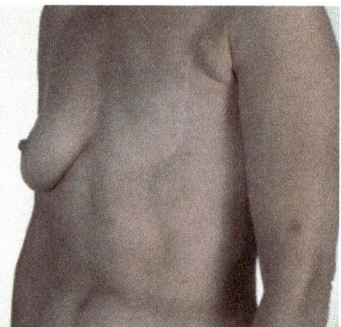
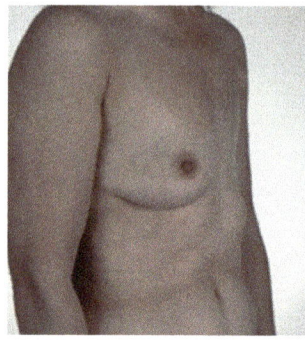

I was fortunate to be able to obtain a huge skin island with the latissimus dorsi myocutaneous flap. And in this case, I placed the flap in the area of the old scar. I used a silicone gel breast implant to obtain the postoperative results below. I "borrowed" the top of the right nipple to make the left nipple and used a split-thickness skin graft for the areola.

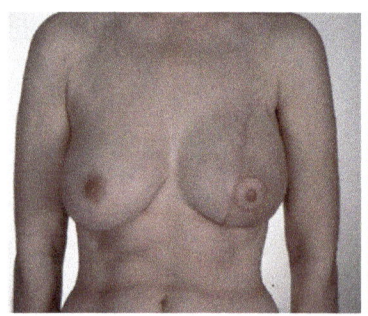
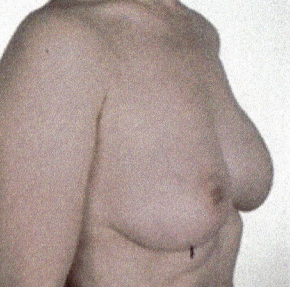
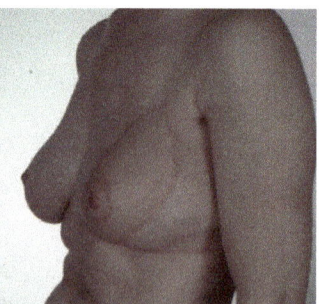

The surgical treatment of breast cancer changed over time. First, modified radical mastectomies that spared the pectoralis major muscle on the anterior chest replaced radical mastectomies. Of course, this made breast reconstruction easier for the plastic surgeon. Still later, skin-sparing mastectomies, which only removed the nipple-areola with the breast parenchyma, replaced most modified mastectomies. This conservative surgery was quite helpful for the plastic surgeon.

The latissimus dorsi myocutaneous flap technique used in immediate reconstruction

"Roberta" is shown preoperatively below with a biopsy scar near the nipple-areola. An immediate skin-sparing type mastectomy was done in her case by the general surgeon. However, he removed all of and the skin between the nipple-areola and the biopsy scar with the breast tissue. Therefore, a significant skin island with the latissimus dorsi myocutaneous flap was needed to replace that breast skin removed. The middle picture below is the intermediate result. The final result on the right is after nipple-areolar reconstruction using the keyhole flap technique and tattoo pigment placement.

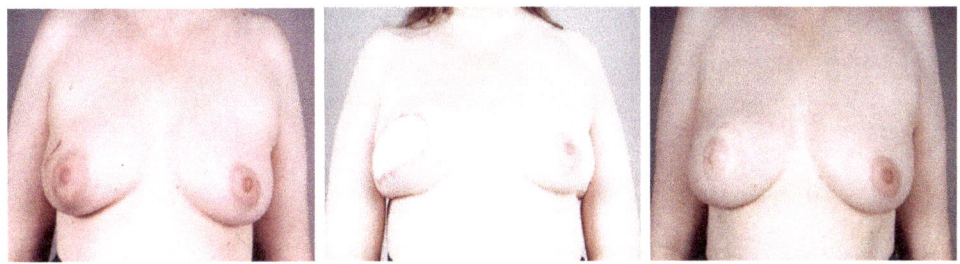

A skin-sparing mastectomy that leaves all the skin of the breasts and only removes the nipple-areola complex together with the breast tissue is probably the most frequent mastectomy done today for breast cancer. Immediate reconstruction pairs well with limited mastectomy.

The diagrams below demonstrate the latissimus dorsi myocutaneous flap in this kind of case. The first drawing below again shows an elliptical island, but in this case, only a circular portion is left intact on the skin island. The rest of the skin ellipse is de-epithelialized so that it can heal beneath the breast skin, adding some bulk together with the flap muscle and subcutaneous fat. The only surface of the flap that needs to show on the anterior chest is a circle that replaces the excised nipple-areola. To add shape and bulk to the breast, the surgeon places a silicone gel implant beneath the flap muscle. Ideally, in reconstructions after skin-sparing mastectomies, there is only a circular scar at the edge of the newly reconstructed nipple-areola. Some examples of cases I have done this way follow.

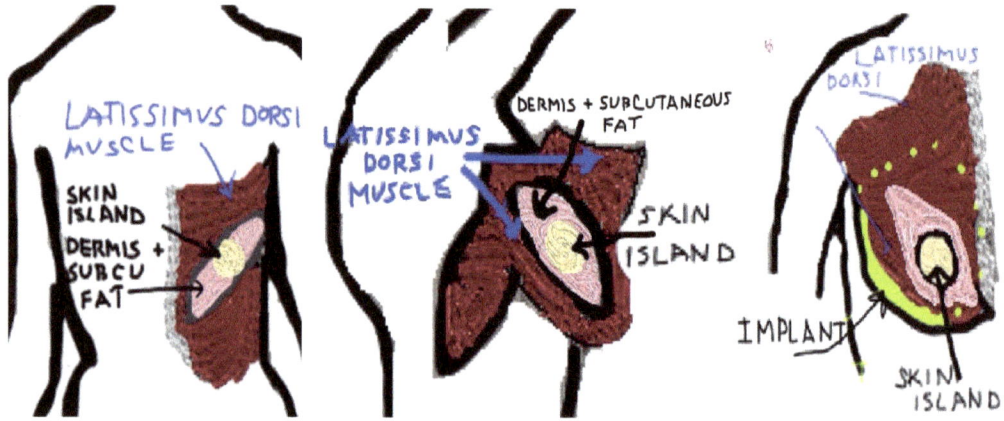

In primary reconstructions after the skin-sparing mastectomies, the orientation of the skin flap is much less critical because the only skin needed is that for replacement of the areola. The lady pictured below "Alberta" had relatively large breasts. She did not want to be a lot smaller. Her general surgeon did bilateral skin-sparing mastectomies, and I performed immediate bilateral reconstructions with latissimus dorsi flaps and silicone gel implants. Her intermediate result is in the center below. At a second operation, I did a nipple-areolar restoration using a keyhole flap technique and a revision to improve the symmetry of the breasts as in the photo on the right.

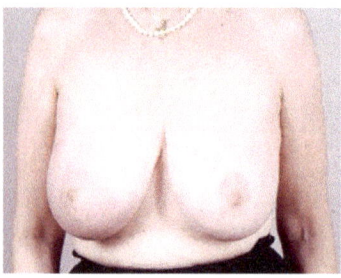 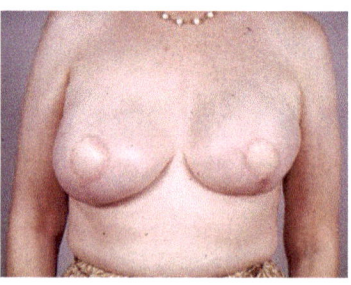

Her lateral view pre and post-op photos are below.

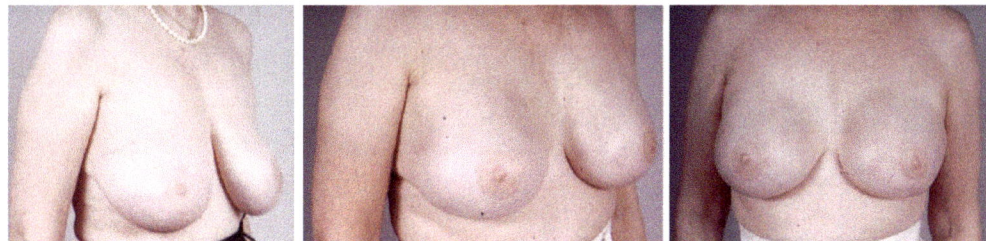

The first two photos below show "Susanna" before any surgery. Her general surgeon did a right skin-sparing mastectomy for her small cancer. I then performed an immediate right breast reconstruction utilizing a latissimus flap with a gel silicone implant. I did the right nipple reconstruction with the keyhole technique. The only scar on the breast is a circle around the nipple-areola. I also performed an augmentation mammaplasty with a silicone gel implant on the left side.

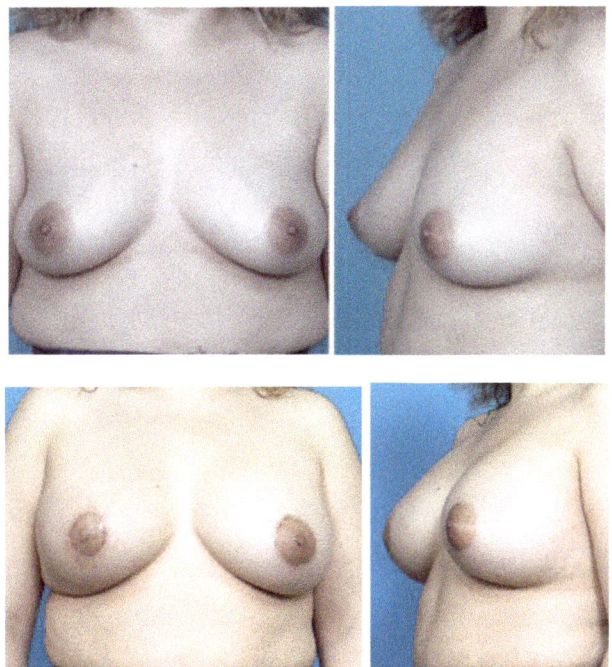

"Queenie" below had a right skin-sparing mastectomy by her general surgeon. I then did an immediate reconstruction utilizing a latissimus dorsi myocutaneous flap and a silicone gel implant (middle picture). At a second operation, I did nipple-areola repair using a nipple sharing technique and tattoo.

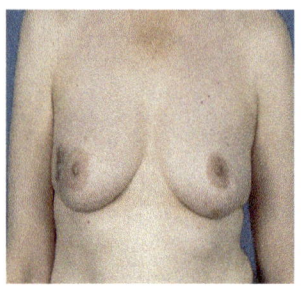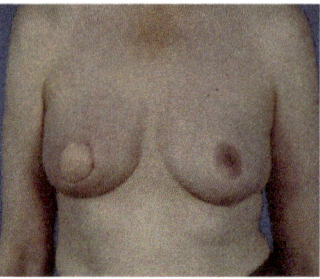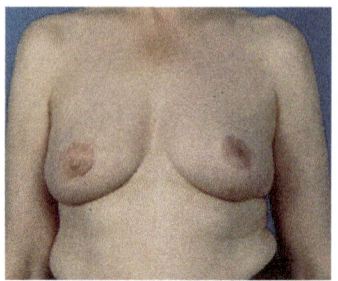

Lateral pre and post-op lateral views are below.

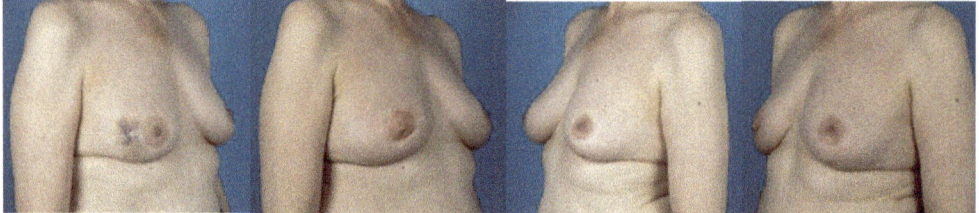

Latissimus dorsi myocutaneous flap reconstruction without an implant

"Nikki" below had a skin-sparing mastectomy by her general surgeon. In my preoperative discussions with her, she expressed a desire for somewhat smaller breasts.

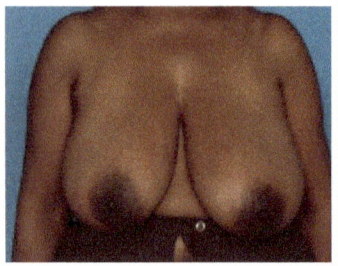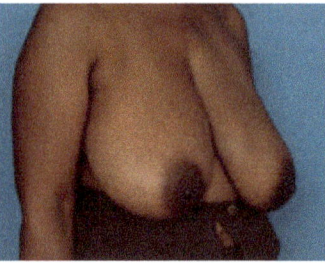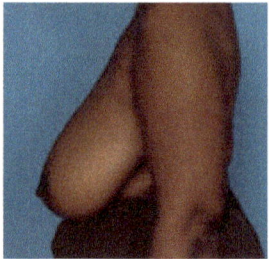

Therefore, I utilize the latissimus dorsi myocutaneous flap differently in her case. Similar to the previous examples, I developed an elliptical skin island on top of the latissimus muscle and transferred this to the anterior chest. However, in this instance, I de-epithelialized the skin island and buried it under the natural breast skin. I had plenty of surface breast skin with which to work. However, I recycled that hidden de-epithelialized skin to add bulk for the reconstructed breast. I adjusted the residual breast skin on the right side for a smaller size breast. I used some of the excess skin to simulate a nipple. At this same operation, I reduced her left chest. Her result after one surgery is below. She declined further areola reconstruction.

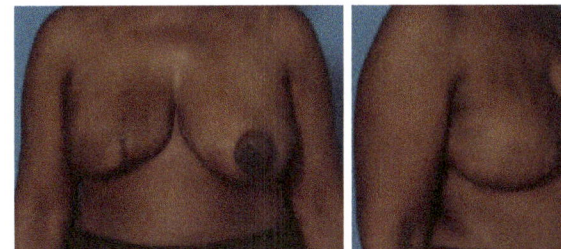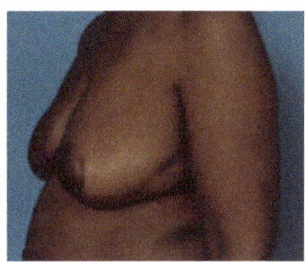

This older middle-aged obese woman, "Janet," had had a left mastectomy, which left a moderate amount of excess skin on the chest. Like the previous case, I again reconstructed this breast using a de-epithelialized latissimus dorsi myocutaneous flap and no implant. I made the nipple with local tissue and tattoo. I performed a breast lift operation on the right side for symmetry. The postoperative result is in the middle photo below. The last picture shows the donor site on the left side of her back.

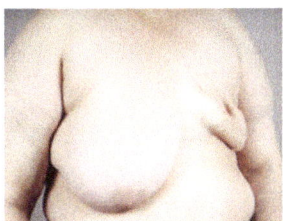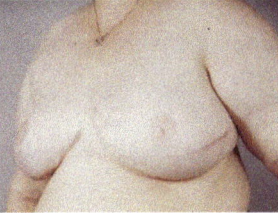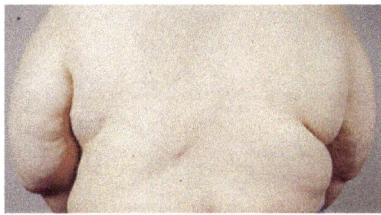

"Tessa" presented after a right modified radical mastectomy. Her general surgeon had diagnosed another breast cancer in the left breast and was planning a modified radical mastectomy for that. This patient had abundant skin and subcutaneous fatty tissue on the back. Therefore, I elected to do bilateral latissimus dorsi myocutaneous flap reconstructions without implants.

On the right side, I placed the skin island in the inferior lateral aspect of the breast. In contrast, on the left, the skin island was completely de-epithelialized and buried beneath the residual breast skin, which was spared by the general surgeon at the time of the mastectomy. She declined nipple-areola reconstruction as do a significant minority of patients.

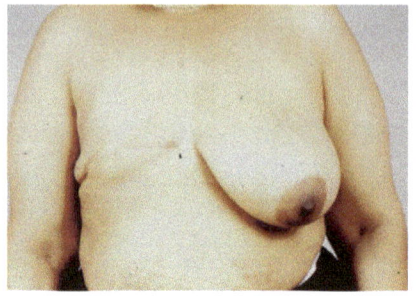
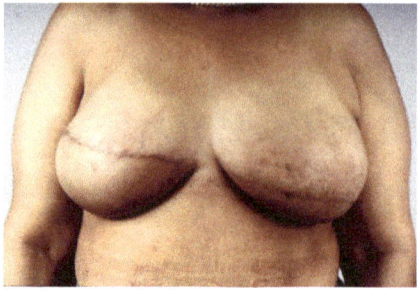

Delayed implant only breast reconstruction

"Clarissa" shown below had a relative skin-sparing mastectomy on the right. She also wished to have somewhat smaller breasts. In her case, I was able to place an implant under the pectoralis major muscle and residual breast skin of the right chest for her reconstruction. No expander was needed, so this was a one-stage reconstruction. I performed a reduction mammaplasty of her left breast for symmetry. She was not interested in a nipple-areola replacement on the right.

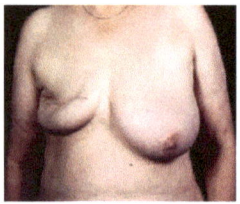
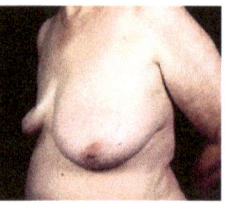
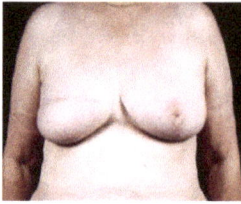
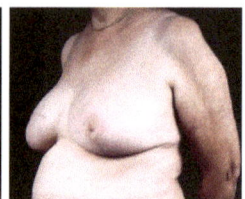

Immediate implant only reconstruction

"Barb" had a needle biopsy, which revealed left breast cancer. She came to see me before her recommended mastectomy to discuss options. As she was to have a skin-sparing mastectomy and had somewhat ptotic breasts, I suggested the placement of a submuscular silicone implant at the time of the mastectomy. At the same surgery, I recommended bilateral mastopexy.

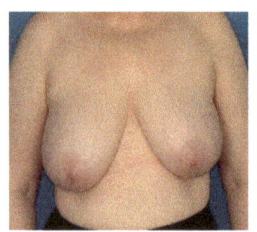
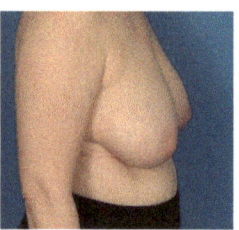
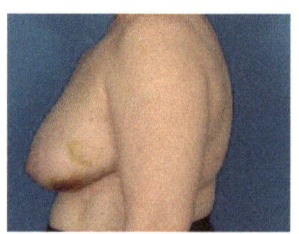

The intermediate result is below.

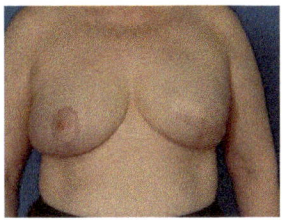

I subsequently did a keyhole nipple reconstruction. Her final results are below.

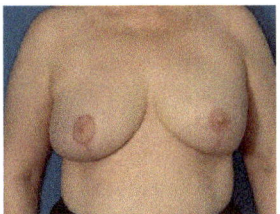 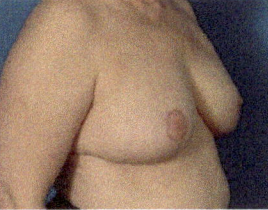 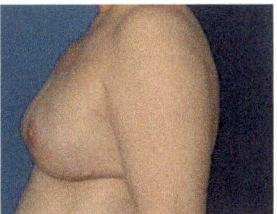

Tissue expander two-stage breast reconstruction technique

In this two-stage technique, the surgeon first places an expander balloon implant beneath the pectoralis major muscle and skin. Postoperatively the surgeon instills saline into the expander via a transcutaneous port with a needle through the skin. I routinely did the injections weekly over five or six weeks, beginning about two weeks after surgery. After waiting a few additional weeks, I exchanged the expander for a regular implant at a second operation.

Besides requiring two stages, disadvantages include it has limited capabilities and requires adequate chest wall skin tissue and usually no previous radiation therapy. Even so, this is probably the most common breast reconstruction technique used today because it does not require additional donor flap tissue. I am less fond of this technique than others. I feel the best reconstructions are those composed with a large percent of the patient's own tissue, with or without an implant.

In this patient "Isabel" below, I utilized a tissue expander with a remote fill port like the one in the second picture. I inserted the expander beneath the pectoralis major and anterior serratus muscles.

The Healing Mission of Plastic Surgery

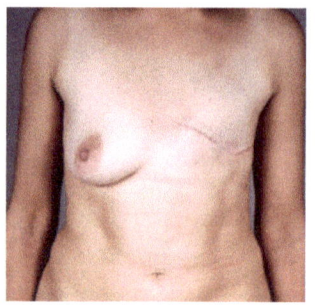 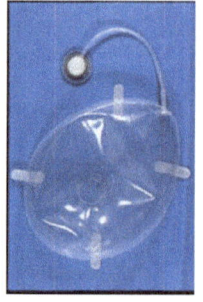 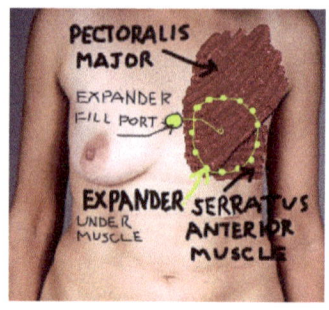

I instilled the expander with saline via needle and syringe (shown below) once a week to gradually over-expand the overlying muscle and skin. The middle picture below shows that I overstretched the surface to allow for later rebound shrinkage. I removed the tissue expander in a second operation and inserted a permanent silicone gel implant. I also did an augmentation with a silicone gel implant on the right. I amputated the top of the right nipple and grafted it to make the left nipple. I tattooed the areolae. The final result is also below.

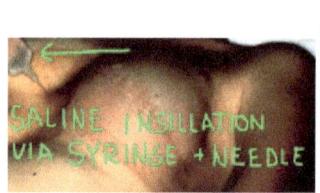 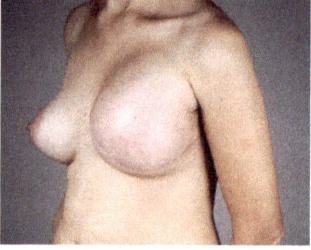 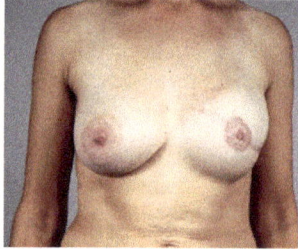

"Hellen" shown below had had a recent open biopsy diagnosis of breast cancer on the right. Her general surgery planned a skin-sparing mastectomy for her. I discussed various types of reconstructions with her. She did not want to have a tissue flap-type reconstruction. Therefore, we planned a tissue expander, two-stage implant only, breast reconstruction. Because she had limited muscle for coverage of the inferior aspect of the implant, I decided to use a dermal matrix product to cover the inferior half of the implant. Specially treated human donor skin produces a dermal matrix that can substitute for living tissue as a sturdy sheet-like layer for various applications. I used the dermal matrix connected to the pectoralis major muscle to cover the inferior half of the tissue expander implant and control the inferior extent of the implant pocket. I used it also to help define the level of the infra-mammary fold.

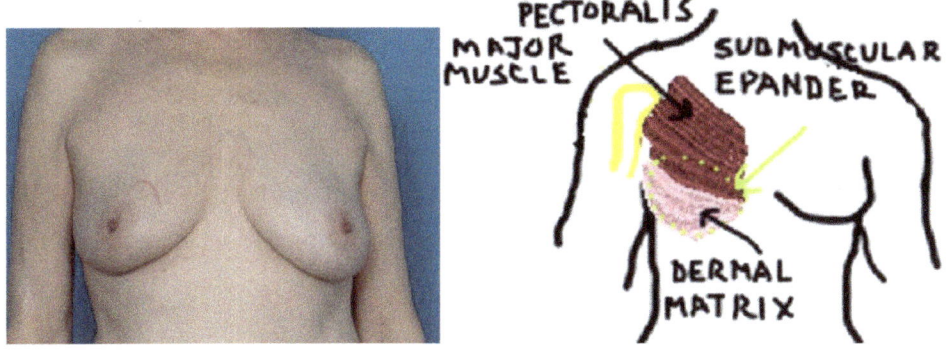

At the second operation, I removed the expander and inserted a permanent silicone gel implant. At that time, I also used injected fat grafts to smooth out some areas of depressions. I performed nipple reconstructions with S flaps (explained later below) together with areola tattooing. Below, post-expansion is on the left and after permanent implant placement and nipple-areola reconstruction on the right.

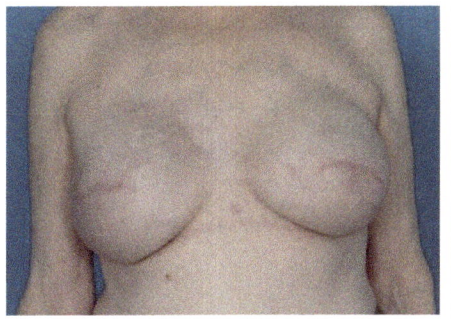
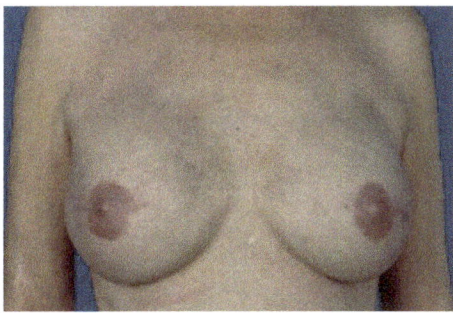

Below the original lateral view pre-op on the left and final result on the right.

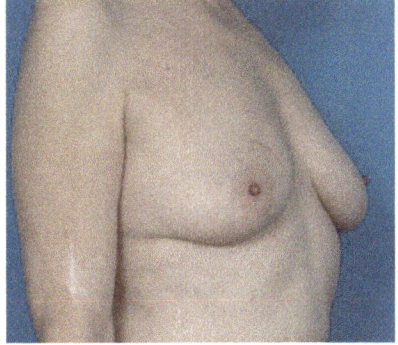
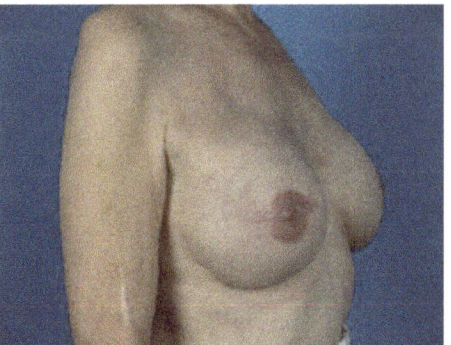

Revision in breast reconstruction

Revisions in breast reconstruction to improve the shape of the breast or to maximize symmetry between the breasts are very prevalent. They may relate to making the inframammary fold position more symmetric or the nipple placement more symmetric. They may involve shaping the chest to make it more attractive or changing the volume. Some of the above reconstructive cases have had small revisions that I did not specifically describe.

The patient below, "Cassandra," is a little different. This patient came to me after she had had several surgeries for breast reconstruction after bilateral mastectomies. She had bilateral silicone breast implants. She wanted a second opinion. Examination revealed bilateral breast reconstructions, which were not very symmetric and not very "breast-like." Also, the position of the nipple-areola complex was questionable. I felt like the left breast could be significantly improved by remaking the pocket and replacing the implant with a larger one. I believed the right breast needed more skin coverage. Therefore, I performed a latissimus dorsi myocutaneous flap to bring additional tissue from the back to the lower portion of the anterior chest. I removed the old implant and inserted a larger implant. I dermabraided the previously tattooed nipple-areolar complexes to obliterate them. I constructed new nipple-areolae complexes using a keyhole nipple technique and adding tattoo pigment.

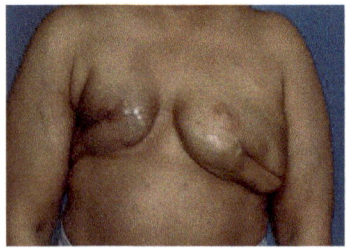 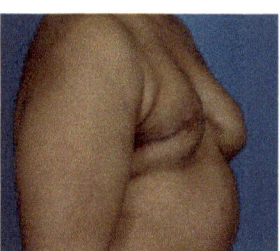 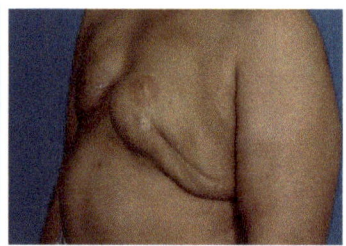

The photo below illustrates the improved shape and position of the breasts and nipples. I believe "Cassandra" was pleased with the result obtained by the revision of breast reconstruction I performed. The hypopigmented areas shown in the final photo should blend in quite a bit over time.

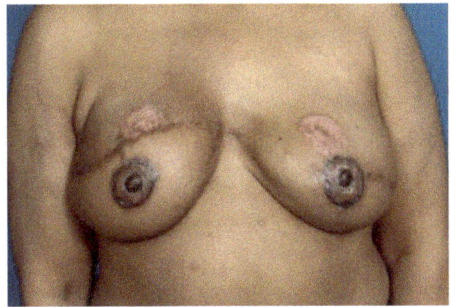

Partial mastectomy cases

Lumpectomy combined with postoperative radiation therapy sounds appealing to many patients instead of a mastectomy. This combination can work quite well for many patients who choose this method. However, when cases are not satisfactory, it often presents awkward problems for both the patient and the plastic surgeon.

The patient below "Antonia" had a partial mastectomy on the right side, which was followed by radiation therapy. She was unhappy because of the significant residual asymmetry, which caused her considerable problems with her clothing.

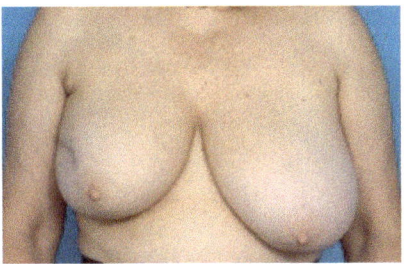 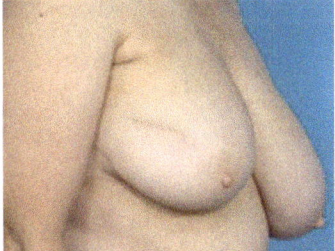

I treated the asymmetry with a mastopexy on the left and a revision of the breast reconstruction on the right with a silicone gel implant and fat grafting by injection. The postop pictures below depict her improved shape and symmetry

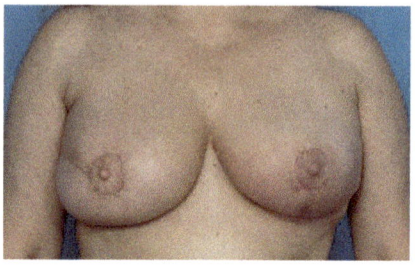 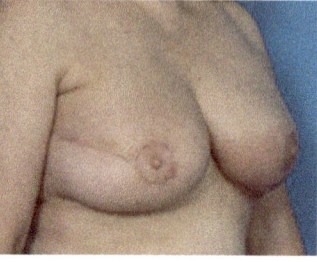

The patient below, "Sarah," had a partial mastectomy for cancer followed by X-ray therapy. One can see significant radiation skin changes. She requested additional surgery to help improve her appearance. After I thoroughly discussed various possibilities with her, I recommended reducing the size of the left breast and revising the right breast to better match the left.

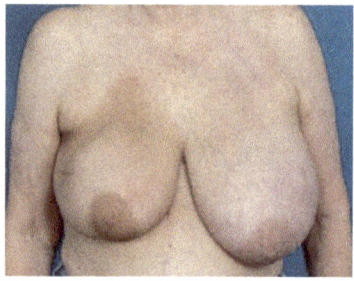 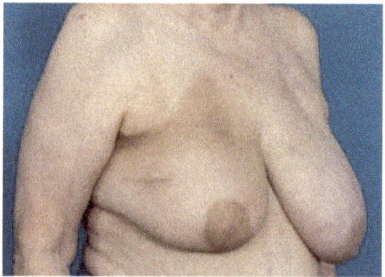

I performed a standard inferior pedicle breast reduction on the left side. I then revised the right breast using a mastopexy technique together with fat grafting in the upper chest to try to improve the damaged radiated skin. The post-operative photos demonstrate some improved symmetry.

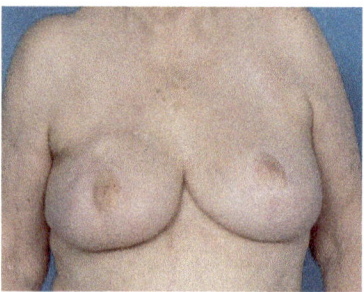 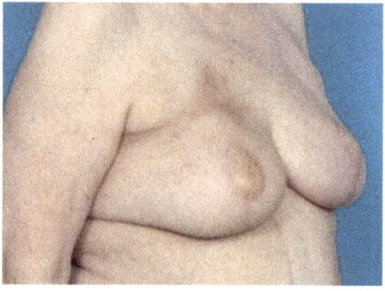

"Mollie" pictured below had lumpectomy and radiation for her breast cancer. She was unhappy with her asymmetry and consulted with me about further reconstruction. For the depressed area in the upper lateral right breast, I recommended fat grafting, together with a small silicone gel implant, to fill out that area and offer increased volume to the right breast. For the left chest, I recommended a mastopexy for improved shape and symmetry with the opposite breast.

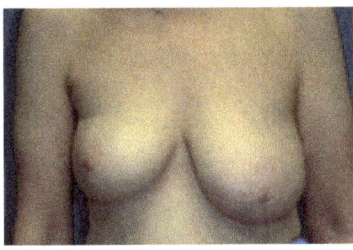 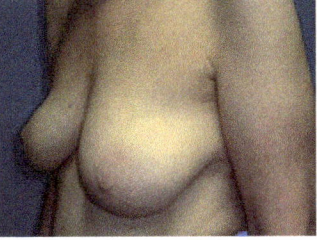 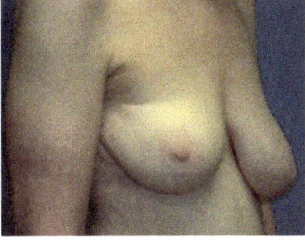

I did perform the fat grafting and implant insertion on the right at the same time as doing a mastopexy on the left. Her post-op photos are below.

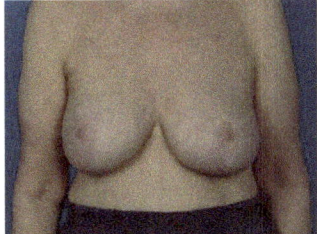 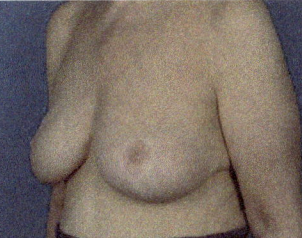 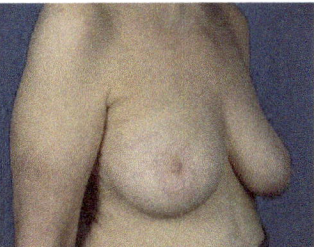

Subcutaneous mastectomy for granulomas after injections

Before the development of modern breast implants, augmentation by injection of silicone liquid or other substances was reasonably common. This phenomenon was especially prevalent in Japan and other Oriental countries. I saw eight or ten such patients who had difficulties with their breasts because of these injections. I present an extreme case in chapter12 Unusual Cases. Most of these patients had indurated lumps in the breasts and mastodynia (painful breasts). Some patients in which the silicone had migrated very superficially into the skin had nonhealing sores, which were uncomfortable and continuously inflamed. Some of these patients needed mastectomies to rid themselves of these hygiene and pain problems. When possible, I did a subcutaneous mastectomy, removing the breast tissue from beneath the skin if it was not involved. I then place a modern breast implant beneath the surface skin or, more likely, beneath a layer of muscle. These patients were quite appreciative of curing their mastodynia yet still having the appearance and feel of breasts. Examples of subcutaneous mastectomies are shown later in this chapter.

Nipple areola reconstruction

More than half the patients who have a breast reconstructed will want the nipple reconstructed also.

The methods include local flaps such as the keyhole and S flap techniques and techniques which share the uninvolved opposite nipple-areola. I used these local flap techniques to make projections for the nipple and tattoo pigment or skin graft for the surrounding areola. When available, I often utilized nipple sharing techniques, as well.

Flap reconstructions

Several small local flap techniques are available. I will show two flaps that I have favored in my practice

S flap nipple-areolar reconstruction technique

The surgeon makes an S-shaped incision and elevates two flaps to facing each other. The surgeon then sews the flaps together to form tissue projection for the nipple. This technique is especially applicable when there is a pre-existing scar across the site for the new nipple, as in the first picture below. The case below shows the S nipple technique used together with a skin graft for the areola. The results shown are 18 months after S flap nipple-areola reconstruction.

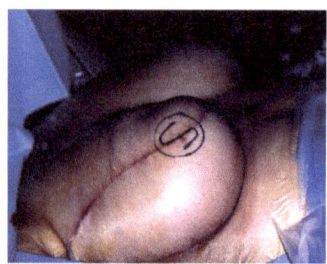 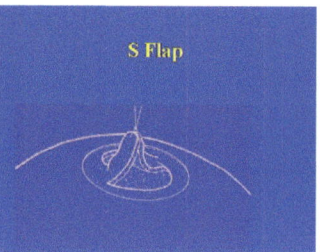 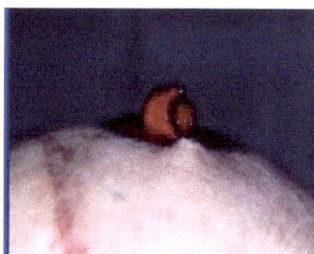

The Healing Mission of Plastic Surgery

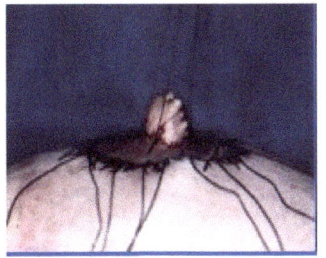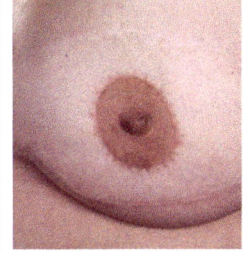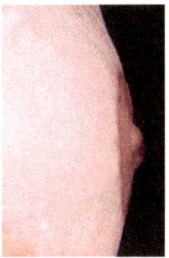

The pictures below show the S nipple used with simultaneous tattooing of the nipple-areola

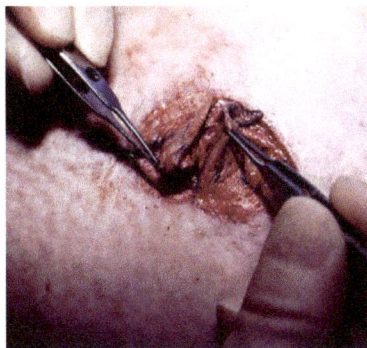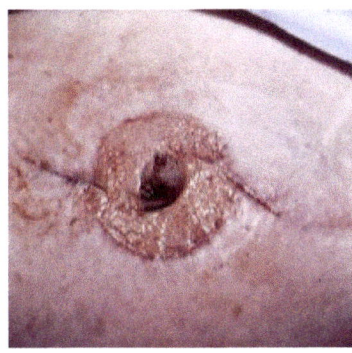

Keyhole nipple-areola reconstruction technique

The keyhole nipple reconstruction technique is a slight variation of previously described methods, such as the "bell" technique. The paper models below show a keyhole -type incision, which creates a flap that is doubled on itself to create the projection. It is essential to produce generous flaps to create a nipple that will resist the natural tendencies for shrinkage and loss of prominence. The surgeon can close the donor site in various ways. The two C points must come together, which creates bunched excess tissue inferiorly. The surgeon can get rid of this dog-ear or standing cone by direct excision inferiorly. The last two pictures below show the incision inferiorly.

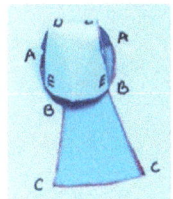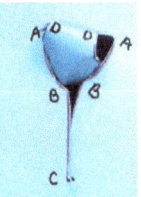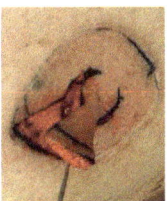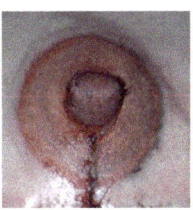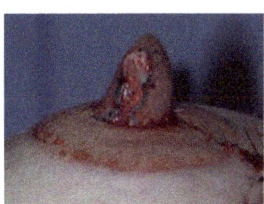

The first picture below is after 18 months. The second one below is post-op 15 months.

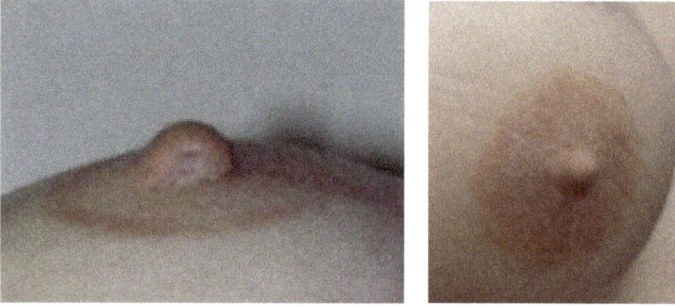

Alternatively, in many skin-sparing mastectomy reconstructions, there is already a scar around the area that will become the areola. In those cases, remaking the circular incision can take care of the dog-ear. So, the scar around the areola may be the only scar left after skin-sparing mastectomy and breast and nipple-areolar reconstruction. Two examples of this kind of keyhole nipple reconstructions are shown below at about a year post-op.

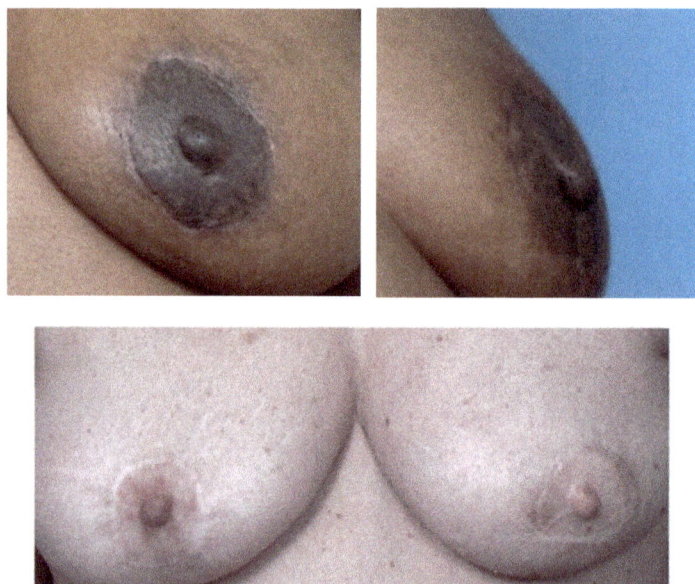

The nipple-areola reconstruction shown below is 15 months after the keyhole technique and areola tattooing.

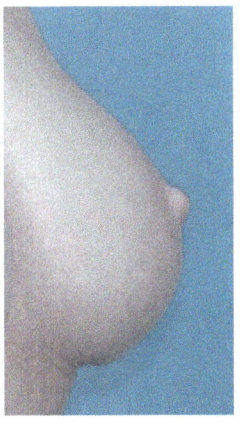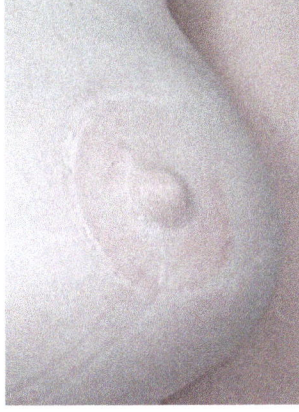

Nipple areola sharing Techniques

When the areola is shared, two areolae can be made from one and still have about 70% the diameter of the original. For example, if the areola has a diameter of 6 cm, then two can be made with a diameter of 4.2cm each.

The conjoined spiral nipple-areola reconstruction technique

In this technique, the incisions are made in a modified yin yang pattern, as shown below, producing two grafts, each with half a nipple and half the areola. Then one graft is replaced to make a smaller nipple-areola at the donor site, and the other makes a new nipple-areola on the reconstructed breast as shown in the second picture.

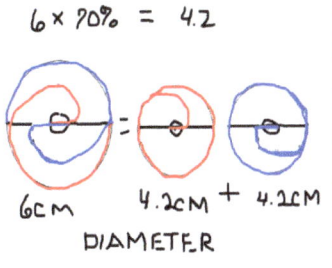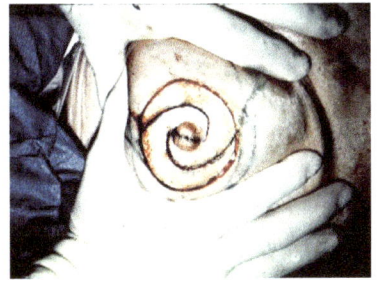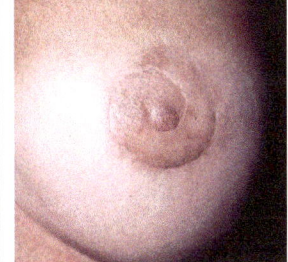

Concentric circle technique

This technique only shares the areola. The surgeon removes a donut-shaped graft from the periphery of the donor areola (blue in the drawing below). He will transfer this graft to the opposite breast for its areola. The case shown below is unusual because I performed a mastopexy at the time of breast reconstruction. Still, because I knew I would like to use areola from that breast at a second operation, I preserved all of that areola temporarily. That is why the areola in the first picture below looks overabundant. The second picture diagrammatically shows the sharing of the donor areola.

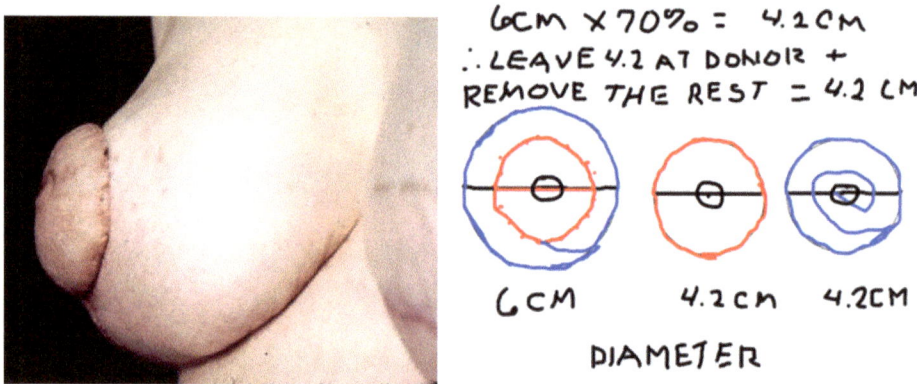

The first picture below shows the marked incisions. This nipple will remain, and the central part of the areola will remain. The surgeon will take the peripheral donut-shaped portion of the areola to make the areola of the opposite breast. The next photo is of the reconstructed breast, which had an S flap reconstruction for the nipple and the grafted areola for areola.

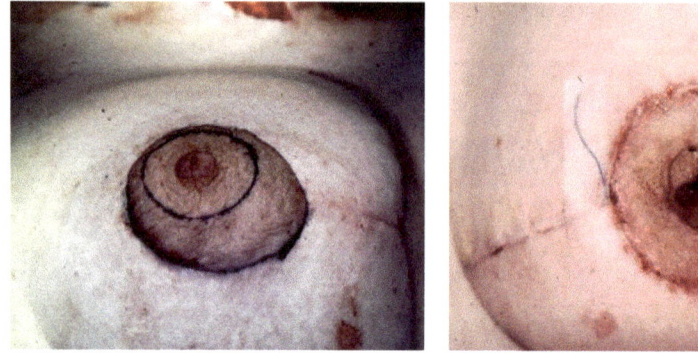

The last photo below shows the right breast, which had a mastopexy and was the donor of the excess areola, which went to the left chest for its areola. I used a latissimus flap and silicone implant for reconstruction for the left breast. I did an S flap for the nipple and used the "borrowed areola from the right breast to make the areola on the left.

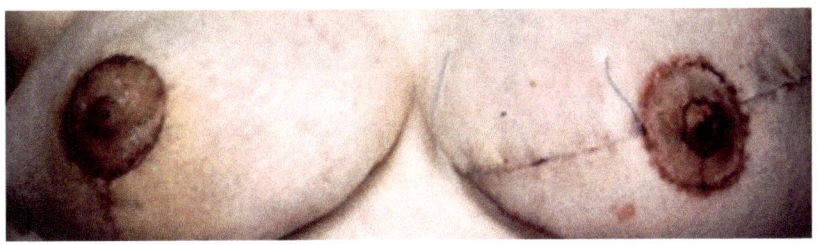

Overall, today, most patients can obtain a satisfactory reconstruction after mastectomy. Patients should have a consultation with a plastic surgeon experienced with breast reconstruction if they learn they may need a mastectomy. Today the most common reconstruction after a mastectomy is with a tissue expander placed beneath the pectoralis major muscle, followed by the exchange of the expander for a permanent type implant at a second procedure. There has been a trend away from pedicle tram flaps to free flaps either with only a small amount of rectus abdominus muscle or without any muscle at all but only skin and subcutaneous tissue and the vascular pedicle. These free flap procedures may have less morbidity and stress to the abdominal wall donor site of the patient.

Prophylactic mastectomy

Prophylactic mastectomy has been a controversial area of medicine. In the past, many general surgeons criticized prophylactic subcutaneous mastectomy (done for at-risk patients without a diagnosis of cancer) as not being radical enough. Now ironically, when a small breast tumor is away from the nipple-areola complex, many general surgeons perform a subcutaneous mastectomy as the total treatment.

I feel vindicated that my long-standing practice of doing subcutaneous mastectomy has been judged sufficient. The presumption is a patient, who has had a subcutaneous mastectomy, has a significantly reduced chance of ever developing breast cancer.

At the Cronin Brauer and Biggs Clinic, we did a high number of subcutaneous mastectomies for breast cancer prevention. In several instances, small cancers were found in the specimens by microscopic examination. These patients needed no further treatment. They were probably quite fortunate in their decision to have prophylactic mastectomies. To my knowledge, there were only a couple of patients who developed breast cancer after subcutaneous mastectomy out of approximately 1000 cases at the Cronin, Brauer, and Biggs Clinic.

Knowing that one of nine women will develop breast cancer in their lifetime, this is quite remarkable. Unfortunately, we never did a scientific review of these cases for various reasons. I performed many prophylactic mastectomies on patients who were likely candidates to develop breast cancer but had no evidence of disease. I routinely performed this procedure through a generous inframammary incision about 10 cm long. I removed the breast tissue except for a small amount immediately beneath the nipple-areola complex. I created a submuscular pocket and inserted a silicone gel implant. I must point out that this procedure is not a cosmetic operation like augmentation mammaplasty. Instead, it is a significant preventative surgery combined with immediate reconstruction. So, if the after photos look as healthy as the before pictures, it is quite a favorable aesthetic result.

"Carolina," whose pre-operative images are below, had a genetically high risk for cancer. Her endocrinologist sent her to me for consultation regarding prophylactic mastectomy.

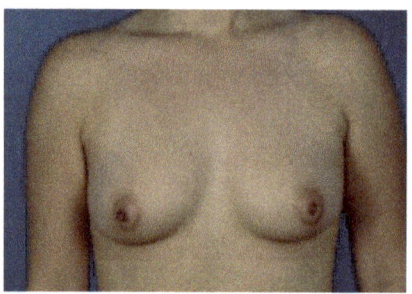 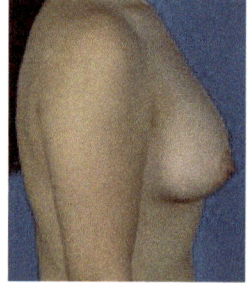

After the thorough discussion, she decided to proceed with prophylactic surgery. I did a subcutaneous mastectomy with immediate reconstruction with silicone gel implants in the submuscular space. Below are her postoperative photos.

The Healing Mission of Plastic Surgery

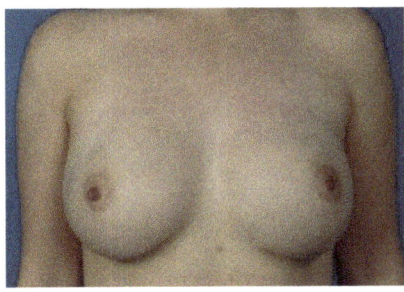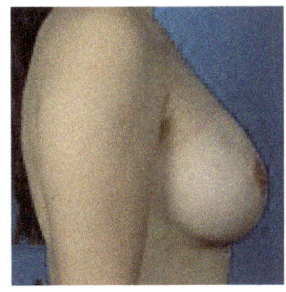

"La Donna" pictured below had had multiple biopsies, a very dense appearing mammogram which was difficult to assess. Physical exam revealed very fibrous and lumpy breasts, which were difficult to evaluate. She also had a strong family history for breast cancer. I did bilateral subcutaneous mastectomies with submuscular placement of gel implants through an incision in the crease under the breast. Her before and after photos are below.

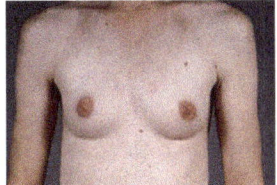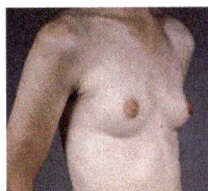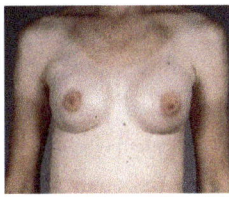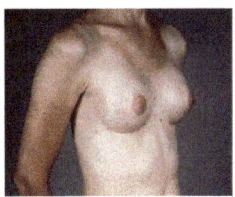

"Rihanna," below, had a strong family history for breast cancer, very lumpy breast tissue, and a difficult to assess mammogram. I performed bilateral subcutaneous mastectomies and inserted silicone gel implants in a submuscular pocket. Her pre-and postoperative photos are below.

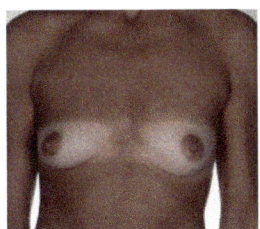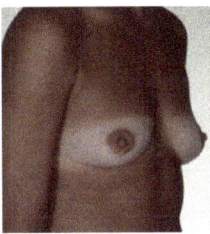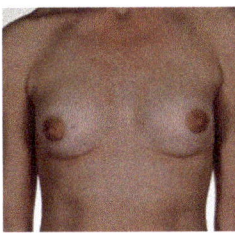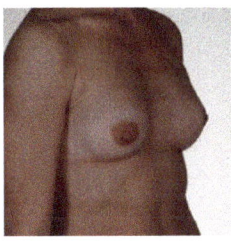

The following patient, "Melody" was a candidate for subcutaneous mastectomy because of high risk for breast cancer. However, she did not want to have an implant. Therefore, I did a bilateral pedicle TRAM flaps, which brought tissue from the abdomen to replace the breast tissue I removed with the mastectomy. She had an excellent result. She also received an improvement in the contour of her stomach.

The Healing Mission of Plastic Surgery

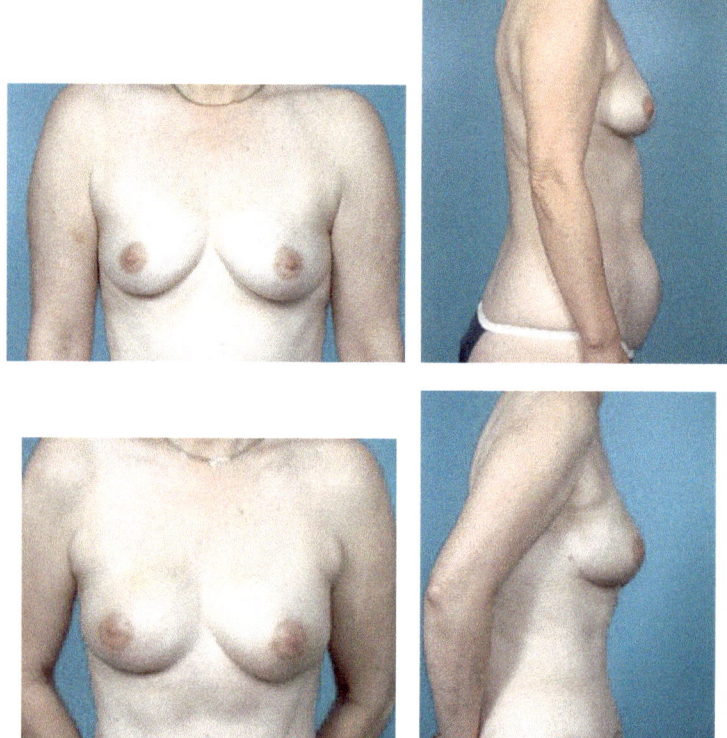

Chapter 10

The French Connection and the Birth of Craniofacial Surgery

In the early 1970s, Thomas Cronin had just returned from a long trip to China. As he was going through his accumulated mail, he found a packet from France sent to him by a surgeon named Paul Tessier. This correspondence contained a series of pre-, and post-operative photographs and an invitation to come to France to watch a unique set of operations. The pictures were of patients with severe congenital cranial facial disorders operated on in recent years by Dr. Paul Tessier.

These were astounding photographs. Dr. Cronin could tell from the photos that Dr. Tessier's work would cause a paradigm shift in reconstructive surgery of the face and skull. So, Dr. Cronin immediately made arrangements to fly to Paris to see the demonstration, which was to occur in only a few days. Dr. Cronin was very impressed with Dr. Tessier and his work. Dr. Cronin invited Dr. Tessier to come to Houston yearly to operate on patients that the Cronin, Brauer, and Biggs Clinic arranged for him. Thus, a long cooperative relationship developed between them.

Each year a consultation clinic was held in which Dr. Tessier would see a few dozen patients. In the first picture below on the left, Dr. Tessier caries on a pleasant banter with a young patient. The second picture shows resident plastic surgeons Drs. Gary Branfman and Hal Mentz studiously overlooking Dr. Tessier as he considers what he will recommend for the little patient they are examining. In the last photo on the right, Dr. Tessier demonstrates a proposed surgical plan to Drs Cronin and Brauer with plaster dental models.

The Healing Mission of Plastic Surgery

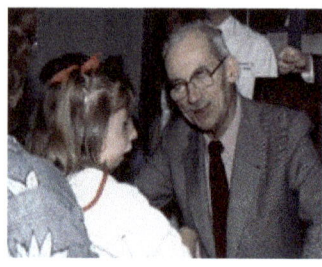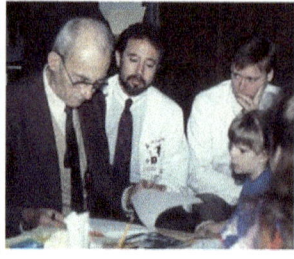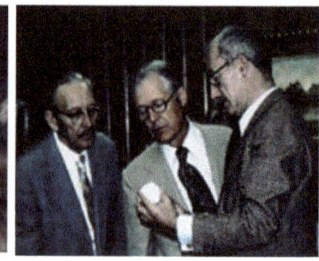

Many plastic surgeons attended this clinic demonstration each year in Houston. There were enough patients for Dr. Tessier to operate on from early morning late into the evening for one week and sometimes longer. A closed-circuit television screen in the surgeon's lounge allowed for observation by numerous visiting physicians. Some of these were cases that no one else in the world would tackle because of their severity and the need for new techniques to treat them. Those were heady days! This invitation to Dr. Tessier to come to Houston to operate became open-ended, and he returned for 17 years in a row. I was very fortunate to be able to participate, starting in 1976 when I was a resident through 1988 the last year doctor Tessier operated in Houston. Each year 15 to 20 patients would have quite complex operations planned and performed by Dr. Tessier. He was a master at analyzing the problems of these craniofacial patients. He was incredibly innovative in creating new procedures.

Below is a view of Dr. Tessier operating at St Joseph Hospital in 1983. Also pictured below are two of the most talented and well-known protégés of Dr. Tessier, Dr. Tony Wolf of Miami, and Dr. Henry Kawamoto of Los Angeles. Each of them visited Houston with Dr. Tessier on several occasions. Both have been advocates of Dr. Tessier's advances in craniofacial surgery and have made significant contributions to this field of plastic surgery.

The Healing Mission of Plastic Surgery

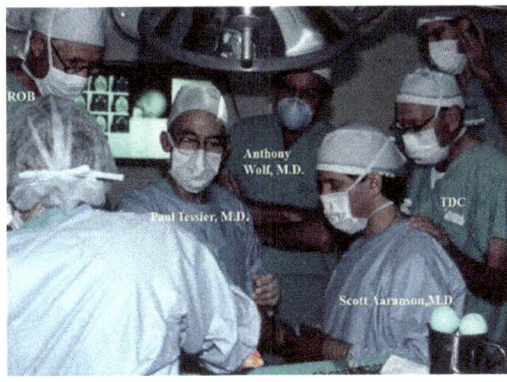 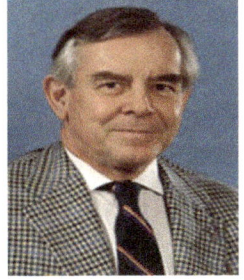 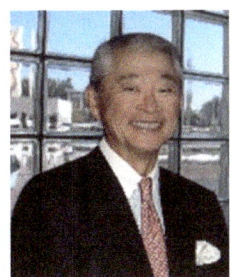

The photo below shows Dr. Tessier in the center together with Dr. Brauer second from the left in the surgical lounge resting between cases and conversing with resident surgeons, Drs Robert Wright, Scott Aaronson, Alfonso Barrera, and visiting surgeons.

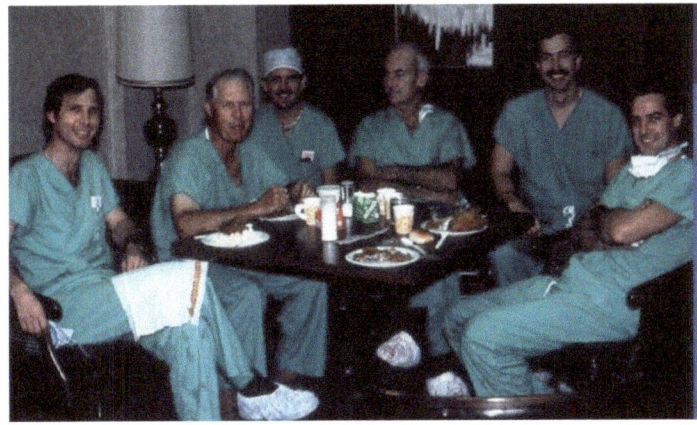

One of Dr. Tessier's accomplishments was his approach to treating patients with Crouzon's syndrome, a congenital problem that previously had no adequate treatment. The drawings below show how from an intracranial approach, he moved the forehead and the upper face, including the orbits, forward without damaging the eyes. He placed bone grafts (yellow) in the gaps created by the forward movement to promote healing and to prevent relapse.

The Healing Mission of Plastic Surgery

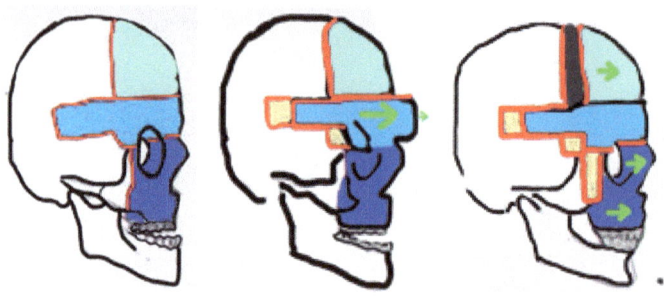

The dramatic transformation shown in the pre and post-operative photos below is of a patient that Dr. Tessier operated on in Houston. This type of life-changing breakthrough surgery catapulted Tessier into worldwide fame.

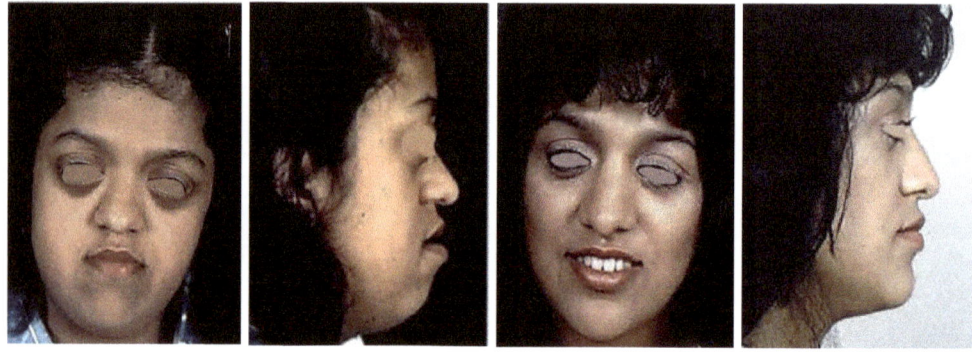

Dr. Tessier developed a numerical classification for rare craniofacial clefts primarily based on his experience with actual patients. It is somewhat different from that expected from general embryologic studies. I made a rough sketch below to illustrate Dr. Tessier's classification with the skeleton on the left and soft tissue on the right.

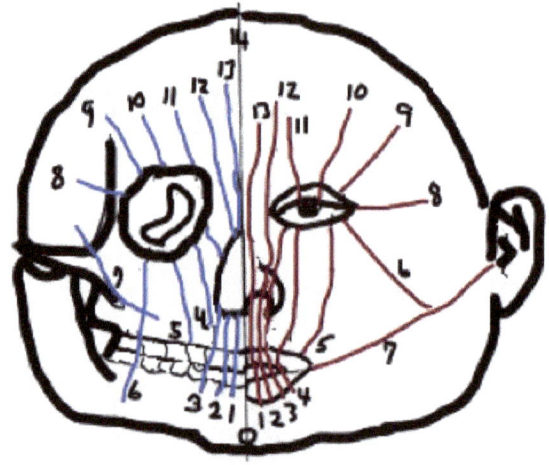

The Healing Mission of Plastic Surgery

The Tessier classification for rare craniofacial clefts is numbered 0 to 14 depending on the relationship to the orbit. The orbit also divides clefts into cranial, superiorly and facial, inferiorly. The cranial and facial cohorts of clefts add up to 14. For example, a number 4 facial cleft might extend to a cranial component, which would be a number 10 cleft or a number one facial cleft might extend cranially as a number 13 cleft. Half of the picture shows the numerical position of the bony clefts, while the other half shows the location related to the soft tissue of the face. Unfortunately, all of these clefts can occur in nature. A few examples given below are illustrative.

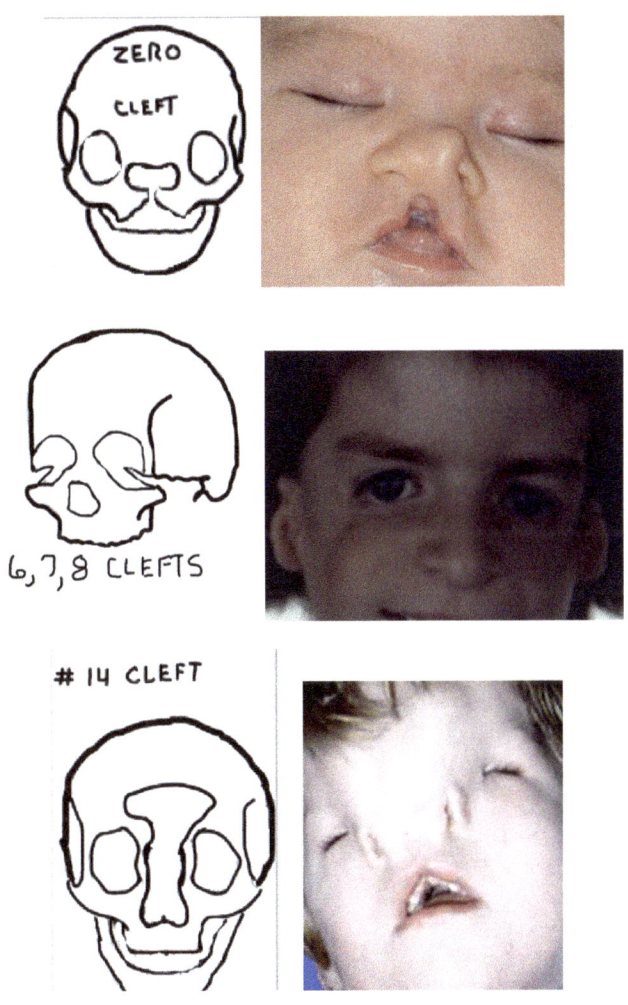

373

The Healing Mission of Plastic Surgery

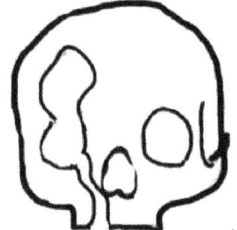
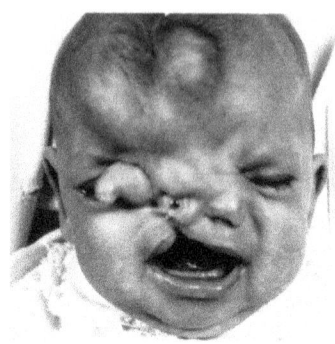

Because of the pioneering work of Dr. Tessier, plastic surgery can help the patients suffering from these rare clefts toward leading an abundant life.

One particular event related to Dr. Tessier's visits I remember acutely occurred when I was a senior plastic surgery resident. We were preparing a patient "Juana" for surgery who had a significant deformity involving the right side of her face. The right side of the jaw was diminutive, and the whole right face was smaller than the left. This kind of deformity sometimes makes it difficult for the anesthesiologist to place a tube through the mouth into the trachea for maintaining the airway during surgery. We had a very experienced anesthesiologist working with us that day, Dr. Fred Thomas.

However, after putting her asleep, he was unable to place the anesthetic tube through the mouth into the trachea. In and of itself, that is not a particular problem because usually, the anesthesiologist can breathe for the patient by compressing a bag connected to the induction mask. However, because of the patient's deformity, her airway was obstructed; he could not force air into the patient's lungs with the bag and mask. His unease was palpable. He said he could not ventilate the patient. Suddenly, the patient turned quite blue then ashen.

I recognized that this was an acute emergency and immediately put on a pair of gloves without going to the scrub sink. (Dr. Tessier and Dr. Raymond Brauer were to operate on her and were waiting to be called to the operating room from the nearby doctor's lounge when the patient was ready for surgery.) I ask the scrub tech for a knife, felt the neck for the thyroid and cricoid cartilages, and made an incision directly over the upper trachea and into the airway. I then placed an anesthetic tube through the trachea into the airway. This procedure literally took 10 seconds. The anesthesiologist could hardly believe his eyes (and neither could I) when I showed him the tube was in place, and he could connect his apparatus to this and begin breathing for the patient.

This emergency procedure could not have gone better. I have always been very proud of saving that young lady and thankful to God. It was one of the most exciting moments in my medical career.

Just then, Dr. Brauer came into the room. I think he was relieved to find I had already alleviated the crisis. After that, we proceeded with about 10 or 12 hours of surgery on several patients that day.

Dr. Tessier introduced me to fantastic new procedures, special instruments of his design, as well as medical devices such as new small titanium plates and screws that replaced wire for holding bones together. I was very fortunate to be invited by Dr. Tessier to visit him in Paris in 1987 and spend the summer working with him in Hospital Belvedere. He had a full-time fellow training with him named Arlen Denney, who is a friendly and competent surgeon. I was able to observe all the cases and to scrub every day to assist Dr. Tessier. I kept a journal of the operations and learned a lot from the variety of surgeries that Dr. Tessier performed. He had a nurse named Elizabeth, who scrubbed for him all the time. She was the best scrub nurse I have ever seen. She usually came with Dr. Tessier to Houston to help with all the cases.

Paris impressed me as a grand imperial city. The large-scale public monuments were designed to be viewed from distant vantage points. Although swamped through the week, on Sundays, I was usually able to take in some of the sites such as the Eiffel Tower, Arch de Triumph, many museums, etc. One Sunday after mass, I was sitting on a concrete stoop in front of a store on the Champ-Elysees. I was dressed casually and was assiduously people watching. Unexpectedly I heard someone say, "Dr. Cronin." I glanced over and observed a young lady and her mother advancing on that promenade with affable smiles on their faces. It turned out they were patients of mine from Houston vacationing in Paris. We had a friendly chat. It was delightful seeing familiar faces while so far from home.

In the last two weeks of my stay, my wife came over to Paris from Houston. We were fortunate in that a physician friend of Dr. Tessier allowed us to use her apartment that week as she was going out of town on vacation. Her flat turned out to be in a 17th-century building in the center of Paris and in the middle of the Seine on Ile de la Cite. Beautiful sites were within walking distance of this location. Over several days, I tried to show Candy the highlights of Paris. We allotted a whole day for the magnificent Louvre, knowing we could only sample its wonders. The Eiffel tower indeed offered a grand view of an imperial city on a crystal-bright afternoon. We visited the oval rooms of Musee de l' Orangerie to see Cloud Monet's impressionist exhibit of water lilies. We took a trip out to the spectacular Palace of Versailles. The hall of mirrors was breathtaking. The mammoth size and grandeur of the palace are overwhelming.

One day we went out to Montmarte and visited the beautiful Basilica of the Sacre Coeur. We had our portraits drawn in chalk by two different artists as we sat next to each other at Place du Tertre. Saint Chapelle was delicate and beautifully colorful, more than a rainbow. The Pantheon is a magnificent sepulcher for distinguished French citizens. Notre Dame was massive and beautiful. One day while visiting that cathedral, there was a choir from the USA performing while the organist from Notre Dame was playing for them- fantastic. The arc de Triomphe de L'Etoile was impressive, the twelve radiating avenues creating a star. Dr. Tessier's office and apartment were near the arch.

The last week, we rented a car and drove to the Solange region, where we stayed the first night in a hundred plus-year-old small French farmhouse recommended by Dr. Tessier's nurse Elizabeth. The next morning our hosts served us fresh bread and jelly. Without a doubt, it was the best bread that I have ever eaten in my life. During one segment of our trip to the countryside, we were on a one-lane road and found ourselves behind a large truck. In a short while began to perceive a pernicious smell. At first, we didn't know where the noisomeness was originating. We then noticed the truck had a sign "Poisson" (fish) on the back. Maybe it was a refrigeration truck that malfunctioned? It took us a long time before we had the opportunity to escape that problem. However, overall, we had excellent luck. We stopped one evening at a little roadway inn in a small town named Ernie. We had dinner in a tiny restaurant. It was remarkably delicious.

We visited the Loire valley and saw the impressive Chateau Chambord and Chateau de Chenonceau. There were a couple of highlights on our road trip. One was Mount San Michel, which is a medieval island town connected to the mainland by a causeway. We had to park the car and walk to the walled island. The only access was one winding pedestrian road going up the mountain. Positioned on the pinnacle was a beautiful and historic monastery. After touring the cloister and gardens, Candy and I walked down a way to enjoy a lovely lunch at a small restaurant with a lovely view. Next, we drove to the charming and picturesque small harbor town of Honfleur. We had to park on the outskirts and walk a bit to find the central square and tiny harbor. Outdoor cafes were ubiquitous and crowded. Again, our dinner was spectacular.

On our way back to Paris, we had planned to see the cathedral at Chartres, but our guidebook recommended we go at a specific time of day to have a tour by Malcolm Miller, an English guide who was the famous "dean" of Chartres cathedral. We would arrive too late if we proceeded to Chartres that day. Therefore, we looked for something else to do. As we were driving along the highway, we saw a sign leading to Solesmes. I had remembered reading something about a monastery where Gregorian chant was prominent.

So, we turned off the highway and drove to that small town to stay the night and made plans to go to Mass the next morning. We got there early before the Mass. The church was beautiful at Saint Peter Abbey, but nothing special when compared to so many of the other churches we saw in France. Faintly we began to hear chanting in the background, which gradually became louder and more precise as about 50 monks processed into the church and took their places on opposite sides of the sanctuary. The mass included antiphonal Gregorian chant pieces, and as the smoke of the incense rose heavenward, it reminded me of the prayers of the saints in the Book of Revelation. It was quite a spiritual experience. Our little side trip to Solesmes turned out to be one of the best most memorable parts of our French vacation.

The next day we did go on to Chartres Cathedral, an important pilgrimage site to the Virgin Mary in the Middle Ages. We were fortunate to meet with Malcolm Miller, who gave a wonderful tour of the church. He explained how the entire structure was a school for religious education and that the visual artwork substituted for the written word for the uneducated portion of the population.

The stained-glass windows have survived from the 12th and 13th centuries. Various medieval guilds sponsored many windows. The window purchased by the shoemaker's guild depicts a cobbler at his trade at the bottom of the window. One window shows an acclaimed image from Bernard of Chartres, a 12th-century scholar. The window has Matthew, Mark, Luke, and John sitting on the shoulders of Daniel, Ezekial, Isaiah, and Jeremiah. Indicating the prophets could see dimly what the evangelists now see clearly. The basilica has abundant instructive sculptures of scenes from the old and new testaments both outside and inside. The labyrinth on the floor is a representation of part of the pilgrim's spiritual journey to the holy land. Chartres Cathedral is an astonishing accomplishment of medieval Christendom.

Candy and I will never forget our beautiful French adventure. The night before we left, we had a gourmet dinner with Dr. Tessier and his wife at his apartment contiguous to his office. He was a very complex man. As we entered the flat, we recognized many elephant tusks lining the hallways. I found out later that Dr. Tessier received the Chevalier de l' order du Merit of the Central African Republic for his work in the preservation of the African elephant. After dinner, he drove us to our apartment. That's when I remembered he had been a race car driver. We sped through the late-night traffic in Paris. Several times his wife yelled from the backseat "se la rouge," letting him know she knew he was running red lights.

As I consider Dr. Tessier, I believe he was one of the most exceptional surgeons of all time. No one was better than Dr. Tessier working with the facial skeleton cutting and repositioning and reshaping the structural parts. He was a master in harvesting and applying bone grafts to the facial skeleton. His pioneering accomplishments won him the title of "father of craniofacial surgery."

No matter how complex the cranial facial problem, he always seemed to have a reasonable solution. Only once in more than a decade of consulting on incredibly tricky cases do I remember him telling a patient, "there is nothing I can do for you." That patient was a young lady whose skull and facial bones were growing thicker and larger so that her whole head was already grossly enlarged. I don't know whatever happened to that patient. She came from somewhere in the northeast United States to have her consultation with Dr. Tessier in Houston.

Dr. Tessier's list of surgical accomplishments is legion. He performed the first genuinely successful Le Fort III osteotomy, and he created the "integral" procedure for Treacher Collins. He developed the bipartition procedure for hypertelorism, the mask facelift, which includes bony structural alterations. He utilized temporalis muscle flaps for intracranial problems. He pioneered various monoblock procedures for severe craniofacial deformities.

Dr. Tessier received innumerable awards including an honorary Doctorate from the University of Lund in 1974, an honorary Fellowship from the American College of Surgeons 1975, an honorary Fellowship from the Royal College of Surgeons London 1984, an honorary Fellowship from the Royal College of Medicine London 1986, an honorary Fellowship from the Royal College of Surgeons Edinburgh 1990, the Chevalier de l' Legion d' Honneur France. He was a candidate for the Nobel prize in medicine. Dr. Tessier showed a skeptical medical community how to correct enophthalmos (a sunken eye) with bone grafts. He was the first to repositioned the orbits up, down, or medially without causing blindness.

Dr. Tony Wolf said, " Tessier is the greatest orbital surgeon of all time"; I would certainly agree and speculate that no one will ever equal his massive experience in this type of surgery. He also demonstrated that sizeable free bone grafts could fill bony defects. Dr. Tessier showed plastic surgeons in the medical community that large segments of cranial and facial bones could be cut and refashion and replaced and maintain their integrity. These innovations enabled him and later surgeons that he trained to take care of many deformed patients that previously were not able to be helped.

Dr. Tessier certainly has left a legacy in the field of plastic surgery and medicine in general. He will always be known as the father of cranial facial surgery. I indeed count him as one of my preeminent mentors as I learned so much from him. The photos below are from one of the last trips he made to Houston. The first picture shows me Dr. Tessier, Dr. Gruber (`orthodontist), Drs. John Smoot and Scott Yarish (plastic surgery residents) and Elizabeth (Dr. Tessier's suburb scrub nurse). The photo on the right is the last time those present were all together.

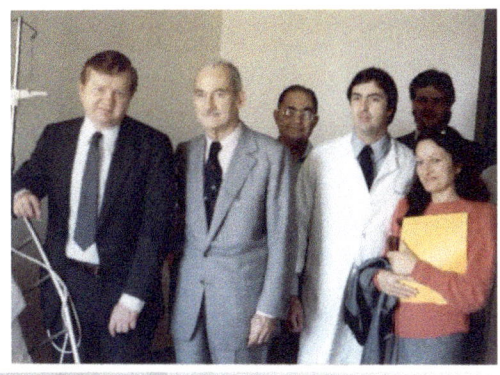

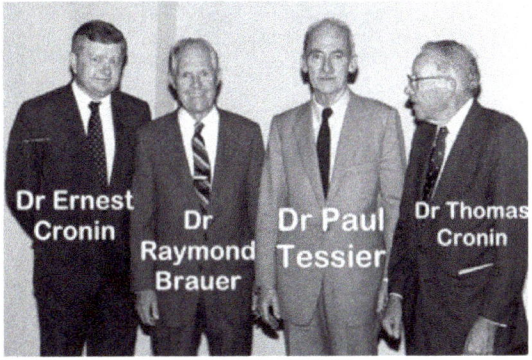

When Dr. Tessier stopped coming to Houston, there were several of his cases that were incomplete. A few of those he continued to follow up in Paris. I inherited several cases from him and will show a few examples of what I did to complete those "Tessier" cases

The patient, "Joe," was born with massive distortion of his skull and face, as shown below. The left side of the nose was absent, and the entire left face constricted, leaving the left eye way lower than the right eye.

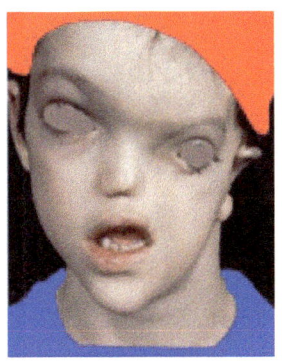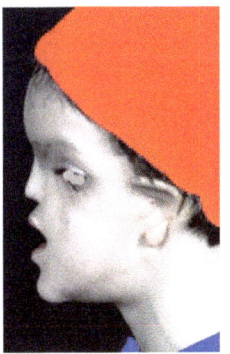

He received terrific results here in Houston from Dr. Tessier. At the time he was reconstructed, Dr. Tessier was probably the only physician in the world who could deliver such results. First, Dr. Hirshberg, a

neurosurgeon, did a craniotomy (heavy red lines) for internal access to the orbits. Then Dr, Tessier performed osteotomies (light red lines) to mobilize the eye sockets. He removed a segment of bone (gold) above the left orbit and moved the left orbit up. He took the bone removed from the left and inserted it above the right orbit to move it downward, thus making the eye sockets more equal. The drawings below illustrate the procedure. The gold segment of bone is moved from above the left orbit and placed above the right orbit.

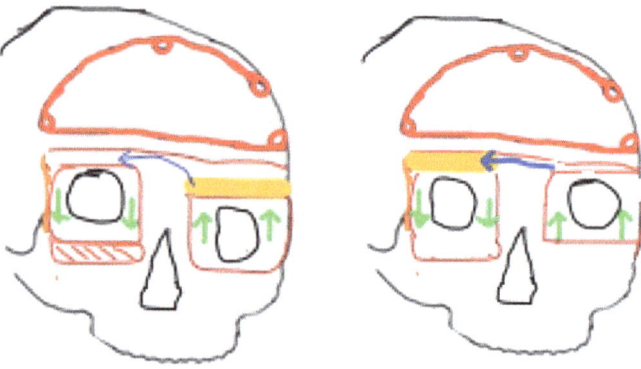

The first intraoperative photo below shows Dr. Tessier cutting the segment above the left eye; the top of the head is to the right. The second photo shows the completion of the orbital osteotomies and space (green arrow) where the bone had been. The third photo shows the left orbit freed, and the forehead and scalp flap turned down.

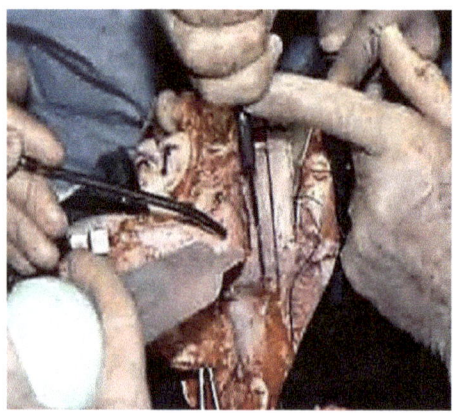
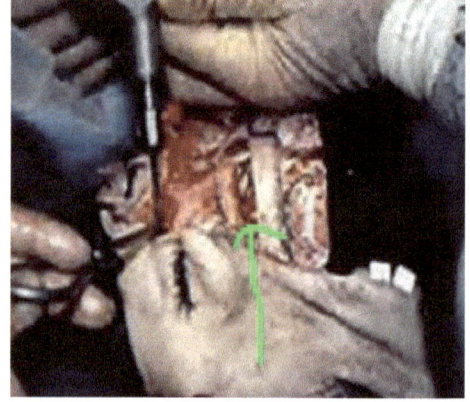

The Healing Mission of Plastic Surgery

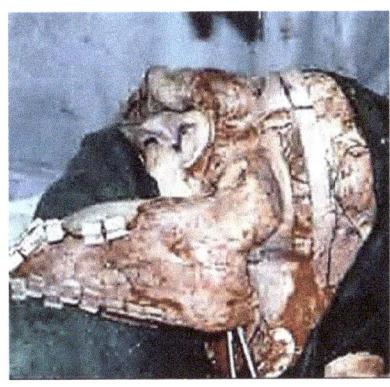

The first intraoperative photo below shows both orbits mobilized. The second photo shows the left orbit being secured upward into its new position.

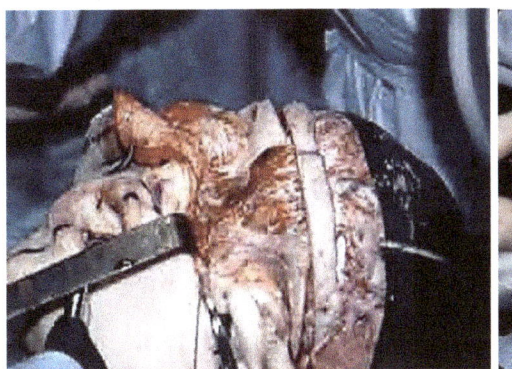 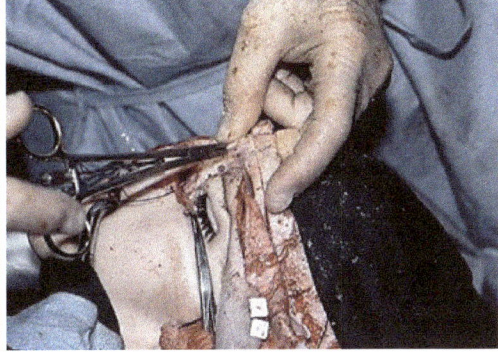

Dr. Tessier has secured both orbits in their new positions the first photo below (top of the head is to the right). The segment of bone from the left supraorbital area is now shown (gold) on the supraorbital area on the right. The photo on the right is oriented with the top of the head superiorly. So Dr. Tessier moved the left orbit up and the right orbit down.

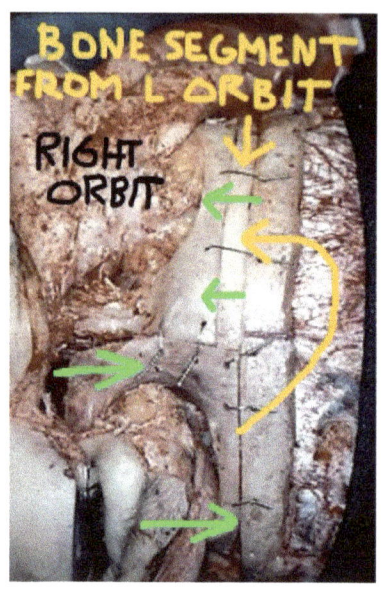
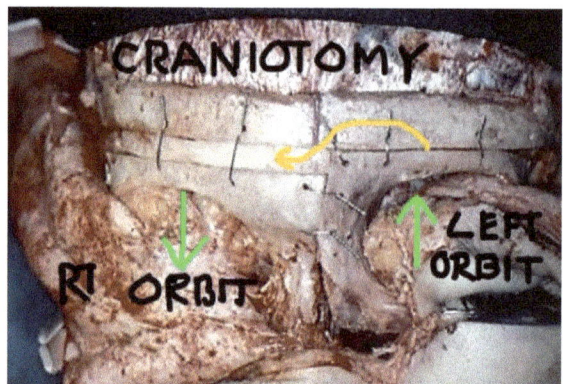

The orbital osteotomies and movement made the level of the orbits more equal. Dr. Tessier also reconstructed "Joe's" left nose with a broad forehead flap, as demonstrated below.

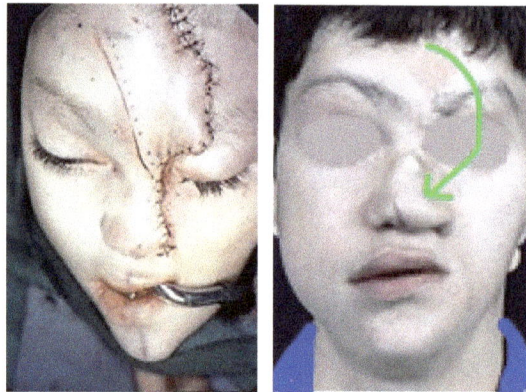

Dr. Tessier recreated the absent sideburn on the left with a hair-bearing flap from the posterior scalp.

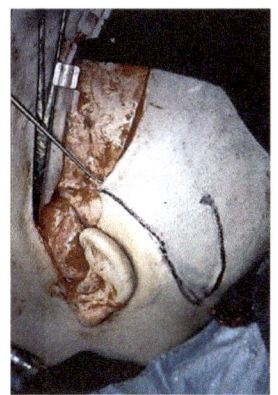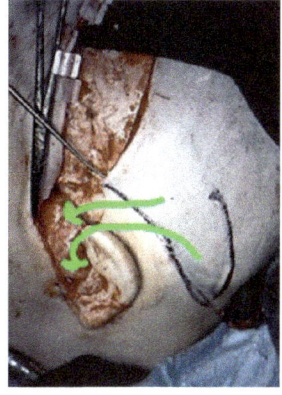

Below photos show the spectacular result that Dr. Tessier was able to accomplish for "Joe," taken at Dr. Tessier's last surgical visit to Houston. The last photo is of Dr. Tessier with "Joe."

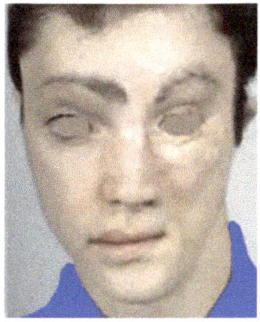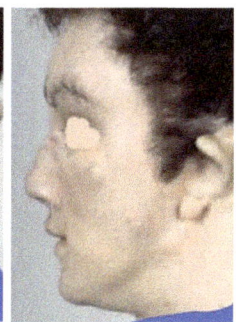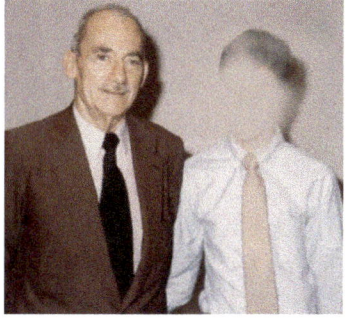

I inherited " Joe's" case when Dr. Tessier no longer came to Houston. I did a couple of relatively small procedures for him. I performed a rhinoplasty to try to improve the nasal shape, including a little more tip definition. I also performed fat grafting to the left side of the face, which did improved symmetry with the right side. His final pictures are below.

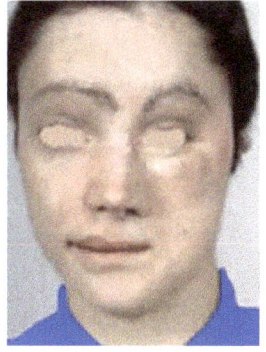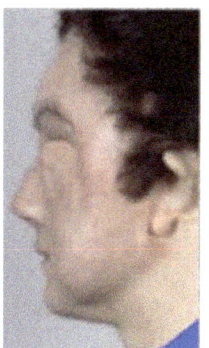

"Annabel" initially presented to our annual Tessier clinic as a three-year-old with the diagnosis of Crouzon's syndrome. Dr. Tessier examined her and felt she would benefit from a craniofacial advancement in a year or so. Dr. Tessier returned the following year and recommended the child undergo a craniofacial advancement. She was then a four -year old with the facial stigma of Crouzon's syndrome. "Annabel" had underdeveloped orbits, which cause her eyes to seem too large and positioned forward. She also had a hypoplastic(underdeveloped) and retruded maxilla.

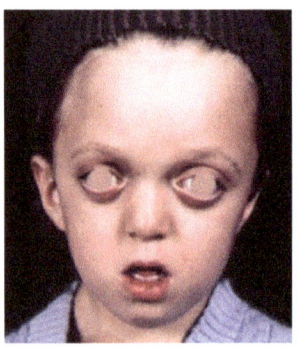 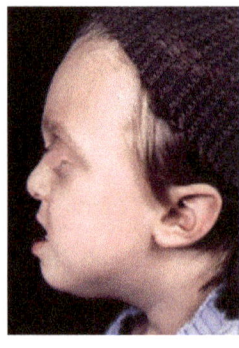 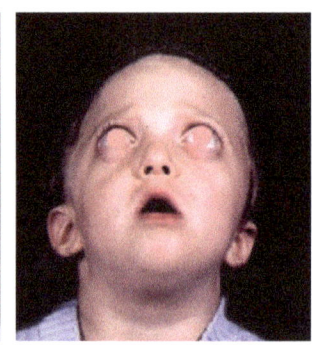

The first portion of Dr. Tessier's operation consisted of a tracheostomy because of the anticipated swelling of her airway. The remaining procedure consisted of an incision across the scalp and incisions under the upper lip. Through these incisions, he exposed the cranium and facial bones. He then made osteotomies or bony cuts to separate the face and the forehead from the remainder of the skull. He then pulled forward first the forehead and then the upper face (maxilla) so that their relationship with the skull was in a more normal position. The relationship between the upper and lower jaw was changed by leaving the lower jaw alone but bringing the upper jaw forward. Dr. Tessier harvested bone grafts from the skull and hip and the lower leg to fill in between the gaps created by the advancement. He secured the segments with wire ligatures as this case was before mini-screws and plates were available.

The surgery went quite well; however, the postoperative course was complicated by a spike in temperature to 106 degrees five hours after surgery, and a cerebrospinal fluid leak was evident. She also had seizures, which were controlled by medication. She was treated vigorously in the intensive care unit. All of these problems responded to aggressive management. She was discharged home in good condition 12 days after her surgery.

It was interesting to note and that the mother took a month or so to adjust to her child's new face. "Annabel" saw Dr. Tessier each year for the next four years in consultation during his yearly visit to Houston

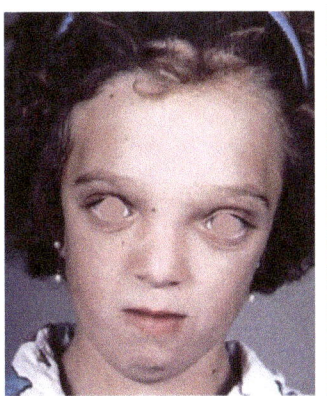
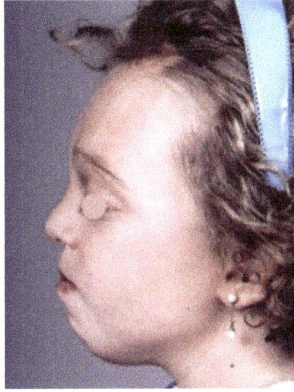
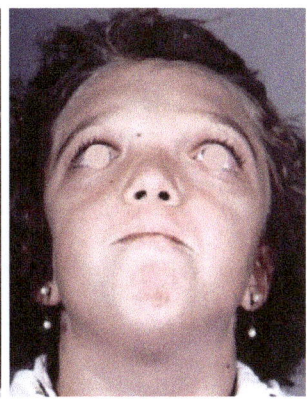

When she was eight years old doctor, Tessier, operated upon her again, placing cranial bone grafts in the orbital region, she did well from this.

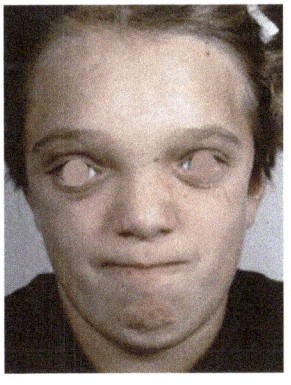
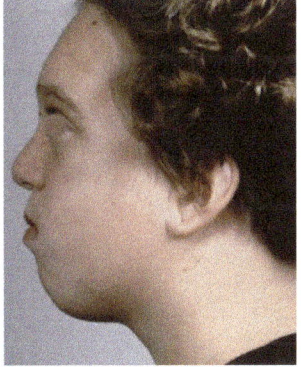

She had no additional surgery over the next several years. After Dr. Tessier was no longer coming to Houston, "Annabel" did return to the clinic to see me. I examined her and noted she had several residual abnormalities, including hypertelorism (eyes wide apart). Also, the chin was vertically very long but not forward enough. Therefore, I proposed another major surgery, which would consist of moving the orbits closer together so the eyes would no longer appear so far apart and moving the chin both forward and upward to improve her lower facial profile. Below is her condition a few years after Dr. Tessier's last procedure and when I took over her care.

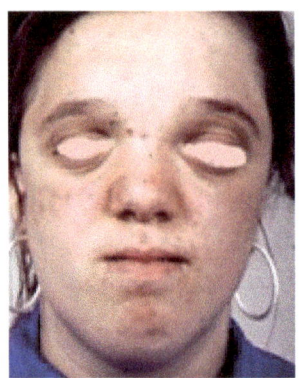
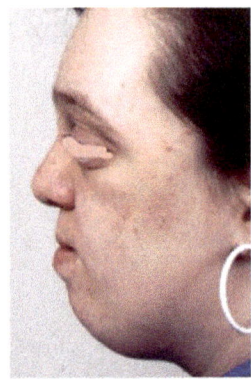

I did her surgery in conjunction with a neurosurgeon, Dr. Hirshberg. He first did a craniotomy, temporarily removing the frontal bones (dark red lines) to give me access to the roof of the eye sockets to make internal osteotomy cuts. I then freed the orbits externally with bony cuts (orange), so I could move them medially after removing some bone between them(solid red). So, in the first drawing below, the red lines indicate the craniotomy. The orange lines indicate the external bony osteotomy cuts that I made to free the orbits. The solid red area is an area of bone between the eye sockets, which I then removed. The drawing on the right shows the orbits before I brought them medially.

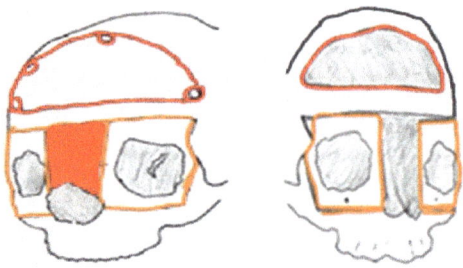

The following intraoperative photos are from another patient who had the same procedure as "Annabell." The intraoperative photo below shows the scalp flap has been turned forward over the face toward the right side of the picture. The bone removed from between the orbits is pointed out by the blue arrow. The yellow E s mark the position of the eyes in the center of orbits on either side. The second photo shows the bony specimen, which came from between the eyes.

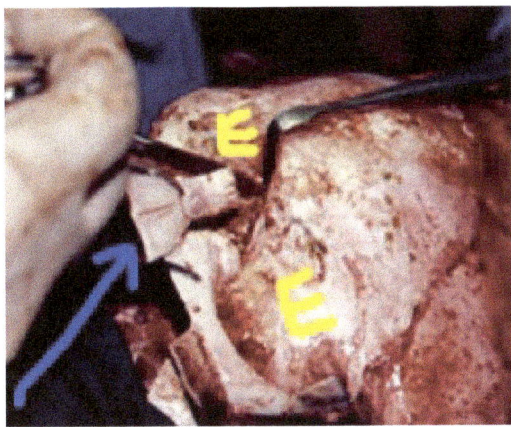
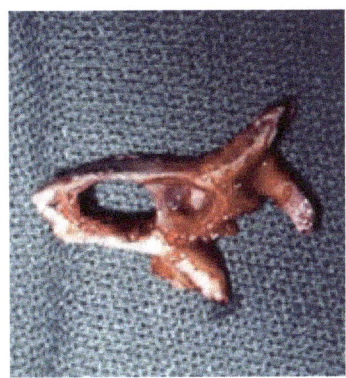

In the first photo below, the yellow Es represent the position of the eyes in the eye sockets. The anterior portion of each orbit has been completely separated from the facial skeleton and is ready to be moved immediately. In the second photo, I have moved the eye sockets medially but not yet secured them in their new position.

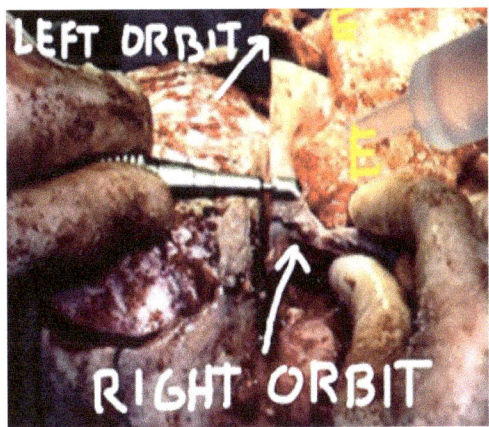
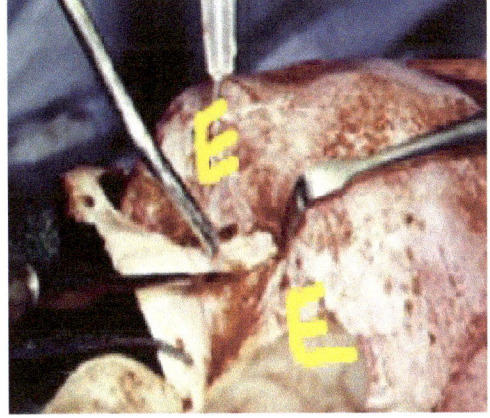

Below the bone from the craniotomy in red has been replaced and secured with plates and screws. The orbits outlined in orange have been brought medially and secured with plates and screws. Areas of bone graft laterally and of the nose are in green. The intraoperative photo on the right below shows I have brought the orbits medially and secured them in place. The center of the eye sockets occupied by the ocular globes is designated by the yellow E's. Next, to complete the operation, I returned the scalp flap to its original position and sutured it into place.

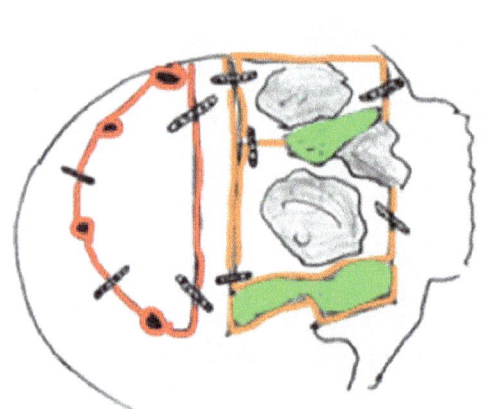 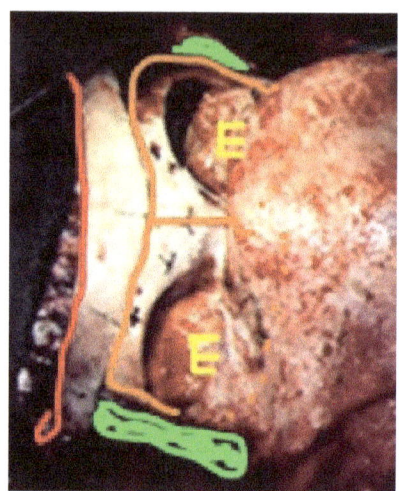

"Annabel's postoperative result is shown below.

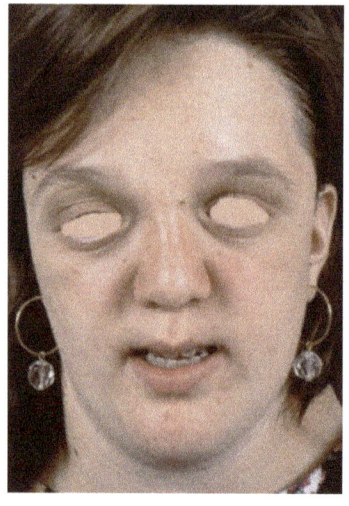 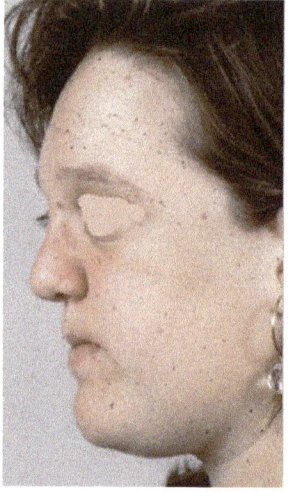

Working with a patient like "Annabel" over decades is something that makes plastic surgery very psychologically rewarding. Seeing this patient first as a three-year-old child and finally it as a young adult knowing all that she had to go through makes me so thankful and that none of my children have had to undergo this type of extensive reconstructive surgery. It also makes me appreciate the indomitable spirit demonstrated by so many of my patients who have had to endure such extensive surgery to try to make them whole.

Another such patient inherited from Dr. Tessier is "Victoria." This patient was born with a severe deformity known as hemifacial microsomia. One side of the face was smaller because of restricted growth, resulting in the bite or occlusal plane being severely tilted upward on the side of deficient growth. Dr. Tessier operated on her several times, placing multiple bone grafts on the right side of the face. He also did osteotomies of the maxilla and mandible to make the facial bones more symmetric. The drawings below simulate "Victoria's" facial form before and after several procedures by Dr. Tessier, each significantly improving her situation. However, she still had several significant issues, including a lack of fullness on the right side of the face and orbital dystopia, with the right lower compared to the left.

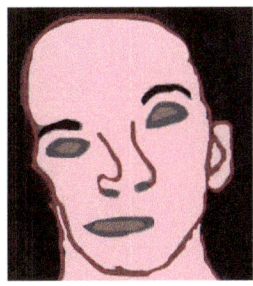 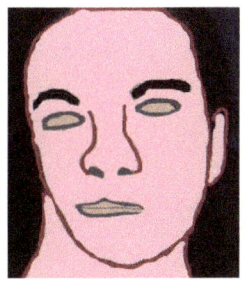

To address the lack of fullness on the right side, I first made a rubber-like model of the shape needed in additional volume, as in the first photo below. I elected to obtain the needed tissue from the abdomen with a free rectus myocutaneous flap supplied by the inferior epigastric vessels. The second picture shows the abdominal tissue I removed and the part that corresponds to the needed tissue(green). The blood supply comes from inferior epigastric vessels shown coming to the flap from below on the patient left. I transferred this free flap of her lower abdominal tissue to the right side of the face and buried it beneath the existing skin. I needed to connect the flap vessels to recipient vessels in the patient's neck. Postoperatively there was increased fullness but also some sagging of the transferred tissue. I still needed to address the orbital dystopia. The right orbit was low, and the left orbit was high, as in the simulated drawings below.

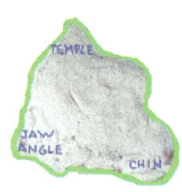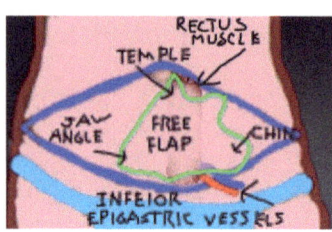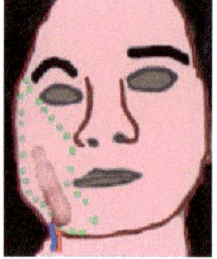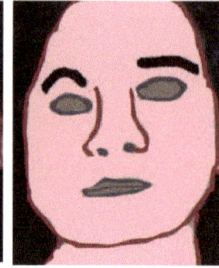

When I did the next major operation to reposition the orbit, I also plicated and elevated the free flap tissue to improve symmetry. The photo on the left below shows the cranium exposed with the scalp flap turned towards the right covering the face. The red lines indicate the bone flap to be removed by the neurosurgeon to give me access to the orbits from the intracranial approach. The orange lines indicate osteotomies I made to remove bone from above the right orbit. The photo on the right shows the right supraorbital bone removed inside the orange marks.

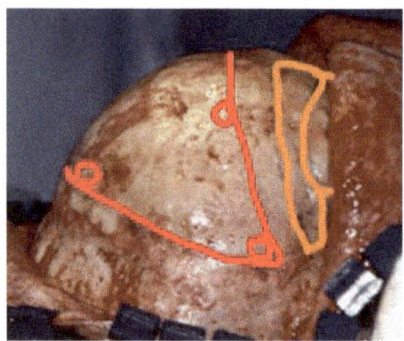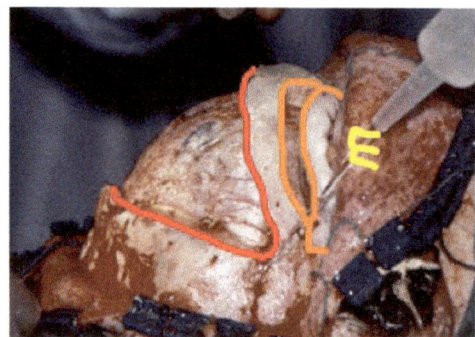

The two following photos below show exposure for the internal orbital osteotomies. The picture on the left shows the view from above working intracranially; the retractor is to protect the eye. On the right shows a retractor in orbit. The yellow E is the position of the right eye still covered by the soft tissue scalp flap.

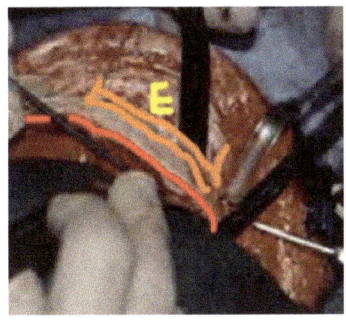 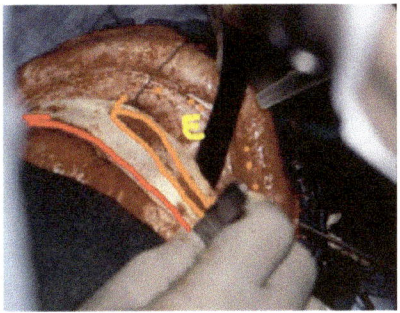

In the drawings below, the red lines represent the craniotomy cuts to remove the frontal bone done for access. The solid red area indicates the bone I removed above the right orbit. The location of the orbital osteotomies is orange. I moved the right eyesocket superiorly into the space created by the removal of the supraorbital bone. The final pictures show the superior portion of the orbit, which has moved superiorly(blue arrows), secured with plates and screws to the skull. Bone graft(green) was also placed below the orbit to support its new position.

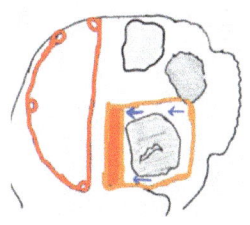 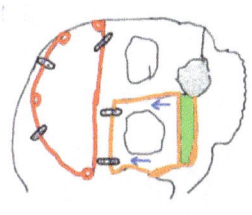 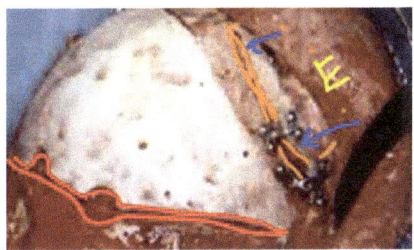

The simulations below represent her original condition, and then after Dr. Tessier did several procedures. The third is after I did the free flap to the right side of her face. The last one is after I moved her right eye higher to correct the orbital dystopia. The patient moved away, and she did not wish to return to Houston for additional surgery. She had the potential for continued improvement with additional surgery, so I hope she was able to obtain that.

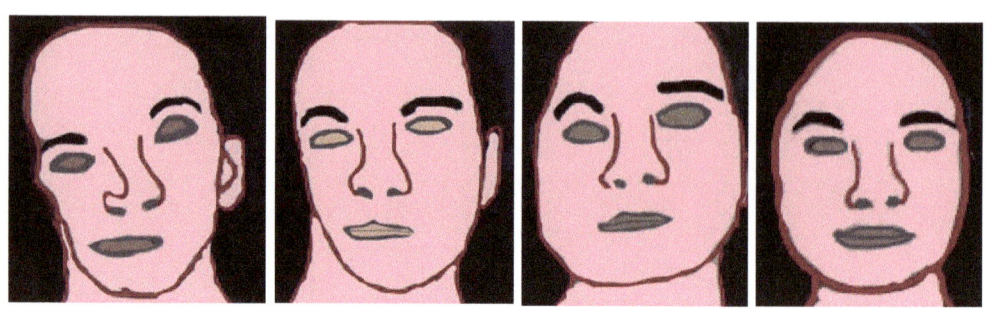

Hemifacial microsomia

A final patient I inherited from Dr. Tessier is "Fernanda." She was born with hemifacial microsomia, with the left side of her face severely underdeveloped. The bones of the lower jaw and the maxilla were smaller, especially in the vertical dimension. Dr. Tessier operated on her to help equalize the facial dimensions. He cut the upper and lower jaw and spliced in bone grafts to build up the smaller side of the face. That surgery was a great success. Several years later, she came to me for some finishing surgery involving her nose. I performed a rhinoplasty that also straightened her deviated nasal septum, which was beneficial for breathing. Last time I saw her, she told me she was involved with a beauty pageant as a contestant. I was thrilled and pleased that she had so much confidence and self-esteem and a comfortable body image, which allowed her to do that.

A patient of mine, named "Brandon," also had hemifacial microsomia resulting in facial asymmetry, a slanted occlusal plane, and a curve of the midline structures. Collaboration with an orthodontist is usually routine with this type of case. He made dental impressions and plaster dental models. We placed them on an articulator and made an acrylic bite split to help guide the positioning of the teeth bearing bony segments.

"Brandon" shown below illustrates these typical findings of hemifacial microsomia. The right face is vertically shorter, and the facial midline curves to the right.

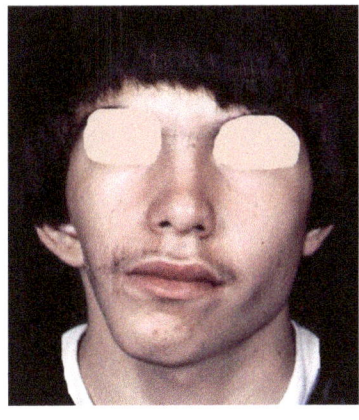
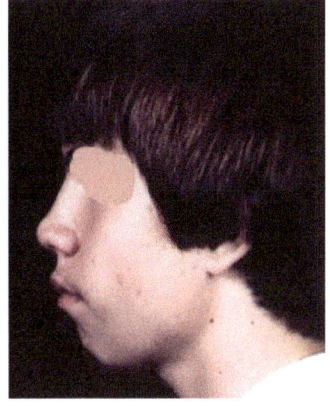

The drawing on the left below shows the osteotomy lines(red), which are made in the maxilla and the mandible to allow the maxilla on the patient's right side to rotate downward and the gap filled with the bone graft (green). The red lines on the lower jaw represent a sagittal split osteotomy technique, which allows the mandible to rotated to the patient's left, improving his facial symmetry. Also, I cut the chin, turned, and moved it anteriorly to obtain better balance and a more pleasing profile. I secured all the osteotomized bones with plates and screws.

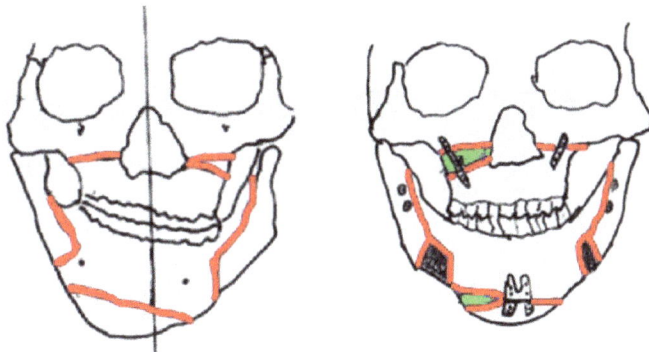

The postoperative photos below show better symmetry, a level occlusal plane, and a better profile.

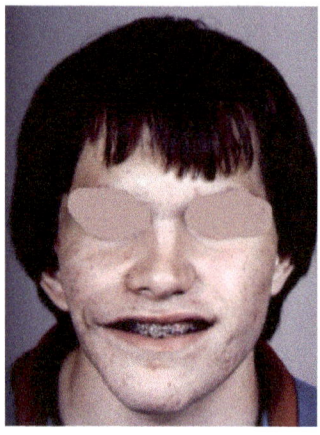
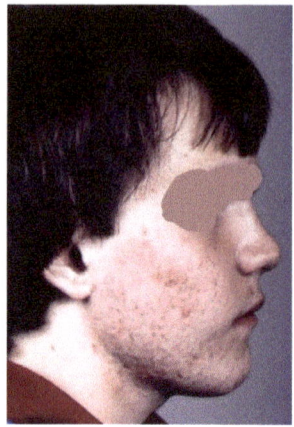

The following case is that of "Rosalind," a child born with Goldenhar syndrome that I first saw as an infant. She had multiple congenital deformities including a cleft lip and palate, a #7 Tessier lateral facial cleft, mandibular hypoplasia with the absence of the ramus of the mandible on the left side, pre-auricular ear deformities, a nasal dermoid mass, and epibulbar dermoids in the right orbit.

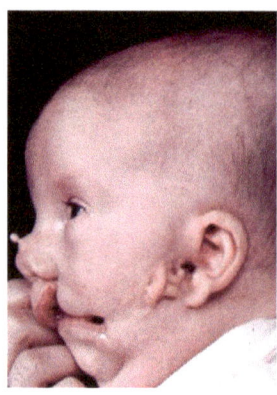
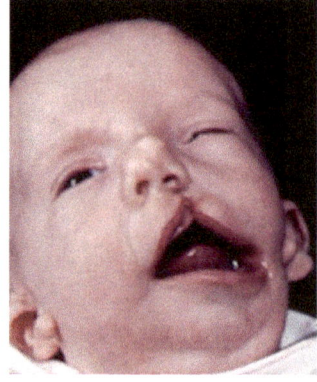

The radiographic image below shows the absence of the ramus and part of the body of the mandible. I multiple operations to repair the above defects. One process involved taking a rib from the patient and using it to reconstruct the missing ramus and body of the mandible on the left side. The middle intraoperative photo shows the rib before placement. I stabilized the graft against the existing jawbone below and the base of the skull above. I did this with stainless steel wires through drill holes in the graft and the extant mandible segment because, at that time, we did not have the luxury of plates and screws of stainless steel or titanium. I have outlined the graft with the red line in the x-ray below.

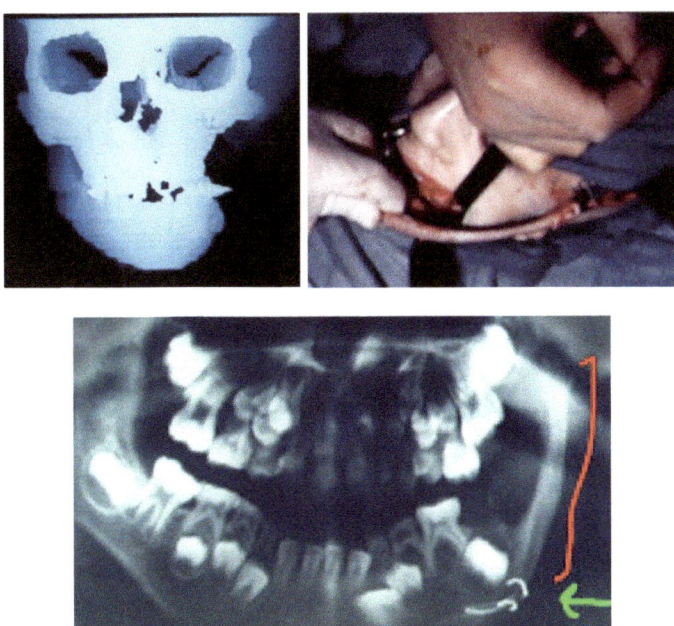

The postoperative photos below show her condition after I repaired her the cleft lip and palate, the left lateral facial cleft, and excised a nasal dermoid (a benign cyst that contains various mature tissues), and excision of preauricular redundant tissue.

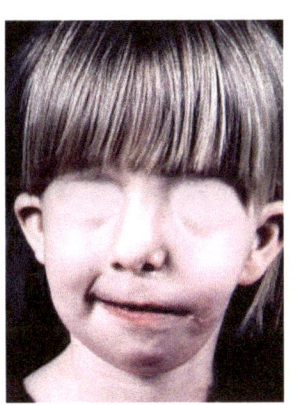 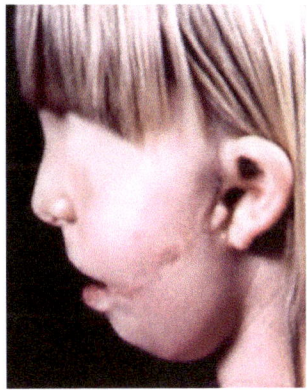

When she was a teenager, I did a genioplasty to advance the chin, which, as you can see from the pictures below, was quite beneficial. The view of the occlusion demonstrates the fact that her rib graft grew with the patient so that her occlusal plane remained horizontal.

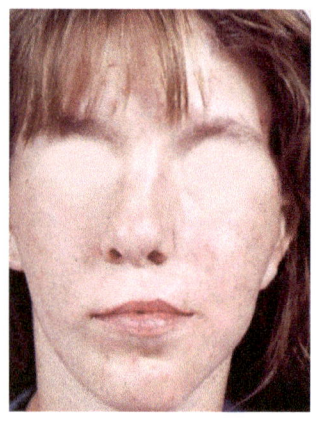 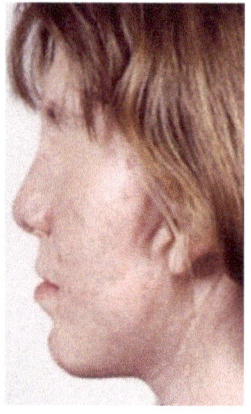 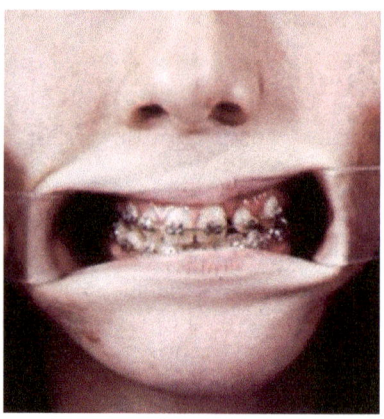

Although we were able to accomplish the bony mandibular reconstruction only using stainless steel wires for stabilization, today, titanium plates and screws make all our skeletal stabilization techniques easier and more secure. The didactic plastic models below demonstrate titanium plate and screw fixation of multiple osteotomy sites such as the mandible, the maxilla, and the chin.

A childhood interrupted.

A 15-year-old boy presented to my office referred by his ophthalmic surgeon. He had significant deformities of the left side of the face, including a non-seeing eye covered by a prosthesis, constriction of the entire left side of the face causing contraction of the corner of the mouth, and the side of the nose. Even the bite plane was pulled upward on the left side.

The very supportive parents explained that the child had a sarcoma cancer at the age of five. He received radiation therapy and chemotherapy for two years. Since that time, he had undergone numerous operative procedures, including skin grafts to the left eye socket region. The radiation caused the deformities. It arrested the growth in the areas irradiated. So, although the right side of the face grew at a usual rate, the left side lagged in growth, leading to the deformities described above and shown in the initial photographs below.

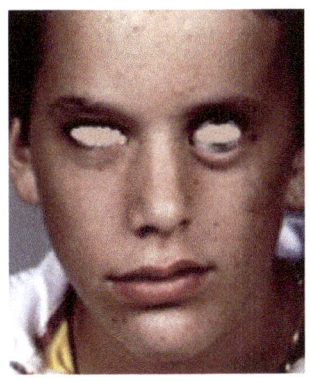 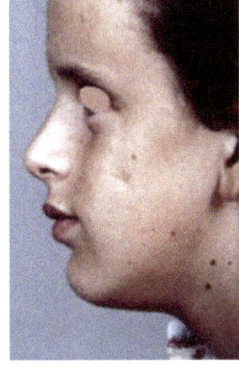 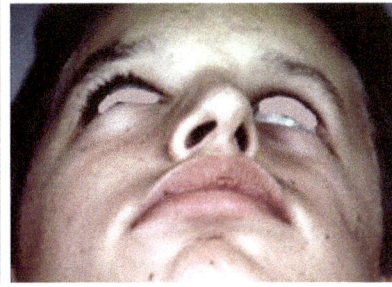

Overall, he had a good result from his therapy having been free of local disease and with no evidence of metastatic lesions for ten years. Over the three or four years after the initial radiation, the eye deteriorated, such that he had a functional loss of his vision. He had problems with extreme dryness, so he had a salivary gland transplant to the eye. Later, he had this reversed because of excess tear formation. He also had had some bone grafts along the cheekbone under the eye.

He had a contracted orbit, and his shell prosthesis did not fit properly. There were scar adhesions between the eyeball and the lower eyelid. The left ear was somewhat shorter than the right one. The left side of the nose was smaller than the right side and was pulled upward towards the eye. Although the teeth fit together reasonably well, the plane of the occlusion was slanted upward on the left side, which caused the mouth to be crooked.

We had a long consultation and discussed the multiple surgeries that would be necessary to obtain an optimal result.

Ironically, before I did any of those procedures, he came back to the office, having had a recent injury. He broke his nose, and it deviated to the left. My first surgery on him was a setting of a broken nose, which did nothing for his primary issues.

Over the next several years, I did many operations on him. The first was orbital reconstruction using some mucosal grafts from the mouth to try to make a better eyelid sulcus for his eye prosthesis. Also, I placed a prosthetic implant under the skin over the cheekbone to build up the contour. He did well for several months and then developed as inflammation of the lower eyelid, which eventually led me to remove that infected implant.

After waiting for more than a year, I was ready to proceed with a major reconstruction for him. I performed an operation in which I made cuts through the mid-face to mobilize the upper jaw and mid-face to reposition the bone and made cuts in the mandible (lower jaw) to reposition both. I did this to straighten the occlusal (bite) plane and change the contour of the left side of the face to be more like the right. I did this surgery after extensive consultation with the orthodontist to whom I had referred our patient. His orthodontist was of great help in dealing with his occlusion. I released a contracture of the left upper lip. He also had to do early stretching exercises to regain the full function of opening and closing his mouth because of some stiffness in the temporomandibular(jaw) joints after the surgery.

Next, I worked on his right orbital area. I harvested skin and fat and inserted this as a dermal fat graft into the upper eyelid. I also placed a cartilage graft from the nose into the lower eyelid and a mucosal graft in the lower eyelid to facilitate a better fit for his ocular prosthesis. He did well after this extensive surgery. He also worked with an ocularist to obtain a new eye prosthesis. He did have occasional inflammatory episodes where some proud flesh or granulation tissue developed inside the upper eyelid requiring a small office procedure to remove some of this proud flesh and treatment with anti-inflammatory and antibiotic eye drops.

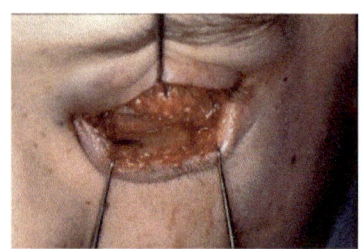 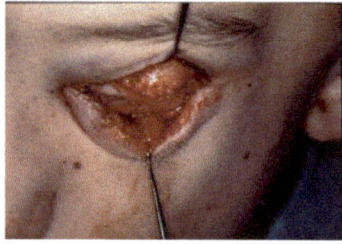 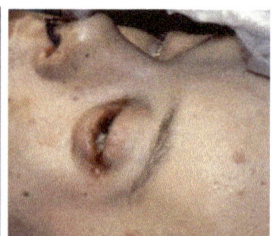

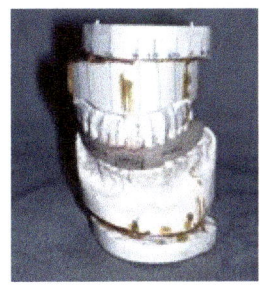
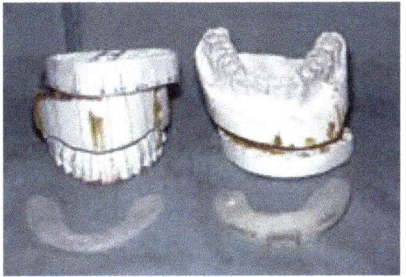

After six months or so, he was ready for another surgery to try to improve his result. I turned over the left temporalis muscle down to build up the left side of the face. I also worked on the nose to build-up and straighten the left side of the nose. Again, he did very well after this surgery.

Periodically, he has had to revisit his ocularist to adjusts his prosthesis. Over a dozen years, I operated on him seven times for significant reconstructive surgery and several other times for minor office procedures.

His was indeed a childhood interrupted by the demon cancer and by my multiple operative attempts to help him. In some ways, he's been fortunate, but he certainly was an excellent and loyal patient who was willing to work with his doctor despite some setbacks along the way. If he had been born in another century, he probably would have died of his cancer. It is incredible how much time, effort, and expense were necessary to try to restore him as close to normal as possible. I followed him approximately 17 years, watching him mature into a nice young gentleman with the constant support of his parents. I was happy when I learned he was engaged and was quite pleased to be invited to his wedding and made a point to attend.

The Healing Mission of Plastic Surgery

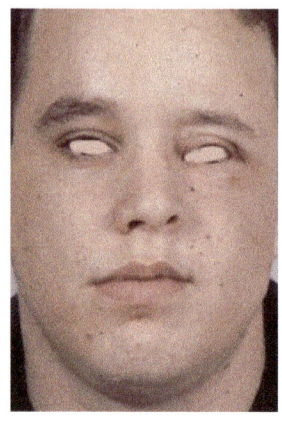
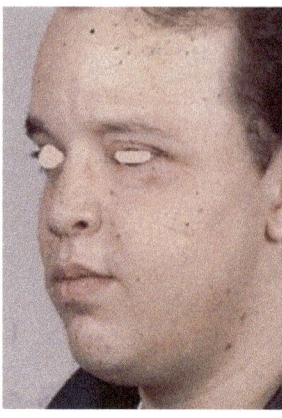

One afternoon as I was seeing patients in my office, I received a telephone call from one of our former residents, an outstanding plastic surgeon in our city. He said he wanted to get a second opinion about a patient of his whom he had operated on several times but was still having problems. We discuss the case briefly and arrange for the man to come to see me later in my office. "Oscar" had been shot by a robber several years earlier as a teenager. He suffered a severe craniofacial injury, including the loss of an eye.

He subsequently underwent multiple reconstructive surgeries, several of which involved placement of implants into the left side of the face in the orbital region. He received considerable improvement from the operations. However, for about a year, he had been suffering from chronic periodic drainage from the right eye socket. The referring doctor decided to ask me to take over this case.

When we examined him, I found that he had drainage from the left eye socket. There was a sinus tract or a little opening through the eye socket that led down deeper towards the bone and towards areas of previous prosthetic material placement. He also continued to have some contour deformity about the left orbit and the left temporal region. We decided that because he had had drainage for about a year, despite multiple treatments with antibiotics that it was fruitless to try to salvage the implants. Therefore, I arranged for exploratory surgery. I removed several facial and orbital prostheses and some infected tissue. Some of the depressed areas of the side of the face probably looked worse, temporarily, but it was necessary before we could proceed with additional surgery. My pre reconstruction pictures of him are below.

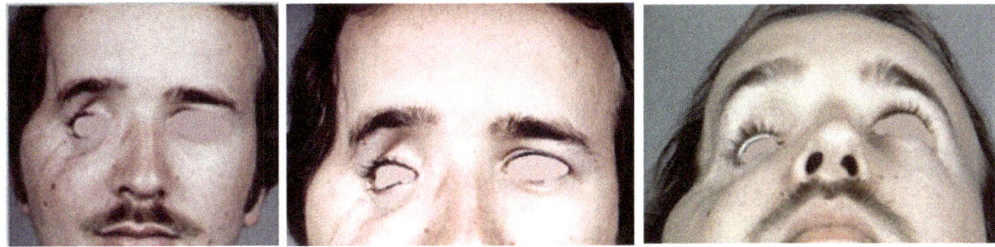

I waited more than six months to be sure there would be no recurrence of the infections. "Oscar's" surgery was a large complex one involving multiple bone grafts. I had a neurosurgeon colleague harvest two full-thickness portions of the skull. I took these to a back table and split each into two parts the inner and outer portion of the cranium. Because I divided it this way, I used half to repair the donor defect and the other half for the reconstruction. The drawing below illustrates this method of harvesting and splitting the skull bone grafts.

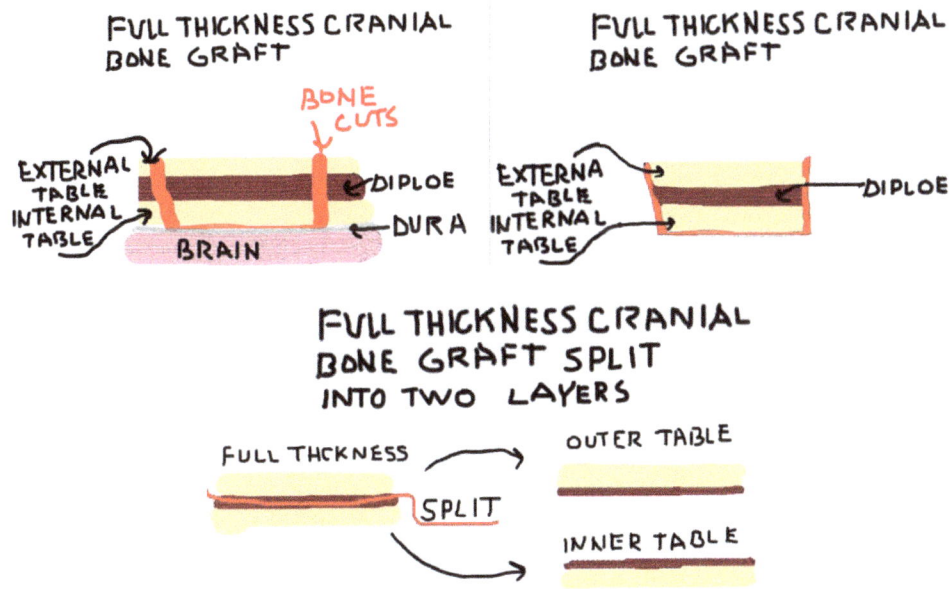

On the left below are the actual four pieces of bone resulting from splitting the two harvested full-thickness graphs into the inner and outer layers. The middle picture shows the right side of the skull with the right ear at the lower edge. I have already replaced two pieces of bone in the donor harvest defect (green). I then fashioned the grafts for the reconstructive needs. The pre-existing temporal defect, which has no bone over the brain, is outlined in blue ink. The orange line indicates the temporalis muscle, which connects the jaw to the skull. I will insert the bone graft beneath the muscle, which I will need to reposition. The zygomatic arch is lower, still hidden beneath the scalp flap to the right of the temporalis muscle. The drawing illustrates the same anatomy, showing the position of the zygomatic arch.

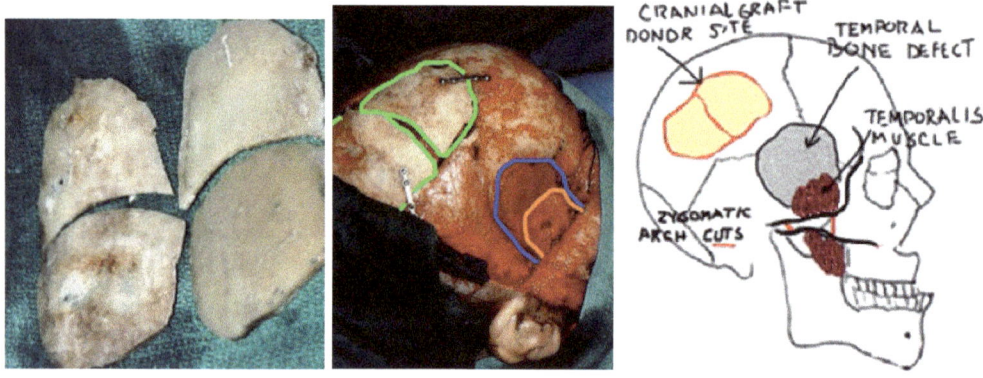

In the intraoperative photo below, the right ear is at the bottom. The blue line outlines the bone graft reconstruction of the temporal area. The orange line outlines the temporalis muscle, which I repositioned and fastened to the large temporal bone graft reconstruction bordered by the blue line. The green lines show the bone grafts I used to repair the donor site. The drawing illustrates the same.

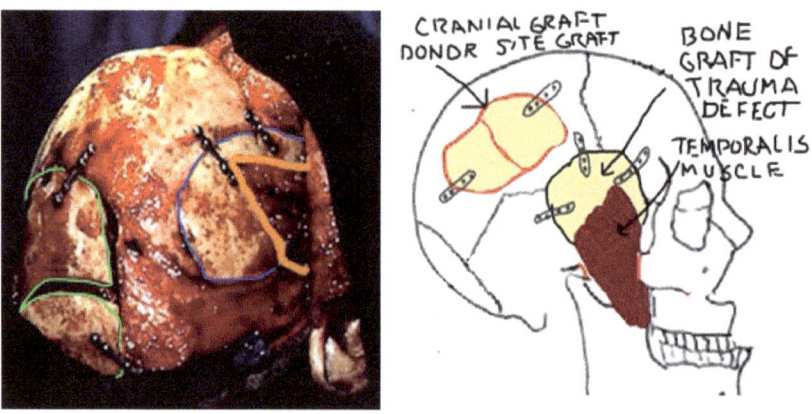

I also placed bone grafts in the orbital floor and lateral orbital wall, the inferior orbital rim, and lateral orbital rim to better support his ocular prosthesis besides the large graft of the right temporal area. I also adjusted the eyelids both medially and laterally to position them more anatomically so that his prosthesis would fit better.

The surgery was effective in restoring some of the normal contours to the orbital and temporal regions. "Oscar" healed well from surgery and several months later was able to have his ocular prosthesis modified to improve his appearance additionally.

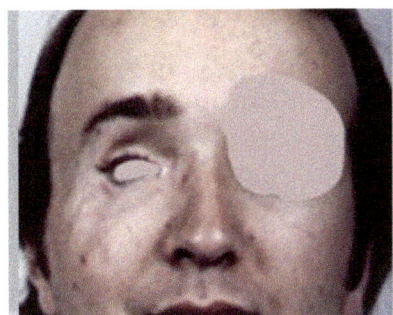
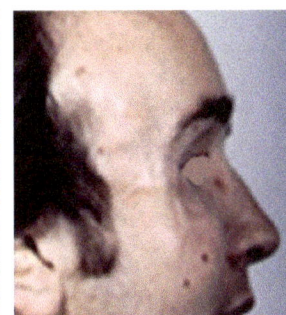

I wanted to do additional surgery for him because I thought he could obtain considerable further improvement. However, "Oscar," said he looked better than he had in eight years, was satisfied and did not want more surgery.

Right unilateral coronal synostosis with plagiocephaly

A newborn's skull is composed of several separate bones, which ordinarily grow a lot in early life as the brain is rapidly growing. Sometimes these growth areas fuse abnormally and stop producing more bone. Distortion of the skull and, in some instances, neurological problems can occur. The child pictured below, "Malcolm," had premature closure of the right coronal suture line between cranial bones resulting in flattening and distortion of the right forehead, as can be seen in the photo and drawings below. The yellow line indicates the premature closure of the right coronal suture. The usual, still open suture lines are in grey.

The Healing Mission of Plastic Surgery

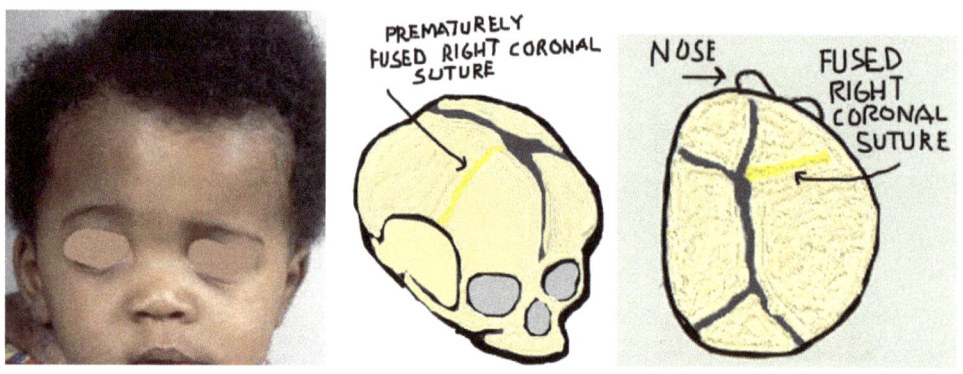

I operated upon him at about five weeks of age. First, the neurosurgeon did a craniotomy removing right and left frontal bones, as in the first two drawings below.

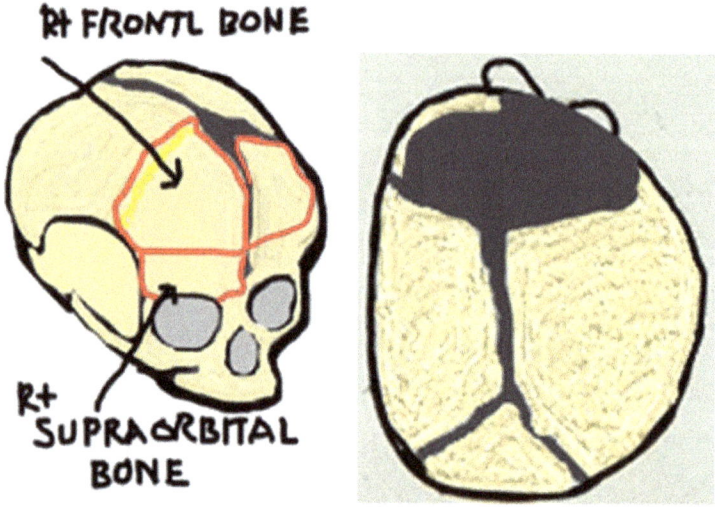

I removed, reshaped, and replace the right supraorbital bone to give him a more normal forehead and orbital contour as indicated by the two drawings below.

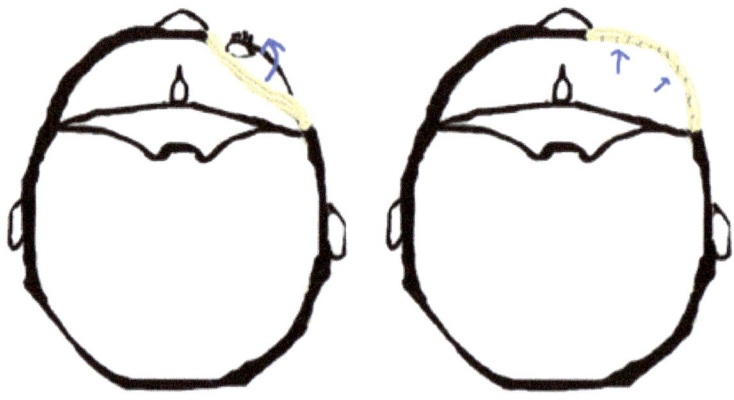

After I reshaped the supraorbital bar and replaced it. I also replaced the frontal bones. I left an area absent of bone to allow for brain growth. New bone formed from the underlying dura layer covering the brain would soon grow to fill in the space. The drawings below illustrate the procedure.

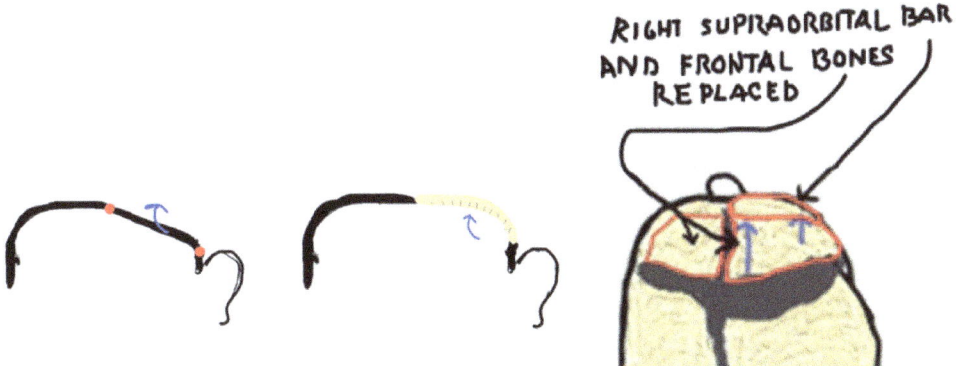

His post-operative result is below.

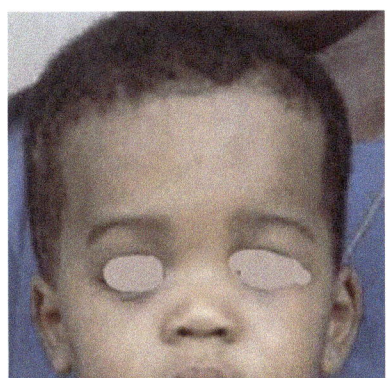

If you would like to read more about Paul Tessier, craniofacial surgeon nonpareil, I recommend *A man from Herrick: The Life and Work of Paul Tessier, M.D., Father of Craniofacial Surgery* by S. Anthony Wolfe M.D.

Chapter 11

Operation San Jose Mission Project

Beginning of OSJ

Operation San Jose is a mission program, which I established in 1983, dedicated to the repair of cleft lip and palate deformities for impoverished children in Latin America. This program came about in a somewhat serendipitous fashion. The visiting head of state from Honduras, President Roberto Suarzo - Cordova, was referred to me for a minor medical problem. In the course of our conversation, we discussed some of the needs and issues of medical care in Honduras. We found that there was a great need in the area of cleft lip and palate care, which was also an area of plastic surgery in which I was quite interested. Cleft lip and palate occur in at least 1in 700 births in the indigenous population of Honduras. There are historical-artistic representations of individuals with cleft lip, like in the picture below, throughout Central America and in the Andes region.

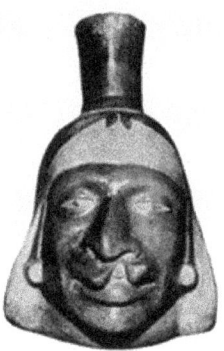

Some societies may have once thought cleft lip was a favorable special touch from a deity, today it can certainly be a burden for those afflicted. As a result of my conversation with president Suarzo, he put me in touch with his minister of health, who was with his group visiting Houston at that time. We arranged to meet and discuss the possibility of a mission trip. My wife and I hosted a small dinner at our home for the minister of health to further discuss the possibility of our making a medical trip to Honduras. We discussed how we might be of some benefit to needy patients in his country.

I then met again in my office with my senior partners and mentors, Dr. Thomas Cronin and Dr. Raymond Brauer. They both had a great experience in cleft lip and palate work and were excited about the possibility of a trip to Central America. After some preliminary planning, I contacted Dr. Cesar Enriquez in Tegucigalpa Honduras. It was my understanding that at that time, he was one of only four plastic surgeons in all of Honduras. I made arrangements for the first trip in 1983. Dr. Thomas Cronin, myself, and two senior residents and one scrub tech constituted the first team for Operation San Jose.

At that time, the only flights to Tegucigalpa were on obscure Central American airlines. The airport had no lights, and because the city was in a valley with small mountains around, it was a little scary landing at the airport in the early evening, just before dark. The plane had to fly low over a highway filled with cars and buses. I remember thinking I was glad none of the coaches was double-decker because we were so low, we might have hit one.

The airport was quite small. We walked down the stairs to the tarmac from the plane into the cramped terminal. At first, we saw nothing of our host. Customs officials pulled us aside and began to open all our luggage. It seems they did not know what to make of some of our equipment and supplies, and they began to spread things out all over. Just at that time, our host Dr. Caesar Enriques arrived. We introduced ourselves to each other, and he seemed to be able to straighten things out with the customs officials quite expeditiously.

Our luggage and equipment were put back in order and returned to us. We were in for a minor shock as we proceeded out to the airport lobby. There was a throng of people immediately outside the doors. We had to push our way through the crowd, which included many small children begging for money. I thought to myself, pickpockets must be everywhere. Dr. Enriques took us in a van to the Mayan Hotel, apparently one of the better hotels in the city. We checked in, and later that night, our host took us out to a typical open-air restaurant where we enjoyed some local fare. It seemed like at every major street crossing was a person in military fatigues with a rifle. The soldier usually looked to be about 15 years old.

The next morning, we went to the hospital, where Dr. Enriques introduced us to some medical students who would be working with us. Below I was photographed with the security detail in the hospital.

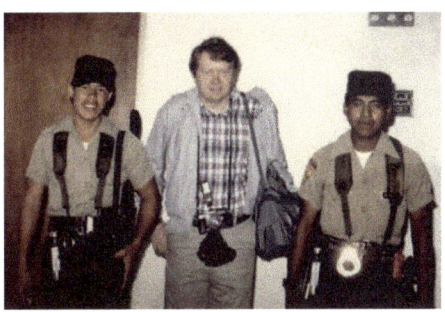

We were shown to a clinic area in the hospital and set up to begin seeing patients. Patients filled the waiting area. Several mothers held babies with cleft lip and palate. Over the next few hours, we saw about 50 or 60 patients. We would first examine the patients, make a surgical plan, and put the patient into a preliminary surgical schedule for the week. We recorded and sketched the findings of the defects in our surgical logbook for the trip. We photographed the patients for whom we scheduled surgery. We saw patients of varying ages from a few months of age to teenage years. Some of these patients appeared to be significantly malnourished. Therefore, we had to turn down some of them for the needed surgery. A few patients had severe cranial type malformations that we could not operate on in that setting.

The next day we began surgery in the early morning and continued to operate on patients until late in the evening. We worked for five operating days in two rooms, most of the time and sometimes three operating rooms. All of the patients we operated on suffered from some form of cleft lip or cleft palate. Many patients were five to eight years of age with complete clefts of the lip and palate, which had never had surgery. We often did quite extensive work on these patients, thinking that perhaps they would not have the opportunity for further follow-up surgery

Many of these cases were orchestrated by my uncle, Thomas Cronin, who would go back and forth between operating rooms, giving direction and advice both to the residents and to me as we worked on these severe cases. We relied on the anesthesia service at the local hospital as had been recommended by our host.

Pictured below are our plastic surgeon host, Dr. Enriques, with Dr. Thomas Cronin and me. The photo on the right is most of our first OSJ team in the hospital from that 1983 trip. From left to right, senior plastic surgery resident Dr. Scot Aaronson, two medical students, Dr. Thomas Cronin, another medical student, myself, and senior plastic surgery resident Dr. Robert Wright. Not pictured is Juana Del Rio CORT, our surgical technician. We judged our trip to be quite beneficial, as Dr. Enriques invited us to return the following year.

1983 Dr. Scott Aaronson, and Dr. Robert Wright senior plastic surgery residents

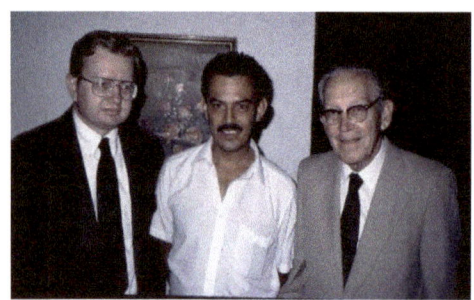
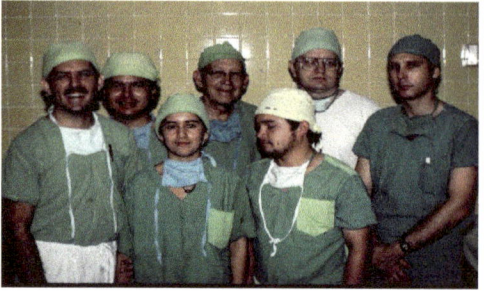

We returned the following year to Tegucigalpa and saw many young patients with cleft lip and palate, as shown in the photo below.

1984 Dr. Alfonso Barrera, and Dr.Charles Stewart senior plastic surgery residents

The photo below shows Dr. Srewart interloping (upper right) into a picture of our preoperative patient group.

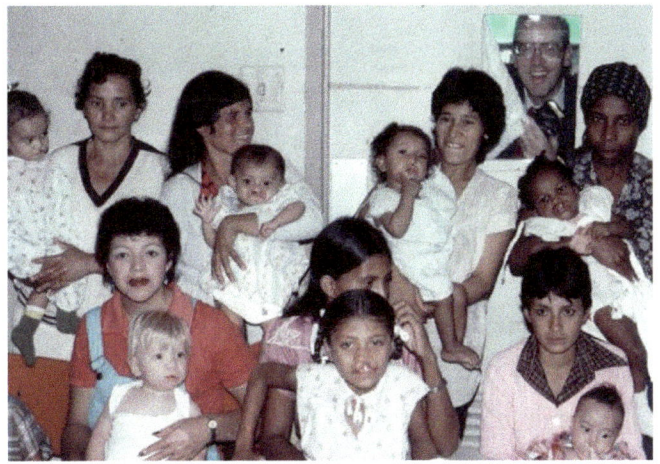

Below Dr. Thomas Cronin directs senior resident, Dr. Alfonso Barrera, in the operating room. Below right, Dr. Charles Stewart and I are performing surgery on a patient while Dr. Thomas Cronin is overlooking from the left side.

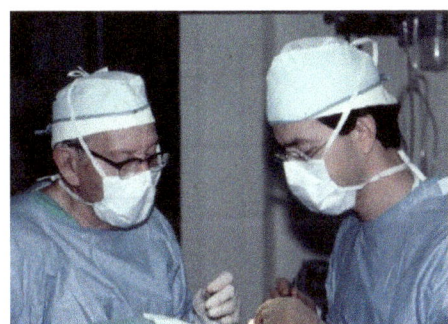 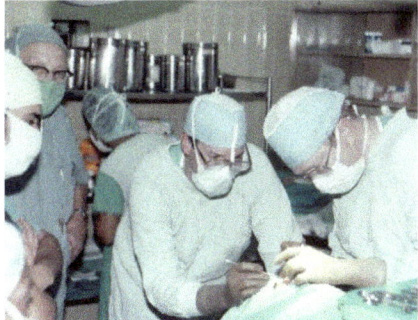

1985 Tegucigalpa, Honduras, Dr. David Humphries, Fred Wilder senior plastic surgery residents

Upon returning to Tegucigalpa the following year, we again had our hospital security detail, as shown below with Dr. Tom Cronin and Drs. Humphries and Wilder.

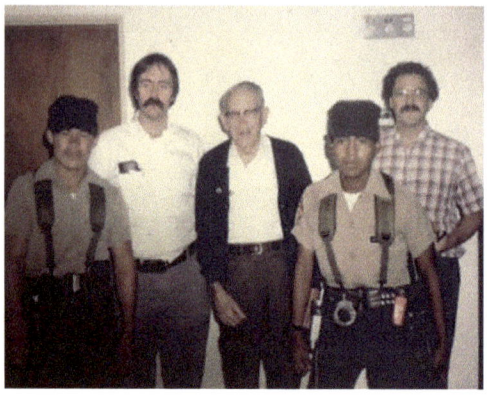

The first group photo below presents some of the patients upon whom we operated.

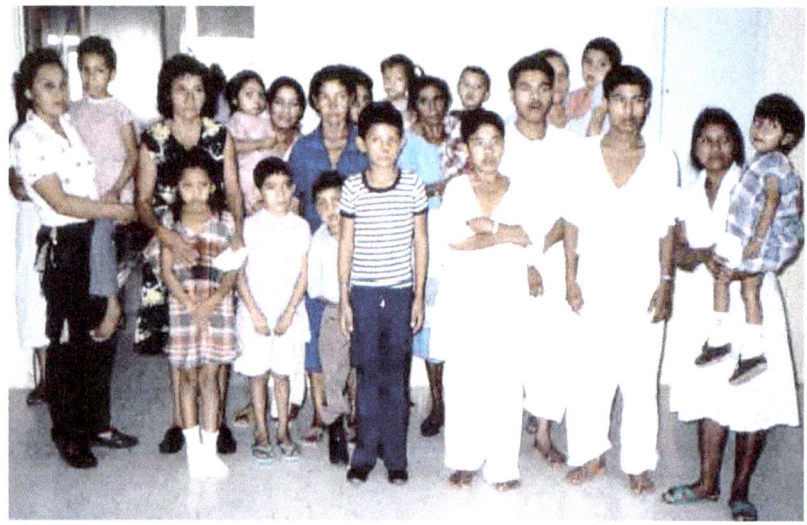

Below is the OSJ team from 1985, which included Angie Silva, CORT, and Dr. Amado Ruiz. Dr. Raymond Brauer was absent from this photo. Dr. Ruiz handled logistic concerns for OSJ beginning in 1985 and for many following years.

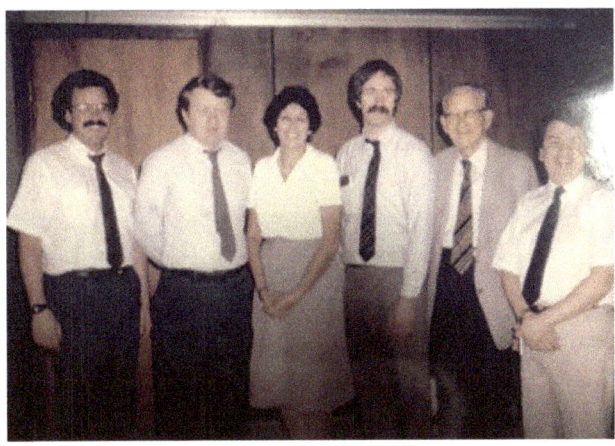

Program evolution

Over time the program evolved and expanded considerably. We began to take our own anesthesiologists to have more control and limit the unknowns.

Dr. Anna Kutka, shown below, was the first anesthesiologist for operation San Jose in Tegucigalpa Honduras. We expanded our team to include recovery room nurses and surgical technicians with us as well as additional plastic surgeons. We became more organized and were able to formalize our mission statement "because every child deserves to face the world with a smile."

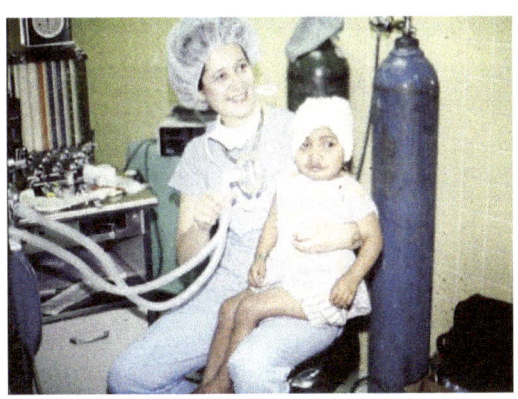
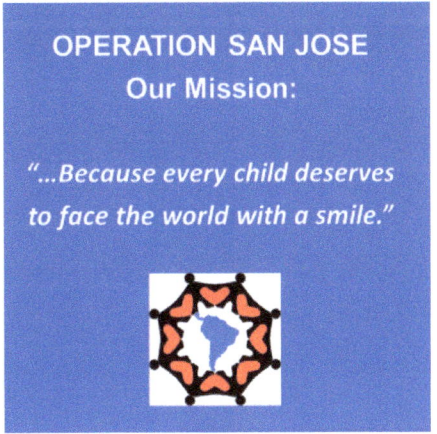

The goals of operation San Jose are: to provide surgical repair for children with cleft lip and palate deformities, facilitate cultural and medical collaboration between the OSJ team and our medical hosts, to teach surgeons in training to refine their skills under the direct supervision of the faculty. We want to have a local medical host, ideally a plastic surgeon working in the area.

Principles of operation San Jose are to make safety paramount, work with local medical people, involve local surgeons and residents when possible, and arrange for postoperative follow-up care. Christus Foundation for Health Care sponsors OSJ, but of course, there is no proselytizing and no religious test for evaluation or treatment.

Operation San Jose provides all the necessary supplies, equipment, personnel, and medications needed to perform the corrective surgeries. Below on the left Father Richard Patrick, the chaplain at St. Joseph Hospital, gives us a sendoff blessing the morning of one of our departures. On the right is a picture in the airport showing more than 30 luggage cases full of medical supplies needed for a typical trip.

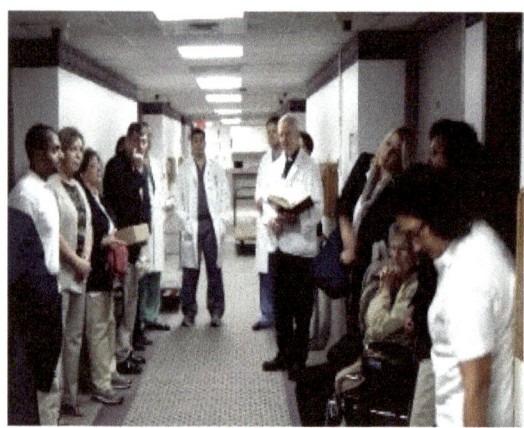 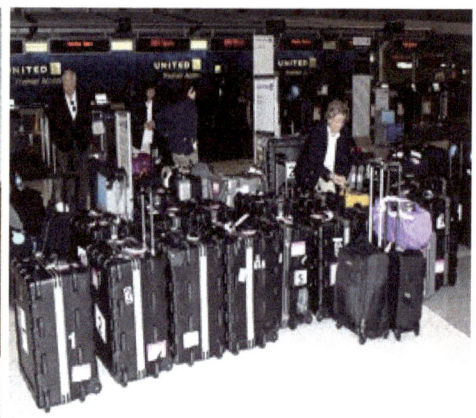

Now the team consists of about 20 professionals, usually three plastic surgeons, two anesthesiologists, a pediatrician, a speech pathologist, two plastic surgery residents, two operating room nurses, two recovery room nurses, three operating room technicians, and other volunteers.

The trip ordinarily lasts about ten days. In most locations, there is no need for particular security detail. Occasionally our hosts have supplied individual security for the team. Below, trip coordinator Veronica Cruz North checks out our security detail in Colombia.

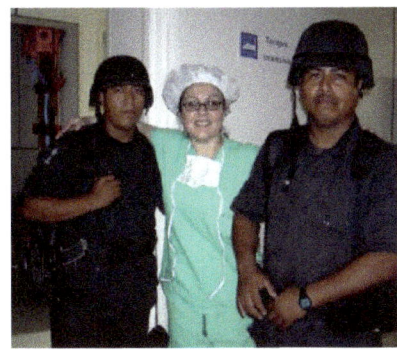

At first, all the participants were from St. Joseph Hospital. Later, we had participants from Methodist Hospital, Texas Children's Hospital, M D Anderson, and other local Houston facilities. For many years Dr. Amado Ruiz, pictured below with a child who has a cleft lip, handled the logistics and organization of the program and did an excellent job until his untimely death. Another person indispensable for most of the past 30 years is Maria Salazar, a surgical tech who, along with many others, has made this program a success. She is pictured below in the operating room.

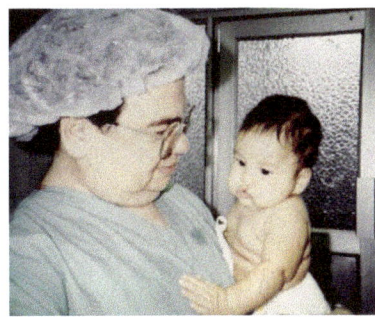
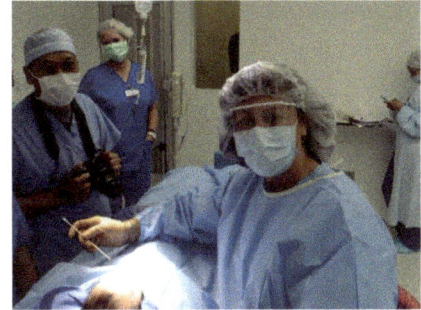

The evaluation clinic

Upon arrival, we unload all of our supplies and organize our supplies in the operating room, recovery room, and in adjacent areas. On the first or second day, we arrange for a clinic to see all the potential surgical candidates in a clinic setting. We often see 80 or more patients in consultation during the clinic time. Many local patients learn of our impending mission through local medical or charitable organizations. Each location has been a little different. Some families have to exert great effort because they live far from the site of our visit. For example, in

Colombia, we had a small child who had brought by her mother, who first had to travel by boat on the Amazon river, then by horse cart and finally by bus to be seen by us for the needed surgery. Below are typical waiting rooms at various locations full of patients for us to evaluate for cleft surgery.

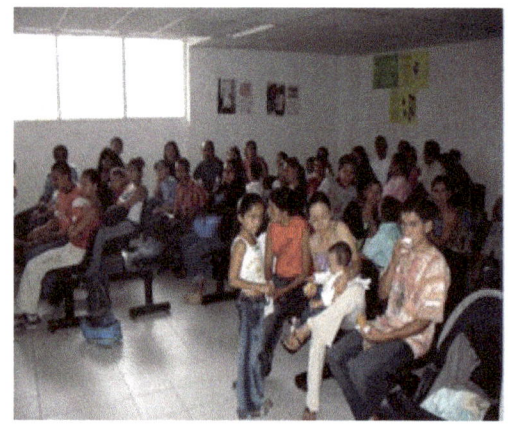
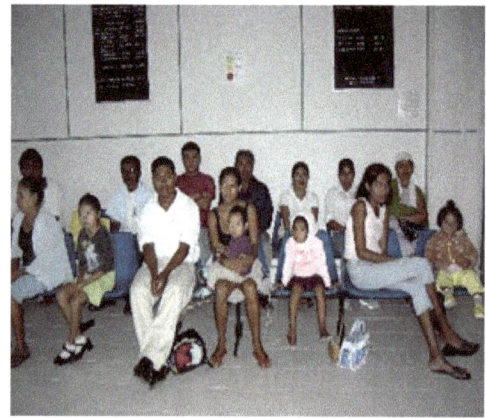
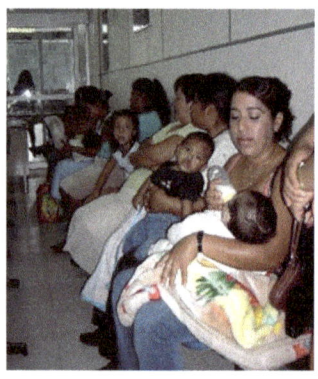
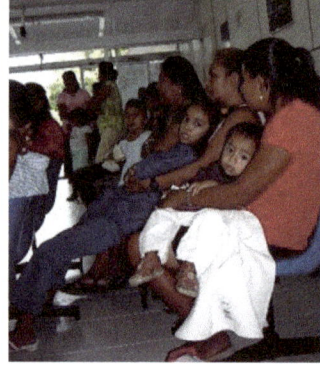
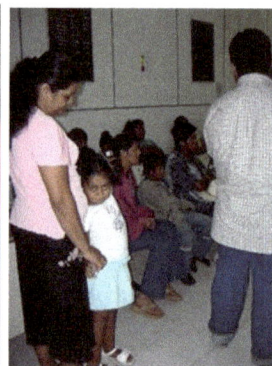

After the clinic, we set up a schedule to operate on about 40 patients over five operating days with two operating tables. We usually see the patients in the clinic on Saturday or Sunday and then work in the OR Monday through Friday. The last Saturday, we have grand rounds, when all of the patients operated through the week are seen back for a post-op evaluation. We make arrangements for any additional postoperative care needed. Finally, we like to get a group picture of our team together with the local hosts and the patients and their families.

Typically, we examined 80 or more patients and selected about half that number for surgery. We will triage patients to be sure they are appropriate for an operation. We will then decide the best surgical approach to their problems. Below are pictures from a representative evaluation clinic. In the first photo, Leticia Lopes OSJ coordinator and Dr. David Bray organize the patients in the clinic. In the next photo behind me is Houston plastic surgeon Dr. Alfonso Barrera who has helped on many trips. The third photo shows me and Juan Cano RN, who has been a great help for many years with operation San Jose. We are evaluating a young surgical candidate. In the last photo, I am getting a close up look at our little patient's cleft problem.

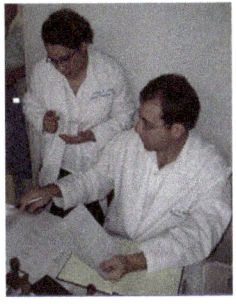 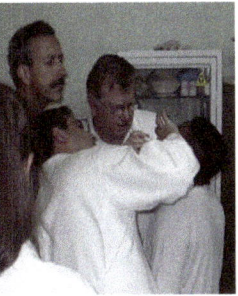 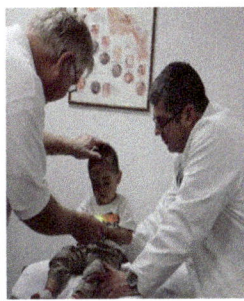 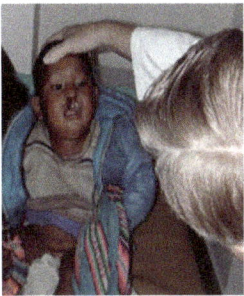

Below, Dr. Donna Fox, speech pathologist, examines a patient to see if she might benefit from additional palate surgery to help her speech. On the right, Dr. Michael Lypka and I are in the preoperative clinic preparing a surgical schedule, selecting about 40 patients, and arranging 8 or 9 cases each day for the 5- day surgical program to follow.

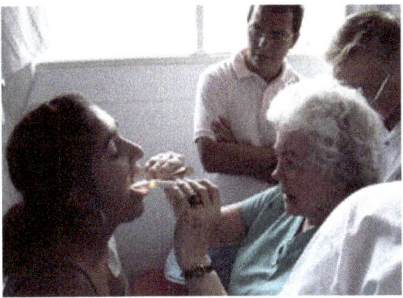 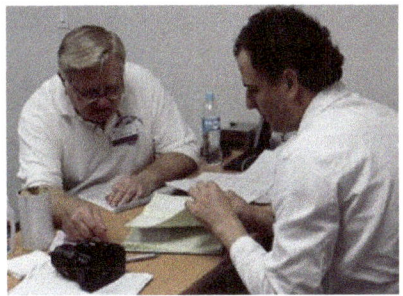

Our pediatrician first clears the patients, like the baby, with the cleft lip below before being scheduled for surgery. Dr. Lozano is discussing a patient's status with his parents in the second photo below. Next, anesthesiologist Dr. Than Tu also clears a patient pre-operatively. Finally, Juana Del Rio CORT entertains a patient waiting for surgery.

The Healing Mission of Plastic Surgery

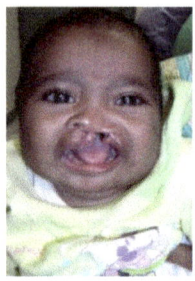 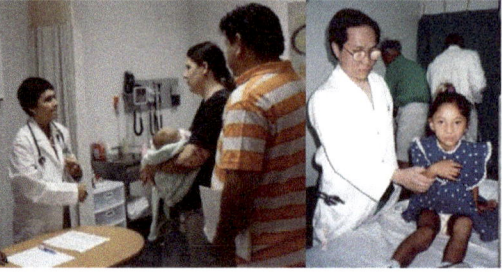 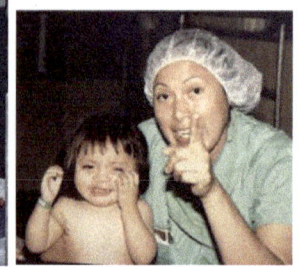

While some of the team are in the clinic examining the patients and planning the surgical schedule for the week, the rest of the group is checking out the operating rooms and setting them up for the upcoming cases. Below doctors, Anna Kutka and Yvonne Cormier, both anesthesiologists, together with Mary Anne Dougherty RN, unpack and organize surgical supplies for use in the operating room. A lot of preparation goes into every case brought to the operating room. On the right below, Liz Marquez CORT, Tina May RN, Debbie Smith-Pierce, and Dr. Mark Hancock move supplies to the operating rooms.

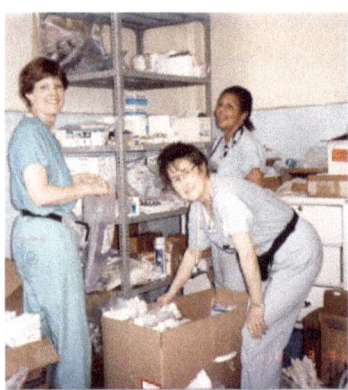 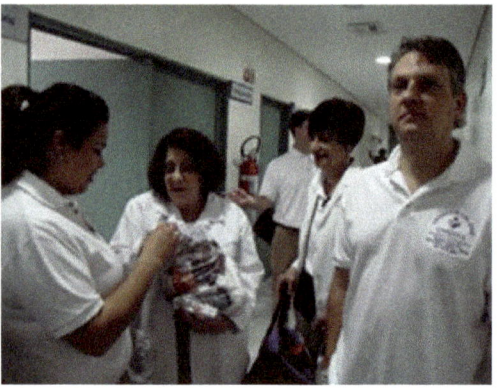

Below left, you see tubing, drapes, and sponges, and other supplies needed for each surgery and a typical set of specialized instruments needed for cleft lip and palate surgery. On top of the cart shown below are about 30 small boxes of specialized suture materials required for our cases. Underneath the cart is additional supplies that may be necessary.

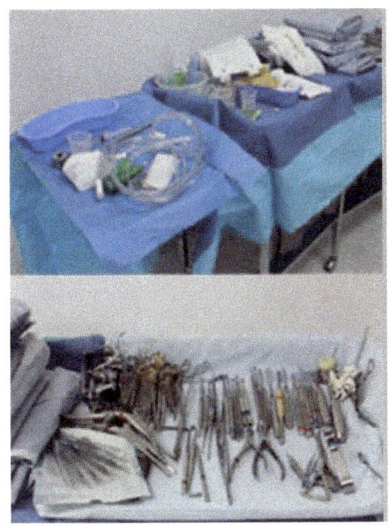
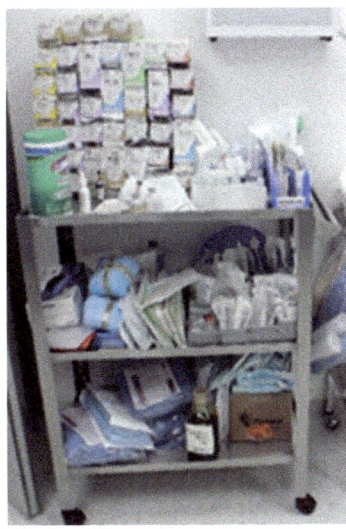

Preoperative holding area

We prepare the patients for surgery in the preoperative holding area. We check the morning of their operation to be sure they have not developed any contraindications such as fever, which would necessitate canceling or postponing the procedure. Candy Cronin reads a story to alleviate anxiety in the preoperative child below who is awaiting palate surgery. In the middle photo, Candy entertains the fasting infant with the cleft lip in the preoperative holding area. Lastly, a father greets his post-operative child in the recovery room while ubiquitous volunteer Candy Cronin looks on.

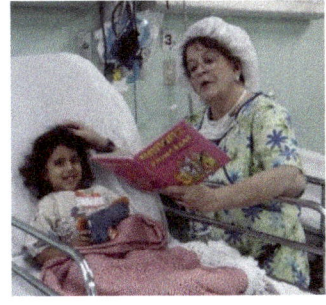
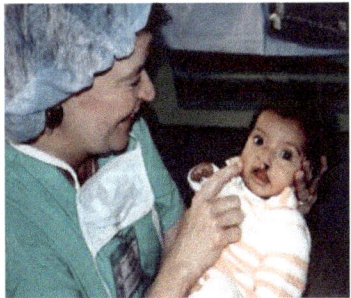
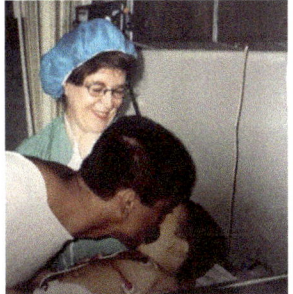

Operating room

Below volunteer, Janine Dubcak brings a child to the operating room and hands her over to the anesthesia team. In the center photo Phil Adamczak, CRNA, carries a baby to the operating room. On the right, Dr.

Paul Sobiesk is beginning to administer anesthesia to a baby scheduled for cleft lip surgery.

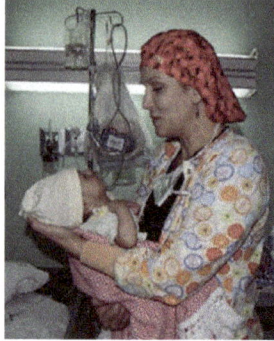 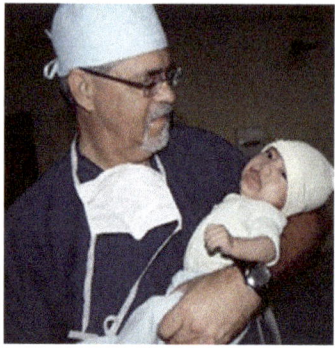 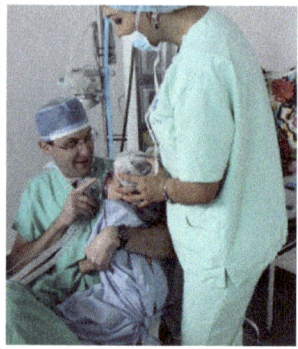

We have been fortunate and are grateful for the volunteer services of many anesthesiologists over the more than 30 years of the existence of operation San Jose. Below, anesthesiologist Dr. Linda Magill has put a patient to sleep in preparation for surgery, while Dr. Paul Hornung is inducing anesthesia for his patient.

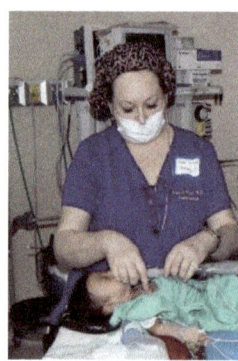 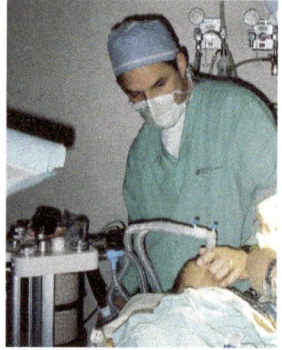

The circulating nurse preps the child below for surgery.

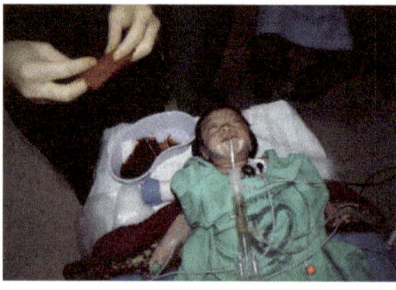 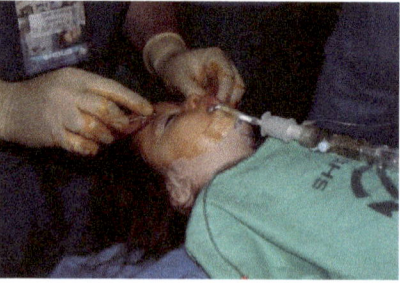

On the left below, I am helping a senior plastic surgery resident Dr. Zafar perform a palate repair. At the same time, in the middle, Dr. Lipka is operating with another senior plastic surgery resident, Dr. Failey, who seems in this picture to have glowing surgical hands. On the right, Dr. Raymond Brauer, a former partner and mentor of mine, is assisting and teaching plastic surgery resident Dr. O'Brien repair a cleft of the lip.

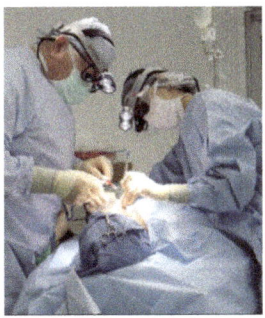 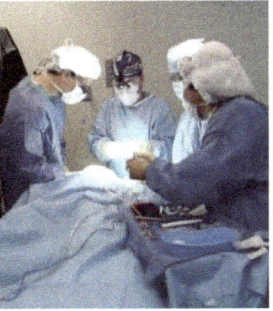 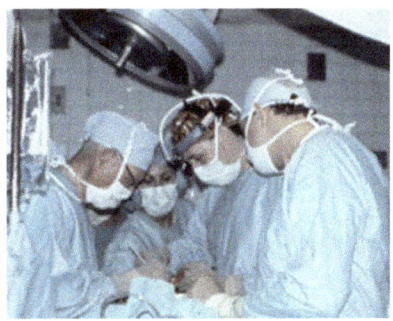

I will next show several typical cases to give you a good representation of the work done by the team. The baby below, "Marcus," had a complete cleft of the lip and palate on the right with severe distortion of the nasal ala on the right. The resident first draws the proposed incisions in blue ink on the baby's lip. The middle picture is the intraoperative result. The last photo is the postoperative result after a few days.

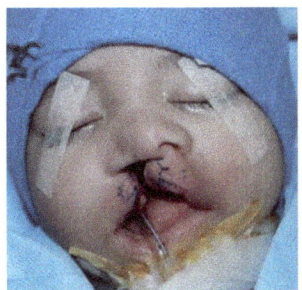 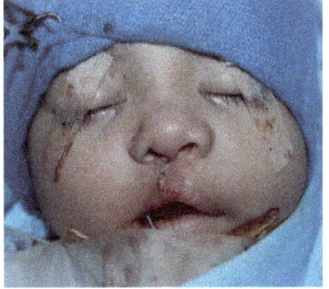 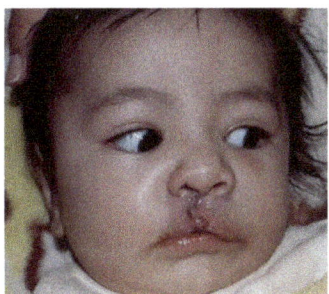

The next case is that of "Vadamir," who had an almost complete cleft lip on the left. The surgeon uses calipers to measure and plan the incisions. The on the table result is on the right below.

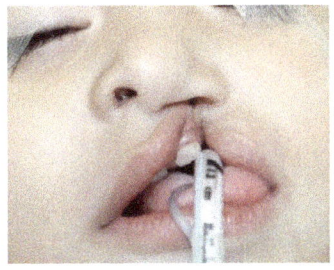 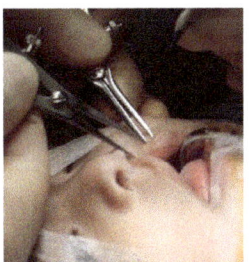 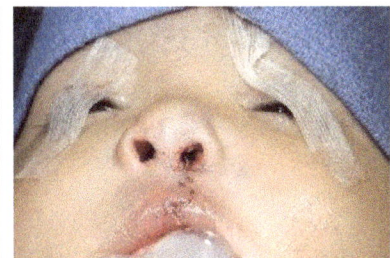

Below, "Tina" is shown with a pre-operative right-sided complete cleft of the lip and palate. There is considerable right nasal ala distortion of the nose. Her postoperative result a few days later indicates the baby has not only a functioning upper lip but also a helpful nasal correction.

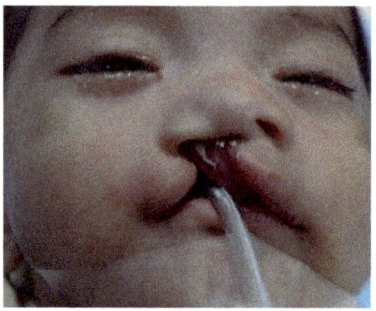
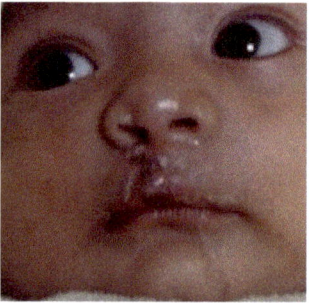

"Jordan" had a complete bilateral cleft of the lip and palate, as shown on the right below. The immediate postoperative result is on the right.

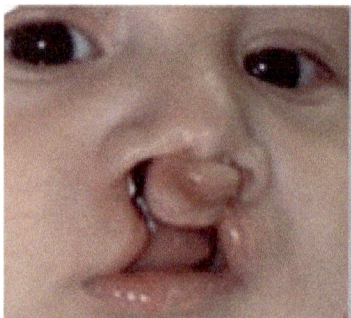
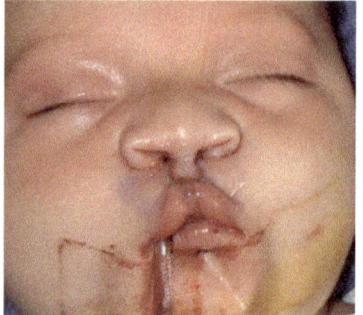

"Miguel" has an incomplete bilateral cleft of the lip and palate. The resident repaired this lip with a straight line modified Cronin technique. His immediate result is on the left below.

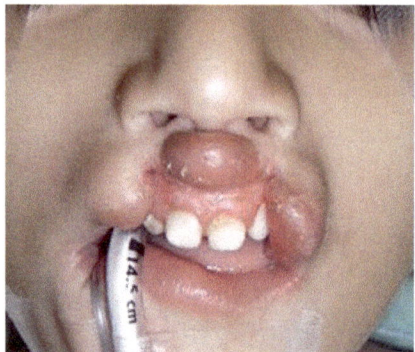
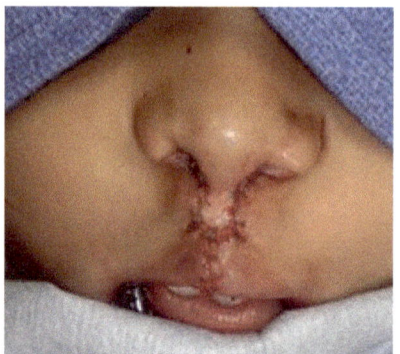

"Roberto" below had a complete bilateral cleft of the lip and palate. Postoperative pictures first with surgical glue on the surface and then after cleaning are shown.

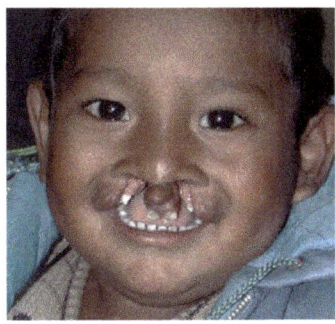 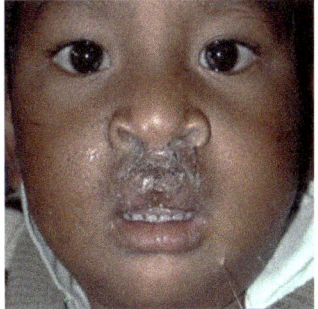 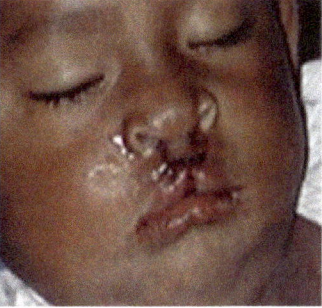

"Virginia," below, had a right side complete cleft of the lip and palate. Her postoperative result a few days later is shown with then-senior resident Dr. Mike Lypka, who as of 2016 succeeded me as medical director of OSJ

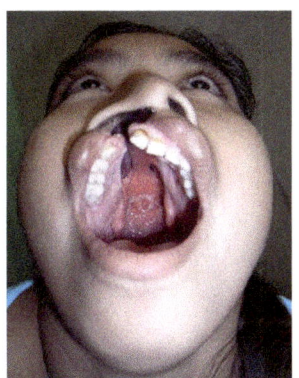 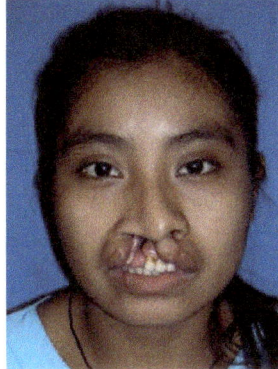 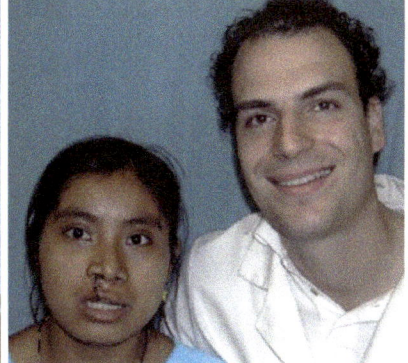

"Graciela" below had a cleft of the palate without a cleft lip. The immediate on the table result is on the right after a two flap palatoplasty.

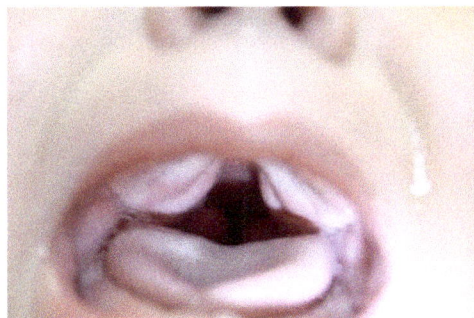 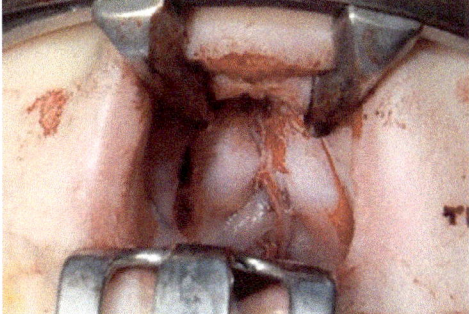

The Healing Mission of Plastic Surgery

The patient below" Maryanne" has a cleft of the posterior palate. When repairing a roof of the mouth cleft, the surgeon works from behind the head of the patient. So, the view is upside down, as in the second photo. In her case, we used a double reverse Z-plasty technique, as drawn in the third picture. The Z plasty not only closes the palate but also lengthens it, so the posterior edge is closer to the pharynx than before the repair.

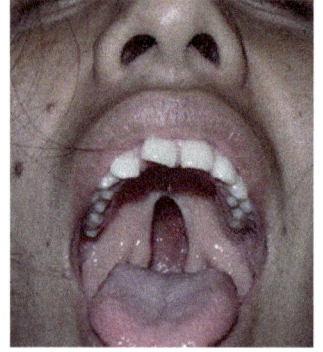
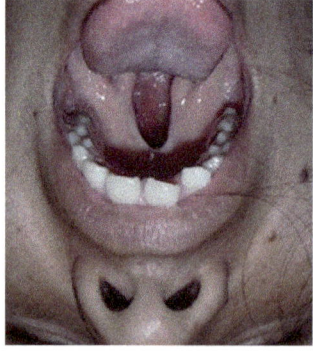
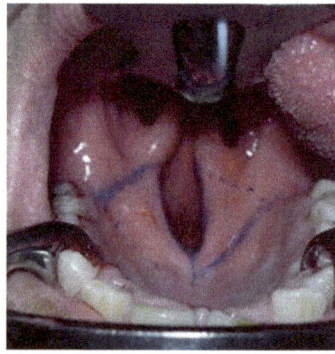
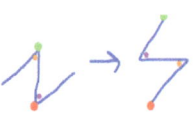
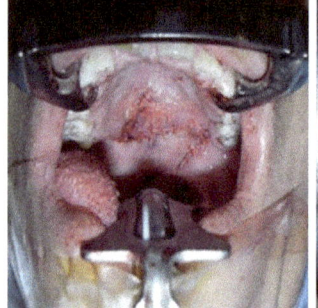
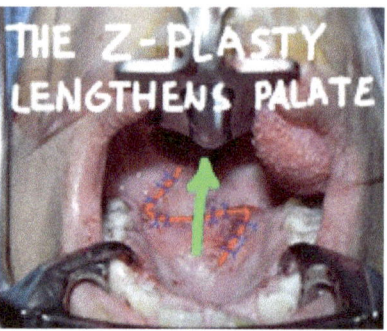

"David shown below was in his 50's and had never had his wide-open palate repaired. He wished to have the surgery to hopefully improve his speech and also to improve his oral hygiene. His intact healing palate is on the right. The early report from our speech pathologist was that he received an immediate improvement in his speech intelligibility because of more natural resonance.

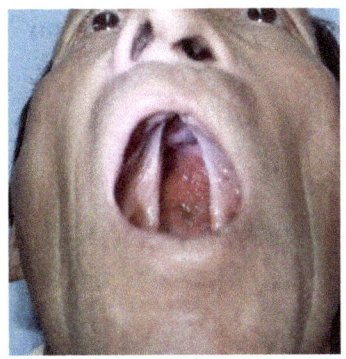 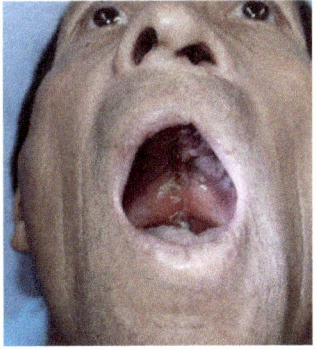

We often encounter patients who have had surgery but could benefit from revision procedures. One such patient was "Juanita" who had had a bilateral cleft lip repaired in childhood. She had some excessive scar and asymmetry, which we revised. Her immediate result is on the right below.

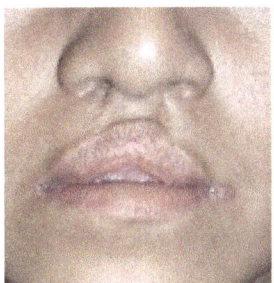 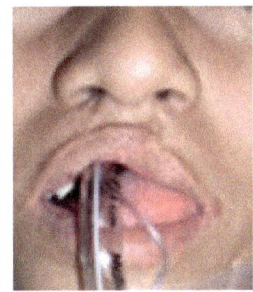 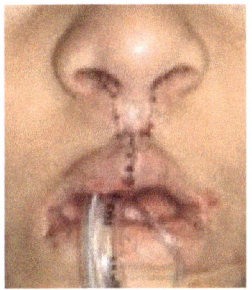

Another patient, "Suanna" below had had bilateral cleft lip repair as a child but desired to obtain improvement in her result with additional surgery. We felt she would best benefit from a two-stage cross lip Abbe flap procedure. Her pre-op pictures on the left show a short lip and no central vermillion. Her on the table immediate result after the first stage demonstrates improved lip length and contour. Although unfinished, one can see the enhanced nasal tip projection and lengthened nasal columella. The final view below shows the improvement in the entire profile. We arranged for our host surgeon to separate the flap connection (blue line) after about twelve days.

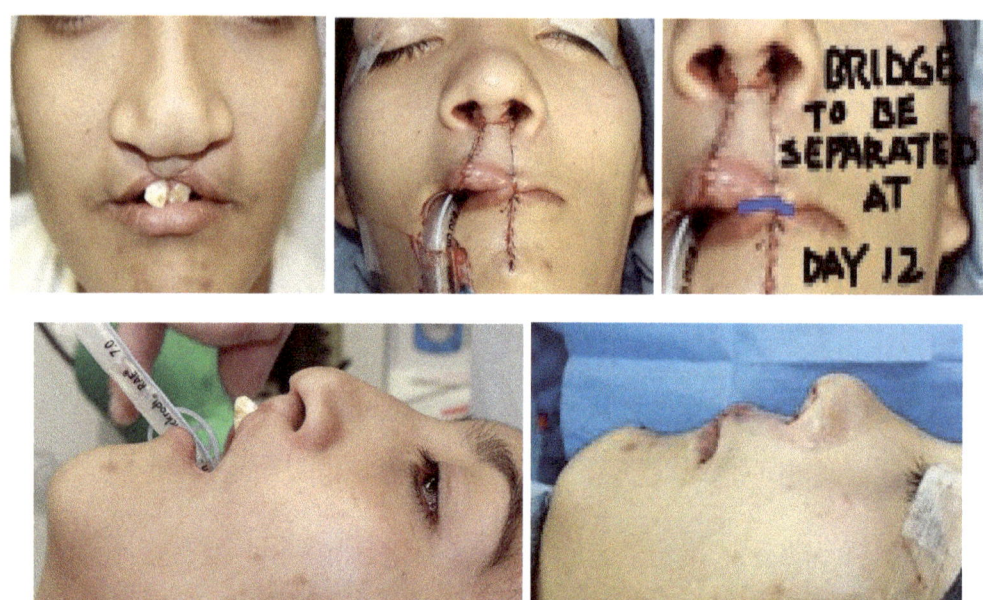

Some of our medical hosts have told us some mission groups will only operate on primary cases, and some even only want to treat cleft lip cases and not palate cases.

The above two cases reiterate that, although revision surgeries may not be as exciting or clean as primary cases, they can be very beneficial for the patients. Therefore, we evaluate all comers and will often do revision surgery. We did many similar procedures with the help of the Houston plastic surgeons in the picture below. Dr. Rafi Bidros is to my right, Drs. Bruce Smith and Leo La Puerta to my left below. I am indebted to them for all their help over many years. Also, I am especially thankful for the expert, loyal, long-serving, and diligent support of Maria Salazar pictured below in the operating room.

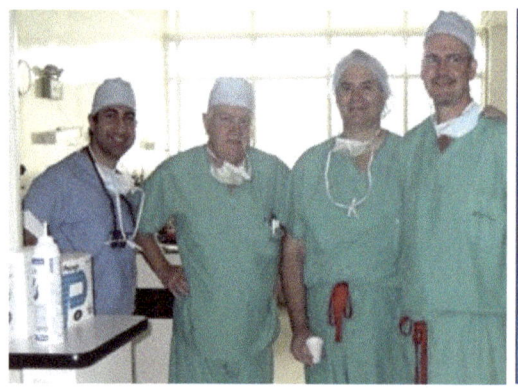
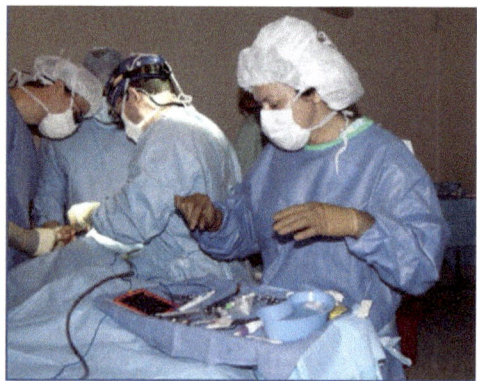

Recovery room

The recovery room is an essential aspect of the care of these patients. On the left below is recovery room nurse Cindy Jones holding her patient, while Dr. Martha Lozano is administering some oral liquid medicine. In the center, the newly postoperative baby receives oxygen via mask from volunteer Candy Cronin. On the right nurse, Tina May does a breathing exercise with a postoperative patient.

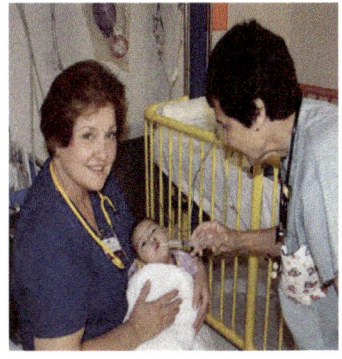 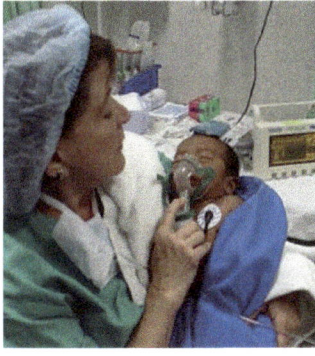 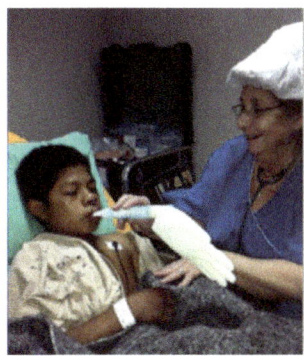

Below left, a postoperative palate patient is being comforted in the recovery room. Most of the cleft palate cases stay overnight in the facility, while most cleft lip patients are outpatients. In the middle, a mother is ready to leave the recovery area with her postoperative child. On the right, a child is doing well, ready to be discharged home from the recovery room after lip repair.

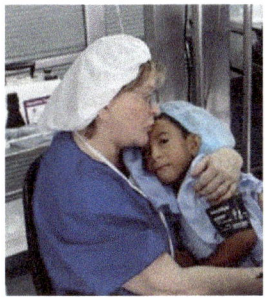 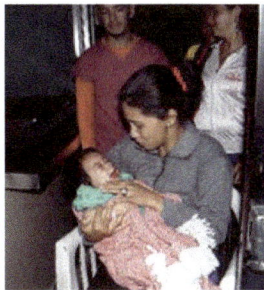 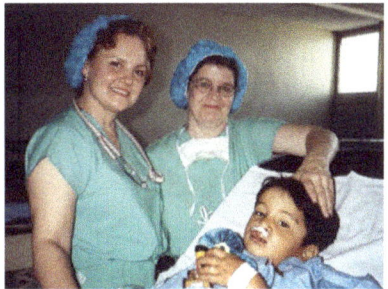

Below are a mother and child ready for discharge from the hospital after an overnight stay. In the second photo, senior resident Alex Colque declares his patient prepared for release. The third photo is Dr. Bidros with his post-op patient.

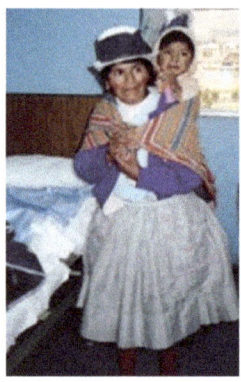 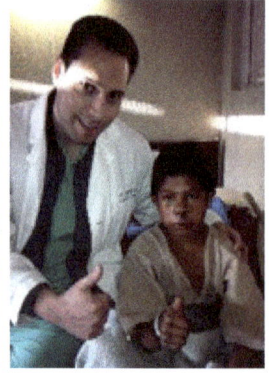 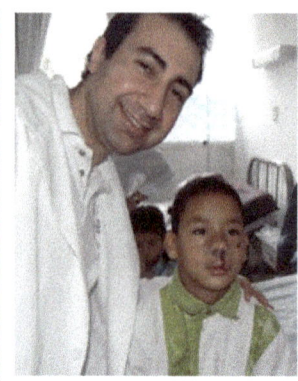

After completion of the Monday through Friday extensive surgical schedule, just when everyone is exhausted, it is time to pack up our equipment that night after the last procedure. Most of the unused supplies we leave for the facility where we worked. Below, Maria Salazar is beginning to organize the packing of our equipment back into our travel cases.

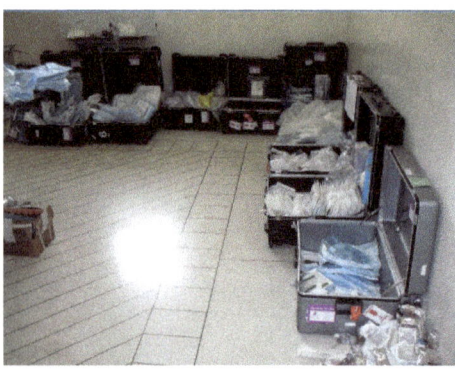 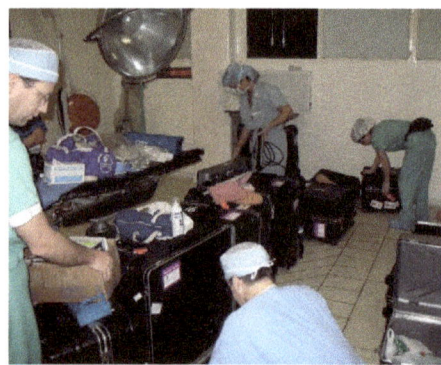

The next morning we have grand rounds when all of the patients operated upon the entire week's return for follow-up. We change some bandages and remove some sutures, clean wounds, and take a lot of photos, both clinical and social. We explain postoperative instructions to families and answer all of their remaining questions. We arrange for additional postoperative visits with our host surgeons as needed. We exchange many thanks and goodbyes.

The Healing Mission of Plastic Surgery

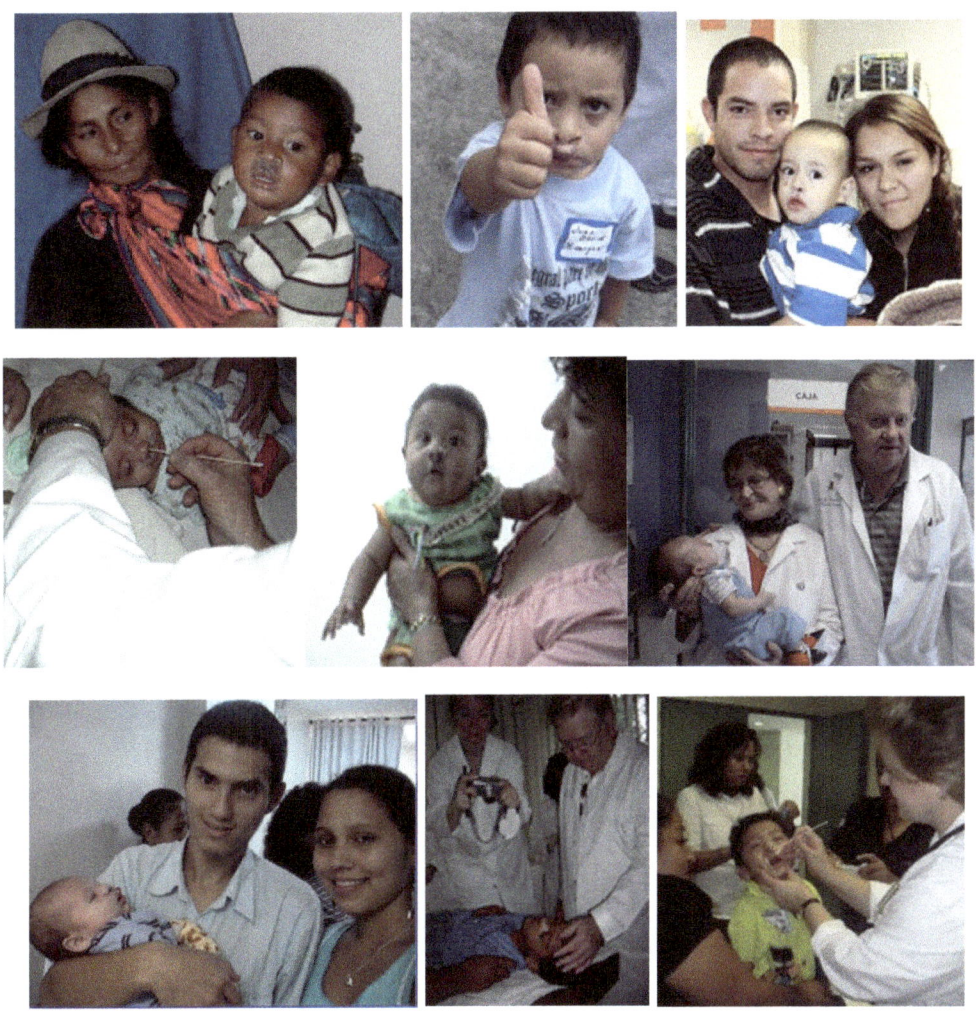

After the grand rounds, we take a photograph of the team together with the patients we have served. Some additional examples of operation San Jose mission trips since 1983 follow.

1990, 1991, 1992 Villahermosa Mexico

1990 Villahermosa Mexico, Dr. Dan Casso, and Dr. Christopher Patronella senior plastic surgery residents

Below, Dr. Christopher Patronella, Dr. Celia Carillo- Perez M.D., I, and Dr. Amado Ruiz pose with patients' families. In the center next to me are anesthesiologist Robert Kavanaugh, TV celebrity and supporter, Marvin Zindler, and Dr. Amado Ruiz. Senior plastic surgery resident Dr. Dan Casso and anesthesiologist Dr. Anna Kutka pose below right.

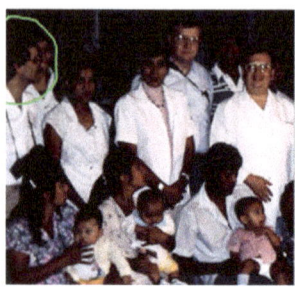 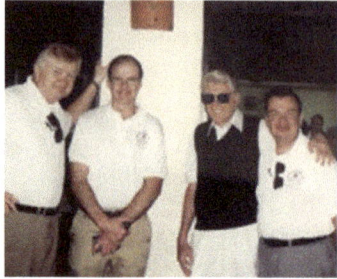 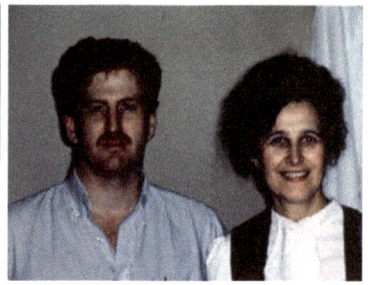

1991 Villahermosa Mexico, Dr. Hal Mentz, and Dr. Gary Branfman senior plastic surgery residents

Drs Gary Branfman and Hal Mentz are on either side of Dr. Brauer on the left side of this photo below from Villahermosa. The picture on the left shows Dr. Branfman with one of his OSJ patients.

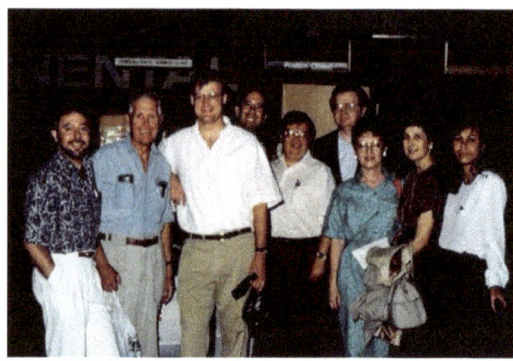 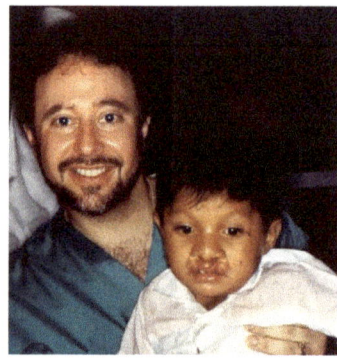

1992 Dr. Clay Moliver and Dr. Bruce Smith senior plastic surgery residents

OSJ visited Hospital Sergio Rovirosa in Villahermosa, Tabasco Mexico, hosed by Dr. Celia Carillo-Perez. The photo below shows part of the 1992 OSJ Team in the surgical suite. From left to right Maria Salazar, CORT, Dr bruce Smith Dr. Ray Brauer Dr. Amado Ruiz, Dr. Clay Moliver, Graciella Angarita, Me, Dr. Celia Carrillo, Dr. Jim Strohmeyer, and Jane Holmes RN

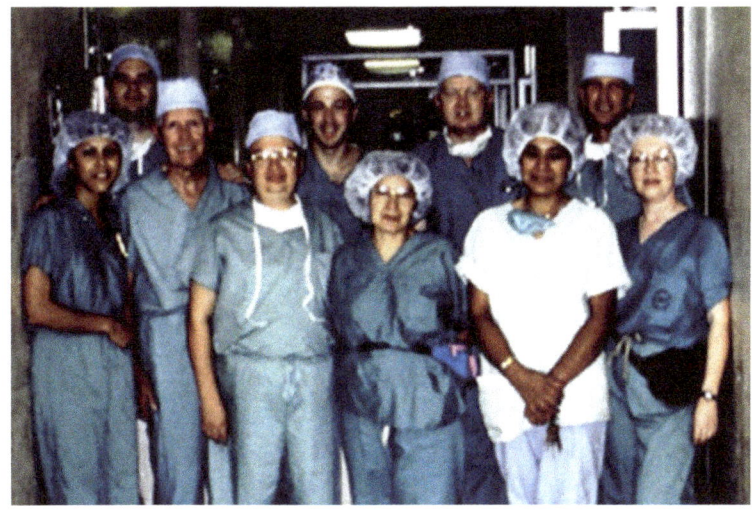

On the right below, Marvin Zindler observes a clinic session. Bob Dows (far right), his cameraman is recording for later use on TV Channel 13 ABC in Houston. On the right below, Marvin Zindler discusses OSJ with team anesthesiologist James Strohmeyer.

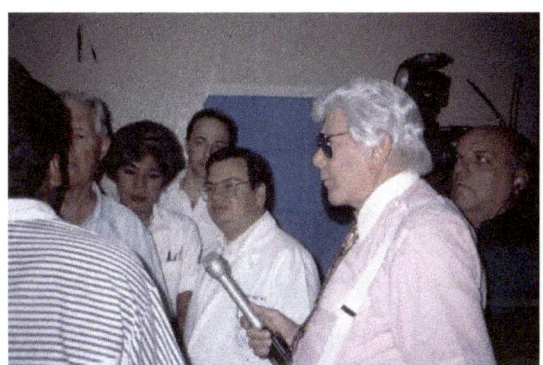 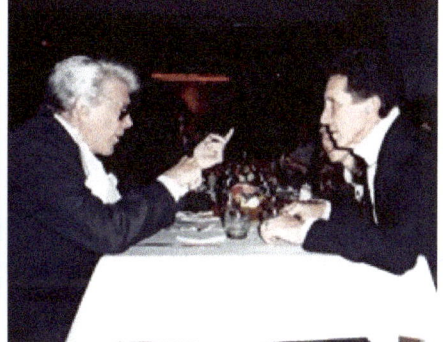

1993 Caracas, Venezuela

1993 Dr. Don Collins and Dr. Herman Newell senior plastic surgery residents

Below is a team picture from the 1993 mission trip to Caracas Venezuela, hosted by plastic surgeon Dr.Jose Ortega Laura. From left to right, Dr. Ben Cohen (my practice partner of 38 years), Maria Salazar CORT, Silvia Brauer, anesthesiologist Dr.Tim Heerensperger(back row), plastic surgeon Dr. Ray Brauer, Dr. Herman Newell (back row), Sarah Cohen, me (back row), Kathy Scrivner RN, Graciela Angarita CORT, plastic surgeon Dr. Don Collins.

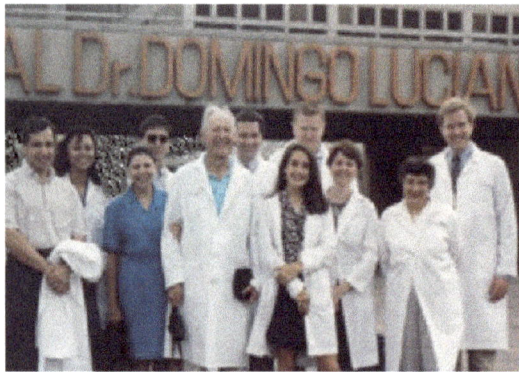
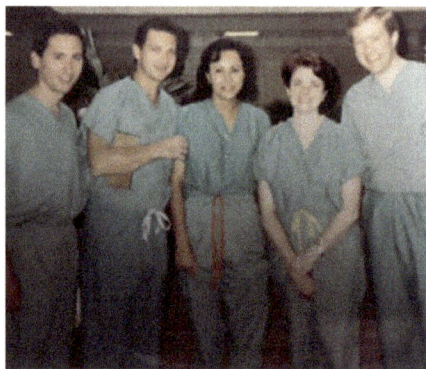

1994 Leon Nicaragua

1994 Dr. John O'Brien and Dr. Tom Weiner senior plastic surgery residents

In 1994 OSJ visited Leon Nicaragua with Dr. Arturo Gomes as our host. The photo below shows from left to right, Dr. Anna Kutka, Dr. Brauer, Maria Salazar Dr. Tom Weiner (back), Dr. Than Tu, a local doctor, Graciella Angarita CORT(front), Dr. John Obrien, Kathy Scrivner RN, Dr. Arturo Gomes, me, and Dr. Amado Ruiz.

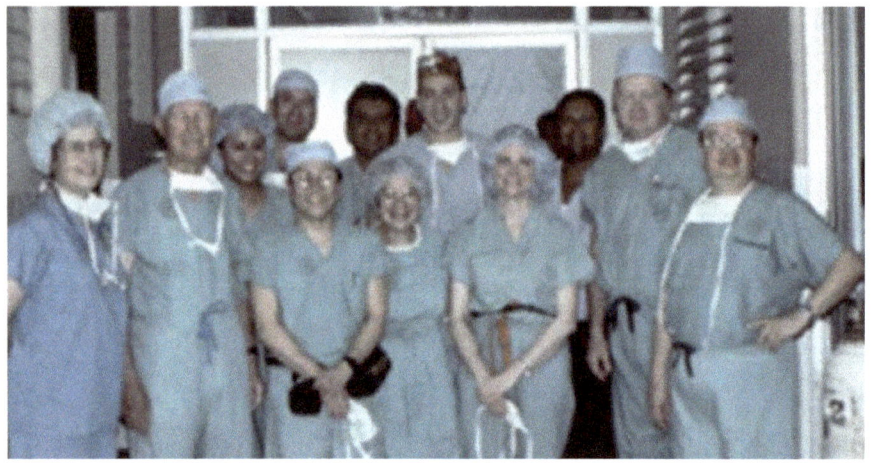

1995 Arequipa, Peru

Dr. Leo Lapuerta and Dr. Joey Haber senior plastic surgery residents

The photo below is of El Misti, the snow-covered volcano of Arequipa Peru. On the right below Marvin Zindler hold a baby who we are to evaluate for palate surgery

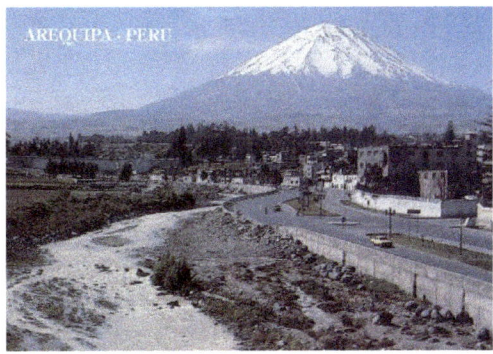 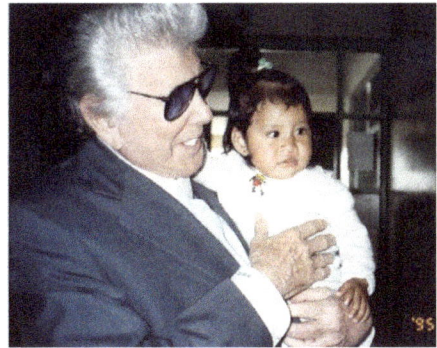

1996 Babahoyo, Ecuador

1996 Dr. Jim Plastis and Dr.Jim Roesel senior plastic surgery residents

OSJ visited the small town of Babahoyo, Ecuador, in 1996 with Dr. Nelson Estrella as our host. The photo below shows from left to right Dr. Jim Plastis, me, Dr. Brauer, Dr. Nelso Estrella, Dr. Jim Roesel, and Dr. Yvonne Cormier anesthesiologist.

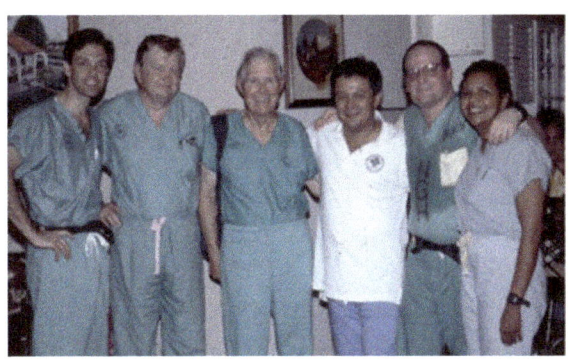

1997 Arequipa Peru

1997 Dr. Phi Nguyen and Dr. Michael Ciaravino senior plastic surgery residents

Plastic surgery residents, Dr. Phi Nguyen, and Michael Ciaravino jest with Dr. Brauer between cases.

The Healing Mission of Plastic Surgery

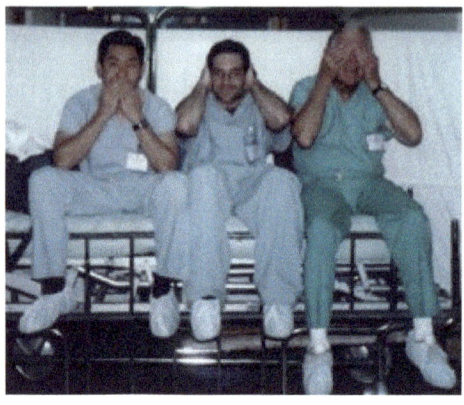

1998 Huancayo, Peru

1998 Dr. Manni Gallas and Dr. Lucien Rivela senior plastic surgery residents

Below, the OSJ team arrives at the hospital in Huancayo, Peru, with about 30 large boxes of equipment and supplies ready to get organized. On the right below, anesthesiologists Dr. Cormier and Dr, Sobiesk interact with a couple of their young patients on the clinic day

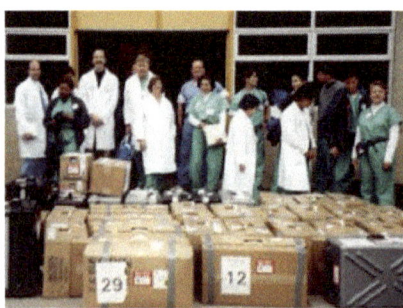
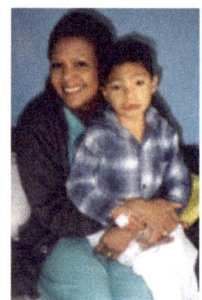
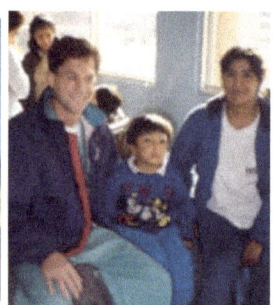

On the left, an indigenous mother and child await evaluation for surgery. In the Middle below, Dr. Ruiz, Dr.Gallas, and Dr. Cormier prepare a patient for surgery. On the right volunteer, Candy Cronin brings a patient to the operating room.

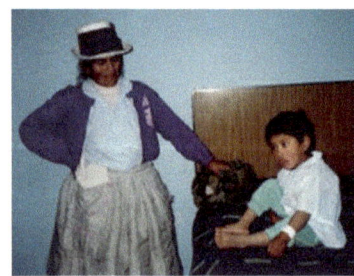
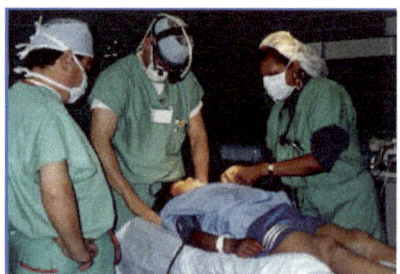
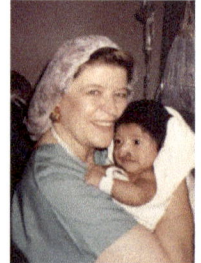

The photo below is of the OSJ team enjoying the view from the roof of the hospital in Huancayo.

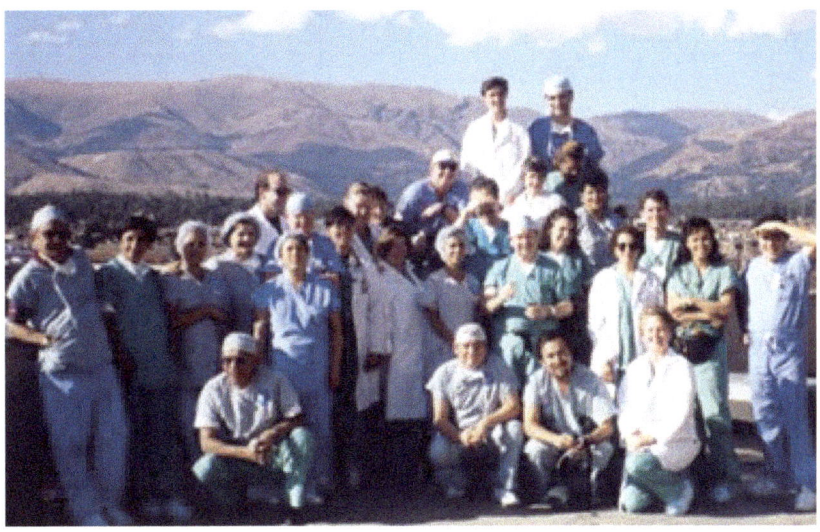

Below, Candy Cronin and Cindy Jones enjoy a short evening break on the hospital roof before returning to the recovery room.

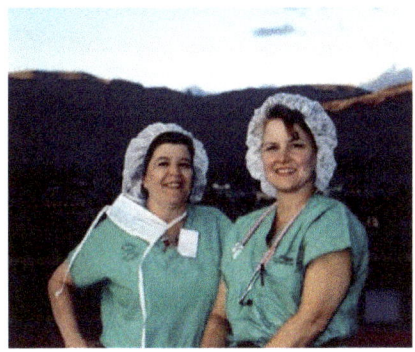

Below, residents Lucien Rivela and Manni Gallas say goodbye to a couple of their post-op patients and family in the post-op clinic on the day of our departure.

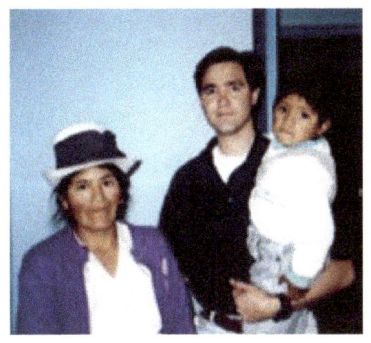 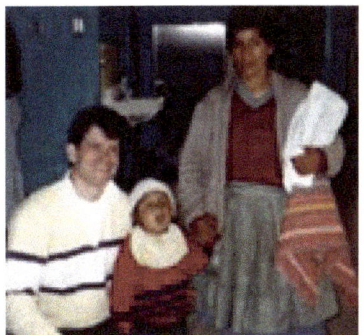

Although we offered to revise the cleft lip on the mother below, she wanted only to have her child operated so that she could devote all her efforts to care for her in the postoperative time. In the middle, this older patient came back to thank us on our final day. Below right is a picture taken from our bus after we had loaded up to leave. Many patients and family members assembled to say goodbye to the team.

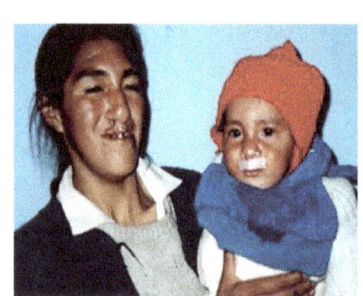 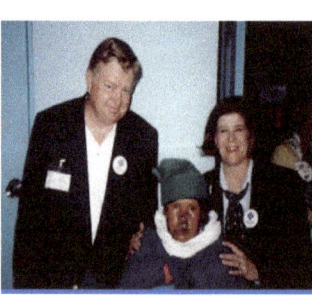 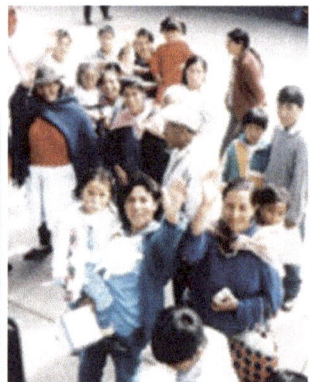

1999 Villahermosa, Tabasco, Mexico

1999 Dr. Jeff Williams, and Dr. Sadri Sozar senior plastic surgery residents

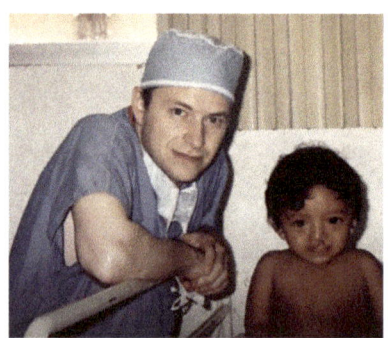

Below the OSJ team from left to right, Dr. Leo LaPuerta, Dr. Jeff Williams, Dr. Jim Roesel, Dr. Christopher Livingston, me, Dr. Sadri Sozar, Dr. Cecilia Carrillo(our host plastic surgeon), Dr. Dr. Amado Ruiz, Dr. Denise Ortiz-Lao, Maria Salazar CORT, Cindy Jones RN, Candy Cronin.

The Healing Mission of Plastic Surgery

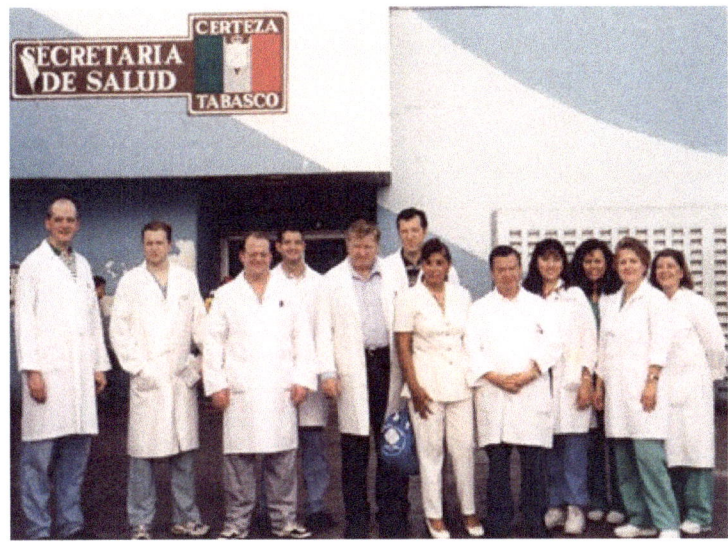

2000 Arequipa Peru

2000 Dr. Lee Steely, and Dr. John Suber senior plastic surgery residents

Below left, Dr. Lee Steely holds a child that he repaired a cleft lip for a couple of days prior.

Below right, Dr. John Suber poses with his cleft palate patient and his happy mother.

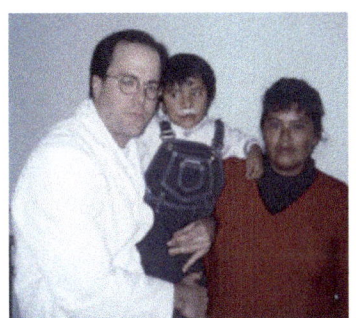
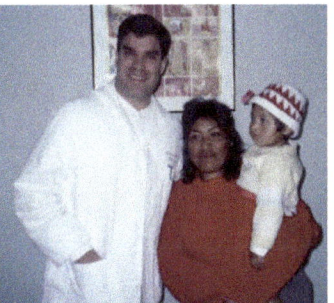
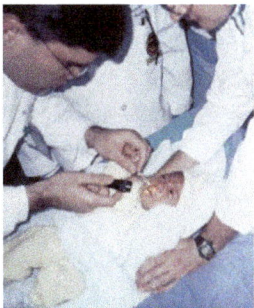

2001 OSJ Mazatlan Mexico

2001 Dr.FranciscoRafolsand Dr. Mark Jabor senior plastic surgery residents

Below, Dr. Mark Jabor and Francisco Rafels(in green scrubs) look on with Dr. Hal Mentz as I examine a pre-operative patient. On the right, Dr. Denise Ortiz-Lao and Dr. Rafels pose with a child this after cleft lip repair.

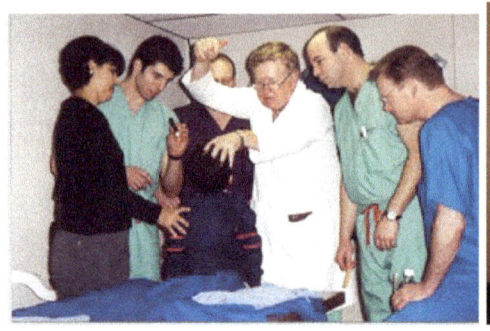 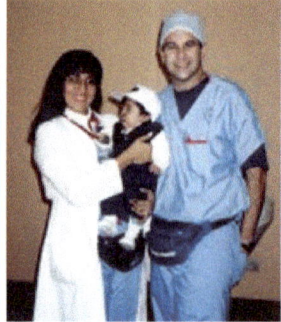

2002 Lima Peru

2002 Dr. Ahmad Ahmadi, and Dr. Camile Cash senior plastic surgery residents

Below the OSJ team in Lima Peru

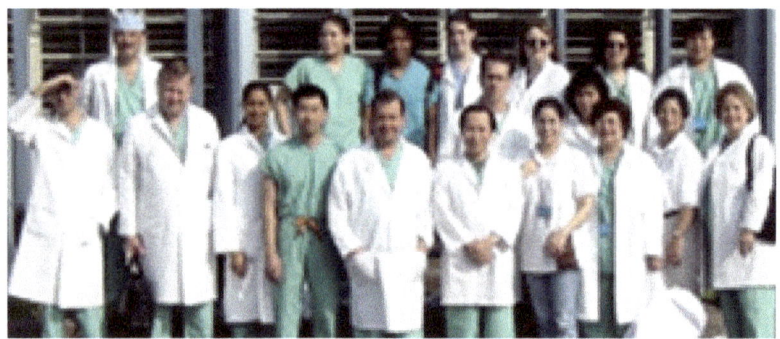

Below, on the left, Dr. Camile Cash is planing a cleft lip repair under the assistance of Dr. Jim Boynton while I am overlooking the procedure. In the middle, Dr. Ruiz assists Dr. Ahmadi. On the right, Drs. Cash and Ahmadi are happy with their contribution to the work of Operation San Jose.

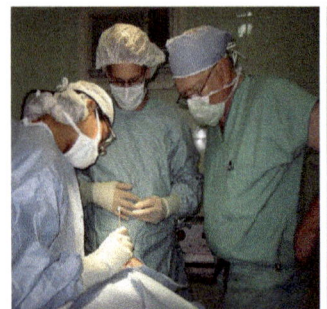 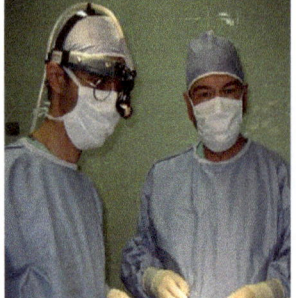 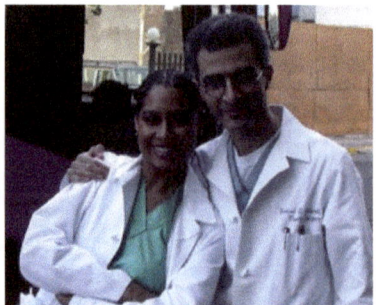

2003 Chihuahua Mexico

2003 Dr. Adam Rubenstein, and Dr. Jon Weinrach senior plastic surgery residents

Below, our host plastic surgeon Dr. Modesto, to my right and the surgical team make hospital rounds a morning after surgery. On the right team members and hosts pause for a photo.

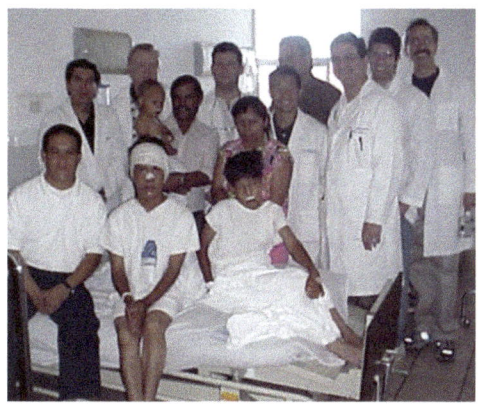 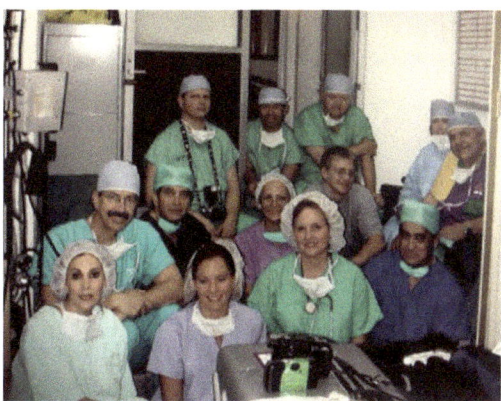

Below, Drs. Mark Jabor, Phi Nguyen, and Adam Rubinstein pose. On the right, Dr. Alfonso Barrera and I examine a patient.

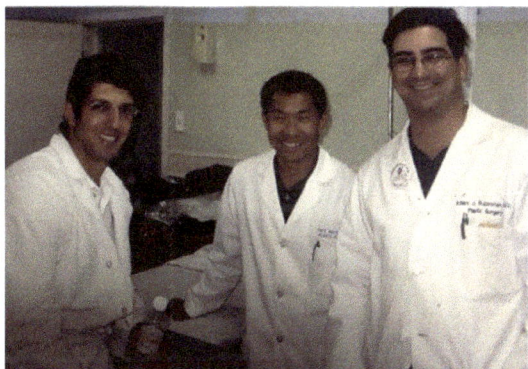 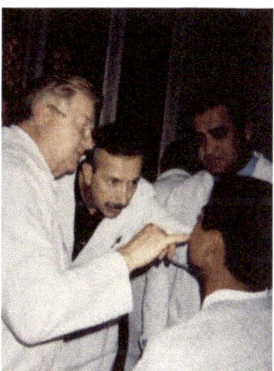

2004 Chihuahua Mexico

2004 Dr. Rick De Splinter and Dr. Arvin Taneja, senior plastic surgery residents.

The Healing Mission of Plastic Surgery

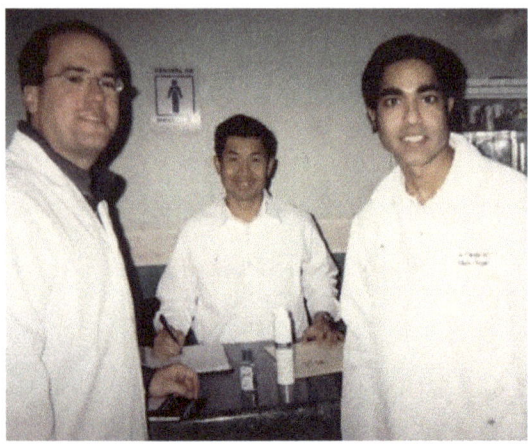 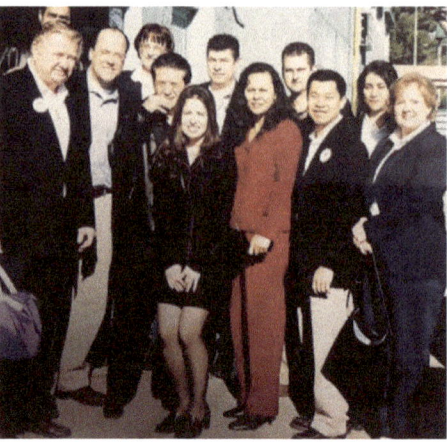

2005 Sucre Bolivia

2005 Dr. Jim Boynton, and Dr. Robert Kratschmer senior plastic surgery residents

Operation San Jose team ready for departure from Houston to Sucre Bolivia via La Paz, Bolivia.

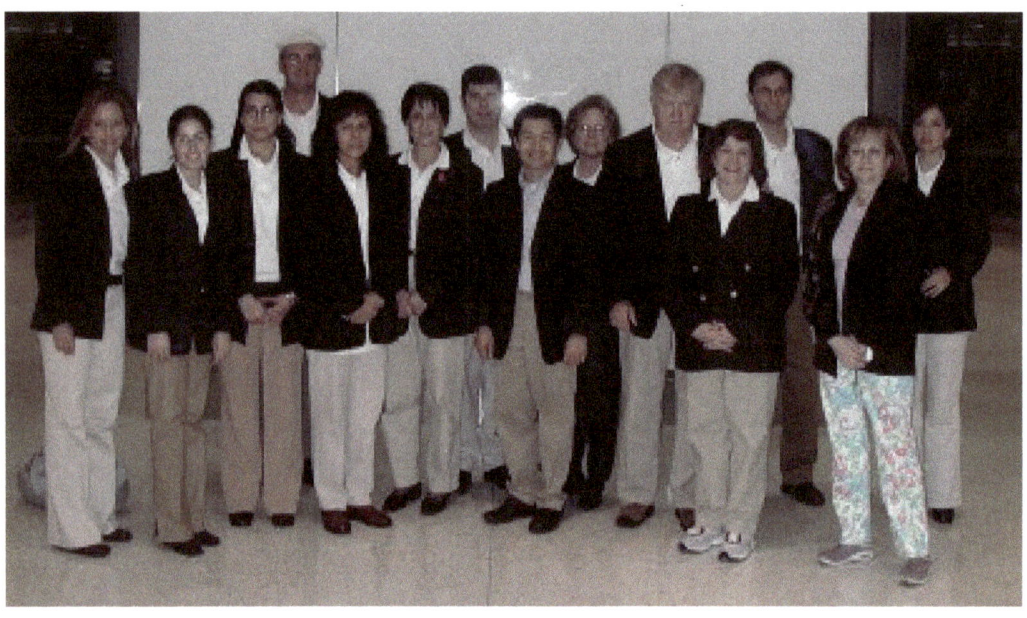

Below left, Dr. Boynton examines a postoperative patient. On the right below, Dr. Kratschmer with one of his post-op patients. Volunteer Alma Lopez with a patient.

The Healing Mission of Plastic Surgery

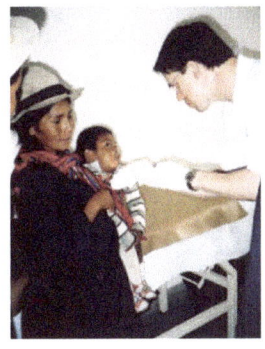 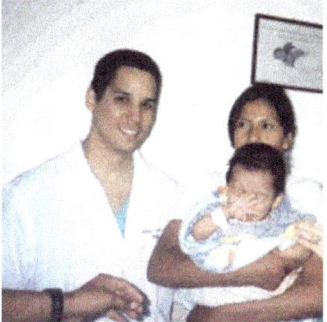 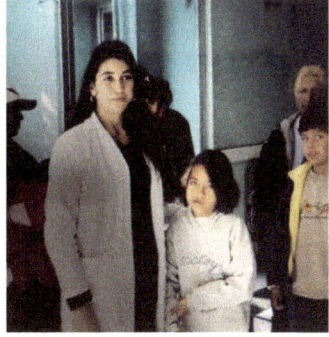

2006 Zihuatanejo, Mexico

2006 Dr. David Bray, and Dr. Virginia Pittman-Waller senior plastic surgery residents

Below Dr. Bray examines his first pre-operative OSJ patient. On the right below, Dr. Pittman-Waller poses with his mother and her child with a cleft lip before surgery.

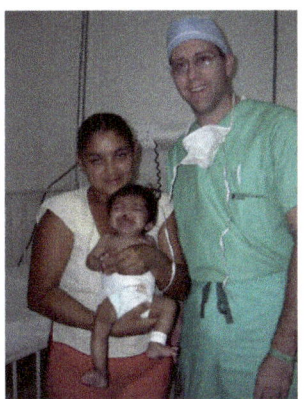 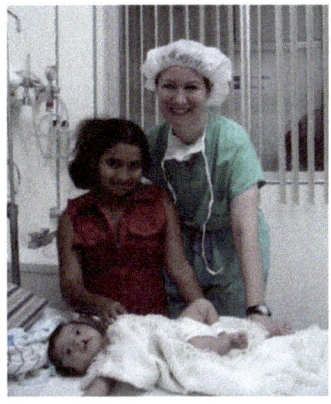

The baby below "Johnathan" immediately pre and post-op.

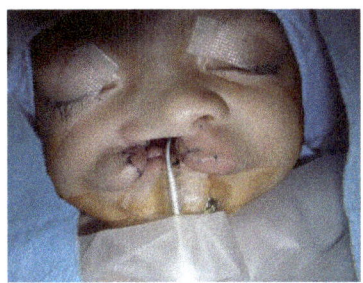 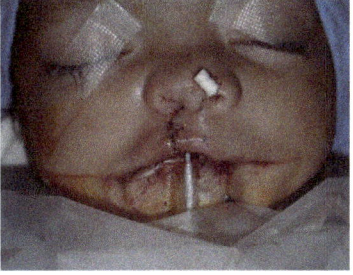

"David," the child below, has an effective plan drawn on his incomplete cleft lip. The view on the right is the immediate post-op result.

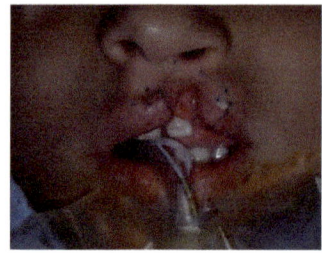 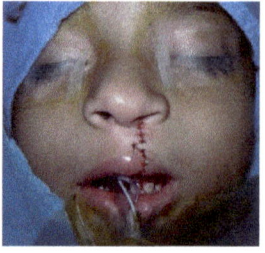

Below left is a patient with a wide-open cleft palate. On the right is the immediate closure in the operating room

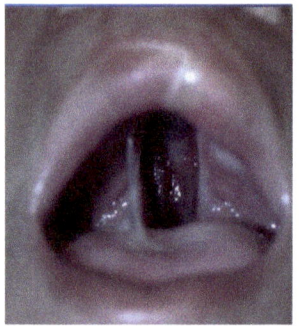 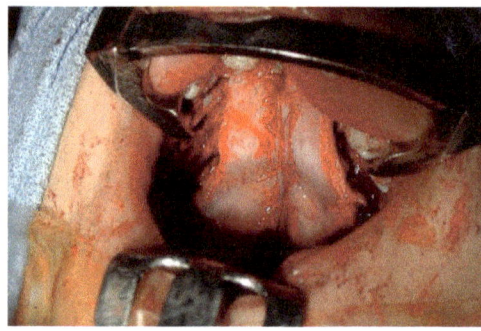

The OSJ team is pictured below with some of our hosts. Standing left Dr. Sanches (Lieutenant& host). Standing right, Dr. Velasquez (Captain & host) OSJ team back row from left, Dr. Alfonso Barrera, Dr. Leo LaPuerta, Dr.Linda Magill, Debi Smith RN, Cindy Jones RN, Juan Cano RN, Maricela Salazar CORT, Dr. Joseph Hornung, Dr. David Bray, Dr. Virginia Pittman-Waller. Front row from left Fernando Barrera, Veronica Cruz North, Kathleen Cronin, Dr. Ernest Cronin, Dr. Phi Nguyen, Tina May RN, Maria Salazar CORT

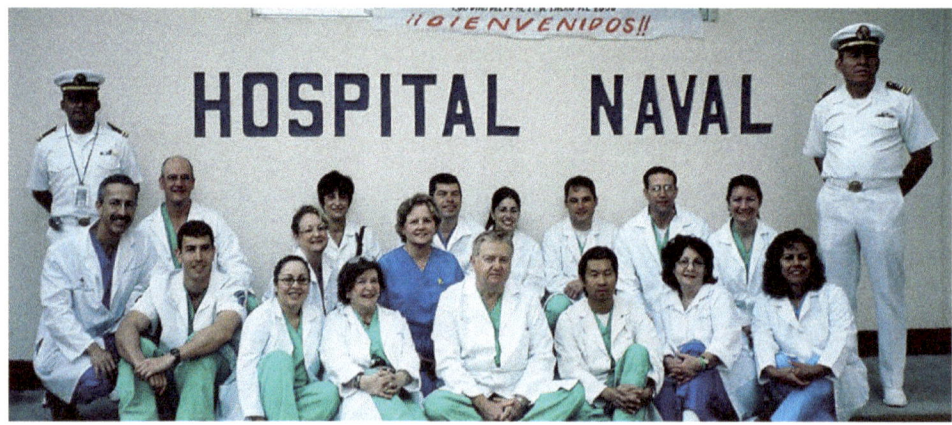

Below are OSJ patients gathered with families on the final day in Zihuatanejo, Mexico, 2006.

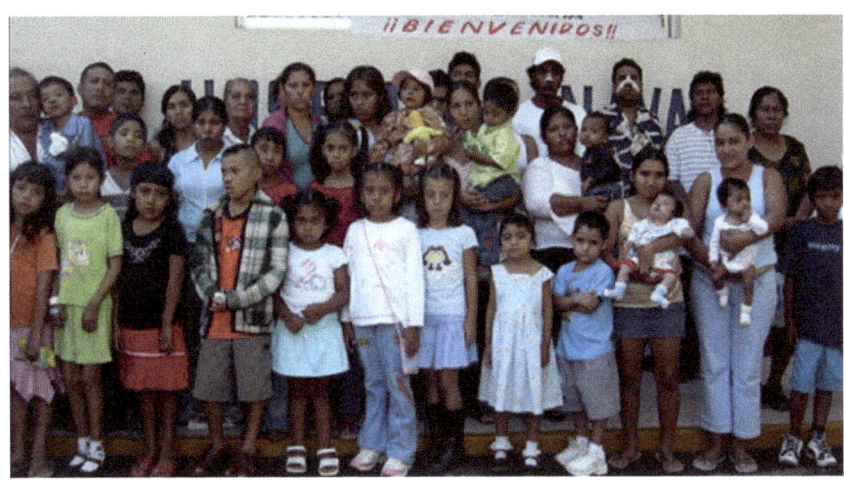

2007 Armenia Colombia

2007 Dr. David Harley, and Dr. Eric Miles senior plastic surgery residents

Drs Harley and Miles are shown below with their newly post-op patients. On the right below is Dr. Cesar Parra, a native of Colombia who served as our pediatrician on several trips.

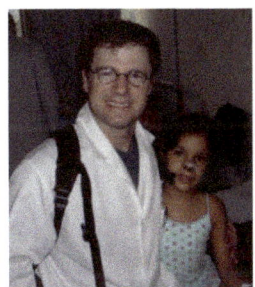 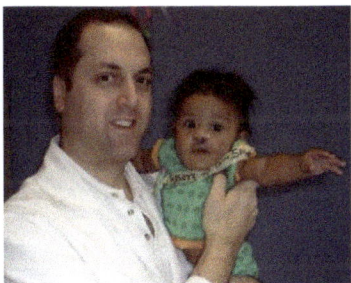 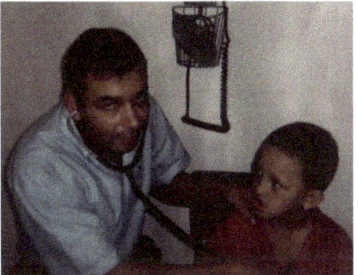

Below is a picture including the OSJ team, patients, and their families after our program in Armenia, Colombia, 2007.

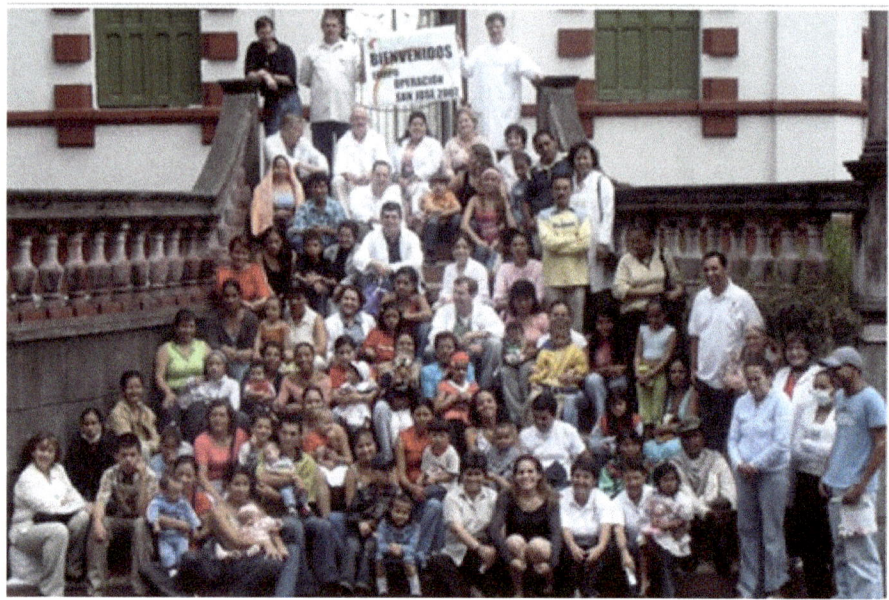

Below is a group picture with both OSJ surgical team members and local hospital staff members.

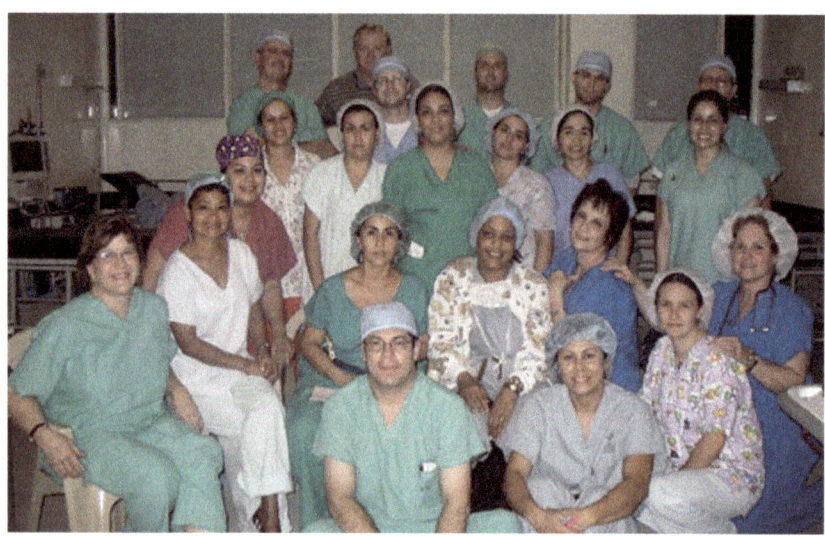

2008 Armenia Colombia

2008 Dr. Rafi Bidros, and Dr. John Nguyen senior plastic surgery residents

Below the team was pictured together with patients and families in Armenia Columbia in 2008

The Healing Mission of Plastic Surgery

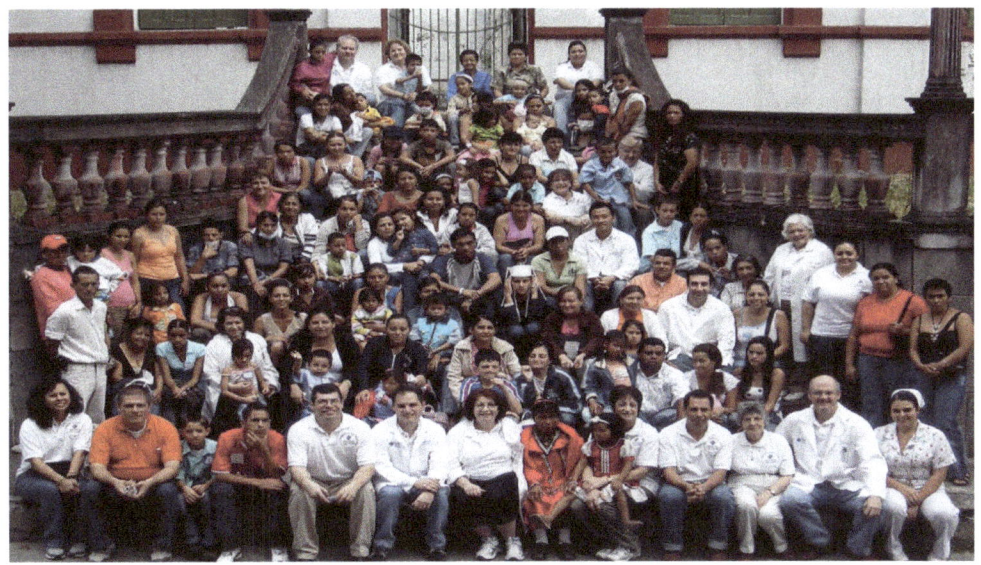

Below, Dr. Donna Fox, speech pathologist, and Graciella Angarita pose with our security team in Armenia. On the right, Dr. Bruce smith and Cindy Jones RN with patients.

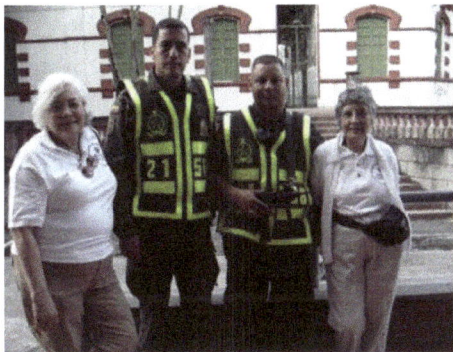
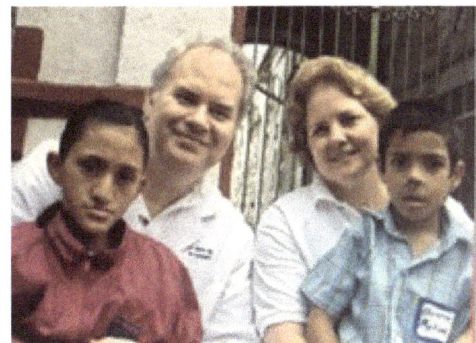

2009 Villahermosa Mexico

2009 Dr. Mike Lypka, and Dr. Mort Rizvi senior plastic surgery residents

Below is a picture of the team and patients in Villahermosa, Mexico, 2009.

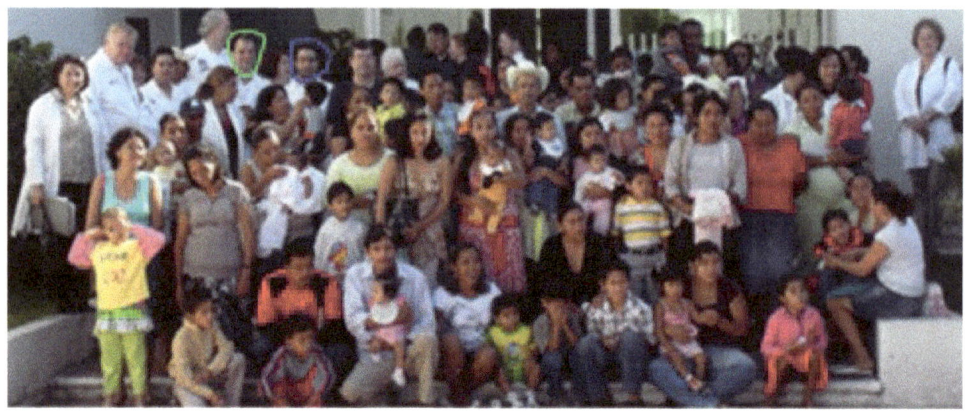

Below, anesthesiologist Mark Hancock and Juan Cano RN prepare for surgery. On the left, Ginger Hancock, RN assists at the operation.

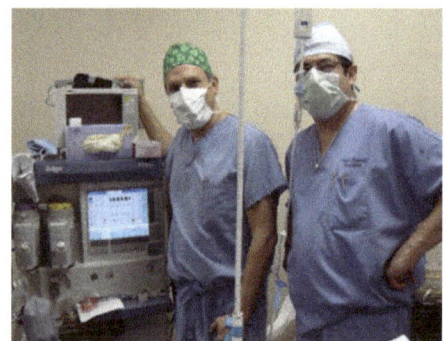 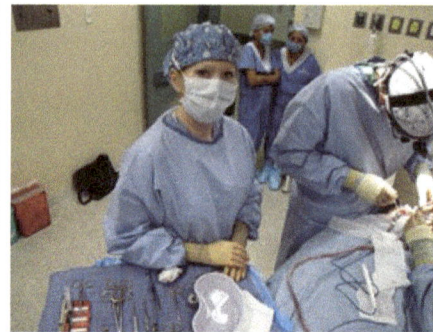

Santa Cruz del Quiche Guatemala 2011

2011 Dr. Alex Colque, and Dr. Peter Fakhre senior plastic surgery residents

Below is a photo of the OSJ team in Guatemala at the start of our program. On the right, a post-op patient is checked the day after surgery in the hospital.

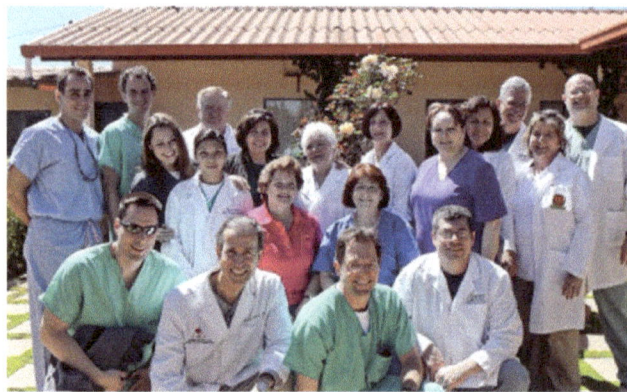 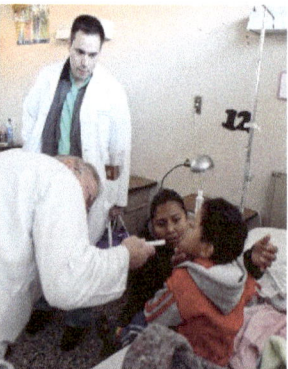

Below, patients have returned on the last day for a follow-up check. Afterward, we took a group picture of both the team and patient families.

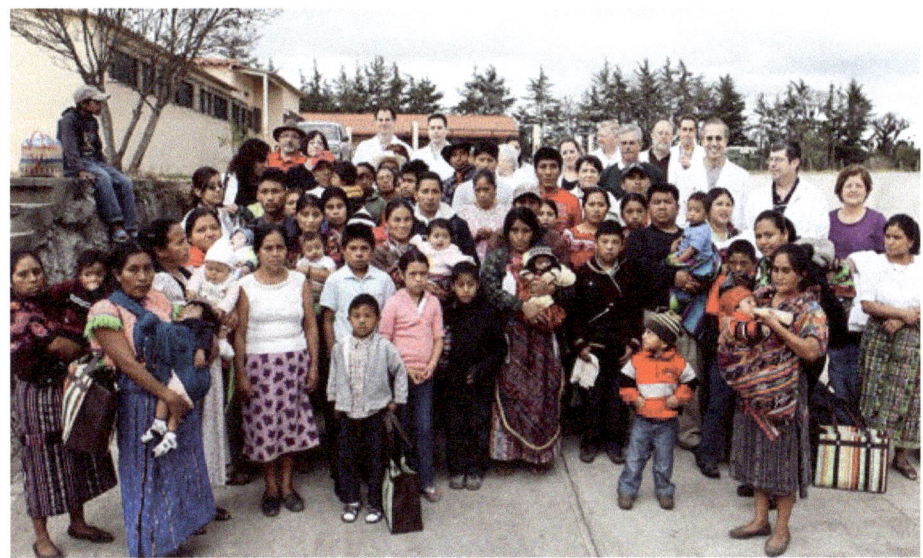

2012 Guayaquil Ecuador

2012 Dr. Colin Failey, and Dr. Ankor Meta (UTMB) senior plastic surgery residents

Below, Operation San Jose team members and patients in Guayaquil Ecuador at the end of our week of surgery. Below that, Dr. Failey and Janine Dubcak admire a post-op patient. Then the two happy plastic surgery residents Drs. Meta and Failey.

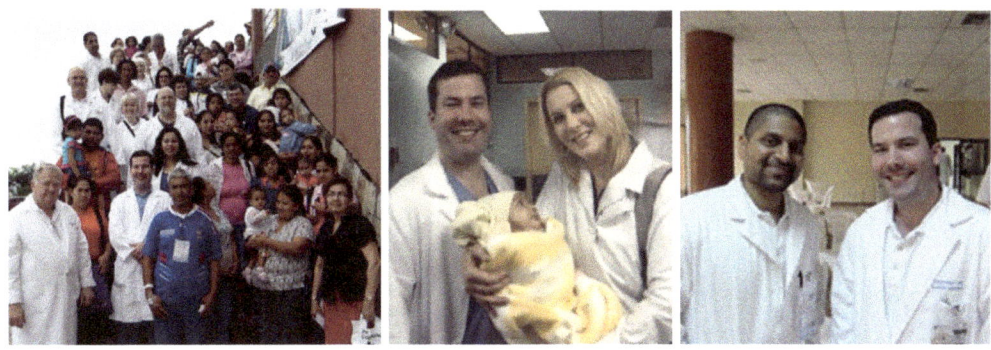

2014 Armenia Colombia

2014 Dr. John McFate, and Dr. Kyle Shaddix senior plastic surgery residents

Below are pictured Operation San Jose team members and patients in Armenia Columbia 2014.

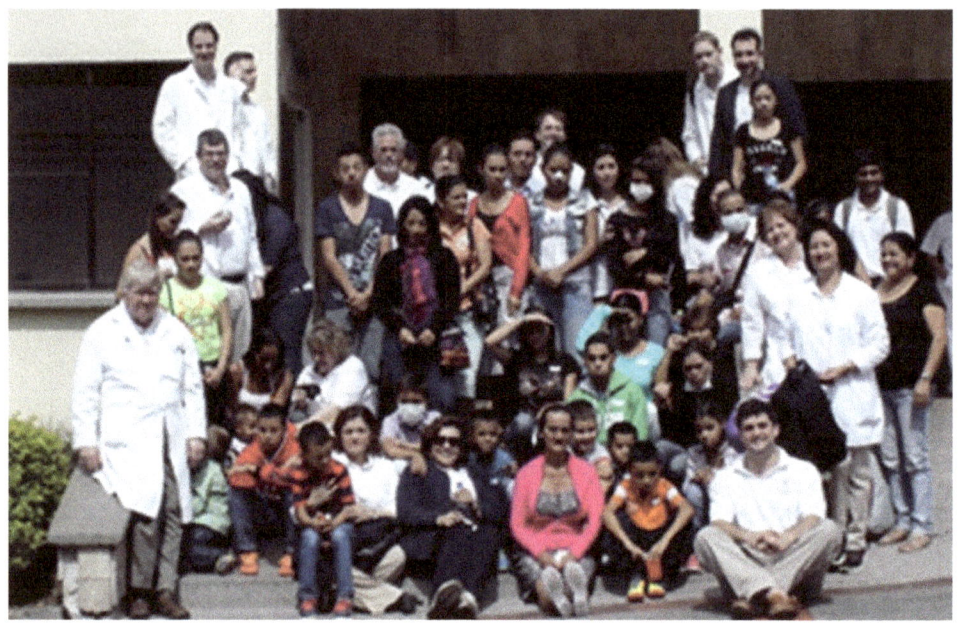

Below, Dr. Mc Fate with a patient. On the right Drs Bidros, Lypka, and next to far-right Dr. Shaddix.

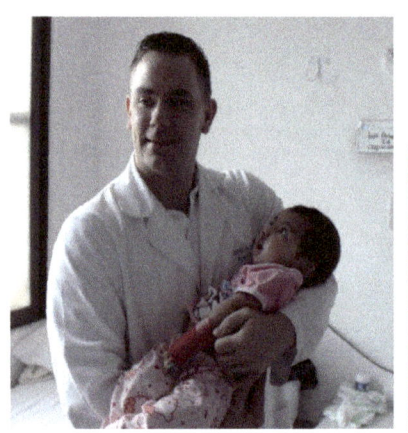
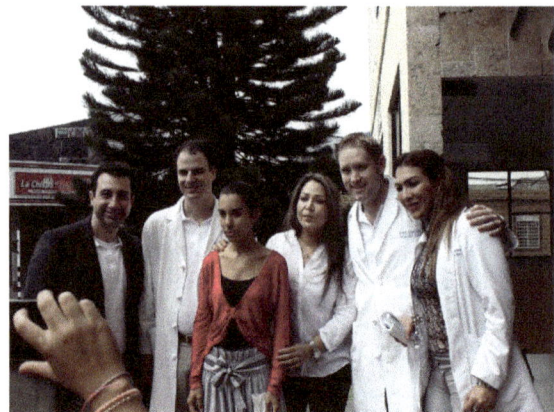

2015 Chihuahua, Mexico

2015 Dr. Hector Salazar-Reyes, and Dr. Sarosh Zafar senior plastic surgery residents

The team is shown below before starting our surgical program in Chihuahua, my last OSJ trip.

The Healing Mission of Plastic Surgery

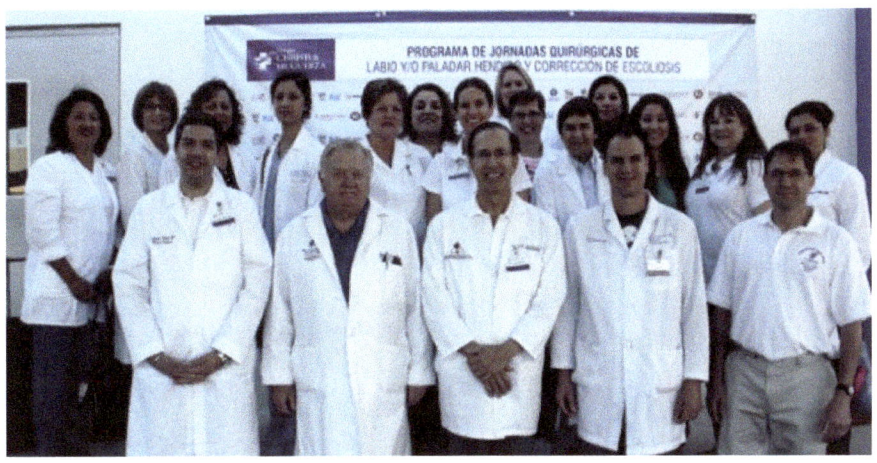

The following list shows sites served by Operation San Jose.

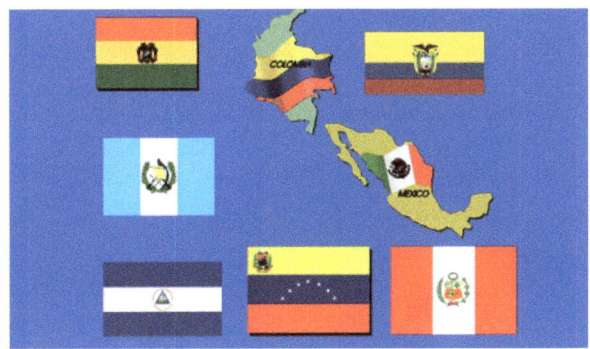

Tegucigalpa, Honduras 1983,1984,1985; Villahermosa, Mexico 1990,1991,1992,1999,2009; Caracas, Venezuela 1993; Leone, Nicaragua 1994; Arequipa, Peru 1995,1997,2000; Babahoyo, Ecuador 1996; Huancayo, Peru 1998; Mazatlan, Mexico 2001;Lima, Peru 2002; Chihuahua, Mexico 2003,2004,2015,2016; Sucre Bolivia 2005; Zihuatanejo, Mexico 2006; Armenia, Columbia 2007,2008;Santa Cruz, Guatemala 2011; Guayaquil, Ecuador 2012; Armenia, Colombia 2014; Chihuahua Mexico 2015; Chihuahua Mexico 2016; Puebla, Mexico 2017; Zacapu Michoacan, Mexico 2018. Monterey Mexico 2019

We have been very fortunate to have had excellent medical hosts on all our trips. Besides our first plastic surgeon host Cesar Enriquez M.D. in Tegucigalpa Honduras, we are especially indebted to Carlos Navarro M.D. and Alberto Bardales M.D. our Peruvian hosts for many visits, and Celia Carillo- Perez M.D., Villahermosa Mexico, who also graciously hosted us for several visits. Other plastic surgeon hosts included José Ortega Lara M. D. Caracas, Venezuela, Arturo Gomez M.D. Leon Nicaragua, Salvador Negrete M.D. Mazatlan Mexico, Dr Barrantes Zihuatanejo, Mexico, Guillermo Modesto M.D., Chihuahua Mexico, Zacarias Crespo M.D. Sucre Bolivia, and Nelson Estrella M. D. Ecuador.

Perhaps the most interesting area we have visited with Operation San Jose has been the Peruvian and Bolivian Andes. There we saw the most colorful native costumes, for example. Some of the patients and their families did not speak Spanish but only native languages. The mother below walked for days carrying "Roberto" from a remote village in the Andes so that he could have his clefts repaired. The lady next to me in the middle picture below has a papoose with a baby on her back. The last lady is also similarly carrying a baby with a cleft problem for us to evaluate.

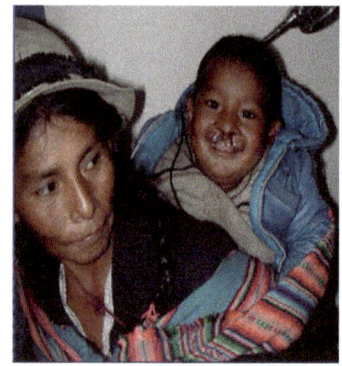 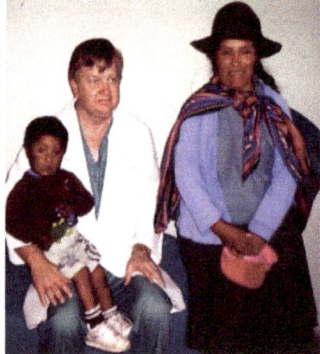 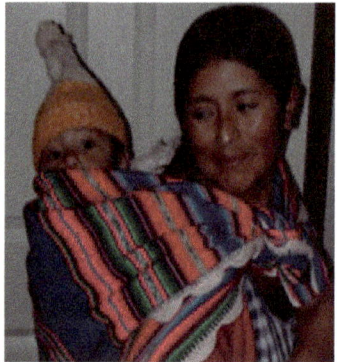

There are always interesting stories associated with each mission trip. In Honduras, in 1985, we examined three brothers, each of whom had a cleft lip and palate. The oldest brother had a complete double cleft of the lip and palate. The younger brothers each had complete unilateral clefts of the lip and palate but on the opposite sides. The boy's father brought them to the hospital from a great distance as they lived in a rural area in the mountains. Fortunately, we were able to operate on all three. The father was beside himself because he was so pleased, he was able to get help for his sons. Their preoperative and postoperative pictures are below.

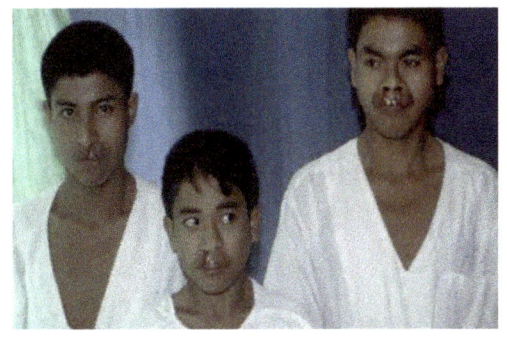 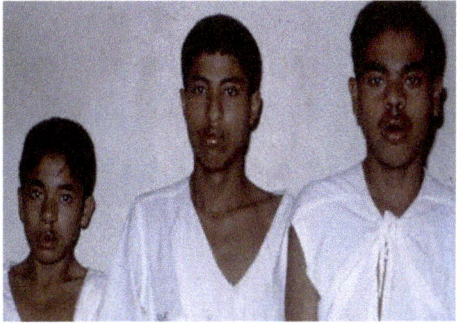

The picture below I took from the front seat of a bus we were riding in on a winding mountainous two-way highway just outside of Tegucigalpa, Honduras. As you might be able to tell, we are approaching a sharp right-hand turn in the road, but this did not deter the two large buses on the left and the Toyota truck from attempting to pass the three vehicles on the right in front of us. Luckily no crashes ensued. And I thought some drivers in Houston were reckless!

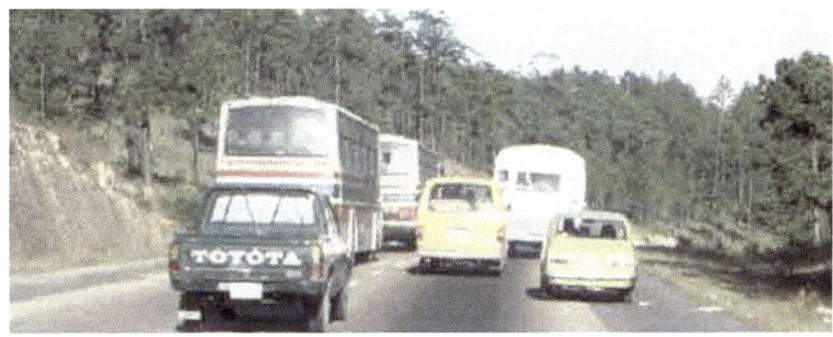

With one exception, the nursing and other hospital personnel have been very helpful and grateful for our efforts. Often a close relationship develops between the members of our team and the host participants. For example, there are often many hugs and tears when our group departs from the host hospital. The only exception was Venezuela in 1993, where there was some friction because the unionized hospital personnel was contemplating a strike. At that particular hospital in Caracas, the nurses were not very cooperative and seemed to be very passive-aggressive and would do whatever they could to thwart productive activity in the operating room. The doctors were accommodating. Because of their help, we were able to get a reasonable amount of work done.

On our 1994 trip to Nicaragua, we first spent a day in Managua, which had large destroyed and deserted areas residual from the massive earthquake of 1972. It seemed to me to be crying out for capital. We took a bus to Leon, where we were to have our program. On the way, we stopped in a remote area at a military checkpoint. An army officer wanted the bus driver to pay a fee to continue. At that time, Dr. Amado Ruiz, a native of Mexico, was our logistics coordinator. When talking with the military officer, all of a sudden, there was a burst of automatic gunfire. One of the soldiers was showing off and shooting into the air.

We were a little uneased but not frightened. We paid the "highway fee" and were on our way in a few minutes. Leon was very different from Managua. It was a relatively clean colonial city with a lot of historical buildings. We stayed at the old hotel shown below. It had no air conditioning but had a sizeable open-air courtyard or atrium with fans. Below, Dr. Ruiz is relaxing in the open-air lobby.

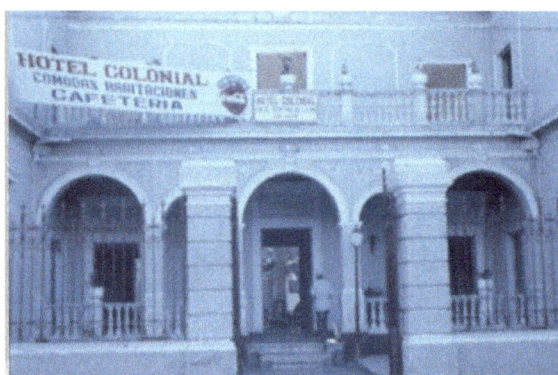
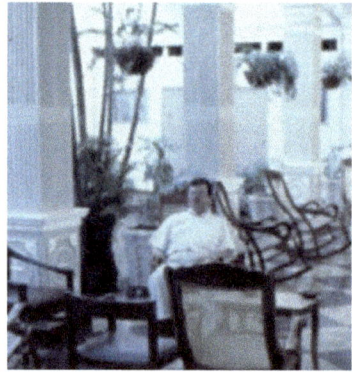

A particularly interesting case was that of a local priest who had a cleft of the lip and palate repaired in childhood. He had a prominent lip scar and residual speech problem with hypernasality. The speech problem caused him a lot of difficulties, especially when he was giving a formal sermon. I revised his lip scar and operated on his palate to try to correct the hypernasality and thereby improve his speech. Even one week after surgery, it seemed his speech was more intelligible.

The Healing Mission of Plastic Surgery

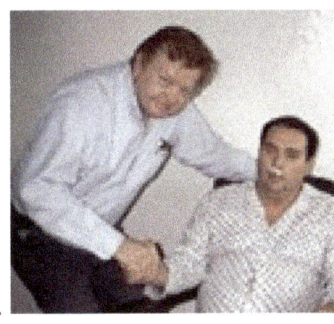

Our first trip to Peru was in 1995 to the city of Arequipa. When we arrived at the clinic where we were to work, the patients were lined up in the halls and cheered and gave us big applause as the team exited the bus and entered the clinic. However, when we checked out the operating room, we had to find a new home for the dog who was living in that space. Below, anesthesiologist Dr. Robert Kavanagh, who helped on several OSJ mission trips, checks out the newer of two anesthesia machines in the Arequipa clinic. Below, Marvin Zindler, Anthony Lucia, a volunteer and benefactor, Dr. Brauer, and Dr. Amado Ruiz discuss conditions.

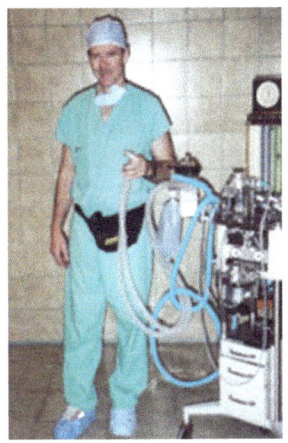 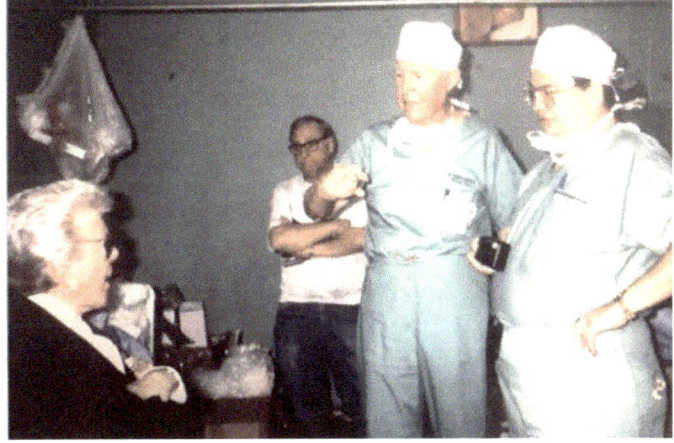

The following year the same clinic had three brand new operating rooms built with the help of a group of Peruvian - American surgeons from the USA. Peru was one of our most exciting destinations because of the cultural aspects of the native population. The oldest cleft lip patient we repaired was a 60 something-year-old lady, "Quesha," shown below with Dr. Brauer and me. After her surgery, there was no space for her to stay overnight, but Marvin Zindler, who accompanied us to Arequipa, to report on our program, paid for her to stay overnight in a local motel. Marvin is on the right below with a younger patient.

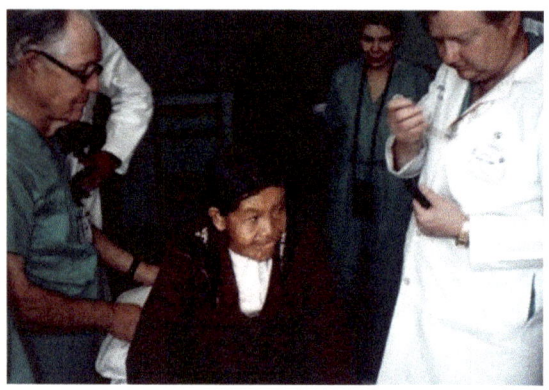 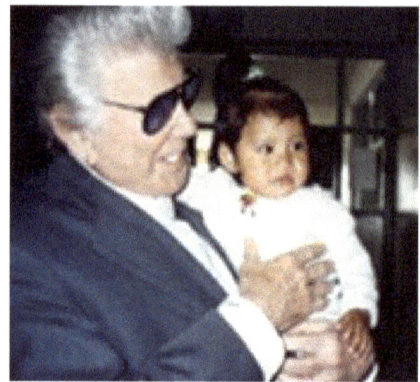

There is an inactive snow-covered volcano called El Misti visible from all parts of Arequipa. It showed no signs of erupting while we were there; however, we did experience a small earthquake while we were seeing patients in the clinic. It was a bizarre sensation to those of us from Houston who had never experienced such before. The locals did not think much of it at all as they frequently occur in Arequipa. There have been many highlights of these mission trips

In 1996 we visited Babahoyo, Ecuador, the smallest town we visited. About half the streets were unpaved. Our hotel was a little strange. The reception area was open to the road without any doors. After getting our keys, we had to go around on the street to another door to enter the hotel rooms. Another strange thing about this hotel was that it had showers with an electric water- heating device on the showerhead. That seemed ok until it seemed that turning on the hot water caused the lights to dim in the room. I took cold showers.

Our transportation from the hotel to the hospital was by a truck, as shown below. Fortunately, it was very close and only took a few minutes.

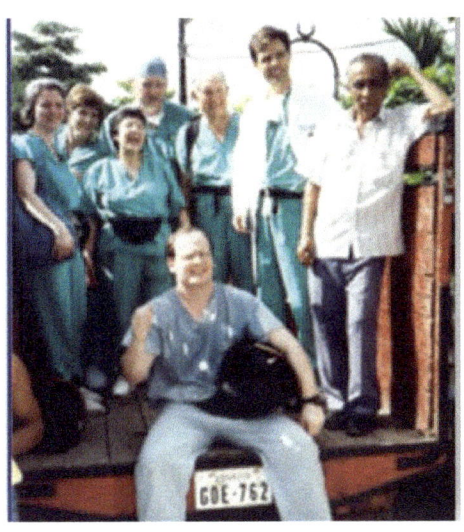

On first entering the hospital, another strange thing happened. We walked into a huge reception room filled with patients. We proceeded to an adjacent, much smaller room where we were to examine the patients. There were about six or seven of us trying to organize ourselves in that smaller ten by 12, foot room. Patients began coming into the room being pushed by those behind them. It was very chaotic for a few minutes. I began to scrutinize the only window in that room to be sure we could escape because I became seriously concerned that we could be crushed right there by the mass of people seeking help. Fortunately, we were able to remove some of the people and close the door temporarily and organized our clinic examination area. After we restored order, we began to see the patients one by one as usual.

Also, in Babahoyo, a grateful parent of a baby who received repair of a cleft lip gave one of our nurses a large paper sack. When she looked in, she found that the gift was a live chicken. I remember hearing from my parents that my grandfather, a general practice physician in Houston, would accept such offerings as payment for services during the great depression. Below are pictured plastic surgeon Dr. Jim Roesel and recovery room nurse Mary Ann Dougherty showing off that gift.

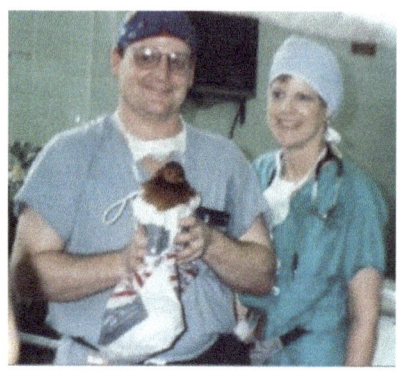

Conditions have been very different in the various hospitals and countries we visited. The most primitive hospital conditions were during our first trip to Peru, but later trips to that country, conditions were adequate. Honduras and Nicaragua generally seem to be the most impoverished countries at the time of our visits.

On one trip to Peru, we planned to operate in Huancayo, which was an eight- hour bus drive from Lima. The bus went over a pass in the Andes, which was 15,806 feet above sea level. Some of our team is pictured below as we stepped out of the bus at this high-altitude. We had oxygen available on our bus, and at that altitude, several of us needed to take advantage of this, as shown on the right below.

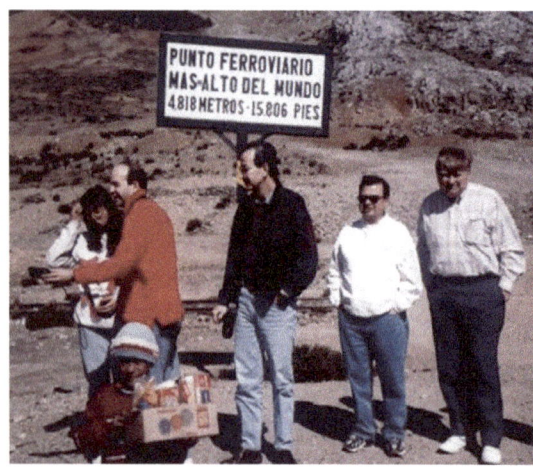 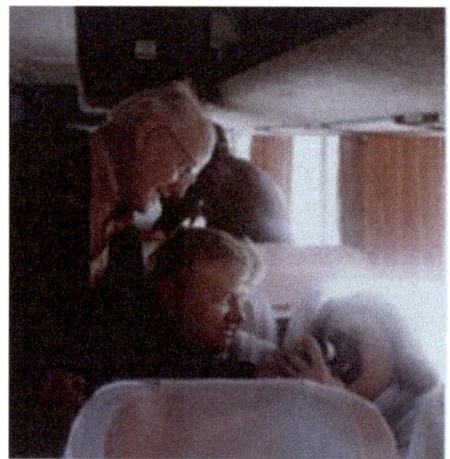

We then descended to Huancayo, which was only about 10,000 feet above sea level. No one had any additional trouble with the altitude there. One thing I noticed in Huancayo was that so many of the indigenous people, including the young children, had wind and or sunburned patches on their cheeks. For example, the mother and newly operated child below have rosy or brown cheeks.

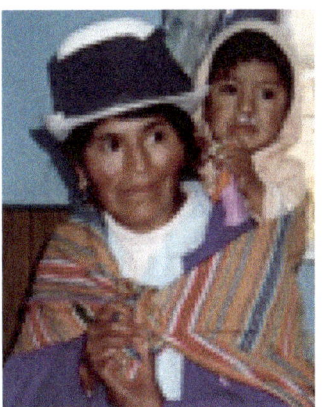

When we were preparing to return on the same highway to Lima after finishing, our program we heard that a day earlier, a bus full of passengers had gone off a cliff, and there were no survivors. We saw no evidence of that on our return.

In Colombia, there was a child whose parents wanted to give him up for adoption because he had a bilateral cleft lip and palate. The young parents had trouble bonding with the child because of the severe deformity. They already had one son about four years old who was healthy. Their social worker was able to convince them to bring the child to the hospital during our visit to see if we can help. The child was healthy despite having a complete cleft lip and palate on both sides. We explained that the deformity was substantially correctable, and they agreed to have us repair the double lip deformity. The surgery went well, and we fixed the lip. The parents were amazed and thrilled; they decided they wanted to keep "Alan."

Although we concentrate on only a lip and palate cases on our mission, we did have an unusual situation in Colombia that involved an injured 17-year-old girl. About three months before, her boyfriend brutally mauled her with a machete and left her for dead in a shallow grave. A passerby heard her cry and rescued her. She had a partially amputated left arm and a severely injured right-hand and prominently scars from lacerations on her face and body. She was mainly concerned with her inability to close her left eye because of the scar contracture. We performed procedures on the upper and lower eyelids, which immediately improved her ability to close her eye. She was quite pleased with the improvement and was understanding that we cannot do more with her scars because they were too immature.

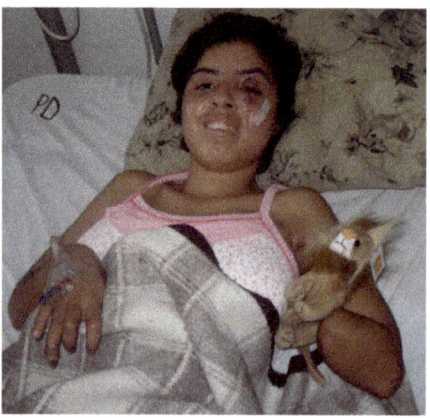

On more than one occasion, some of our equipment did not make it onto our plane. Sometimes as we looked out the airplane window, we could see several of our distinctive luggage cases did not make it on board.

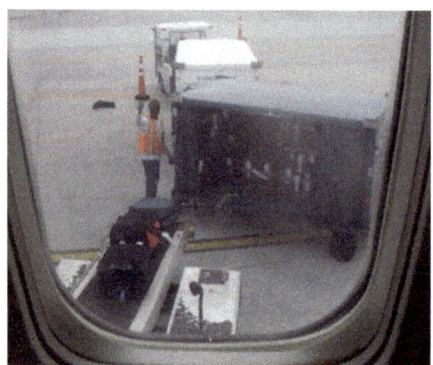

However, we always received our supplies in time the following day. Of course, this was stressful as we did not want to be unable to complete our mission. On our 1995 trip to Arequipa Peru, while we were transferring our luggage at the airport on the return in Lima, someone stole Bob Dows's expensive cameras. During our trip to Guatemala in 2011, one of our doctors decided to go for a jog and found himself in a rough neighborhood, where ruffians robbed him of his cell phone. He was upset but unhurt.

On several occasions, we received some local news coverage in the host country. OSJ had several local newspaper articles written about it. We participated in a couple of local TV programs and had some radio announcements of our mission and its schedule.

At the end of our 2012 trip to Guayaquil Ecuador, we were given a dinner reception by the Rotary Club of Guayaquil. They provided all the team members with locally made "Panama" hats, which are a symbol of Ecuador. We are proudly wearing the hats below.

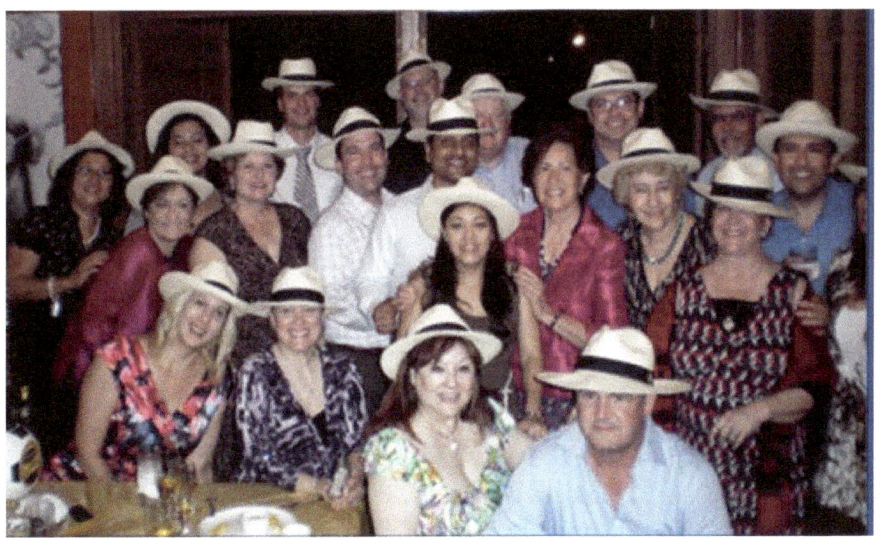

I would like to recognize and list all the participants in operation San Jose from 1983 to 2015, which was the last mission trip that I led. I apologize to any volunteers I have failed to acknowledge.

Operation San Jose participants as of 2015

Faculty plastic surgeons

Alfonso Barrera M.D., Rafi Bidros M.D., James Boynton M.D., Raymond O Brauer M.D., David A Bray Jr, M.D., Benjamin E Cohen M.D., Ernest D Cronin M.D., Thomas D Cronin M.D., David H Harley M.D., Mark A. Jabor M.D., Leo Laporte Jr M.D., Michael A. Lipka M.D., Henry A Mintz

III M.D., Phi P. Nguyen M.D., James M. Platis M.D., James F. Roesel M.D., Amado Ruiz-Razura M.D., Bruce K. Smith M.D., Robert L, Steely M.D.

Faculty anesthesiologists

Yvonne Cormier, M.D., Mark Hancock, M.D., Tim Heerensperger, M.D., Joseph Hornung, M.D., Robert Kavanaugh M.D., Anna Kutka M.D., Linda G.S.Magill M.D., Paul Sobiesk M.D., James Strohmeyer M.D., Than Tu M.D.

Faculty pediatricians

José Jesus Diaz M.D., Stacy Gallas M.D., Denise Ortiz - Lao M.D., Cesar Para M.D., Martha Lozano M.D.

Surgical staff

Philip Adamczak CRNA, Graciela Angarita CORT, Juan A. Cano RN, Vicki Contreras CORT, Marisela S. Corpuz CORT, Julie Couvillon RN, Deborah Davis RN, Juana Del Rio CORT, Mary Ann Dougherty RN, Rosalinda Elizalde CORT, Ruby Federico RN Ginger Hancock RN, Jane Holmes RN, Cynthia E Jones RN, John Kirkland RN, Elizavet Marquez CORT, Tina C. May RN, Betsabe Quezada CST, Maria T Salazar CST, Kathy Scrivner RN, Angie Silva CORT, Debbie Smith-Pierce RN, Bjorn M. Sundet RN, Teresa S. Torrance RN, Adriana Vides RN, Cora Wilson CRNA

Speech pathology

Donna Fox Ph.D., Branden Rabe CCC-SLP

Trip coordinators

Amado Ruiz M.D., Alma Lopez, Leticia Reyes Lopez, Veronica Cruz North, Elsa Olivera

Photographers

Jaclyn glaze, Isha E Lopez, Natalie B Shelton, Armando Federico

Volunteers

Fernando Barrera, Sylvia Brauer, Paola Chavarria-Lehman, Sarah Cohen, Claire Cormier-Thielke, Brendan Cronin, Kathleen Cronin, Alice Diaz, Bertha A. Diaz, Janine Dubcak, Jessica Edquist, Alma Lopez, Anthony Lucia, Natalie Magill, Donna Mc Dowell, Angel Jesus Parra, Jose Miguel Parra, Christy Raines, Narainsai K. Reddy, Brit Sobiesk, Susan Strohmeyer,.Andea Zararte Nikki Devine Zindler,

Senior plastic surgery resident participants

Scott Aaronson M.D., Ahmad H Ahmadi M.D., Alfonso Barrera M.D., Rafi S. Bidros M.D., James Boynton M.D., Gary S Branfman M.D., David A. Bray Jr M.D., Camille G. Cash M.D., Daniel Casso M. D., Michael Ciaravino M.D., Donnell R Collins Jr M.D., Alex P. Colque M.D., Richard DeSplinter M.D., Colin Failey M.D., G. Peter Fakhre M.D., Mennen T. Gallas M.D., Joseph L Haber M.D., David H. Harley M.D., David H. Humphreys M.D., Mark A. Jabor M.D., Robert C Kratschmer M.D., Leo Lapuerta Jr. M.D., Michael A. Lipka M.D., John McFate M.D. Henry A. Mentz M.D., Ankor Meta M. D., Eric Miles M.D., Clayton L. Moliver M.D., German Newell M.D., John T. Nguyen M.D., Phi Nguyen M. D., John J. O'Brien Jr. M.D., Christopher Patronella M.D., Virginia Pittman-Waller M.D., James M. Platis M.D., Francisco J. Rafols M.D., Lucian J. Rivela M.D., Murtaza Rizvi M.D., James F. Roesel M.D., Adam J. Rubenstein M.D., Hector Salazar -Reyes M. D. Kyle Shattix M.D., S. Ozan Sozer M.D., Bruce K. Smith M.D., Robert L Steely M.D., Charles Stewart M.D., W. John Suber Jr. M.D., Arvin Taneja M.D., Jonathan C. Weinrach M.D., Thomas C. Weiner M.D., Alfred Wilder M.D., Jeffrey L. Williams M.D., Robert Wright M. D. Sarosh Zafar, M. D.

Micro-surgical fellows

James Boynton M.D., J Timothy Katzen M.D., Christopher Livingston M.D., Kaiulani Morimoto M.D., Francisco J Rafols M.D., S. Ozan Sozer M.D., Thomas C. Weiner M.D.

Media representatives

KTRK TV channel 13(ABC News)

Bob Dows, Lori Rheingold, Marvin Zindler

KXLN TV channel 45 (Univision)

Maria Teresa Farfan, Edgard H. Hinojosa

KTMD TV channel 47 (Telemundo)

Claudia De Champs, Mauro L. Peña

Bob Dows, Lori Rheingold, and Marvin Zindler, pictured below, were particularly special people that we appreciated very much.

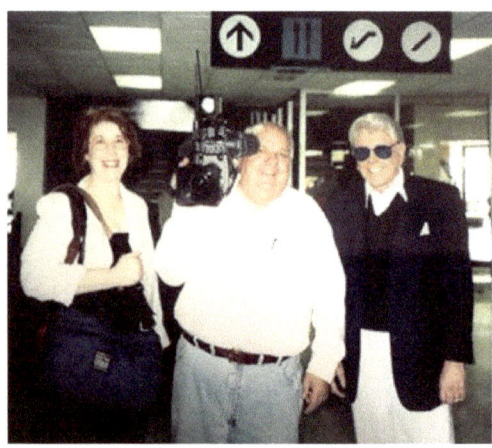 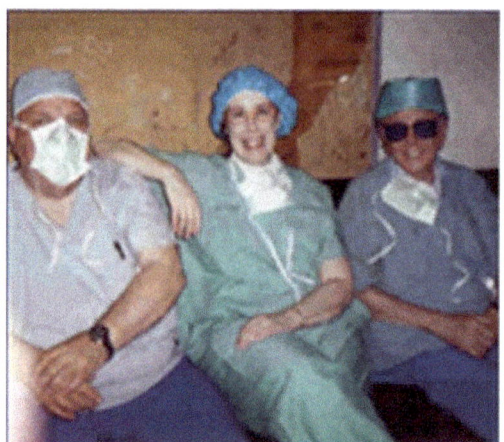

Marvin Zindler was a top-rated TV personality consumer advocate in Houston for many years. He obtained tremendous notoriety when he investigated the brothel "Chicken Ranch" in La Grange, Texas. This confrontation led to the famous stage play the Best Little Whorehouse in Texas. I'm very grateful for his support. Marvin gave the program significant positive publicity on his Channel 13 news program.

I remember distinctly at the end of the first trip we made to Arequipa Peru; while we were getting ready to take our transportation to the airport, he pulled Dr. Amado Ruiz and me aside. Then he said that, after first-hand observation, he knew this organization was a worthy cause, and he wrote out a donation check to Operation San Jose. After the first trip to Arequipa Peru in 1995, he featured Operation San Jose on five consecutive shows entitled "The Mask of Arequipa."

His producer, Lori Rheingold and his photographer Bob Dows were great. The three of them were an informative and entertaining team. Although Marvin was the celebrity, he relied very much on his team. Lori Rheingold organized everything. She and Marvin would banter about anything. Usually, Lori would prevail, but occasionally Marvin would put his foot down and veto her suggestions. Bob Dows was a gentleman and a great cameraman. Below Marvin visits an orphanage in Arequipa, Peru.

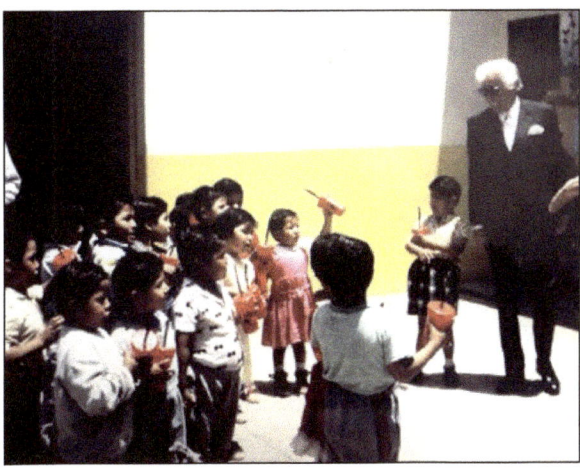

After my retirement in 2016, I enlisted the help of Mike Lypka, MD, who practices in Kansas City to take over running the program. He was one of my former residents and already a participant in the program. He has done an excellent job. He has enlisted the help of some of his colleagues in Kansas City, although most of the participants are still from the Houston area.

Operation San Jose continues to be an outreach program of the Christus Foundation for Health Care. (Houston). Private donor contributions to Operation San Jose through the Christus Foundation for Health Care to ensure the continued success of this project. We are particularly indebted to the Christus Foundation for HealthCare (formally, the St. Joseph Foundation) and the Dunn Foundation for support. Also, Mr. Anthony

The Healing Mission of Plastic Surgery

Lucia and Mr. Eugene Malloy, who gave seed money for specific funding of the Operation San Jose Project. Also, we are deeply appreciative of the generosity of Bob Devlin of American General Insurance Co., who was an influential early supporter of the program.

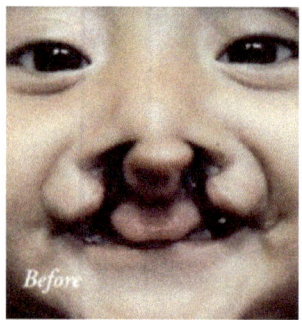
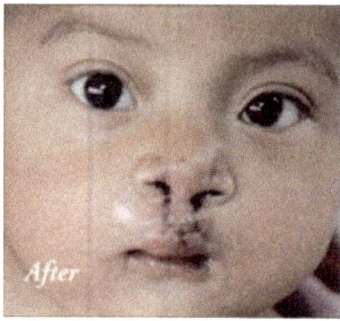

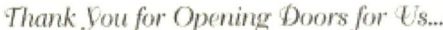
Thank You for Opening Doors for Us....

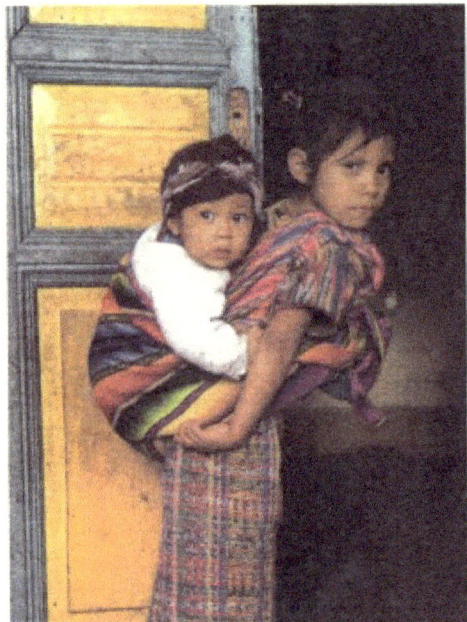
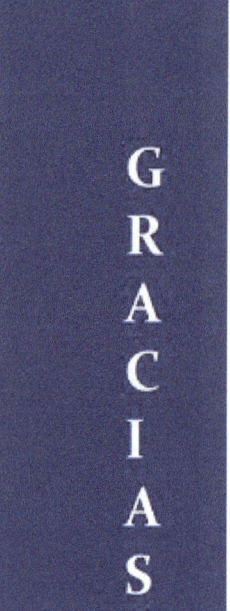

THANK YOU   GRACIAS

Chapter 12

Unusual Cases

I was seeing patients one afternoon in my office when a nurse came and said Dr. Thomas Cronin had a patient whom he would like for me to examine with him in another exam room. The patient was a young man who was an old patient of Dr. Thomas Cronin. We inspected his upper thighs and groin area. I could tell this patient's problem had required several complex surgeries. He previously had flap transfer of tissue locally in the area. I later learned this was for the closure of open, ulcerated wounds caused by radiation burns. He had done well for many years and was now returning for relatively minor scar build-up, causing tightness in the area.

Dr. Thomas Cronin did recommend and later performed a minor surgical revision for him. After the consultation, I learned the rest of the story. The boy's parents divorced when he was a child, and the boy would spend time with each parent as they had joint custody. Over several months he developed wounds in the groin area with no apparent reason. The mother took him to see many doctors, but no one could find the cause for the painful sores. Finally, his family doctor referred him to my uncle to see if he could do anything to heal the wounds, which persisted no matter what the previous doctors prescribed.

When Dr. Tom Cronin first saw these wounds in this little boy, he recognized the characteristics of radiation burns. There was no way the boy should come in contact with such radiation. Dr. Cronin notified the authorities who investigated the case. They discovered that the father had access to radiation pellets in his work. It turned out that the father placed these radioactive pellets near his son's groin while he was sleeping in bed. The father was later convicted for this mutilation of his son and sent to prison. Years later, I understand there was a movie about this case. It is challenging to comprehend how a father could commit such a premeditated assault

Unusual pressure sore

I discuss pressure sores or decubitus ulcers in some detail in chapter 14.

One unique patient developed bilateral ischial ulcerations because he was in a catatonic psychotic state. He sat without moving for hours on end. However, with the proper psychiatric medications, the patient's affect became normal; he "woke up" and began to interact socially and ambulate normally. I excised the wounds and repaired them with local rotation flaps. The patient readily healed and had no more difficulty in this regard. He presented an ideal circumstance for a favorable outcome in what usually are more difficult postoperative environments because his prescribed medicine cured the reason that he developed pressure sores.

Double lip deformity.

This patient presented with a deformity, which was somewhat minor but of considerable concern to the patient. On both the upper and lower lip, he had a redundancy of tissue, which he said made him look like he had double lips. Correction of this deformity was straight forward excisions, as outlined in blue ink on his mouth, and then tailoring of the residual lip tissue. I did his surgery as an office procedure under local anesthesia. The patient was quite pleased with the result and said he wished that he had known about the possibility of this surgery years ago.

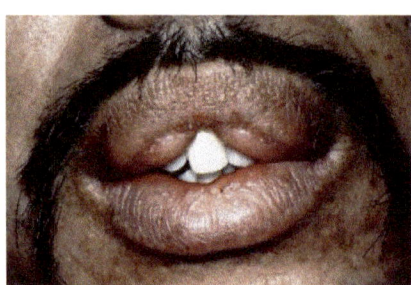 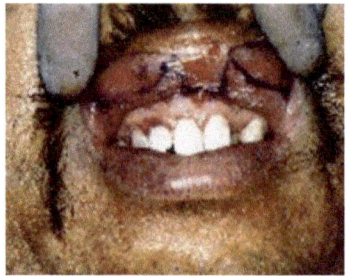

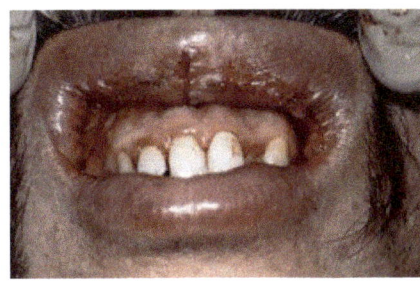 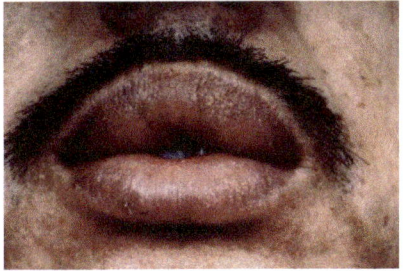

Leather Chest

"Dawn" was a 50-year-old lady who was in a category of our own. I received a call from an emergency-room doctor about 30 miles away. He said he had a patient with a unique problem of the chest, which involved significant infection and drainage. He said she would need substantial surgery and wanted to refer her to me.

"Dawn" apparently received injections of some liquid into the breasts more than 20 years ago in Japan. Over the past several years, she had suffered from multiple sores and draining areas in the breasts and chest wall. I never saw any breast injection injury as severe as this before or after. The entire anterior chest from the clavicles to just above the belly button was dark, almost black, and of a leathery consistency. The breasts were shriveled prunes. There were multiple areas of draining opens sores. I believe she had been quite miserable with this problem for many years. We admitted her to the hospital and began to administer intravenous antibiotics and local wound care to clean up the sores.

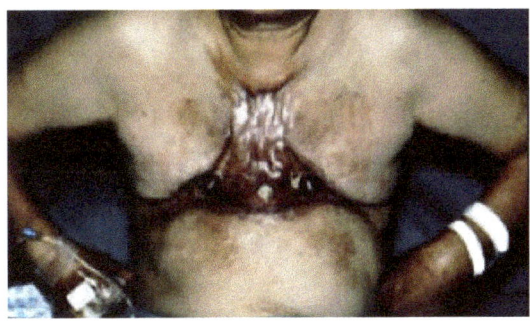 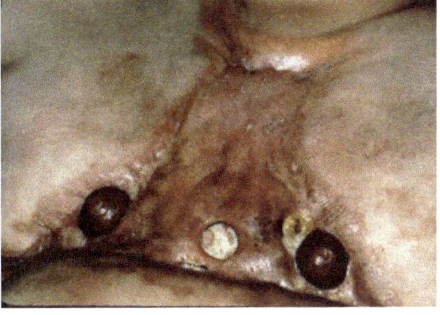

After a few days, I was ready to take her to the operating room. I removed the entire involved skin of the anterior chest wall, including the remnants of both breasts, as in the first photograph below. I performed a large rectus abdominis flap with both horizontal and vertical components. The primary blood supply was from the superior epigastric artery via the rectus abdominis muscle, as shown in the second two pictures below.

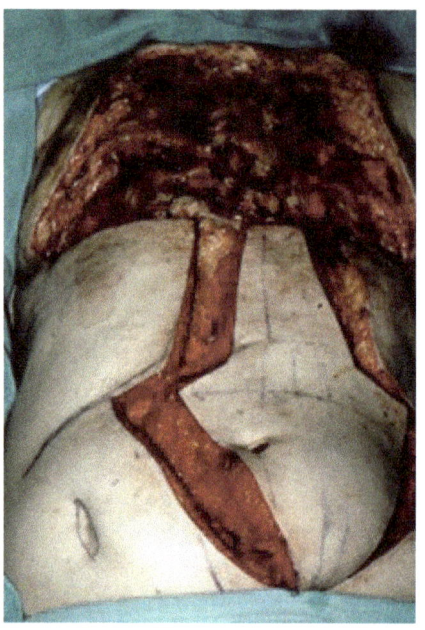

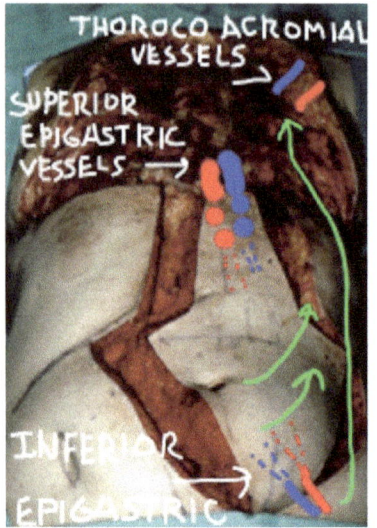
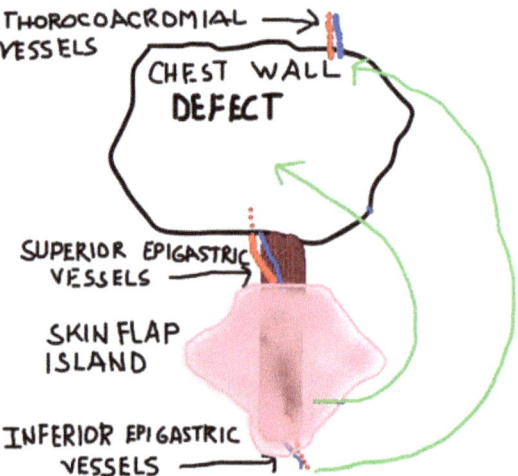

Because of the size of this flap, I "supercharged" it by connecting the inferior epigastric blood vessels from the flap (schematically represented by small red and blue lines at the inferior aspect of the flap), to recipient thoraco-acromial blood vessels in the left upper chest (also schematically represented by small red and blue lines). The thoracoacromial artery provided additional blood flow into the flap. The primary blood supply was coming through the rectus muscle from the superior epigastric vessels. I was barely able to close the flap under a little bit of tension.

This flap similar to the flaps we use for breast reconstruction. However, in this instance, we need a larger than standard flap to just replace the surface skin of the anterior chest without any attempt to reconstruct breasts. The post-op photo below shows I turned the flap 180 degrees to close the chest wall defect. This reorientation also facilitated the anastomoses of the inferior epigastric and the thoracoacromial vessels. The superior epigastric vessels remain intact as the primary blood supply.

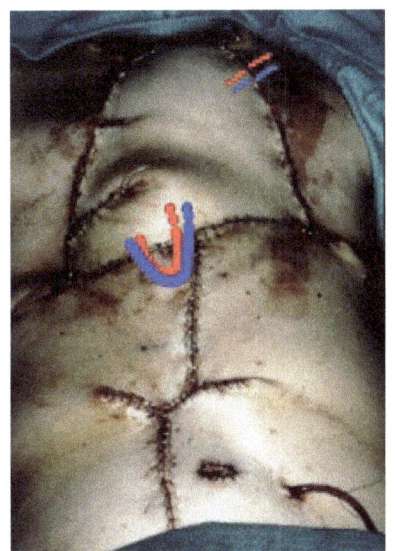
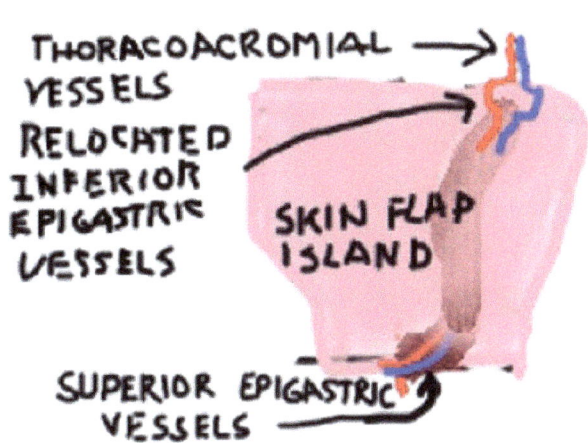

Fortunately, no infection ensued, and the wounds healed nicely. After about a week, she was able to return home more comfortable than she had been in years. I later discussed with her the possibility of building her breasts from flaps of tissue from the back, but she declined.

Factitious arm wound

A 20-year-old girl "Helen" came to the office because of an injury of the wrist, which she said occurred because she fell and scraped it against the sidewalk. It seemed like keeping the wound clean and applying some antibiotic ointment would be sufficient for its cure within two weeks. I rechecked her in two weeks, but the injury seemed to be even slightly more profound. On the other hand, there did not seem to be any abnormal drainage or infection. I made a slight change in the recommended regimen of local wound care and had her come back again and two weeks.

At that time, the wound looked about this the same as it had on the previous visit. I questioned "Helen" about the care, and she said she'd been doing just as we told her. Although the patient was utterly oriented, quite normal in appearance and speech, she did seem a little high strung and fidgety. On a hunch, I decided to treat her not with just a small dressing on the wound but with a bulky dressing and a plaster cast covering her hand and forearm. I left the cast in place for 3 ½ weeks. When I removed the cast, I saw a completely healed wound!

She never admitted fiddling with the injury, but I think that it had not improved on its own previously because she had picked at the wound either consciously or subconsciously. I occasionally dealt with such factitious wounds. Usually, they were in patients who received a secondary benefit from not being well. They may have been able to not go to work or may have received sympathy for their problem.

Foreign body

One afternoon during my E N T residency, I was in the clinic seeing patients. A mother brought in a four-year-old child who was complaining of pain in the left ear. On inspection of the ear, something was blocking the canal. I used a small ear forceps to remove the obstruction. The foreign body appeared to be a decaying bean. Everyone was relieved when we found out what the problem was. It is quite common for small children to put small foreign bodies in various orifices. In this case, it just so happened as I completed the examination looking in the right nostril. I saw a little red plastic disk. I said to the mother, you might be interested in this also, as I pull the tiddlywink out with a small pair of forceps. This occasion was the only instance I removed two dissimilar foreign bodies from two orifices in the same patient. I have removed small plastic beads from the ear, insects from the ear canal, coins from the esophagus, a fishbone stuck in a tonsil, etc.

Neurofibromatosis

The photo below shows a typical presentation of multiple soft, fleshy growths along small nerves on a patient's trunk. I have seen several patients with similar or lesser involvement. I have sometimes removed bothersome lesions, but there is no cure for this disease. "Rebeca" was a young woman with neurofibromatosis type I, commonly known as von Recklinghausen disease. It is genetic and occurs in about 1: 3000 births.

Sometimes the tumors can be malignant. Besides several similar tumors like the ones in the first photo, "Rebecca" also severe manifestations because of intracranial tumors, which also distorted her forehead and pushed the left eye downward and forward. Because of erosion into bone, her eye throbbed with her heartbeat. Her intracranial tumors were considered inoperable from a neurosurgery standpoint. I operated on her a few times, debulking the large neurofibroma of the forehead and orbit to try to improve the contour of her forehead and the position of her eyelids, knowing that these interventions would only provide her limited benefit.

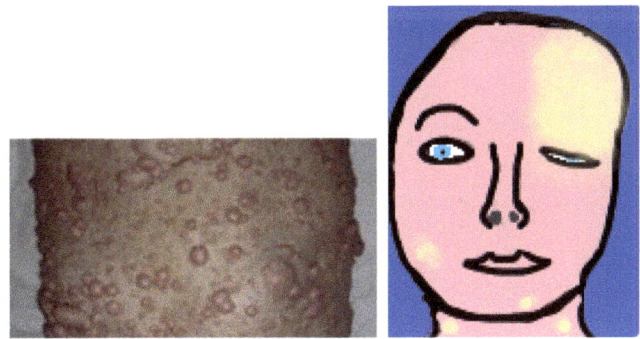

Medicine ball leg

A quite unusual case presented to me in my office one afternoon. "Barbara" was a middle-aged lady, overweight, although she had undergone a stomach bypass procedure. It seemed her upper body was not unusually large, but her hips and legs were quite large. The striking thing was the posterior aspect of the lower extremities. A large tissue mass each about the size of a medicine ball one might use in the gymnasium was present on either posterior thigh. It was amazing that she could walk at all. These masses certainly made it quite difficult for her to get around. The cause of these masses related mainly to her obesity and to abnormalities in lymphatic drainage from her lower extremities. She told us that previously a surgeon had attempted removal of the masses but abandoned the procedure because of bleeding from large veins in the tissue. Her pre-operative photos are below, right lateral, left lateral, posterior, and anterior views.

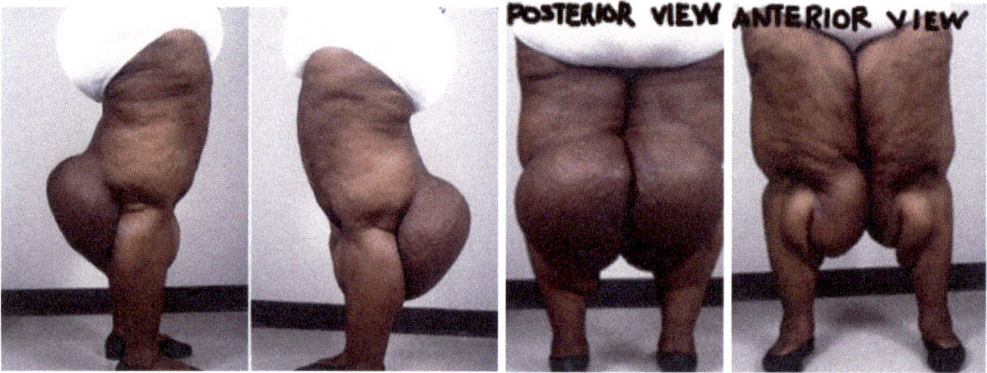

The photos below were taken in the operating room immediately before the excisions.

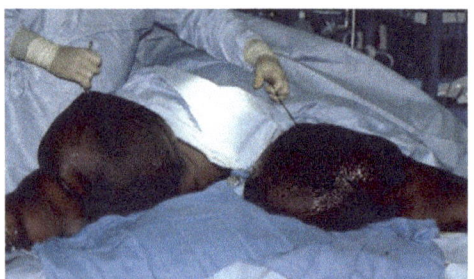
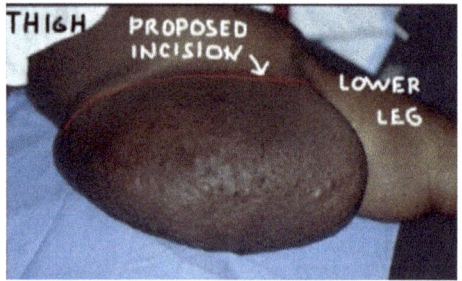

I removed these bulky masses taking great care to limit the blood loss from the dilated veins, several of which had diameters as large as a finger. All of the tissue was read by the pathologist as benign, with some dilated lymphatics and large varicose veins. As might be expected, she had persistent swelling for a long time, and she did have some minor delay in the healing of the wounds. She went on to heal entirely and was much improved, as can be seen from the postoperative photographs below.

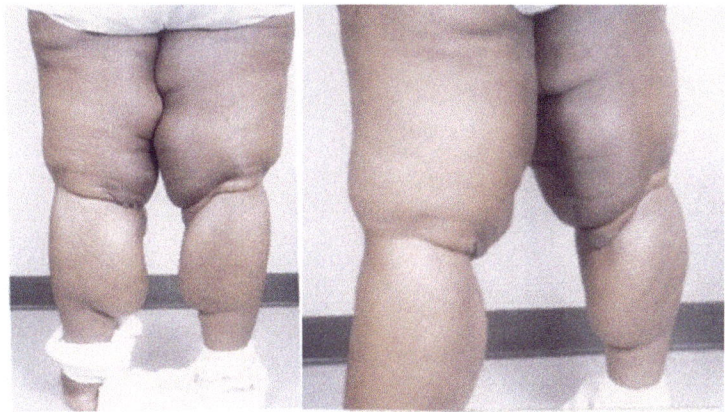

Strange scalp lesion

An elderly patient came to see me, brought by her daughter, who had noticed a large lesion on her scalp. I thought this was probably skin cancer either a squamous cell carcinoma or a basal cell carcinoma or perhaps even a keratoacanthoma. A keratoacanthoma is a skin lesion that often has a significant amount of dry skin and keratin built up to create a mass. These can be confusing for pathologists to differentiate from squamous cell carcinoma.

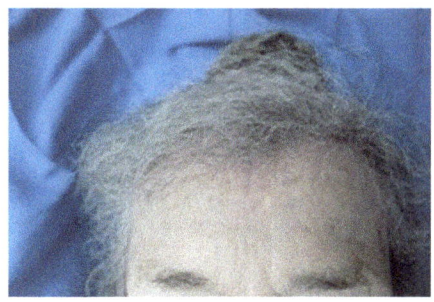
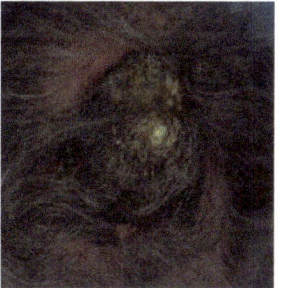

Because she was easily agitated, I took her to the operating room to further evaluate the lesion and obtain biopsies. I easily scraped off a large mass of keratin from the surface of the scalp, as shown in the photos below.

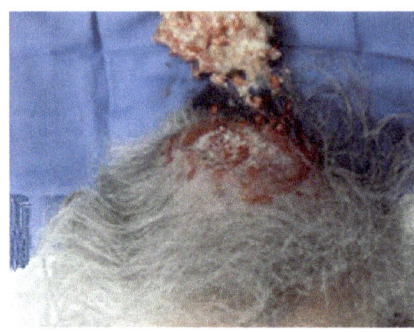

At this point, I thought she had a squamous cell carcinoma. However, rather than excising the entire lesion, which was a significant part of the scalp, I did multiple biopsies of the area. To my surprise, no severe pathology was evident from the frozen section microscopic examination, so I was happy that I had not excised the whole thing. I, therefore, "scraped off" the lesion in its entirety. It was apparently an area of neglected severe seborrheic dermatitis. The final photo shows the healing scalp three weeks later.

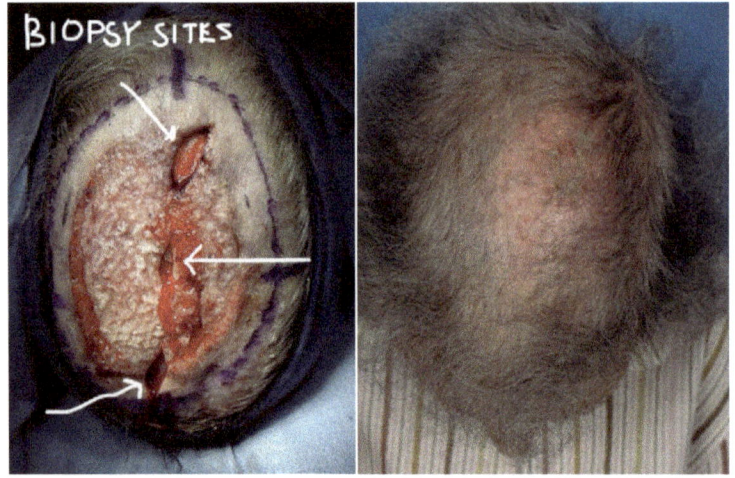

IV infiltrate

"Dante" was a premature infant in the neonatal intensive care unit who suffered a devastating IV infiltration injury to the left lower leg. This type of injury was once common in Neonatal ICUs but has become less so as more "central lines" have made it possible to avoid small veins in these infants' tiny extremities. In Dante's case, the infiltrate was caustic. It caused circumferential necrosis of the skin of the lower leg from the ankle almost up to the knee. I had to excise all that dead tissue.

Then I needed a skin graft for replacement. In a tiny infant like this, blood loss needed to be minimal. Harvesting a sizeable split-thickness skin graft would have resulted in significant bleeding. Therefore, I devised a technique to take full-thickness skin (FTSG) from the abdomen. A full-thickness skin graft would also be less likely to contract and scar than a split-thickness graft. I pinched together the needed abdominal skin and sutured what would become the edge of the excision after removal of the full-thickness skin. I did this before taking the graft! The pre-suturing eliminated all the loss of blood that would've taken place if I had excised the skin before suturing it together. I diagrammatically show the procedure in the drawing below.

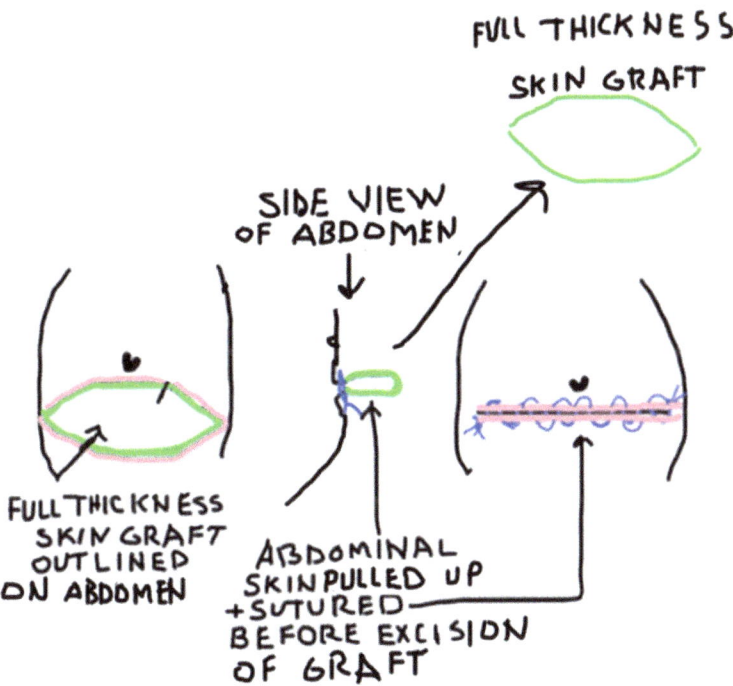

I placed the full-thickness skin graft circumferentially on the raw surface I had created by excision of the dead skin of the lower leg. Fortunately, the FTSG took 100%, as shown in the second picture below. Notice the small size of the leg as compared to the adult fingers holding the leg. The final picture shows the grafted leg healed several months later.

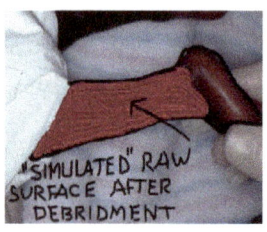 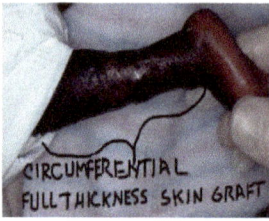 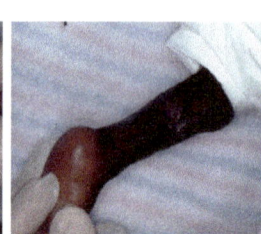 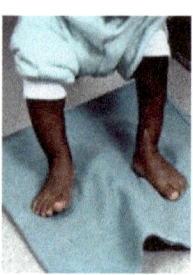

Fibular free flap jaw reconstruction

One particularly stressful case was that of an elderly gentleman "Frank" with a large cancerous tumor of the lower jaw and floor of the mouth under the tongue. He had multiple medical problems, such as partial renal failure, hypertension, and cardiac disease. I was asked by another surgeon to see this patient in consultation regarding facial reconstruction. I was happy to see him. He was an older veteran who had developed a large tumor of the jaw over several months, which was beginning to protrude from the gum.

The tumor extended from the jaw to the floor of the mouth towards the underside of the tongue. The visible cancer was about the size of a large plum. Commonly, tumors in the mouth of this size would have already spread to regional lymph nodes and perhaps would have already metastasized to distant areas of the body. However, "Frank" had no evidence of spread to the neck or symptoms of distant spread. Therefore, although he was an older man with medical issues, it seemed reasonable to approach his tumor aggressively by surgical excision and reconstruction of the defect. After consideration of various types of restorations, I decided on a fibula free flap reconstruction which involved taking a large portion of the fibula, (the smaller of the two long bones in the lower leg), together with a contiguous large ellipse of skin, and a small portion of a muscle.

After considerable pre-operative planning, the day of his surgery arrived. Instead of the usual 30 minutes needed to prepare the patient and put him to sleep before beginning the surgical incision, this case took us an hour and a half to place all the intravenous lines and prepare the multiple surgical sites. The head and neck surgeon and a resident began the ablative surgery in the neck by elevating a large skin flap to expose the jaw and the tumor (red). In anticipation of an extensive mandible resection, they bent a long, sturdy stainless- steel plate so that it conformed to the jaw. They drilled several holes to temporarily fasten the plate on either side of the planned resection of the jaw and then removed it from the mandible and sterilized for later use. The surgical resection of the large tumor of the mandible and lymph nodes on both sides of the neck proceeded.

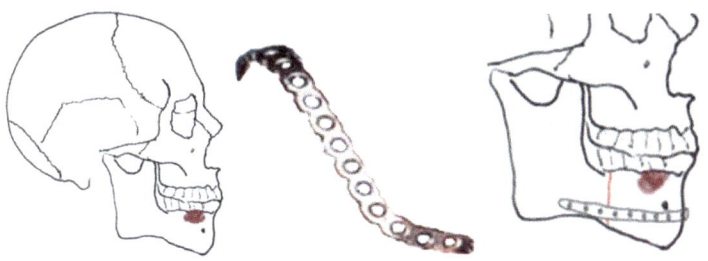

The anterior jaw resection can result in the potentially horrendous Andy Gump type deformity demonstrated below.

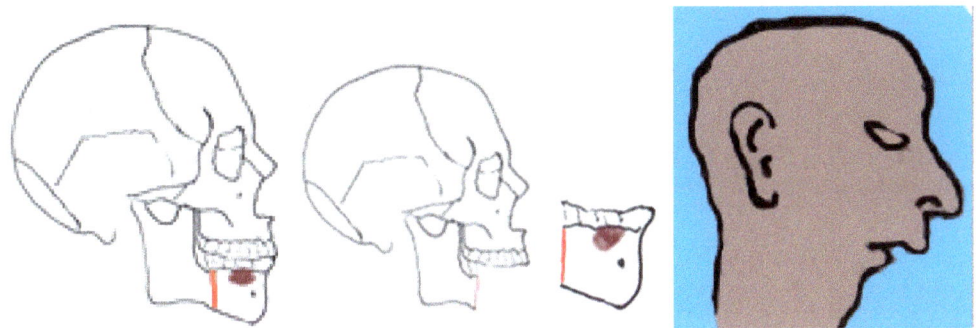

Simultaneously my resident and I began working on the patient's lower leg. I marked out a large ellipse of skin in the proper portion of the calf using anatomic landmarks. I identified and preserved the peroneal blood vessels to this tissue so that they could later be connected to large blood vessels in the neck to resupply blood to this composite graft of bone muscle and skin.

The dissection of this flap from the lower leg is quite tedious. After we dissected the skin, subcutaneous fatty tissue, and a portion of muscle surrounding the fibula, it was time to saw through the fibula. A significant length of fibula more than 20 cm was cut free on either end. We identified the artery and veins carrying the blood supply to this tissue. The vessels were made ready for later use.

The pre-shaped stainless- steel mandibular plate was then brought to the leg so that I could fashion the fibula to fit it. We needed to make several additional cuts through the fibula so that I could curve the bone to fit against the plate to mimic the shape of the excised mandible. It would have been easy to slip a little when cutting the bone and mess up the blood vessels, thereby making the whole reconstructive effort a failure. So that maneuver was quite stressful itself. Below left is a diagram of the fibular flap and its vascular pedicle. On the right is a drawing of the flap after shaping it to conform to the pre-bent plate and securing it with screws.

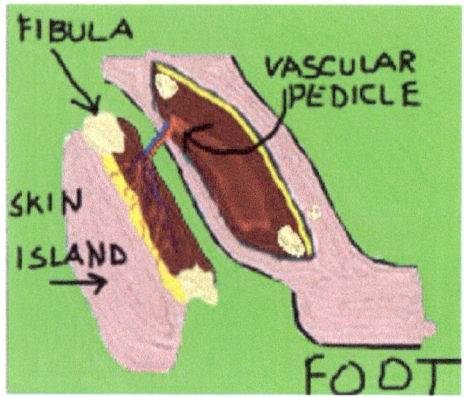
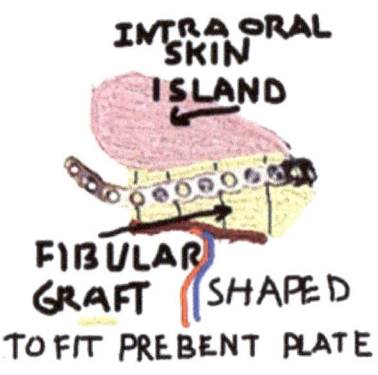

The stress continued when we were ready to transfer the tissue from the calf to the face. Once we disconnect the blood supply of the flap from the leg, we have a limited amount of time to reconnect the blood vessels, to restore the blood supply so that the tissue would live. This anastomosis process of sewing the vessels together seemed to go well in this case initially. However, after a few minutes, the blood flow stopped, so we cleaned out clots from the area and redid the anastomosis. It worked for a little while, but then the blood supply closed down again.

Therefore, we had to regroup, find some new, slightly larger vessels in the neck. We took down the first anastomosis and redirected the artery and vein of our flap all over again to different, marginally larger vessels we had prepared. All this is going on while the clock is ticking because we know we must reestablish the blood supply in short order, or the entire flap will die. This time, we restored the flow, and it remained functional. We were then able to suture the rest of the flap into position and close the wounds and complete the reconstruction as indicated by the drawings below.

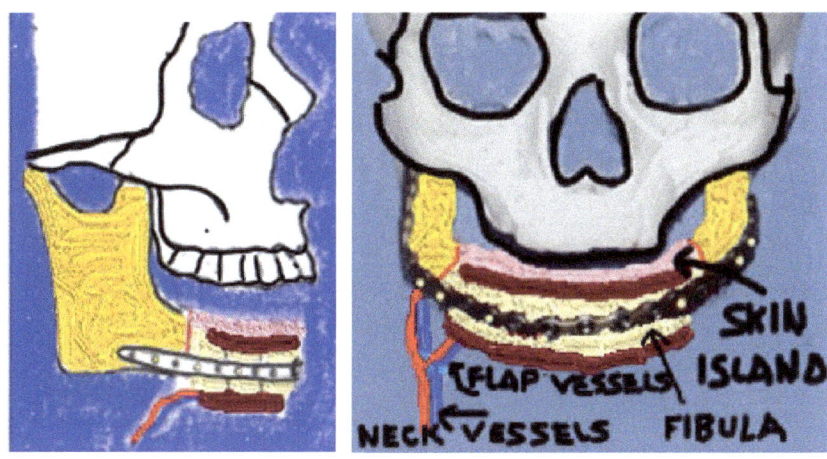

As I have described, it takes more than one individual surgeon, and in this case, preferably a two-team approach for the best expeditious care of the patient.

We did not complete the surgery until late in the evening. I remember not being able to sleep well that night, worrying about the patient. After completion of the operation, however, the stress does not end. If the vessels clogged within the first few days after surgery, we would lose the flap unless we re-operated and restored the blood flow.

In this particular case, the way we monitored the blood supply to the flap was by periodically sticking a needle in the skin portion. I specifically remember the morning following surgery going into the patient's room in the intensive care area with some apprehension as to how the flap would look. I was impressed that the contour of the jaw was almost like the preoperative state. However, when I inspected the skin of the flap in the mouth, it did not look perfect because it had some dried saliva and blood on the surface. I got a large needle and stuck the flap. I was extremely relieved when some red blood emerged from the site. Fortunately, throughout the post postoperative course, the blood flow was adequate, and the flap went on to heal uneventfully. The operation was a success! There are several other methods of monitoring such flaps continuously now. I regret that I have been unable to find

photographs documenting this surgery.

Shoulder Grooves

A pleasant middle-aged lady came in for a somewhat routine reduction mammaplasty consultation. She complained of common symptoms of back and neck pain. She also complained of deep shoulder grooves from her bra straps. Besides the reduction mammaplasty, she was extremely interested in trying to correct the appearance of the shoulder grooves. She said, "can you just but some tissue there." So, we talked about options for that. We decided that fat grafting by injection might be beneficial, especially if she were able to limit pressure to that area after her reduction mammaplasty.

I had never done fat grafting for that purpose. The initial results were fantastic. The patient also had a special pad that she placed on her bra strap to bridge the area to eliminate most of the pressure that otherwise would have been there. Of course, because breasts were smaller after the reduction mammaplasty, there was less pressure in the area postoperatively. The results were good several months later. It is usually helpful to listen to the patient as he or she might have some good ideas. I could not find her pictures.

Unusual otoplasty

I recall a unique case that was a self-performed otoplasty. An elderly gentleman came to see me and said that he had prominent ears and wanted to do something about it. However, as I looked at him, it seemed his ears were quite flat against the side of his head and not prominent at all. So, I asked him to him show me what he was interested in accomplishing. It was only then that he reached up and gently pulled his ears away from the side of his head. And they were prominent with lack of the anti-helical fold. He had been super gluing his ears to the side of his head for years. He had become quite adept at this. However, he was tired of this daily process of a self- performed otoplasty. I recall that I did operate on him, using sutures to define the anti-helical fold better and bring the ears closer to the side of the head.

Nasal Cleft

This child " Alfred" had a very unusual congenital deformity with multiple clefts of the nose without cleft lip. There is a cleft through the left nasal ala, another cleft with a significant absence of tissue at the base of the right nasal ala. "Alfred" was the only case even similar to this that I saw during my more than 40 years in medicine. Unlike cleft lips, there is no standard approach to a situation like this. I needed to customize his treatment. Using basic plastic surgery techniques, flap development, and rearrangement of tissue, I planned multiple small procedures for correction.

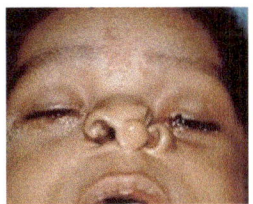 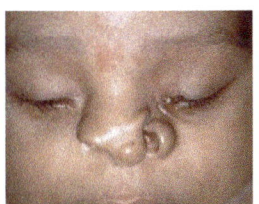 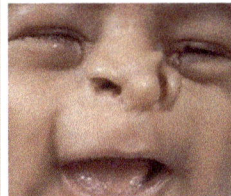 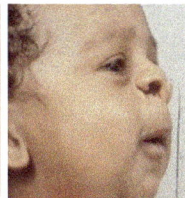

For example, the second and third photos below show the right ala freed by the red incision and brought inferiorly towards the lip to put it in a normal position while leaving a raw surface gape from where the ala came shown in the third picture. Tissue from the cheek is designated to fill the defect created above the ala by its rotation downward.

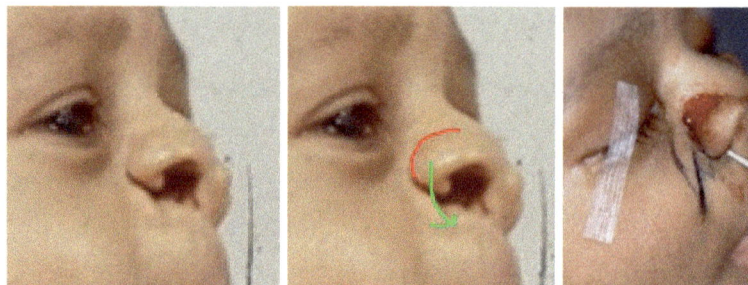

This procedure is an application of a very valuable and standard plastic surgery procedure known as a Z- plasty. In his case, I transposed the two flaps with one another. I gained tissue for vertical expansion while borrowing tissue and tightening laterally.

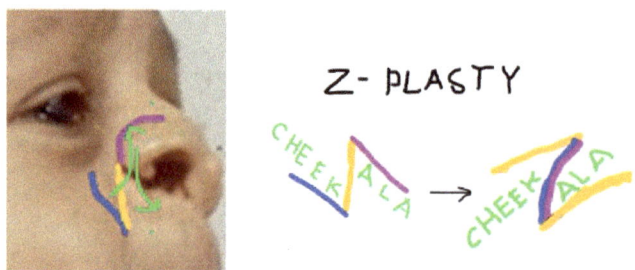

I performed four separate small procedures on this patient over a few years. The immediate intraoperative result and the result a few years later are shown below. When I last saw "Alfred," I was impressed that he was a well - adjusted, polite young man. I wish him the best.

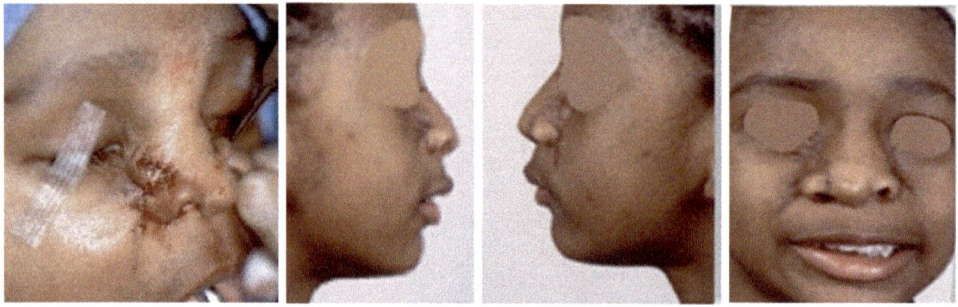

Pharyngeal stenosis

"Judy" was a 31-year-old schoolteacher referred to me by an ENT specialist. She complained of difficulty sleeping and hypo nasal speech because of scar tissue in the pharynx, stemming from a tonsillectomy at age 7. Examination of her mouth and throat showed an excess of scar tissue between the palate and the side and back walls of the pharynx. The opening from the oral pharynx to the nasal pharynx was only the size of a number two pencil eraser. Such a complication is rare from a childhood tonsillectomy alone. I have seen a few similar cases related to more extensive surgery done for sleep apnea, which included excision of a portion of the palate and the tonsils. That palatopharyngoplasty procedure often does help enlarge the airway and improve sleep for selected patients. However, if excessive scar tissue develops, it can cause a contracture that further constricts the airway, making the problem worse. Fortunately, this is unusual. The two drawings I made below show the scar tissue between the soft palate and the posterior pharyngeal wall, nearly obliterating the air passage between the oral and nasal pharynx.

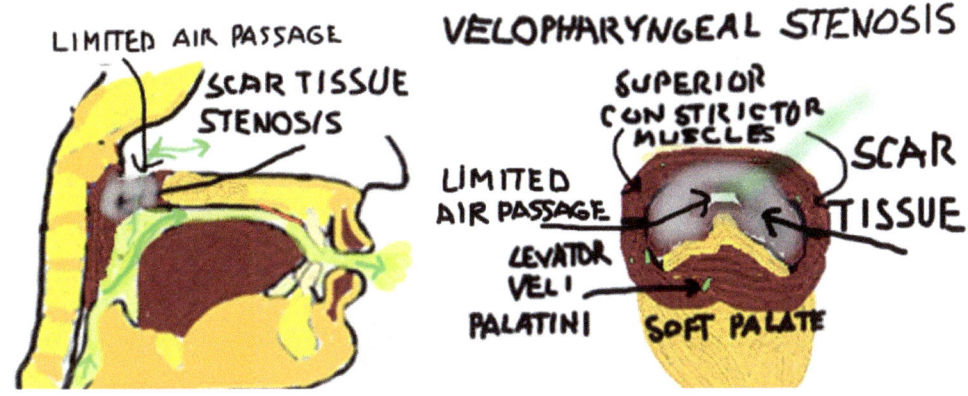

"Judy" was willing to have surgery to try to enlarge the opening to improve her breathing through her nose. This surgery involved making Z-plasties at the perimeter of the opening to widen the air passage, as shown below. I designed the closing incisions at right angles so that scar tissue shortening would discourage a circular constriction. She tolerated the surgery well and went home after an overnight hospital stay. I made the opening large because I knew there would be a tendency for some relapse of the scar contracture. A few weeks later, after healing was complete, she had improved. The opening was several times larger than the preoperative state, although not at all normal. Her speech was improved, although she still was not sleeping as well as she would like.

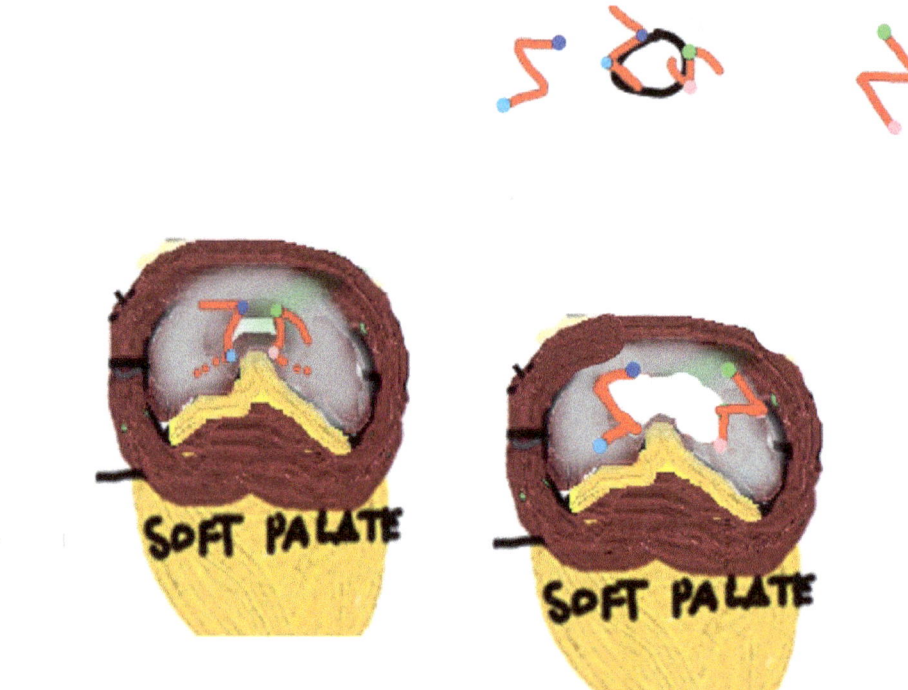

No Palate

Over the 38 years of my plastic surgery practice repairing cleft palates, one little girl's problem was unique. I believe "Shirley" was about four years old when her single mother brought her to me for a consultation. She had several other congenital problems, including significant deformities of the hands as well as an abnormal gait. "Shirley" had an enormous congenital palatal defect. She had an upper alveolar ridge but virtually no hard palate. There was residual soft palate tissue that was widely cleft. My drawings below illustrate her nearly absent hard palate and limited soft palate.

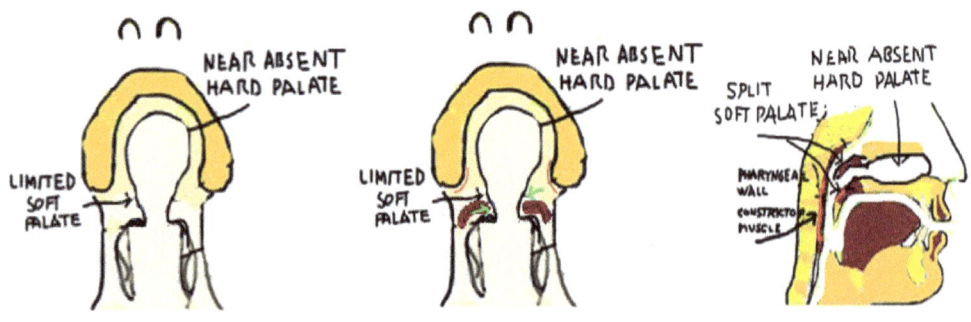

Her mother reported that another physician had taken her to surgery to repair the palate. However, he aborted the procedure when appreciating the full extent of the defect. Usually, the surgeon rearranges adjacent palate tissue to close closing the palate cleft. (see chapter 7). In this case, I needed to get additional flesh from other areas. Eventually, I was able to close her palate, but it took extraordinary procedures.

First, I did a soft palate only repair, hoping that this would allow for some stretching of the tissues, and perhaps the tension would narrow the cleft over a little time. I made relaxing incisions laterally(orange) to allow the soft palate to move to the midline for repair. The repair included the levator palatini muscle needed for speech. I illustrated this initial operation in the two drawings below. The patient photo below shows the massive defect of the palate residual after soft palate repair

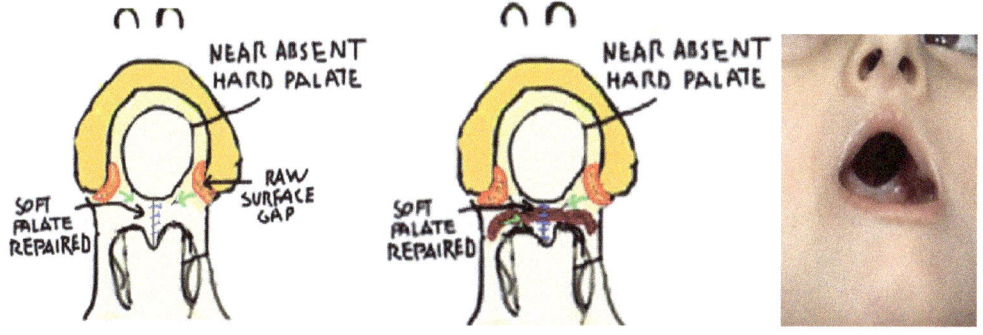

I diagrammatically show the residual cleft after soft palate repair from the sagittal view below. The entire hard palate area is still open.

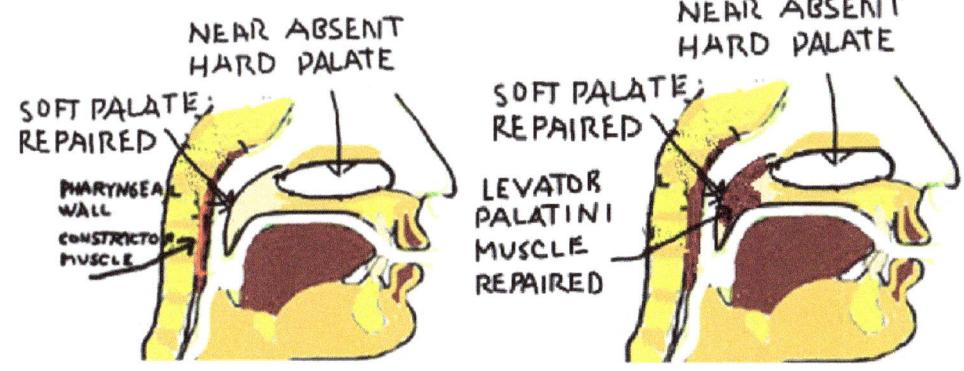

Next, I performed the superiorly based posterior pharyngeal wall flap illustrated below. I occasionally use this flap of mucosa and muscle to

correct speech problems of velopharyngeal insufficiency after palate repair (see chapter 7). Typically, the flap remains attached to the posterior pharynx, so it acts as an obturator to prevent abnormal nasal air escape during speech. However, in this unusual case, I used the flap differently. I turned it forward and attached it to the anterior edge of the previously repaired soft palate (green dots) instead of the posterior margin. Below the flap is outlined in blue ink on the patient's posterior pharyngeal wall.

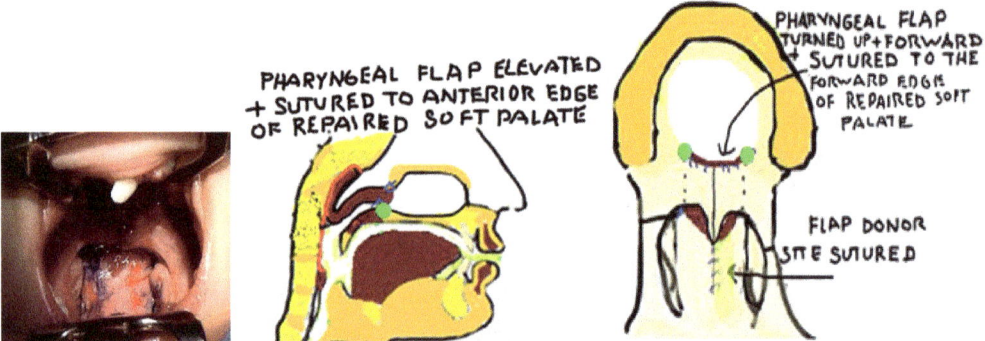

Then after two weeks, I did a second stage where I cut the base of the pharyngeal flap from the pharynx, leaving it attached to the anterior edge of the soft palate (green dots). I then took the pharyngeal flap from the posterior pharynx and turned it forward and attached it to the hard palate cleft (blue dots) while it was still attached to the soft palate. "Shirley's" is the only case in which I did this type of pharyngeal transfer. The repositioned flap closed most of the hard palate defect, but there remained a significant anterior opening in the hard palate. In the first drawing below, the green dots are where the pharyngeal flap was attached to the soft palate. The blue dots are at the base of the pharyngeal flap. After cutting to release the flap, the area of the blue dots was turned and brought forward to close most of the hard palate. The blue dots move to the anterior part of the hard palate.

The Healing Mission of Plastic Surgery

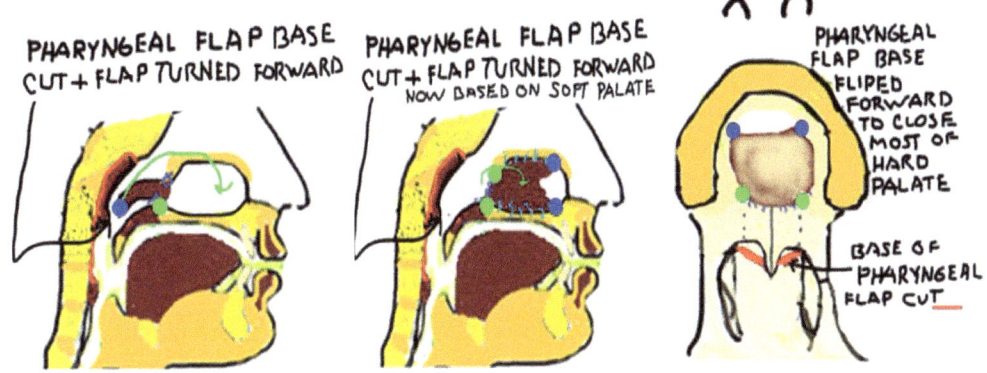

Now "Shirley" was still left with an opening in the hard palate anteriorly that was large enough to cause significant speech problems with nasal escape. Therefore I devised another flap to address this residual opening. I planned a large anteriorly based tongue flap, which was incised and brought up to the roof of the mouth and sewn to the edges of the residual anterior hard palate cleft to complete the hard palate closure. The completed hard palate closure eliminated the abnormal opening between the oral and nasal cavity. I illustrate the first stage of the tongue flap procedure below.

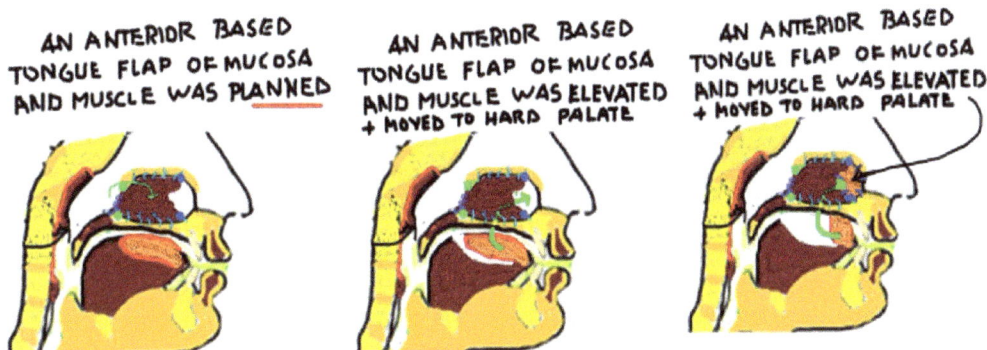

The second stage illustrated below was needed to cut the base of the tongue flap, which left tongue tissue to obliterate the anterior hard palate opening. I then sutured the cut base back to the tongue donor site.

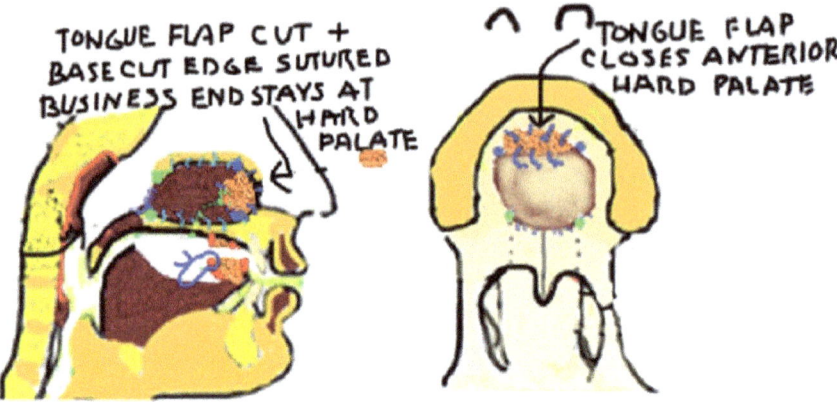

This two-staged tongue flap was able to deliver a significant amount of tongue tissue to the hard palate, as shown in the first photo below. The second photo shows another view of the healing roof of the mouth.

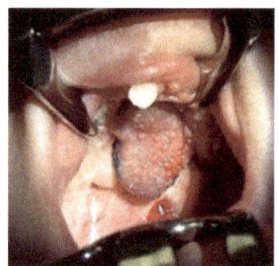 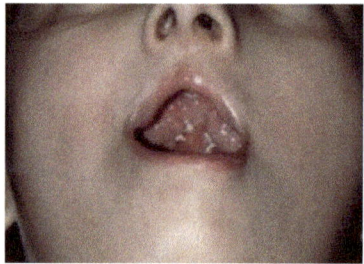

These procedures enabled the patient's speech to go from unintelligible to intelligible, although not normal. I regret that I was unable to complete all my operative plans for this patient because of my unplanned retirement. She was an exceptional patient. When I saw her in the office, she always ran up to me and gave me a big hug. She sometimes brought me a card saying, "I love you, Dr. Cronin." She had a lot of issues facing her, and I worry about her future. Fortunately, she seemed to have a very loving and supportive mother. I pray that she will thrive.

Another cleft patient that I regret not being able to complete reconstruction for is "Tommy."

His situation was very different. He was one of several patients I treated over the years adopted from Russia or Ukraine. Both of his adoptive parents were very engaged in his care. I first saw him when he was about eight months old and had an unrepaired bilateral cleft of the lip and palate with a firm very protruding prolabium and premaxilla.

I first did a bilateral lip adhesion procedure followed a few months later with a full lip repair and palate repair. As I treated "Tommy" during his first few years, it became evident that he was brilliant and also gregarious. He obtained normal speech after his palate repair, which made his sophisticated vocabulary seem almost cosmopolitan. He was taking Latin in grade school and greeted me with "salve, Dr. Cronin." Although he had the misfortune of being born with bilateral cleft lip and palate, I feel like he is off to a great start in life and should do well. I pray for all of my cleft patients.

Large wood splinter

One afternoon I was called to the emergency room to see a carpenter who had injured his hand. He had been cutting some large boards with a saw. A shard of wood split off from the board and skewered part of all four fingers of his right hand. It was quite remarkable to see this long thin piece of wood connecting the fingers as in the preoperative photos below. I was amazed to find he had sensation at all the fingertips.

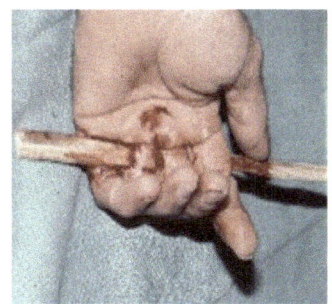 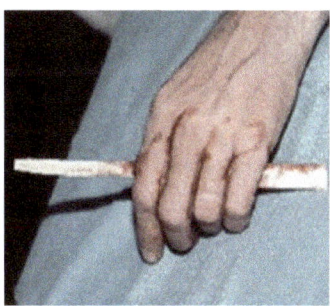 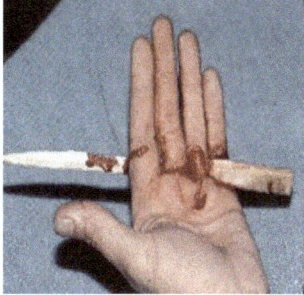

I took him to the operating room. After cleaning and prepping the area, I carefully remove the large splinter by cutting the wood between each finger and carefully pulling out each piece so as not to have to drag more wood through the fingers.

Each wound was then carefully explored to be sure that the nerves and blood vessels that run on each side of the palm side of the fingers were intact. Since the wood passed on the palm side of the bone of each finger, I had expected severe damage to several of the neurovascular bundles, but to my delight, that was not the case.

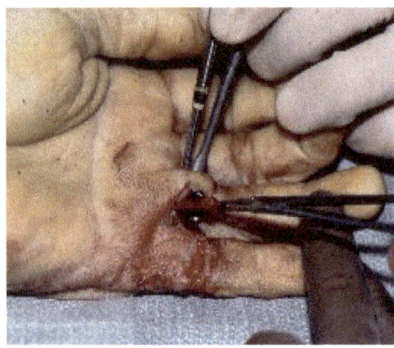 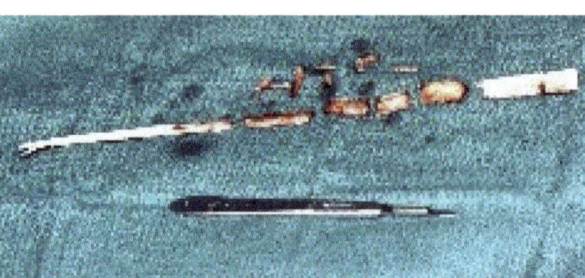

I repaired the wounds, and this carpenter made a full and rapid recovery. His postoperative photos are below.

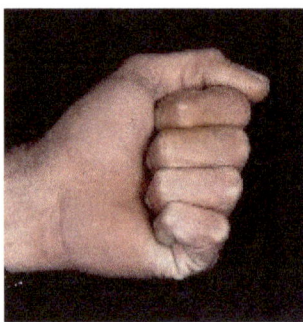 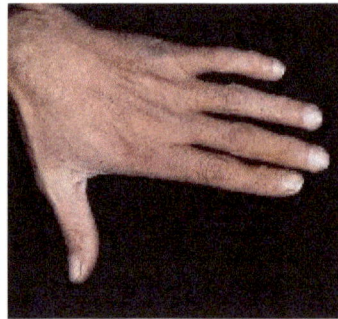

Pierre Robin Sequence

A special circumstance

The Pierre Robin sequence is a particular congenital problem that sometimes includes a cleft of the posterior (secondary) palate. It occurs in about 1:10,000 births. Micrognathia (small jaw) or retrognathia (posteriorly positioned jaw) characterizes this condition. The etiology is unknown. It may be genetic but is probably related to intrauterine pressure and the flexed position of the embryo's head and neck during development, which may result in a very high arched palate or a cleft in the palate. The tongue tends to fall back and obstruct the airway (glossoptosis).

The severity of the condition varies greatly. In minimal cases, no treatment may be necessary. In more involved examples, the child will struggle to breathe and have difficulty feeding. In mild cases positioning the child in a prone position might be enough to alleviate the struggle to breathe. The first diagram below shows that the tongue can fall back against the pharynx and obstruct the airway, especially when the infant is in the supine position. Moving the tongue forward by whatever means tends to open the airway, as indicated in the second drawing.

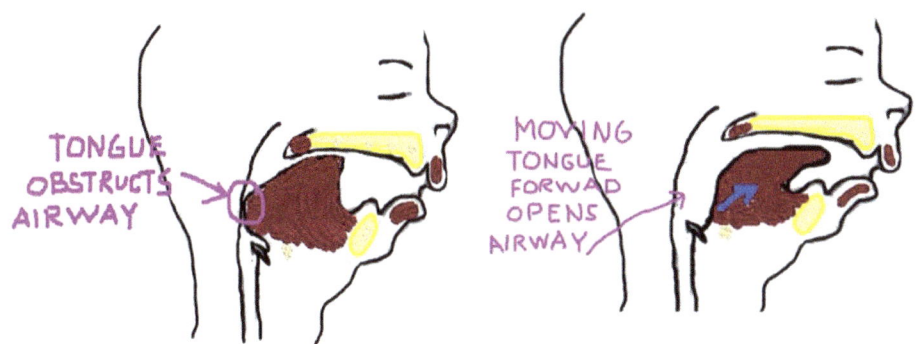

In more involved cases, the child will eventually die from exhaustion and airway obstruction if no surgical intervention occurs. One effective treatment is to short circuit the area of airway blockage with a tracheostomy. A tracheostomy opens an airway in the neck directly into the trachea, as demonstrated in the drawing below.

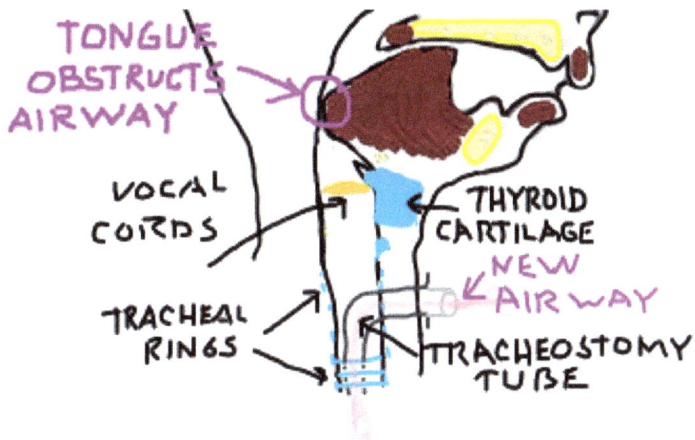

A tracheostomy can thus be lifesaving. However, it does add a level of care that can be a burden to the parents. Occasionally a child will die of airway obstruction because the tube is dislodged or becomes clogged. As the child grows and becomes more robust, he will be able to overcome the problem with the tongue obstructing the airway. He can often "outgrow" the problem. Once created for this problem, a tracheostomy will probably need to stay at least one year.

The traditional mainstay treatment for many years was a tongue - lip adhesion. This procedure involves moving the tongue forward and suturing it to the lip. This operation will usually alleviate the problem and will allow the child to thrive and grow stronger and develop without the need for a tracheostomy. Often in six months or a year, the tongue-lip adhesion can be taken down without ill effect.

The following drawings diagrammatically illustrate the tongue lip adhesion procedure to treat Pierre Robin Sequence. It is a little complicated to understand and may take an attentive study of the pictures. In the first drawing, the red lines indicate incisions in the tongue to develop a flap of tongue tissue and also an incision on the inner side of the lower lip to form a lip flap. Two connections are then made by sewing tissue together. Suturing the leading edge of the tongue flap to the edge of the incision made to develop the lip flap creates a lower connection, and suturing the leading edge of the lip flap to the cut edge of the tongue creates the upper attachment. The drawings below illustrate the tongue and lip fusions. Following the blue suture connections will help to understand the way the flaps interact.

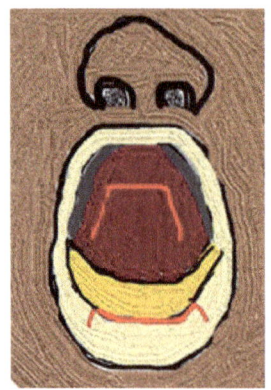 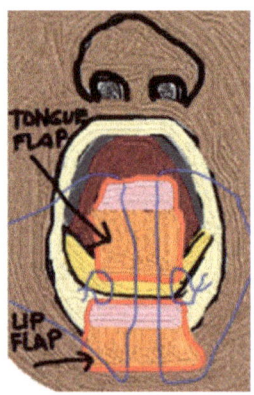

The first two drawings below illustrate the same tongue and lip flap adhesion from a sagittal perspective. These flaps are colored orange to also correspond to the flaps in the above illustrations.

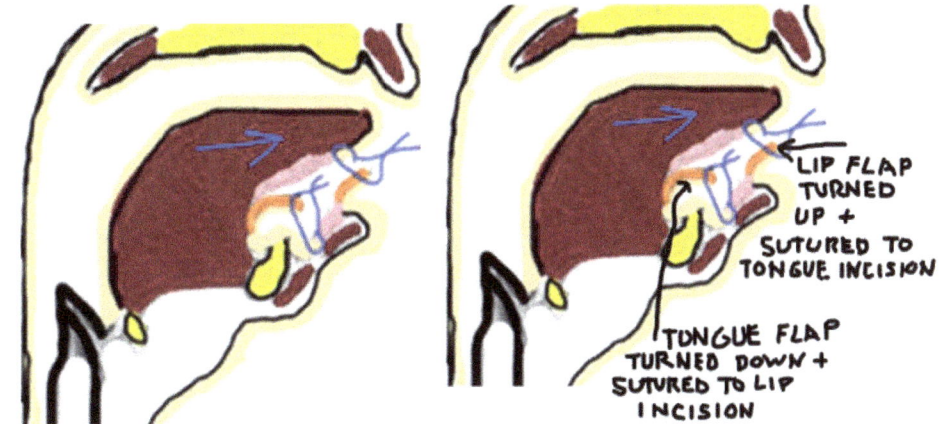

The final drawings below show a large suture from the chin going around the mandible to the base of the tongue to promote the forward movement of the tongue and to take tension off the healing tongue-lip adhesion. A button (brown) at the back of the tongue keeps the suture from pulling through the tissue. The button under the chin is also to prevent the large stitch from pulling through the skin. After healing, the adhesion, indicated by the green line, holds the tongue forward, so it does not obstruct the airway. At that point, the surgeon removes the buttons and heavy ligatures.

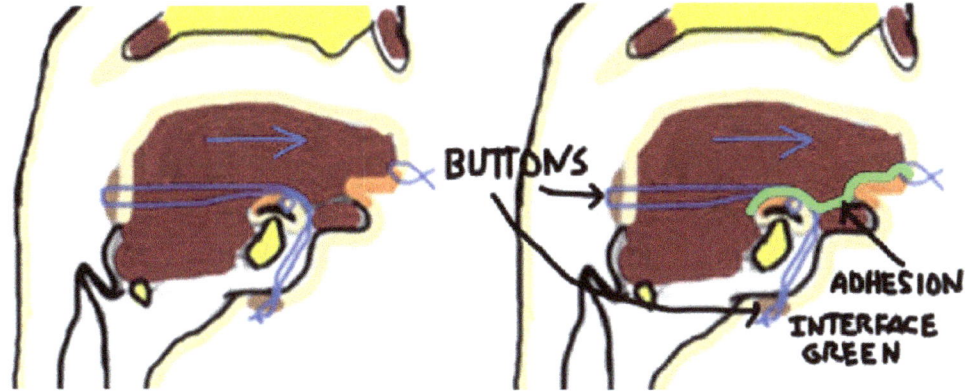

After the child has grown stronger, the surgeon will take down the adhesion, and the child will breathe normally.

Occasionally the tongue lip adhesion will not solve the problem, and it may be that the surgeon must do a tracheostomy

More recently, surgeons have used the mandibular distraction technique with success in severe cases. Moving the jaw forward also moves the tongue forward and alleviates the airway obstruction. This procedure is similar to the deficient chin mandibular distraction case "Pete," which I presented in chapter 2. In the drawing below, the surgeon cuts the mandible and secures a distraction device to either side of the cut. A ratchet on the device slowly pushes the bones apart, allowing new bone production to occur. When the desired lengthening has occurred, time is allowed for bony solidification before removing the device.

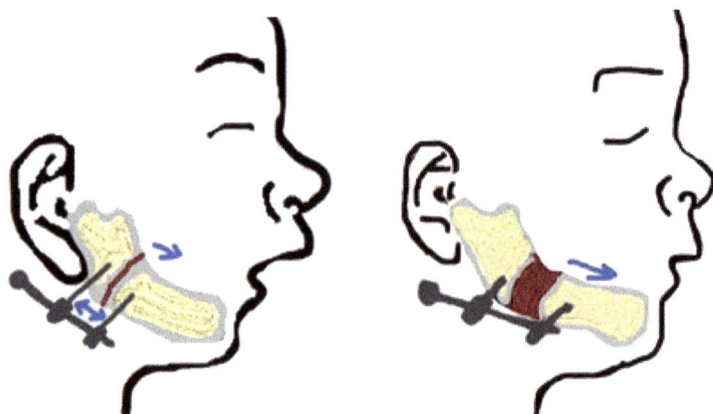

"Gregory" came to the cleft palate clinic when he was about ten days old because of a cleft of the posterior palate. He looked thin and was in some distress with labored breathing. He had a small, retruded mandible. The mother said she was having trouble feeding the child. This child was in trouble. Without intervention, he would continue to deteriorate, weaken, and finally succumb to respiratory failure.

I arranged to admit him to the hospital, where he was positioned to relieve the obstruction. I also had a nasogastric tube placed that held the tongue slightly forward and allowed for small areas for breathing on either side of the tube. The next morning, I performed a tongue-lip adhesion. He did well postoperatively. He began to feed better and gain weight. He was able to be discharged a few days later. I repaired his posterior cleft palate at about eight months of age when he was in good nutritional shape. I was able to take down the lip adhesion at about 11 months of age. He did well after that. If this child had not been seen in the cleft clinic that day, he might have had a disastrous outcome.

Traumatic enophthalmos with secondary upper eyelid ptosis

"Olga" shown below had a traumatic orbital injury with enophthalmos. Enophthalmos is a condition in which the globe is too far back or too inferior. She had an orbital floor fracture, and the eyeball receded posteriorly and inferiorly. She was especially bothered by the left upper eyelid ptosis, evident in the first photograph. Unlike other cases of ptosis correction (see chapter 14), this patient did not respond to the regular operation because of the abnormal position of the globe. The second photo shows the postoperative result after I performed a standard ptosis type procedure. She received minimal benefit from the method.

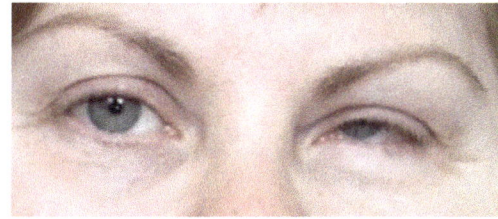 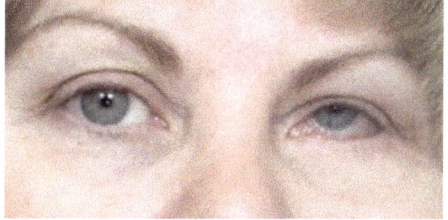

After reassessing her situation, I decided that I needed to make the orbit smaller to reposition the globe forward and up. Therefore, I re-explored her eye socket. The first two intra-operative pictures below show exposure of the orbital floor, while the third one shows the exposure of the orbital roof.

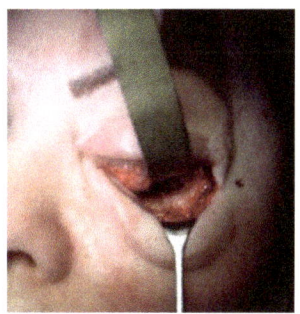 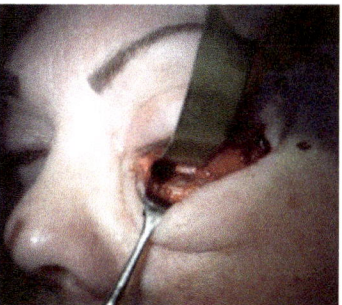

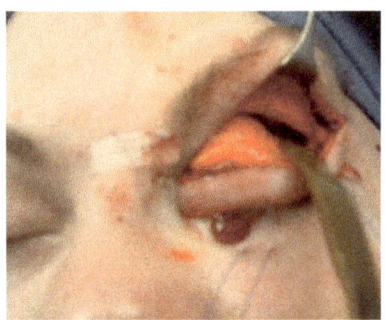

I placed several implants in the eye socket to reposition the globe. The first intraoperative photo below shows one of the white synthetic implants ready for placement in the medial portion of the eye socket. Correcting the globe position in the orbit allowed the ptosis correction to be much more effective, as shown in the final picture.

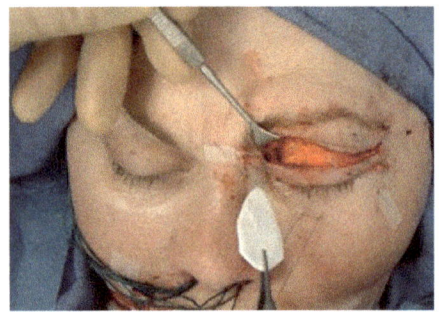
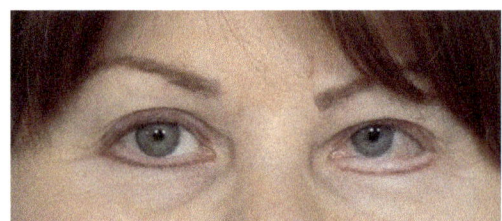

Unusual frontal bone injury

"Roseanne" had a strange, slightly pointed traumatic fracture in the glabella when she hit against a sharp cornered piece of furniture. I explored the wound and found no other injury. I repaired this by replacing the displaced fragment of the frontal bone and securing it with a microplate and screws. This injury probably would have healed well even without the plating.

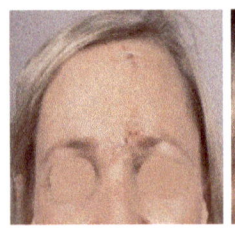
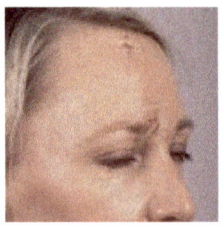
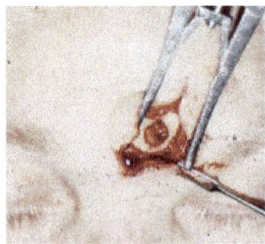
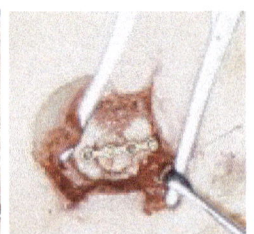

Nasal Cyst

"Helena" presented with a complicated history of previous trauma and multiple surgeries, including a bone graft to the bridge of the nose. The first two photographs show a bulbous mass on the bridge of the nose. The previous surgeon used an incision on the nasal dorsum to introduce a bone graft. I marked the scar with a blue line.

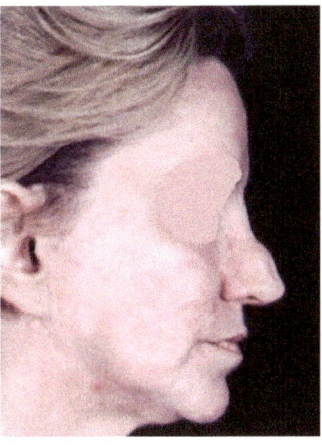
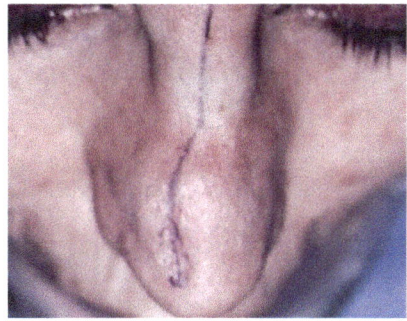

Upon exploration through that incision, I found a cystic area filled with mucus material. I cleaned this cyst out. In the second photo below, one can see residual of the previous bone graft and a notched area where the cyst had eroded into the bone graft. The final photograph shows the result after I reshaped the graft.

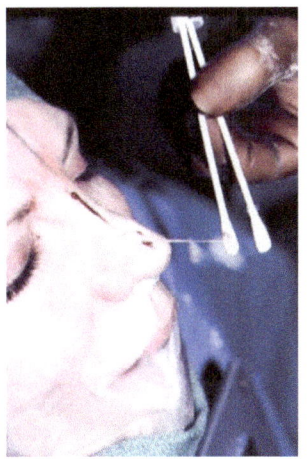
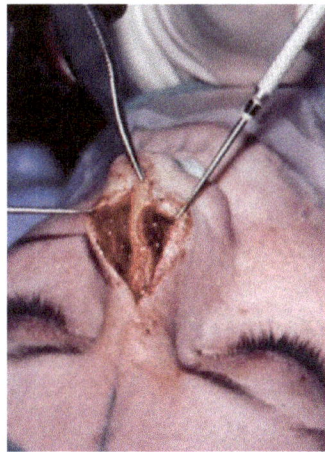
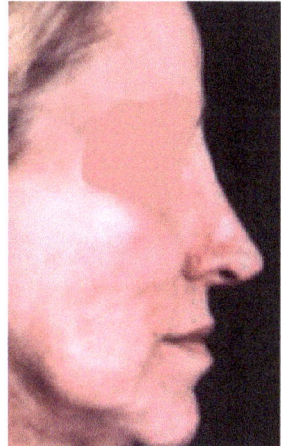

Fatal augmentation

It seemed a little unusual from the beginning. The lady was older than the average patient coming in for augmentation mammaplasty. She had some preexisting medical problems. She came in with a boyfriend who was probably a little younger than she. Although she seemed fairly strong-willed, it did seem that the impetus for the surgery came from the boyfriend. Both the patient and the boyfriend were Hispanic and spoke somewhat limited English. The consultation was in English with translation in Spanish as needed.

Although I thought she was not the best candidate, she and her boyfriend were undeterred. We brought them back for the second consultation, covering risks benefits and alternatives of procedure. I got feedback from some of my staff who felt the boyfriend was "creepy."

I went ahead with the procedure which she tolerated well. However, a few days after surgery, she did develop a hematoma in the left breast. Was this spontaneous? Or had they been too active too soon? A hematoma is a blood collection under the tissues which occurs about 2% of the time in augmentation mammaplasty. I took care of this complication, and she did well. She obtained an excellent result, although the boyfriend wanted her to be still more abundant.

The last time we saw her in the office, she was doing quite well, and I documented this with postoperative photographs.

A few months later, we heard about a common-law husband arrested for the murder of his wife. She turned out to be our patient. She had gone missing, and some of her neighbors called the police. The man was living in the house, which belonged to the woman. At first, he said that she had gone to Mexico to visit relatives. However, the police were quite suspicious and dug up the newly built patio in her backyard and found her body.

The man claimed that she died of natural causes but, because he was afraid the police would blame him, he tried to conceal findings by burying her in the backyard. I believe he's serving the time in prison.

Litigious event

One day in the office, a patient came to see me for whom I had done an augmentation mammaplasty a few years previously. The breast augmentation controversy was raging then. Malpractice suits in Texas named surgeons along with the implant manufacturers. Apparently, in many other states, the surgeons were not named in these lawsuits. My understanding is as long as the doctor's name stayed on the suit for a year and a day, the plaintiff's attorneys could keep these cases in state court rather than federal court. I believe the plaintiff's attorneys felt they had more leverage in the state courts of Texas.

When I looked at her chart in preparation for going into the examination room, I seem to remember that her name was on the list of patients who had filed breast implant lawsuits. I checked this with my secretary, and sure enough, her name was on the list of patients who were suing because of alleged problems with their silicone breast implants. I was not exactly sure how I should handle this situation.

I went into the room and greeted the patient as I usually would. I asked her how she was doing. She said everything was fine and she was quite pleased with the result and was having no problems. The nurse then gave her a gown so that I could examine her. I then returned the examination room with the nurse and examined her. She had an excellent result from the augmentation mammaplasty, which I had done with silicone gel breast implants.

At the end of the visit, I asked her if she knew that she was suing me. She was taken aback and looked as if she might faint. She said, "No! No doctor, Cronin, I'm not suing you". I told her she was on the list of patients that we had received notice on, who were suing me. She then said that she had gone to an attorney to check into the matter because of all the publicity in the news about silicone breast implants and lawsuits about silicone breast implants. She said she never gave the attorney permission to sue me. She was very apologetic and said she was quite upset with the attorneys and would check into it. We ask her to return each year as we had in the past. She never came back. Eventually, a year or so later, I received notice of a summary judgment dropping the suit.

Only a short bicycle ride

A significant part of my practice was breast reconstruction after mastectomy for cancer. Some of my most grateful patients are breast reconstruction patients. I remember a particular patient who was quite young when she developed breast cancer. As a 30-year-old, it is quite a shock to be told that you have breast cancer and need to have a mastectomy. My patient was a very outgoing, vivacious young woman with young children. We planned to do an immediate reconstruction at the same time she had her mastectomy. After discussing various methods with her, we selected a way that used an abdominal flap made of skin, subcutaneous fatty tissue, and muscle from the lower abdomen. I planned to bring this tissue to the mastectomy site and fashioned it into the shape of a breast.

She did exceptionally well with the surgery and was in the hospital for a few days and then was discharged home to be followed a few days later in the office. To put this in perspective, most women who had this particular operation were in the hospital about four to five nights as they're very restricted in their activity and need to walk around slightly hunched over because of the tightness and discomfort in their abdomen. Minor exercise might begin at three weeks, but vigorous exercise would have to wait six weeks, and particular vigorous exercise using abdominal muscles would have to wait about three months.

Her first visit back to the office after discharge from the hospital was at about the 9th or 10th-day post-surgery. I ask her how she had been doing because it seemed like she had had an excellent preliminary recovery while in the hospital. She stated, "I was doing fine until I fell off my bicycle." Well, I nearly fell off my examination stool when she said that. She said I told her she should not drive an automobile until we said it was okay. Her husband had to go out of town, and she said she needed to go from her home to a nearby bank to conduct a transaction for them. She went on to relate how she took a little spill on the way back from the bank but was not hurt. After examining her, we found no injuries, and she continued to recover well, and she went on to obtain a lovely breast reconstruction result.

Unfortunately, this lady was one of the unlucky ones who developed metastatic disease. She died of her breast cancer a couple of years later. She was a brave young woman, and I was happy that I was able to attend her funeral and graveside service. This experience served to remind me that life is fleeting, and we need to take advantage of the time we do have here on this earth.

Like any surgery with cosmetic overtones, if we look at a series of breast reconstruction cases, most will have a satisfactory result. A few may have extraordinarily excellent results, and some may have relatively poor results or even suffer some significant difficulties. It may seem a little strange, but some of my most appreciative patients have been those that initially had some complication. However, I do recall an unusual case in which a patient had a lovely result but was unhappy and even angry and told me I should have been able to give her a "perfect" outcome.

Dog Bites

Over the years, I have treated many patients with dog bite wounds, including some nieces and nephews. Unfortunately, most of these were small children. In adults, the most common areas I saw were the hands and arms. I remember one elderly lady, "Maggie," who had two dogs, which she said would periodically fuss with one another. She commonly had to break up their feuding. I met her one night in the emergency room because of multiple lacerations to both hands. These wounds had to be cleaned up and irrigated with antibiotic solution copiously and then repaired. These went on to heal uneventfully.

However, several months later, I was called to the emergency room to see the same lady. This time her injuries were much more significant. She had fractures of the metacarpal bones in her right hand from the severe dog bite. This time I had to take her to the operating room, where we cleaned the wounds, pinned the fractures, repaired the lacerations, and put her hand in a splint. The recovery from this injury took months. She had some residual stiffness in her knuckle joints, even after physical therapy. Incidents like this and many others I have always been a little leery of dogs around my children.

Accidental skin peel

One day I received a call from the pathology laboratory at St. Joseph Hospital because a middle-aged female laboratory technician "Barb" had suffered flash burns of her face when a chemical with which she was working ignited. I was able to hurry over to the lab, which was in the building adjacent to my office. Fortunately, she had no damage to her eyes. She suffered superficial second-degree burns of the entire face in a reasonably uniform manner. She singed her eyelashes and eyebrow hairs. This lady was quite fortunate.

After a two- week treatment with antibiotic ointment, the sloughed superficial layer of skin had been replaced with new pink epithelium. "Barb's" healing was similar to what one might experience from a medium depth, chemical, or laser peel of the face. Although she had had a frightening experience, the effect was a significant rejuvenation of her facial skin. The cosmetic result was excellent.

Rhinophyma

Rhinophyma is a bulbous growth of the nose that can distort its typical features. It occurs in patients with severe rosacea, a granulomatous inflammatory infiltration of the skin of the nose. When severe, it can be improved by tangentially cutting the bulbous growth and allowing the skin to heal secondarily. In "Horatio's" case, shown below, I shaved the bulbous growths and let the wound heal. The patient developed some scar but was much improved, as shown below.

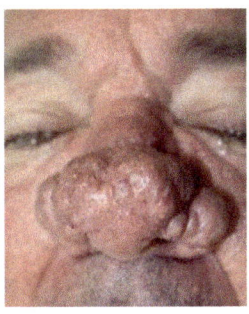 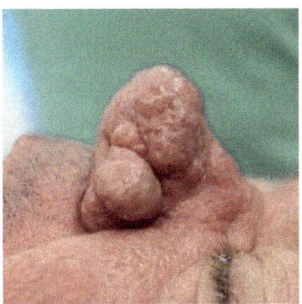 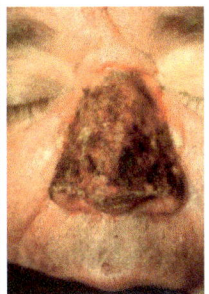 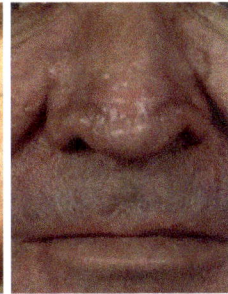

Gumbo Burn

The patient "Michael" was a 90-year-old man whose grandson found him sprawled on the floor of his kitchen where he had fallen. He had been cooking a huge pot full of gumbo, which turned over onto him as he fell. At first, it may sound funny; however, he suffered extensive third-degree burns to a large portion of his lower extremities as well as spotty areas of his trunk and upper extremities. His injury was a severe injury that could have been fatal. The thick gumbo tended to stick to his skin more than just boiling water would have, thus increasing the depth of the burn wounds. I performed several surgeries to debride the skin and some deeper tissues. He required extensive skin grafts as well. His hospitalization lasted about two months, but when I discharged him, he was ambulating again and returned to his home.

IV drug use

Another unusual and alarming case I observed was that of a lady with an IV drug abuse problem. She injected intravenously illicit material, which caused spasm and thrombosis in the arteries supplying blood to her left hand, which necessitated amputation. It seems like knowledge of such tragic consequences of drug use and drug overdose deaths would tend to quell the deadly drug and opioid crisis occurring now in the United States.

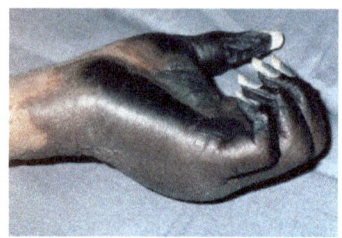 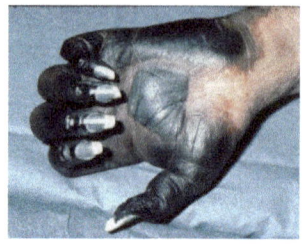

Cocaine Nose

The following patient was referred to me by a plastic surgeon colleague who had recently done some cosmetic surgery for her. She complained that her nose was collapsing because of her long history of cocaine use. She had snorted cocaine into her nose, which has an effect of constricting the blood vessels locally. With frequent chronic use, it can cause necrosis of the mucosa and even the cartilage of the nasal septum and surrounding tissues, as in her case. Her septum partially necrosed, resulting in a sizeable septal perforation and collapse of the nasal tip because of a lack of support. The angle between the columella and the upper lip became abnormally sharp as her nasal tip fell. After obtaining assurances of "being clean," I agreed to operate on her. The pictures below illustrate the preoperative condition.

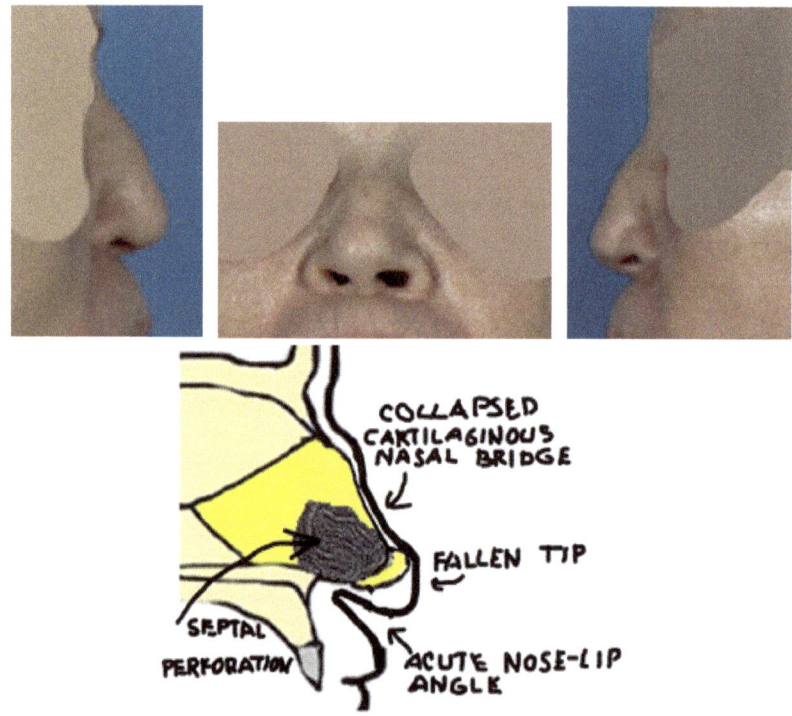

Although I had successfully closed several septal perforations, I felt it was not likely I would be able to close the hole in her septum because of its size and the generally poor condition of the surrounding septum. However, I surmised that I could restore support for the nasal tip with cartilage grafts. In her case, I used irradiated donor cartilage. I placed grafts to build up the bridge of the nose. I used an additional columella graft to elevate the tip. Together they then constituted an L shaped cartilaginous reconstruction as illustrated in the following three drawings.

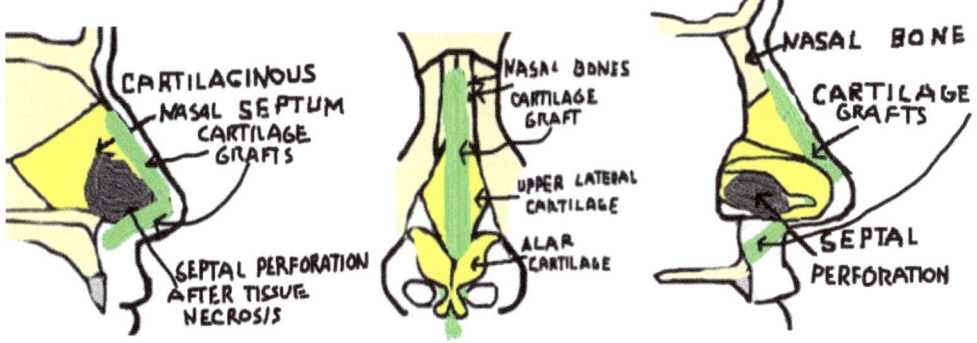

Her post-op photos are below.

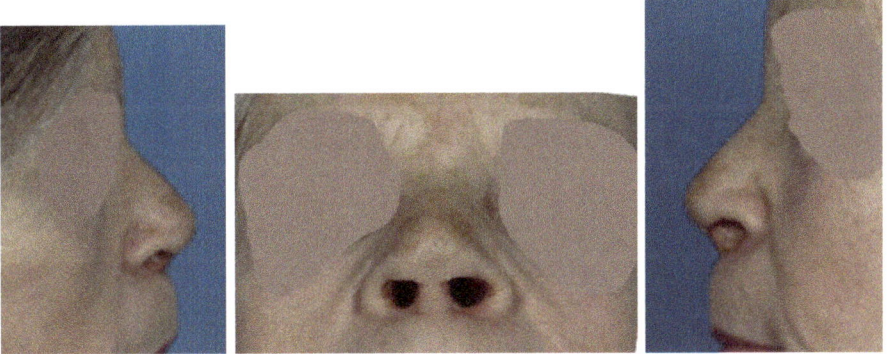

Hidradenitis Suppurativa

Hidradenitis Suppurativa is a chronic inflammatory disease that is manifested by small lumps under the skin, which can suppurate and spontaneously drain pus. It develops in intertriginous hair-bearing areas like the axilla groin, breasts, buttocks, and perineum. It tends to be progressive and can tragically influence physical and emotional wellbeing. It is not contagious. The cause is unknown but may be related to hormones and the immune system. The source is not an infection or poor hygiene.

The areas often become secondarily infected and even noisome. Antibiotics are helpful during flareups. Abscesses require incision and drainage. Other medicines sometimes used are corticosteroids, oral retinoids like Accutane, hormones like birth control pills, or drugs known as biologics such as adalimumab (Humira). The most common presentation that I saw in my practice was involved underarms. I had a few patients with severe issues that got better after wide excision of the entire hair-bearing skin and coverage with a graft or flap.

I took care of a particularly pleasant but unfortunate lady "Mary" who had extensive disease. The first drawing below illustrates the preoperative condition in the perineum. Both axillary areas were involved, the groin and breasts. I treated infection with antibiotics and drained several abscess sites multiple times. It seemed that the only thing that cured an area was the complete excision of the involved skin. I performed many excisional operations for her and used split-thickness skin grafts and flaps to reconstruct the areas. She epitomizes the fundamental reason patients go to see doctors. She sought relief for her distress.

The case below shows a patient with severe hidradenitis suppurativa of the vulva. I treated her most recent flareup with antibiotics, and the area was relatively quiescent. The first photo is pre-op; the second shows the removed specimen; the third shows the wound after I completely excised all the affected tissue. The fourth picture shows a "meshed "split-thickness skin graft I placed on the wound. The last photo shows the healed wound.

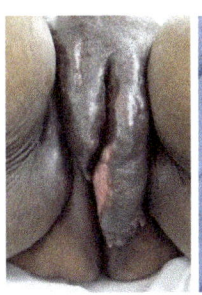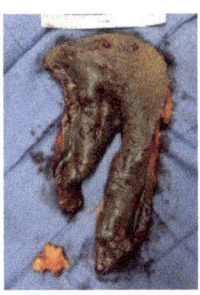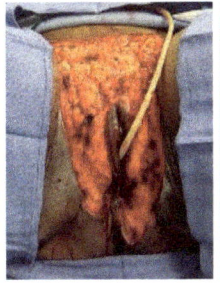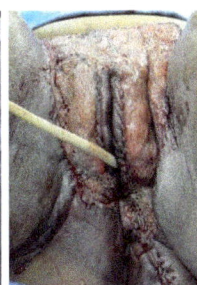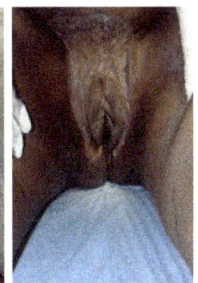

A meshed split-thickness skin graft is one that has run through a roller, which causes multiple small cuts in the graft. The purpose of the meshed graft is twofold. It is to allow any drainage or blood to cross through the graft without accumulating beneath it, and this is quite effective in preventing graft failure from fluid lifting it up or from infection. The other use of meshed grafts is to stretch the area coved as the slits in the graft allow it to expand. The drawings below explain "meshed "split-thickness skin grafts.

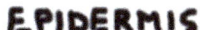
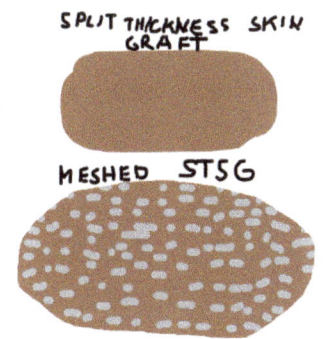

Nasal speech without cleft palate

The mother of a cleft palate patient referred a six-year-old boy with nasal speech. "Robert" had severe speech difficulty. His adoptive parents said "Robert" had severe nasality and could not be understood the majority of the time. When he was three years old, the boy and his younger sister were abandoned in a hotel room by their biological parents.

The adoptive parents arranged for an office visit. The boy was cute and well behaved, but his speech was very nasal and very difficult to understand. He was quite smart and had an appropriate vocabulary for his age and displayed quite proper sentence structures. Other pertinent information was that the boy had a history of asthma, although he had been free from attacks for more than a year. He had had an adenoidectomy at one-year of age which can some- times cause velopharyngeal insufficiency. He also had a tonsillectomy several months before this visit.

On examination, his palate seemed quite short relative to the depth of the nasal pharynx. The mobility of the soft palate(velum) was excellent, but it could not reach the posterior pharynx. Therefore, breath abnormally escaped from the nose with some speech sounds

I arranged to see the boy back in our cleft palate clinic so that we could get consultations from our speech pathologist and other members of the team. I also ordered a special study called a videofluoroscopy. This moving picture type x-ray shows the movement of the palate and pharynx during speech. Our speech pathologist, together with an experienced radiologist, did these studies together and obtained excellent results, which helped us decide the best method of treatment.

The speech pathologist confirmed our diagnosis of velopharyngeal insufficiency. The videofluoroscopy documented a large gap between the palate and the back of the throat with speech sounds that should have caused the velum (soft palate) to move up and back and close the nasopharynx and prevent nasal air escape. The options were a pharyngeal flap, a pushback palate lengthening procedure, or augmentation of the posterior pharyngeal wall. After discussing options with the parents, we selected a pushback palatoplasty

This operation lengthens the soft tissue portions of the palate so that there is less distance for the soft palate to move to the back of the throat. The child did well with this surgery and stayed one night in the hospital.

This surgery resulted in improvement in his speech; however, he remained slightly nasal. Therefore, he was again studied with a videofluoroscopy and found to have a small residual gap between the palate and nasal pharynx with speech. I took him to the operating room a second time, and I placed a synthetic implant made of polytetrafluoroethylene in the back of the throat beneath the muscle layer. This implant brought the pharynx a few millimeters forward so that the palate had less distance to move back and upward before it would reach the nasopharynx and complete the normal sphincter action. Once he healed from this surgery, Dr. Fox, our speech pathologist, judged his speech to be within normal limits. We all know how vital normal speech is in everyday life. It made me feel great that we were able to take this boy from virtually unintelligible speech to normal speech.

Stria after augmentation mammaplasty

An unusual complication of breast augmentation with a silicone gel implant occurred in one of my patients, "Sylvia." She was a 20 something young woman who had very little breast development. She sought augmentation because she believed that would give her more confidence in interpersonal relationships.

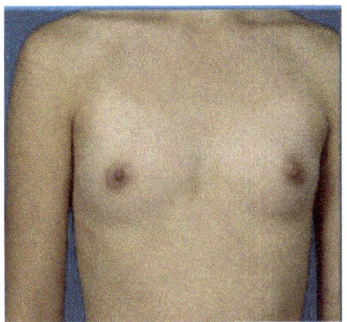 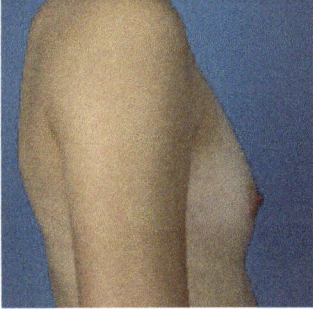 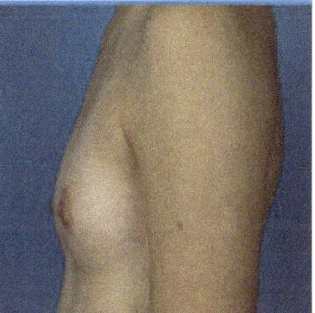

I performed an augmentation mammaplasty, placing a moderate-sized silicone gel implant in a subglandular pocket through an inframammary incision as an outpatient. She did well; however, a few weeks after surgery, she developed pink stria in the central part of her breast, as shown in the post-op photos below. Over time the pinkness faded, but the stria remained. I believe she was the only patient of mine that had this complication.

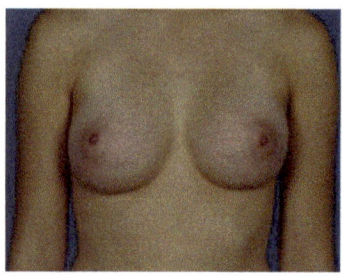 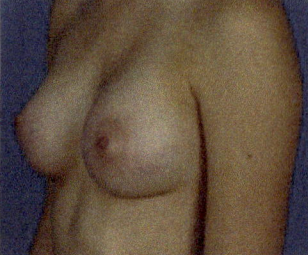 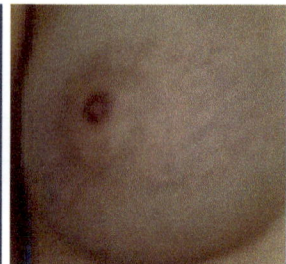

Lipomatosis

A lipoma is a benign fatty tumor that commonly occurs in the subcutaneous fat layer but can occur in other areas. They are often without symptoms' they may be unsightly or can cause problems by pressure on adjacent structures. Sometimes they are painful. I have seen a few patients with lipomatosis, with numerous lesions as the patient below demonstrated. "Jack"

the man shown below had countless small subcutaneous lipomas all over his body. At his request on one occasion, I removed a couple of dozen lesions that were bothering him. You can see these lesions below.

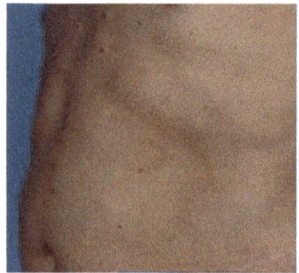 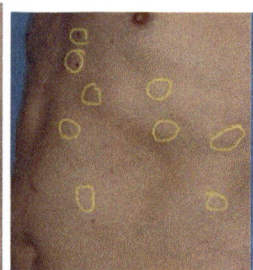 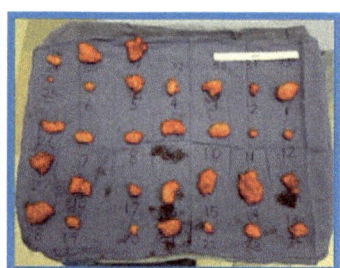

Nasal tumor-Delayed Dx

A middle-aged lady, "Gladys," came to see me at the insistence of her internist. She had been having a nasal problem for many months and had seen her ear nose and throat physician for nasal congestion, but he had not made a specific diagnosis. Her nose had begun to change shape with the tip becoming deformed. I took the pictures below when I first saw her. I could immediately tell that this was serious. I surmised a squamous cell cancer was eating the nasal septum and collapsing the nose. If not that, it was a lethal midline granuloma, a rare type of lymphoma that presents with epistaxis, nasal congestion, rhinorrhea, and pain. I performed extensive biopsies that revealed squamous cell cancer. A large part of the nasal septum was involved. After confirming she had cancer, her primary physician referred her to M.D. Anderson Cancer Center. She needed a total rhinectomy and prosthetic reconstruction.

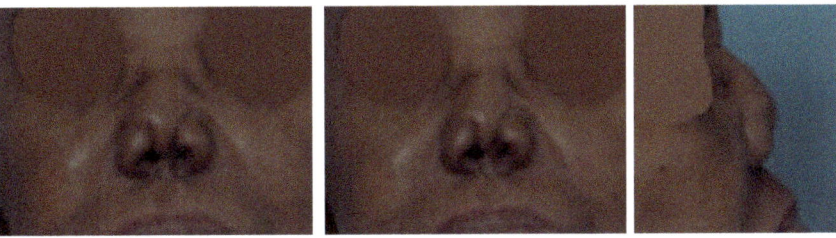

Small head

My uncle had a very unusual patient whom I got to meet and observe. He had been treated as a child with radiation therapy to the head. As a result, his head had not grown in proportion to the rest of his body. He had an average size and appearing body except for his head. Although all his facial structures were proportional and symmetric, his entire head was disproportionally small for his body. This patient also had developed multiple skin cancers of the head and neck region because of early radiation therapy. I realize that this sounds far-fetched. If I showed a photograph of this man the observer's first impression might be that it was photoshopped

Patient of courage

I was fortunate to have a patient with multiple facial clefts come to me for additional surgery. She had bilateral # 4Tessier rare facial clefts. She had had numerous previous well-performed surgeries. She did have significant residual deformities. Over a few years, I performed several additional surgeries for her, including an Abbe flap lip switch procedure, in which I moved tissue from the lower to the upper lip (as in the patient "Jim" from chapter 1). I remember that she was charming and brought gingerbread houses to me during Christmas time. Although she continued to have significant appearance differences despite the multiple surgical interventions, she was very positive. She became a clinical pediatric nurse, and at the time of the last contact I had with her, she was working in a large pediatric hospital. She represents the inspirational attitude of many of the patients I was fortunate enough to try to help during my plastic surgery career.

Meningococcal Meningitis

One of the saddest cases I had was a child with meningococcal meningitis. He had the sudden onset of high fever and disorientation and later developed large areas of necrotic tissue all over his body. His treatment with large doses of antibiotics had assuredly saved his life at another hospital. When I first saw him, however, he was still in considerable danger because of all this dead tissue from the "flesh-eating bacteria." We had an excellent pediatrician to help direct his overall medical care.

Soon after first evaluating him, I took him to the operating room to cut away the dead tissue and further assess the injuries. There were areas on his face, trunk, and upper extremities, but by far, the worst areas were his lower legs. After a few debridement sessions, it was evident that the damage was both extensive and profound. I asked an orthopedic surgeon, Dr. Brad Urquhart, to consult on the case. We decided that, unfortunately, the amputation of this child's lower legs was necessary. We would have liked to have done this at the level below the knee. However, significant infection and dead tissue extended to the knee joint of both legs.

Therefore, the amputation had to take place at the level of the knee. Multiple skin grafting operations followed, but eventually, after perhaps a dozen surgeries, all the wounds were healed. The child had no permanent neurologic damage. He had multiple skin grafts and scars from the healing of the various areas of damage from this flesh-eating bacterial infection. The most devastating blow was the loss of both lower legs. After the wounds healed, he went to a rehabilitation hospital for further help in securing prosthetic limbs. It is interesting to note he was able to walk on the stumps of the amputated legs.

The last time I saw him was about three years later; he was having what seemed like some minor problems of irritation of the stumps from the prostheses. I then lost him to follow up. I indeed wonder how this young man is getting along now. I feel good that we work so hard and helped to save this boy's life. Yet I feel bad that we were not able to prevent his losing his lower legs.

It is interesting that as I was writing about this case, one of my daughters sent me a little video clip by e-mail of a young mother taking care of her infant. It showed the mother changing the baby's diaper, holding him, and playing with him. The young mother had no arms, so she did everything with her feet. She was a significant inspiration to everyone who knew her. My patient seemed to have spunk similar to this young mother, so I hope he has pursued his happiness and is a useful member of society.

Amblyopia–Hemangioma

I consulted on a baby "Candy" born with a severe capillary hemangioma of the soft tissues of the right side of the face and around the right eye, including the upper and lower eyelids. The lesion was a thick raised, blotchy, strawberry red tumor that seemed to be getting more significant daily. This type of non- malignant blood vessel tumor is frequently present at birth as in "Candy's" case or appears in the first weeks of life. The natural history of a hemangioma is rapid growth for about six months, then a stable period usually followed by involution by age seven.

Therefore, they are often treated with "benign neglect" because they get so much better on their own. About 70% of these tumors will involute, sometimes leaving no residual of the original tumor. However, most of the time, even though the lesions involute, there are residual changes such as thinning of the skin and subcutaneous tissue, which might require surgical revision. If a baby has such a growth, which blocks vision, amblyopia can result. Amblyopia is a disorder of vision due to the eye and brain not working well together. If a hemangioma blocks one eye for even a period, as short as a few weeks, permanent visual damage can result. So, blocked vision is a condition that mandates intervention with removal or steroid injection of the hemangioma to try to restore the line of sight in the affected eye. I took "Candy" to the operating room and removed an overhanging mass of hemangioma from the upper lid, which was blocking the right eye. I did this very carefully to avoid much blood loss. At that same setting, I injected steroids into the upper and lower eyelid hemangioma to try to reduce the visual blockage further. The remaining hemangioma began involuting after the child was about a year old.

I remember another giant capillary hemangioma in an infant that was problematic because of periodic bleeding from this forehead lesion. In that case, baby "Gregory" had a lesion that was present at birth and was increasing over the first few weeks of life. The hemangioma developed a central necrotic area, which bled several times. Because of this bleeding, the parents had to make frequent dressing changes.

So, I began to treat this lesion with pressure, both for the hemostatic benefit and to induce further involution. Over several weeks, a pressure bandage prevented repeated bleeding episodes and seemed first to halt the progression of the lesion and to promote involution. The central necrotic area healed, and the hemangioma was no longer growing, so I then discontinued the pressure therapy. The hemangioma continued to involute over the next few years. Systemic corticosteroids or systemic propranolol are now often used to try to induce early regression of these hemangiomas.

Progeria

Progeria is an extremely rare autosomal dominant mutated genetic disorder characterized by premature aging. The average life expectancy is only about 13 years, so it is rarely inherited. Signs of the disease, such as growth delay, small face, and short height, are usually present by the first year of life. There is no effective treatment. I saw "Juanita" when she was about six years of age. The mother wanted to know if there was anything I could do for her child. "Juanita" seemed somewhat small for a six-year-old. Her face looked emaciated, although she was not malnourished. Her eyes seemed sunken.

The bony structure around the orbit and cheeks seemed abnormally prominent because of the thin skin and lack of subcutaneous tissue of her face. Veins in the upper face and forehead were prominent, not because they were full and bulging but because the blue coloration penetrated through the pale, thin, skin. Her nose seemed prominent and overly mature. Her ears seemed abnormally large and prominent because her face lacked the fullness of a child. I briefly wondered whether I might make some improvements with fat grafting techniques, which we used by this time for many applications. But with just a little reflection, it was apparent that it would only be meddlesome. I had to tell the mother I had nothing to offer her child. There was little I could say to encourage the mother. "Juanita" was a delightful child, which made the experience, all the sadder, knowing the natural history of this disease.

Xeroderma pigmentosum

Xeroderma pigmentosum is an autosomal recessive genetic disorder that renders those affected hypersensitive to skin damage by ultraviolet light. Those afflicted cannot repair microscopic DNA damage caused by sun exposure. About half of these patients die of their disease in childhood. I help to take care of two patients with this disorder early in my career. They were siblings, a girl "Maria" about eight years old and a boy, "Jose," about six years old from Central America who were severely affected by xeroderma pigmentosum. Dr. Bardwill, a head and neck surgeon, asked me to examine them regarding their care. They still lived in Guatemala and came to Houston for medical care. They wore protective clothing but did not have the resources to avoid sun exposure. A dermatologist treated them with topical agents such as 5 FU (5 Fluorouracil).

Both had severe skin pigmentation issues and multiple skin cancers, especially of the head and neck area and severe bilateral cataracts. "Jose's" nose was gone, having been completely eaten away by cancer, as was his left ear. The boy was more affected than his sister. If the patients are entirely sheltered from ultraviolet light exposure, beginning at an early age, the prognosis is improved. They were already severely affected and had multiple squamous cell carcinomas. They were both incurable.

However, it seemed reasonable to remove some cancers that were open ulcerated wounds and cover these with split-thickness skin grafts. "Jose" had a prosthetic left ear and a nose fabricated for him as he was not a candidate for reconstruction. I saw both of them only on a couple of occasions about a year apart for ablative surgery. Each time they returned to Guatemala. I'm sure that within a few short years of that, sadly, both "Maria" and "Jose" succumbed to their disease. In the future, perhaps, genetic engineering techniques will be available to cure patients, such as these two unfortunate children

Amniotic Band Syndrome

A newborn child "Roger" had bilateral cleft lip and palate. Besides the bilateral cleft lip and palate, the physical exam also revealed the absence of the left lower leg, the complete lack of the right arm, and the absence of the second and third phalanges of the right foot. Although this case only goes back to 1999, it is interesting to note that prenatal ultrasonography recognized the cleft lip and palate but failed to appreciate the limb abnormalities!

Plastic surgery resident Dr. Mark Jabor and I studied the literature and concluded that "Roger" probably suffered from a manifestation of amniotic band syndrome. It occurs in about 10% of stillborn infants and between 1in 1200 to 1in 15000 live births. It occurs sporadically. The most accepted pathogenesis is the rupture of the amnion resulting in the formation of amniochorionic mesodermal bands. These strands may entangle and strangulate digits and limbs. These amniotic bands may also be pulled into the mouth of the baby causing cleft deformities. Other theories implicate vascular disruption as causative. The drawing below represents the likelihood the amniotic strands were causative in "Roger's" case.

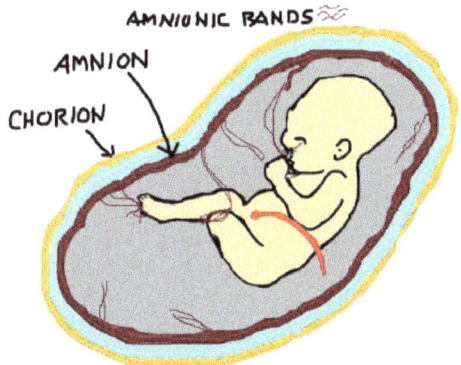

Amniotic band syndrome may now be detected by ultrasound as early as 12 weeks gestation. In the vast majority of cases, ABS is not treatable until after birth. Partial constriction can be relieved by plastic surgical interventions such as multiple Z plasties. I repaired "Roger's" cleft lip and palate, and an orthopedist got him a leg prosthesis. Unfortunately, he was lost to follow up when his mother moved.

Chapter 13

Frustrations and Joys of Plastic Surgery

General regrets

I would have to say I wish some things had turned out differently. For example, I wish that the Cronin Brauer and Biggs Clinic had not broken up in 1988. I think there was more potential for doing good through that organization than was the case after it dissolved. I regret the Sisters of Charity of the Incarnate Word sold St. Joseph Hospital, my main hospital. I regret that working with the administration and even spending time as Chief of Staff of the hospital, I was not able to help bring about a renaissance of that fine institution. I regret that I was not able to convince the hospital to continue and upgrade its pediatrics services. Therefore, I eventually needed to take the Cronin Brauer Cleft Palate Clinic to another venue, Shriners Hospital, for Children Houston, which has worked out nicely. The Cleft Palate Clinic is discussed further in chapter 7.

Frustrations

Everyone has problems. There are problems in every human endeavor. Some of the frustrations I have encountered in plastic surgery were only annoying, others more serious. It is very frustrating to find that the results of your surgery are less than you expected. Sometimes a routine case, one like many others that have turned out very well, does not turn out so well. As a surgeon, I feel bad for the patient, and pride being what it is, selfishly feel bad also for myself. I wished that I had hit a "home run" for every patient upon whom I operated.

Although seeing patients in the clinic can be delightful, on occasion, it can also be frustrating. For example, as strange as it may seem, sometimes people want you to work for nothing. I've had numerous patients who come to see me who have had surgery from other doctors and are unhappy with the result. Some have said, "I've spent thousands of dollars on my surgery, and I don't want to spend any more." It is as if they think I should try to correct or improve someone else's surgery for nothing.

Sometimes the surgery seems to have been good and sometimes less so. Rarely was it grossly inappropriate or incompetent. Every type of plastic surgery on occasion could benefit from revision surgery. Indeed, many times, I did revision surgery on my patients without charge, depending on the circumstances. There were even a few examples in which I "helped out" surgeons who were good friends of mine by doing some minor surgical revision on their patients without charge. In most instances, when I did secondary surgery on my patients, I did charge them at least a nominal fee.

Most patients are understanding; some have even expressed empathy toward me, knowing that I was disappointed for not producing the result that we both desired. It is only the occasional patient who seems unreasonable. One reason we went over many potential problems with patients before surgery and tried to document their problem or issue photographically is so we can reference that later if needed. Complications that can occasionally occur in almost any type of surgery are infection, bleeding, or hematoma (a blood collection beneath the skin). Some patients recognize these unusual occurrences are part of the risk they have agreed upon before embarking upon surgery. Others look for a specific mistake the surgeon may have committed, to blame for the complication.

Volumetric breast surgery, such as breast augmentation or breast reduction, occasionally requires revision. Both involve a change in the size of the breasts. Although usually, the results were quite acceptable to everyone involved sometimes, the augmentation patient feels like she is either too large or remains too small after the surgery. Similarly, on occasion, the breast reduction patient may feel she is too large or too small. It is hard to please everyone all the time, and that can be frustrating for both surgeon and patient.

Worry and stress

During my practice from 1978 to 2016, with the one exception of visiting Dr. Tessier in Paris in 1987, I was never away on either vacations or medical trips for more than a week or ten days. Usually, after three or four days, I would get antsy to return to my practice so that I could follow up on my patients. I have spent many sleepless nights worrying about my patients. I might be concerned about potential bleeding in the patient whom I had difficulty with hemostasis during surgery.

Sometimes it might only be an apprehension that fastidious patients will not be satisfied with my efforts at correcting their problem with surgery. For example, one night, I was worried about a breast reconstruction patient upon whom I had operated. The flap I brought from the abdomen I knew would be ok; however, the survival of the natural breast skin, which the general surgeon had saved, was a little doubtful. At surgery, I needed to either sacrifice that skin or save it to use for the reconstruction. I remove a small amount of the worst looking skin to see if the edges of the remaining skin would bleed. They did; therefore, I buried the abdominal flap, which I brought to the breast area under the natural breast skin. The next day, when I went to see the patient, I was encouraged that the natural breast skin was going to be OK by its improved appearance.

Sometimes under similar circumstances, a portion of that skin might die, which would then cause either a significant delay in healing for the patient. Or perhaps the need to do more surgery to remove the dead tissue and revise the reconstruction.

From time to time, even without any particular complication, results are less dramatic and mediocre. Such effects can be an emotional drain and disappointment for the surgeon, as well as the patient he wishes to help. Stress is part of the human condition. I felt a lot of psychological weight in the practice of plastic surgery. Sometimes this was because I utilized a free flap procedure that depended on anastomosis of small blood vessels.

They could quite easily clog up, thereby depriving the transferred flap tissue of its necessary blood supply. This risk diminishes over time. However, it is worrisome for several days after performing one of these free flap procedures. If the vessels clogged off, one must quickly return the patient to the operating room and try to relieve the obstruction, or the free flap will fail.

Cardiac arrest

A particularly stressful event occurred with one of my trauma patients. She was a young woman, about 20 years old, who fractured her jaw in an automobile accident. I had treated her at the time by realigning the fractures of the mandible and wiring her teeth with arch bars to keep her mouth closed with her bite correctly aligned.

After a few weeks, I removed the elastics that had kept her mouth shut. Everything was healing well, and the occlusion was proper. Now it was time to remove the remaining hardware from her mouth. She did not want to have this done under local anesthesia, as I often did. So, I took her to the operating room for a short general anesthetic as an outpatient for that purpose.

On induction, she had a sudden cardiac arrest. Her airway tube intubation was smooth, so a lack of oxygen was not the cause of the arrest. We immediately initiated CPR with chest compressions. After 15 minutes or so, there was still no response. A supervising anesthesiologist, who had come into the room to help my anesthesiologist, said we better start thinking about abandoning the CPR. I was distraught. Kyrie Eleison, Christe Eleison, Lord have mercy; Christ have mercy. Mercy! Mercy! Mercy! was all I could think. Finally, after several tries with the defibrillator paddles and intracardiac injections of epinephrine, the original anesthesiologist asked me if we should stop.

Almost precisely at that time, suddenly, the straight line converted to a normal cardiac rhythm. The entire room and sighed relief and gratitude. I removed the hardware. The patient went to the recovery room and woke up without any neurological deficit. She did have a sore chest. Because of her other injuries, she completed her treatment in a physical rehabilitation hospital. This type of experience probably significantly ages everyone who feels responsible for the care of the patient.

After the fact, we analyzed this almost catastrophic event. The cause of her cardiac arrest pointed to a muscle relaxant drug given intravenously by the anesthesiologist. In recently traumatized patients, the agent might cause excess potassium in the bloodstream, leading to a heart stoppage. I am forever grateful for God's mercy in this incident.

Frustrating insurance issues

Insurance issues seem to increase over the decades of my plastic surgery practice. Early in my practice, fee-for-service with usual and customary fees predominated. Although this seemed to work well for the Cronin Brauer and Biggs practice and me, I did hear of many circumstances where physicians abused this situation and charged exorbitant fees, probably a significant factor why this method of payment is no longer standard.

In the era of managed care, insurance companies have successfully ratcheted down reimbursements for most functional and reconstructive surgeries. Initially, one of the ploys of insurance companies was the promise to steer an increased volume of patients to surgeons who signed up with them at "discounted" prices. Once contracted with the insurance company, the physicians would receive new contracts each year with lower and lower reimbursements. Of course, physicians could decline to sign up with insurance companies. So, when large companies contracted with individual physicians, the companies won.

Another ploy of insurance companies, I believe, was to separate procedural activities such as surgery from cognitive activities usually associated with specialties like internal medicine. In this way, they divided medical professionals. So, when insurance companies reduced surgical fees, they would entice, if not support, at least complacency from the "cognitive" specialties by the promise of better reimbursement. With medicine less united, it just made it that much easier for insurance companies to ratchet down fees across the board. As I may lament these developments, I realize the public does not have sympathy for "rich doctors." I recall a line of Robert Burns, "Oh would some power the gift to give us to see ourselves as others see us."

When organized medicine was coerced by the Federal Trade Commission beginning in the mid-1970s to no longer restrict its members from advertising, the slide from professionalism to commercialism began. On the other hand, there was an inability of the AMA or any other organized medical group to advocate for physician financial interests successfully.

Local physician organizations like, in my case, the Harris County Medical Society and the Texas Medical Association, are outstanding organizations that are beneficial to physicians and the public alike. Restraint of trade issues prevents physicians from collaborating in setting fees. It sometimes seems that physicians have become laborers for management (large insurance companies or hospitals) without the practicality of unionization. More recently, many physicians now work for hospitals. The field of plastic surgery, which has a significant fee for service aesthetic surgery component, is partly shielded from some of these problems. However, this has led some practitioners to abandon many vital areas of plastic surgery to concentrate only in the field of cosmetic surgery for economic reasons. I never wanted to do that.

An especially egregious problem I remember from my last decade in practice involves large self-insured companies. On numerous occasions, we received from third-party administrators, letters approving specific proposed procedures. However, after we completed the surgery and billed the company through the third-party administrator, our claim was denied. When we go to the State Commissioner of insurance, we get no help because these self-insured companies are outside of the jurisdiction of the state because of federal ERISA laws.

Commercial hype

Lasers

Various vendors bombarded practicing plastic surgeons with advertisements for materials and equipment. Lasers were a particularly frustrating area. Plastic surgeons typically use lasers for skin resurfacing, treatment of vascular lesions, removal of tattoos, and amelioration of scars. Lasers can be quite beneficial for all of these uses. They also can be configured as surgical cutting instruments; however, when I retired, they still did not seem to offer advantages compared to other conventional cutting techniques. My chief complaint regarding lasers was that the promotion for successive lasers was always overblown. The results never seem to live up to the expectations created by the vendors selling the instruments.

Fillers

There has also been some disappointment with injectable fillers. Surgeons must take claims of no complications for long-acting injectable materials with a grain of salt. Fillers such as hyaluronic acid are beneficial, safe, and effective. I will not attempt to sort out for you here, this area of continuing evolution.

Medical failures

Medical failures will occur if one practices medicine. Doctors are only human. Having practiced medicine for more than 38 years, I certainly have accumulated a list of failures. Human nature being what it is; I probably mentally suppressed others. However, I will mention a few to give the reader an idea of the kind of things about which I am talking.

It is seldom that I have not obtained a satisfactory breast reconstruction result even in severe cases. When I was first learning breast reconstruction as a resident, often, we had radical mastectomy cases. Today general surgeons don't perform such radical surgery, so less severe defects make breast reconstruction easier.

I remember one particular patient who had a modified radical mastectomy on the right side and no surgery on the left side. The opposite breast was huge, making it very difficult to try to match the breast. She was extremely lopsided. I decided to do the reconstruction by splitting the huge left breast, leaving half on the left, and taking the other half to the mastectomy site to reconstruct the right chest. Older plastic surgery literature described this operation. However, it was not a typical operation because other procedures had superseded it for most applications.

I moved half the tissue from the left breast to the right chest in two stages to ensure blood supply to the tissue. Unfortunately, this procedure did not work very well. The transferred tissue was not very healthy. It scarred excessively and never looked much like a breast. The patient who was not strongly motivated to obtain a breast reconstruction became discouraged and essentially gave up, so that was one breast reconstruction I was never able to complete.

I remember another nice lady who needed an implant as well as flap tissue. She repeatedly developed severe scar contracture around the implant, which distorted the breast's shape. I was never able to get her a satisfactory result; she may have sought further treatment elsewhere.

Infection occurs about 1% of the time with breast implant use, which usually leads to the removal of the implant. This complication is very devastating to the patient and upsetting to the surgeon. Since I have placed many hundreds of breast implants, I do have some patients in whom this happened for whom I feel bad. In most instances, after the complete resolution of the inflammation, a new implant can be successfully placed. Over the years, with various reconstructive procedures using flaps, etc. occasionally, they did not work well; flaps died, extensive revisions were needed, etc.

I recall a particularly nice elderly gentleman that I treated several times for a recurrent squamous cell carcinoma of the forehead just above the brow. I initially operated on him, removing the area of recurrent tumor which extended over this superior orbital rim into the orbit. I obtained many frozen sections of the margins and believed I had removed all the cancer. It was necessary to bring a flap of tissue into the area to close the defect. Because of its extensive nature and knowing that persistent tumor or recurrence was certainly a possibility, I advised the gentleman to have postoperative radiation to the area. I discussed this case with a radiologist back in his hometown. I explained the area of concern was underlying the flap of tissue used for reconstruction. Some months later, I saw the patient and discussed his radiation therapy with him. I was dismayed to find out that it was not concentrated in the area I intended. To make matters worse, he had a recurrent tumor and eventually needed nucleation of his eye because of the persistent tumor.

One cordial but very persnickety patient whom I was unable to satisfy was an engineer who had relatively minor jaw asymmetry. He brought drawings he had designed of the implant he thought was needed on one side to correct the facial asymmetry. I placed a corresponding polyethylene implant that did not accurately correct the problem, probably because I failed to get it in the precise position intended. I went back and revised that surgery. The placement was proper, but this time he had a weakness of a branch of the facial nerve. He thought I had cut a nerve, but retraction of tissues to get exposure during the procedure had stretched the nerve. This weakness cleared in about six weeks. Unfortunately, neither of us was elated with our interactions.

I recall a nice man for whom I had done a carpal tunnel operation. He did well and came back for a release on the opposite wrist. A resident and I did this case together; unfortunately, he did poorly after the surgery. I later went back and explored his wrist and found that we had injured his median nerve, which I then repaired. This complication should be rare. It should not have happened. He was forgiving and empathetic with our disappointment in his result.

Malpractice Threats

Another area of stress is the threat of malpractice lawsuits. Fundamentally, most surgeons tried to do the right thing by doing for their patients what they would do for one of their family members.

Litigation

During the time of breast implant controversy in the 1990s, Houston was a real hotbed for litigation, partly because this was where the silicon implant originated and was so popular. But perhaps more importantly, because Texas was such a favorable state for plaintiff's attorneys. To keep these implant cases in Texas state court, the plaintiff's attorneys included the implanting plastic surgeon in each of these lawsuits.

Usually, after a year or so, the doctor would be dropped while the manufacturer would remain in the suit. Apparently, in some states, the plastic surgeon was not named in these suits, but only the implant manufacturers. To show how crazy things got, one day, I was getting ready to enter an exam room to see the next patient. I looked at the chart and noticed it was an old implant patient who was on the list of implant patients suing me. I checked to be sure and then went into the room to see her. She was very cordial and just wanted a follow-up check as she was doing fine. After I had finished the exam and I answered her questions, I said: "did you know that you are suing me"? I thought she was going to faint; she was so taken aback. She said, "No. I did go to a lawyer, but I never gave him permission to do anything."

During my 38 years of private practice in plastic surgery, I never lost a malpractice case. I have been sued for malpractice about 40 times. However, three dozen of those suits were breast implant cases that arose out of the controversy as to whether silicone made people sick. Although the implant crisis was very disconcerting and took about ten years to resolve, eventually, I was dropped from all those cases. Other litigation issues were more specific and personal.

Vocal cord paralysis

I was named in a suit by a patient who suffered a vocal cord paralysis after a thyroidectomy done by a general surgery colleague of mine. Vocal cord paralysis is a known but unusual complication of thyroidectomy surgery. I did not participate or assist in any way in the thyroidectomy. However, at the same operating session, I did a small dermabrasion procedure on the patient's cheeks. Even though this dermabrasion had nothing to do with vocal cord paralysis, the plaintiff's attorney sued me. I consider this to have been a frivolous and unjustified suit. About a year later, they dropped me from the case. Of course, I had the bother of dealing with my defense attorneys and medical records, etc.

Congenital facial reconstruction

In another case, I had done multiple operations on a patient born with severe congenital deformities. One of these procedures involved taking a rib from the patient and placing it to construct a large missing part of the lower jaw. She obtained a very nice result from all of these procedures. I thought I had a good relationship with this patient and the family. I did remember they had sued the manufacturer of an anti-nausea medication widely used in pregnant women. Anyway, I received notice of the suit, which stated that I had reconstructed her jaw" backward." This action on their part personally hurt me. However, this ludicrous suit never caused me much worry because I knew she had gotten such an excellent result. My defense lawyer got this case dropped within a few months.

Infected breast reconstruction case

I had a patient in the early 1990s when the implant scare began on whom I performed a flap reconstruction with a silicone gel implant for additional volume. She developed an infection around the implant a few days later, and I had to remove the implant. She and her husband became angry and went somewhere else for care. They sued the implant manufacturer and me. About a year later, they dropped me from the suit. I felt terrible and was sorry she had this complication.

Malocclusion

I assisted Dr. Paul Tessier in a case that involved the repositioning of the upper and lower jaw on a patient who had some facial deformity. Postoperatively the midline of her occlusion was slightly off compared to the soft tissue—a resulting suit named Dr. Tessier and me, although I had a minor role in this case. The process lasted more than a year. Eventually, there was a nonsuit.

Bedsore

The family of a patient who developed a bedsore in the hospital sued the hospital and all the doctors who were involved in the patient's care. The patient's primary care doctor asked me to treat the patient's bedsore. I performed local debridement and cleaning of the wound and redoubled the precautions for avoiding pressure. The problem developed before I was involved with the case. They eventually dropped me from the suit. However, the process was disconcerting because it did cost me time and effort and the resources of my malpractice carrier. I believe this was another example of a frivolous lawsuit.

I was fortunate to never go to trial for any malpractice suit since I went into practice in 1978. Also, I never had to settle any malpractice suit from my 38 years of private practice.

Lost Finger

However, there was a case going back to my senior year of training as a plastic surgery resident, the year before I went into practice. I took care of a small child about six years old who had his hand crushed between his mother's car and a tree as she was backing her car out of the driveway. The injury was significant, with fractures of a couple of fingers and significant soft tissue injury.

I saw the patient in the emergency room and ascertained he needed to go to the operating room for surgery. I notified my on-call staff surgeon, who told me to go ahead and take the patient to the operating room and call him back. Today, this would not be allowed; residents now have to have their staff surgeon present in the operating room. However, back in 1978, things were much less regulated. After reviewing x-rays and getting the patient to the operating room and looking closely at the injuries, I called my supervising staff back. He told me to go ahead and pin the fractures and close the wounds. So, I pinned the fractures and close the wound and put on a dressing with a splint the next morning when I saw the patient one of the fingers look like it had limited blood supply but would probably survive. If I had recognized the vascular compromise at that time, I still would not have been able to do anything to cure that situation.

Microsurgery for traumatic vascular finger injuries was in its infancy. When I saw the patient back in the office a few days later, it was apparent that one finger was not going to survive because it lacked adequate blood supply. I needed to take the patient back again to surgery a few days later and amputate the dead finger. Sometime later, I was named in a malpractice suit and, after consultation with my defense attorney, agreed to settle this case for a nominal amount, which I believe was $3000. I don't think that I did anything wrong with this case except underestimating the severity of the crush injury. If I had prepared the parents for the inevitable result, which was caused by the original injury but not fully appreciated in a timely way by myself, there probably would have been no suit. During my 38 years of private practice, I never lost or had to settle a malpractice suit with any payment.

In 2003 a reform of Texas law regarding malpractice suits called proposition 12 limited non-economic recoveries from malpractice suits. This law seems to have had a significant effect on lowering the number of malpractice suits, especially those which might be termed frivolous.

Death

One thing that is often wrong about our current medical system is medical personnel aggressively performing too much futile care on patients during their last days. Often such aggressive care is at the instigation of the patient's family. Often a patient, who would be best off, dying at home with friends and family nearby, is brought into the hospital placed in the intensive care unit and is subjected to multiple tubes and lines that only delay the inevitable while making it more challenging to come to peace with his loved ones, and God. I believe that it is essential that the treatment be proportional to what we are treating. Although, as a specialty, plastic surgery deals with death, less frequently than many other fields of medicine, I had some insight into such cases because I was on the ethics committee at my hospital. In that capacity, I came to appreciate the guidance given by *The Ethical and Religious Directives for Catholic Health Care Services.*

Unfortunately, over 38 years of extensive practice, I encountered the stress, frustration, and feeling of hopelessness dealing with the death of patients. One particularly sad case was that of "Victoria." She was born with giant congenital hairy nevi. The largest one covered her upper chest and back like a T-shirt, as in the pictures below.

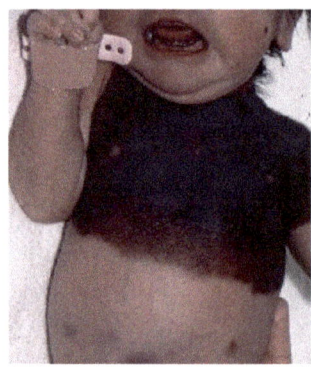
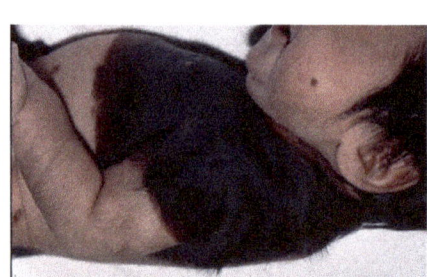

Besides, it's obvious disfigurement this entity also presents a medical dilemma because these nevi can degenerate into melanoma. The rate of such transformation is probably proportional to both the size of the nevus and the amount of pigment, especially how dark it is. With this in mind and with cooperation from the baby's mother, we embarked on a long process involving multiple surgeries to remove this and other darkly pigmented lesions she had over her body.

Many of the procedures included tissue expansion with expandable balloons placed under adjacent healthy skin that were then injected with saline over time to stretch the surface, just as a woman's abdominal skin stretches in the last months of her pregnancy. After obtaining more skin this way, I surgically removed sections of the primary lesion. I repeated this process several times. Because of the size and nature of the nevus, I also used split-thickness skin grafts as well. Although I excised the majority of the congenital nevi, some remained.

Despite this aggressive treatment, this child developed melanoma as a teenager. Her oncologists treated her with both surgery and chemotherapy. She did well for several years and had one child herself. However, the melanoma was relentless and spread throughout her body. In her last days, she received hospice care at home with her family. I visited her with two ladies who worked in my office and had become close to her. It was heartbreaking to see a young life brought down that way by metastatic melanoma. I believe she was glad to see us come to her home to visit. She died shortly after that. I reflect on John Donne's 17th meditation. "God's hand is in every translation, and his hand shall bind up all our scattered leaves again. … so this bell calls us all,". and "No man is an island, entire of itself."

Another patient, "Marshal," was a cardiac surgery patient who had an infection of his operative site, causing a non- healing wound of his sternum (breast bone) and rib cage after coronary artery bypass surgery. The thoracic surgeon had gone back to try to close the open sternum, but it again failed to heal. The thoracic surgeon asked me to see him in consultation to help close the wound. When I first saw the patient, he was quite ill with somewhat unstable vital signs. After removing the dressings from the chest, I could see his heart beating in the depths of the wound.

I decided to do several days of dressing changes, packing the wound with gauze to try to get it as clean as possible. I waited for several days to optimize "Marshals" medical condition. When he seemed to be in as good shape as possible, I proceeded with the surgery. He was the patriarch of his family and fought very hard to get well. He had extensive family support throughout his ordeal.

I performed multiple muscle flaps taking both pectoralis chest muscles, as well as one abdominal rectus muscle. I used these flaps to fill in and repair the defect in the chest wall. The operation seemed to go well; however, in the postoperative course, the patient developed an abnormal bleeding problem. He began to bleed from all the wound surfaces. It was necessary to transfuse him with several units of blood. I took him back to surgery to remove all the blood clots and to control the bleeding better. I consulted extensively with his thoracic surgeon and with a hematologist.

I remember that I had planned to go to San Antonio to see the Pope and attend an outdoor Mass but had to send my family without me because I needed to tend this sick man. His condition deteriorated over several days. His heart was not healthy enough for the trauma involved in his surgeries, and he died while still in the intensive care unit. His death was a sad defeat for everyone.

"Xavier" was a Nigerian physician who had been in prison at home because of political oppression. He escaped and immigrated to the U S. He was not able to practice medicine because of licensing issues. He presented to my office with a large mass protruding from the right side of his scalp. The lesion was five to 7 cm in diameter and about 2 centimeters thick. There was some ulceration in the center, and a small amount of bleeding had occurred. He said that it had only been present for about three weeks. If the history was accurate, this had to be a very aggressive tumor.

There was no evidence of the spread of cancer to lymph nodes in the neck nor any sign of distance spread. After getting some preliminary tests and laboratory work, I talked about the possibilities and our course of action. I took "Xavier" to the operating room and removed the mass with a two to 3 cm margin of the normal-looking scalp. Unfortunately, the pathologist reported the lesion was an angiosarcoma, and all the margins were involved with tumor on frozen sections! Angiosarcoma is a very aggressive tumor, which is usually rapidly growing and fatal; they are notoriously difficult to cure.

Initially, getting a free margin around the cancer is often impossible. The cure rate is only about 5%. I persisted with additional much more extensive excisions until the pathologist reported the final specimens were free of tumor. By then, the scalp defect was more than 6 inches in diameter and down to a thin layer over the skull.

I took a sizeable split-thickness skin graft from his thigh and placed it to repair the raw area of the scalp. His initial postoperative course was very smooth. However, we recommended consultation with both the radiation therapist and a medical oncologist as he might need both radiation therapy and chemotherapy. A few days later, the permanent pathology report arrived. Tragically this report differed from the frozen section report I received at the time of surgery. It indicated residual cancer at the margins of my resection.

Again, postoperatively I discussed therapeutic options with my patient. Postoperatively I recommended he obtain consultations regarding chemotherapy and radiation therapy. He did get several second opinions but did not want to begin additional treatment immediately. Within a few weeks on a follow-up visit, the tumor was so aggressive that there were several small growths visible around the periphery of the previous excision. This cancer was swift-moving!

He was placed on multiple chemotherapeutic agents, which caused the tumors to regress for a while, but did not cure him. Throughout his ordeal, he would come back to our office every week or so to let us know how he was doing. He became very friendly with all the staff in my office, and I believe he received encouragement and some emotional strength from that interaction. Eventually, the tumor spread to his lungs and other distant locations. He ultimately succumbed to this terrible form of cancer.

I remember quite well a teenage cleft lip and palate patient "Thomas" from another large city in Texas. I performed significant surgery on him, including a rhinoplasty, movement of the jaw forward, and a genioplasty, which also brought his chin forward. He obtained greatly improved aesthetic results. The profile view went from a very abnormal retrusion of the midface to a standard facial profile configuration. After one of his surgeries, he had cardiac arrhythmia for a short time, which we treated. He was able to leave the hospital after a couple of days. We followed him postoperatively, and he healed nicely.

About a year and a half later, we got a call from his mother who wanted to let us know that since the surgery, her son was the happiest he'd ever been in his life. She attributed this to the improvement he experienced in his self-image after the surgery. However, she sadly told us that while he was in a classroom at school, he had a sudden cardiac arrest and died. Everyone in the office knew this boy to be a very nice young man, and we were all taken aback and very sad.

I remember "Mrs. Smith," an octogenarian who initially had breast cancer, was treated by surgery and radiation, and later developed a sarcoma because of the radiation. Her oncologic surgeon asked me to help him with the closure of a wound after he was going to resect a recurrent sarcoma of the left chest wall. She was a rather frail older lady with a very attentive daughter-in-law. I explained our part in the proposed surgery. The general surgeon removed the recurrent tumor, and I designed a rotation flap for closure of the wound. The extirpative operation was palliative, not curative.

She did well for a couple of days and left the hospital only to come back a few days later because a small portion of the wound had pulled apart. At the bedside, I added some additional sutures under local anesthesia to close the wound. She did fine, and I discharged her home to New Braunfels, a small town about 150 miles from Houston. I saw her in the office periodically over the next few months when she came to see the surgical oncologist.

Although she healed from her surgery, she seemed to be growing weaker each time I saw her. Her oncologist had nothing more to offer for her. It was summertime and quite hot all the time. Every summer, my family goes to New Braunfels for a family reunion, so I arranged to go by and see Mrs. Smith during my vacation. I brought her a CD of very soothing Gregorian chant music. Her daughter in law showed me to her room where she was in bed but alert and conversive. She seemed very happy to see me, although we certainly did not know each other all that well. It was a small effort to go by and see her. I was pleased with her response. A few weeks later, the daughter-in-law called our office to let us know Mrs. Smith had peacefully passed away. I'm so glad I went by to see her.

Another failure that I will never forget involves an older man who was a heavy smoker and drinker. He came complaining of a chronic sore throat. I found no mass or ulcer to explain the pain. He did have some redness in the back of his throat, and I was suspicious of cancer. I did take him to the operating room and, under general anesthesia, scrutinized the pharynx and obtained multiple random biopsies. He had a chronic inflammatory picture, as might be seen in a heavy smoker. The biopsies were negative for cancer but showed some mild pre-cancerous changes. I saw him a few more times over several months but eventually lost him to follow up. A few years later, I found out that he had developed throat cancer and had passed away. Perhaps if I had been still more persistent with additional biopsies, I might have made the diagnosis sooner, with a different outcome.

Another patient was a coach in a nearby high school. His history was notable in that he had had a liver transplant 14 years earlier. Because of that, he was on immunosuppressant medications, which was why he was developing many skin cancers. On initial examination, he had some conspicuous skin cancer lesions of the scalp. I ordered a CAT scan, which did not show any bony involvement. I took him to surgery and excise multiple squamous cell skin cancers of the scalp. I, therefore, had to reconstruct his scalp with a split-thickness skin graft. He also had several lesions on the cheeks, forehead, and temporal regions, which I removed. It was only about six months later that several new skin cancers popped up.

These lesions were proliferating because of his depressed immune system. He repeatedly returned for additional surgery for squamous cell cancers on the scalp and facial area; I had about six major surgical sessions with him to remove significant skin cancers. He always healed well from these surgeries. Finally, after I took care of him for about five years, he had to go to another location for medical care because of a change in his insurance coverage. About ten months after that, his family notified us that he had developed cancer of the kidney and died.

There was a young African-American woman "La Kesha" with extensive inflammatory breast cancer. Her oncology surgeon referred her to me to help close the wound after a proposed mastectomy. Inflammatory breast cancer is far more aggressive than other types. When I examined her before her surgery, she had a large mass of the breast, which was growing out through the skin. Her surgeon planned an extensive excision and wanted me to close the wound without reconstructing the breast. At the time of surgery, the surgeon kept having to get wider and wider margins, which left a significant defect. I brought a TRAM flap up from the abdomen to cover the wound. However, within a matter of several weeks, there was evidence of recurrent cancer on the surface of her chest. She died a few months after her mastectomy surgery. The surgery was probably not really of any benefit to her. These cases are tragic. It's hard to figure out why some people have good luck and others such bad luck.

I remember fondly a middle-aged lady "Mary" I saw in consultation for a rhinoplasty. Apparently, since her teenage years, she had been unhappy with a large hump on her nose but was afraid to have surgery. Later in life, she finally garnered enough courage and had the means to address this problem. I performed a reduction rhinoplasty, which was quite successful and gave her significant satisfaction. A few years later, I was happy she came to see me for a facelift. I performed a rhytidectomy on her, and she did quite well. Unfortunately, a few years later, her daughter called to let our office know that "Mary" had developed pancreatic cancer and died within six months of her diagnosis.

Incomplete Cases

Because my practice was cut short by illness, I was not able to finish a few complex reconstructions which I had begun on some of my patients. One such patient is "Sue" shown below. She had an absent eye on the left, with distortion of the left face and forehead. She had a cleft lip and palate on the right. She had a vertically short maxilla and mandible on the left and a low set ear.

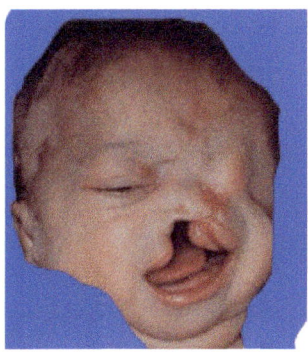 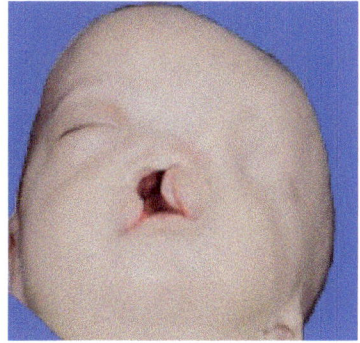

I repaired the cleft lip at about three months of age and the palate at about a year. Those procedures helped "Sue" functionally with eating and initiating speech. Her status, after lip and palate repair, is below.

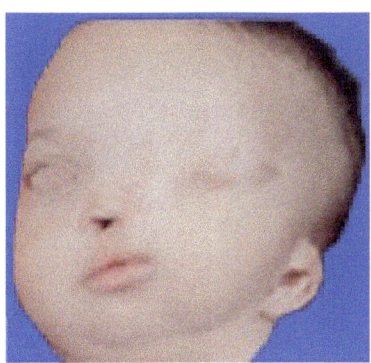 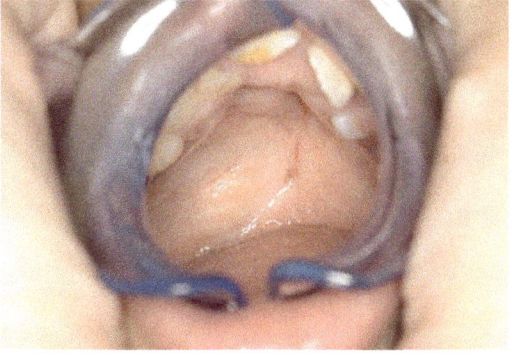

At her next operation, I placed a silicone sphere into the inchoate orbit on the left. The purpose of the sphere was to stimulate the growth of the bone around the orbit. The presence of the ocular globe creates part of the stimulus for orbital bone growth. This procedure was repeated a few times with successively larger spheres in anticipation of eventually utilizing an eye prosthesis on the left. Intermediate stages are below.

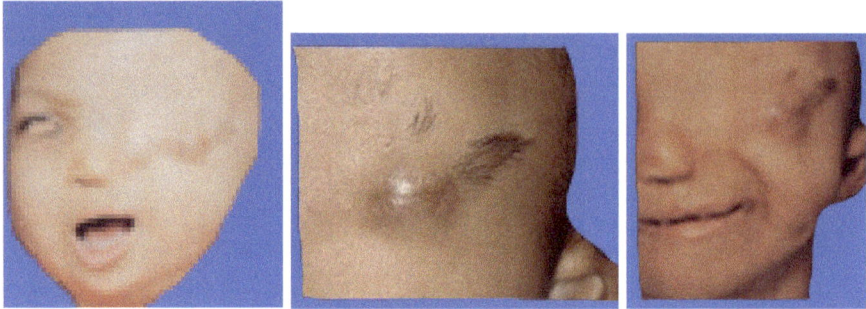

Next, I did a hemi-nasal reconstruction with a forehead flap (as with "Charles chapter 6) and rib graft to the nose. In the pictures below, she has only a right-sided nose.

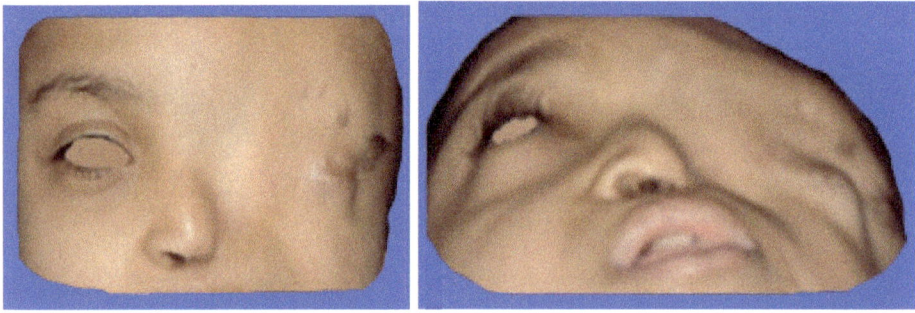

Below are postoperative photos after the three-stage forehead flap hemi-nasal reconstruction.

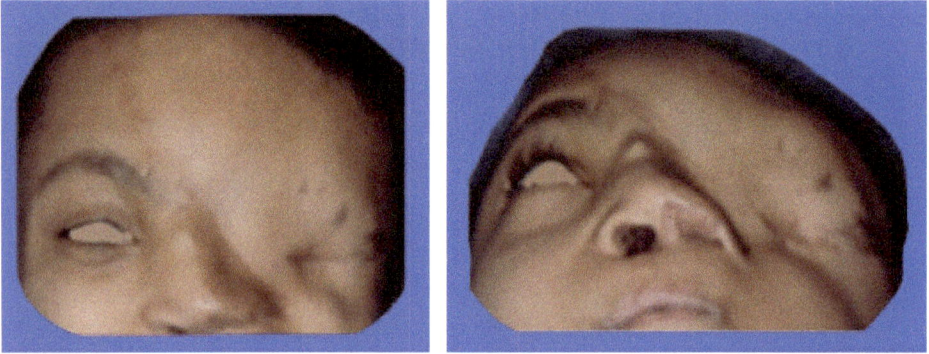

At this point, I had repaired the cleft lip and palate repair, a hemi nasal reconstruction, and some orbital expansion. She will need additional major procedures over several years, including reshaping of the forehead, osteotomies, and bone grafts of the upper and lower jaw to lengthen the left side of the face vertically, a genioplasty to bring the chin forward, and an ocular prosthesis and ear reconstruction. She seems to be a happy child. She has tolerated her difficulties better than may have been expected. I regret that I am unable to help her reach her fully reconstructed potential.

I also had another patient, "Bobbie," who was born without a left eye and had only a hemi right nose. He had a large cleft of the palate and a severely constricted left face. He had had some previous surgery for closure of a facial cleft. I was able to perform a forehead flap for left nasal reconstruction. I also did an Abbe flap to expand the upper lip. I also place orbital spheres to expand the left orbit. When I retired, he still needed significant major surgery to complete his reconstruction. "Bobbie" would routinely ask when we would be finished with his operations and more poignantly "when will I look normal, doctor Cronin." Unfortunately, I never had a satisfying answer for him.

Fame and fortune

The late 70s and 1980s, when I was a young surgeon, were heady times in plastic surgery at the Cronin Brauer and Biggs Clinic, the premier plastic surgery group in Houston. The group ran the independent plastic surgery residency program at St. Joseph Hospital. The clinic was well respected, and we had frequent visitors of plastic surgeons from all over the world, including most Latin American countries, England, France, Germany, Japan, China, etc. They came mainly to visit with Dr. Thomas D Cronin, Raymond O Brauer, and Thomas Biggs.

Many were well known or famous, while others were inchoate, adding to their education by visiting prominent practices. Dr. Thomas Cronin was avuncular but extremely inquisitive. He invited erudite surgeons to visit Houston, so we all could learn and welcomed nascent surgeons as well. Those were halcyon times before some of our current issues with managed care, unrestrained advertising, and defensive medicine were so prominent. I recall that we had two visiting doctors from China who showed us a presentation of free tissue forearm flap reconstructions. This new technique, unknown to us before then, impressed us. Subsequently, this flap has become quite useful and part of the standard plastic surgery operative armamentarium.

Besides working with my well-known mentors, I was privileged to participate in the yearly visits of Dr. Paul Tessier, who was probably the most famous plastic surgeon in the world at that time. I assisted Dr. Tessier in most of the cases he did from 1978 to 1989 in Houston. I was very fortunate during my career to work with many famous plastic surgeons. I may occasionally have felt jealous of some of the renowned and well accomplished plastic surgeons with whom I met. However, when I think of two American plastic surgeons, quite renowned and famous, whom I knew personally, unfortunately, I am reminded of Edward Arlington Robinson's poem "Richard Cory." That's when I know I must count my blessings and also that we never know the full story of others with whom we may be envious.

Joys of Plastic surgery

One of the blessings I truly appreciate has been working with so many wonderful sisters, nurses, surgical techs., residents, and ancillary personnel and even administrators at St. Joseph Hospital.

The practice of medicine is a privilege granted by the state to individuals who have fulfilled the prescribed requirements. The specific practice of plastic surgery is not so directly regulated by the state as it is indirectly by hospital privileges and by quasi-governmental agencies such as the American Board of Medical Specialties and the American Board of Plastic Surgery. I feel grateful every day for the opportunity of having practiced plastic surgery for more than 38 years. It is a wonderful field. I was fortunate to treat a tremendous variety of patients and perform a powerful array of procedures.

I would never have been able to get through medical school and seven years of residency to prepare myself for the field of plastic surgery if it not been for my wife, Candy. I am totally indebted to her. Having a stable situation to come home to after experiencing the vicissitudes encountered daily in the practice of medicine has been incredible. Many of my classmates were married during medical school only to have their marriages end in divorce soon after graduation or during the trying times of residency training.

Once I had proven myself, through medical school and prerequisite surgical training, having the support and encouragement of my uncle Thomas Cronin was a real blessing. Training with him as a resident for two years was exciting and enlightening. Joining him in practice was a great honor. I was lucky enough to be able to practice with him and doctors Brauer, Biggs, Wolf, and Cohen for the following ten years. It was an exciting and dynamic time for the development of the field of plastic surgery. Such things as microvascular surgery, myo-cutaneous flaps, lasers, and liposuction became part of the field of plastic surgery during that time.

When our practice split up in 1988, it was quite satisfying that no attorney was involved. We accomplished an amicable resolution to all the complex issues with only the aid of our accountant. Since that time, I have been quite fortunate in having a partner with whom I am so compatible. Dr. Benjamin Cohen is a highly accomplished plastic surgeon, totally ethical and trustworthy. He and I formed a new group as the former one dissolved. It was a real joy for us to have our partnership for more than 25 years. We were fortunate from the start as we searched for new employees. We interviewed two young ladies, one for the position of insurance clerk and one as the receptionist. They seem so good we hired Janine and Elizabeth on the spot. After a few years, the receptionist became our office manager and held that position for more than ten years. The lady, who was the first insurance clerk, succeeded as the office manager later and was still in that position when I retired.

My partner and I have been very fortunate with our office staff. We have always tried to cultivate a pleasant working environment. We have been relatively flexible at times with life situations such as pregnancy leave, the need for flex scheduling, and the need for dealing with family issues of our employees. In turn, our employees have been most loyal and ethical.

Grateful patients can make the surgeon's day joyful. Patients appreciate friendly and respectful treatment. Sometimes it is hard to understand the reaction of patients to plastic surgery. Some patients are inherently optimistic and positive thinkers. They tend to react well, no matter what happens. They seem to be understanding when things do not work out as well as expected. Patients are quite appreciative and thankful for the excellent results we usually obtain for them. It's easy to use a proverbial baseball analogy for the judging results of plastic surgery. It is exciting when I hit a home run by obtaining a particularly good result from surgery. What is especially joyful is that circumstance when the patient also recognizes that they have been the recipient of such a home run result.

I've been quite fortunate to have excellent colleagues with which to work. Originally Dr. Thomas Cronin and Dr. Raymond Brauer and Dr. Tom Biggs were my mentors and colleagues. They were gentlemen wonderful with which to work, always professional with the best interests of their patients foremost.

Because of our residency training program, I worked closely with a nucleus of young plastic surgeons. Doctors Bruce Smith, Don Collins, and Leo La Puerta were core faculty for our residents. Also, we had an adjunct faculty of outstanding, competent plastic surgeons, including Doctors Alfonso Barrera, Camile Cash, Rafi Bidros, Robert Kratschmer, Lee Steely, Jim Boynton, and others.

Another gratifying and positive aspect of my practice of plastic surgery has been working at St. Joseph Medical Center with St Joseph/Methodist

Residency plastic surgery residents. Every year two new plastic surgery residents came to the program, and two would graduate and go out into the private practice of plastic surgery or possibly to do some additional fellowship training.

They are usually quite appreciative of what we were able to teach them.

Most residents were eager to show their mettle and to learn everything they could about plastic surgery. It has been great to work with residents as they were often very enthusiastic and brought new ideas with them from which I undoubtedly benefited. I was also fortunate to be able to work with residents from the University of Texas Health Science Ctr., Houston, and the University of Texas Medical Branch at Galveston, who would rotate to St. Joseph Hospital.

Another source of great enjoyment was working at Shriners Hospital. After several changes at St. Joseph Hospital, I decided to move the Cronin and Brauer cleft palate clinic to the Shriners Hospital for Children Houston in 2014. The Cronin and Brauer Cleft Palate Clinic merged with the existing cleft palate program at Shriners Hospital under the direction of Dr. Steve Blackwell. This merger produced a program with an expanded team of specialists and services available to the cleft palate patient and family. For about 2 1/2 years, I was able to do cleft lip and palate surgery at the Shriners Hospital and enjoyed very much working with residents there.

Honors

Some of the joy of plastic surgery personally was being recognized for my professional work.

I was delighted that my co-authors and I received first place at the 113th annual session of the Texas Medical Association scientific exhibit for "Reconstruction of the Breast after Mastectomy" Houston 1980. It was an honor to serve as President of the Houston Society of Plastic Surgeons 1993 – 1994.

Also, I received the Irish Houstonian Award from The Shalom Center of the Diocese of Galveston Houston in 1995. I recall a priest who worked at the center made the presentation. He took my hands, thanked me, and then spoke eloquently about the duty, responsibility, and privilege of using them to help my patients. In 1995 my family received the St. Martin de Porres award from the Southern Dominicans for Service to the Church, Family Values, and Medical Care for the Indigent. I was also very fortunate to be recommended for the Jefferson Award by a former breast reconstruction patient of mine. My wife and I traveled to Washington DC, where I received a Jefferson Award presented by Texas Sen. Kay Bailey Hutchison (a lovely lady!) in the capital building in 1998. The experience was unforgettable.

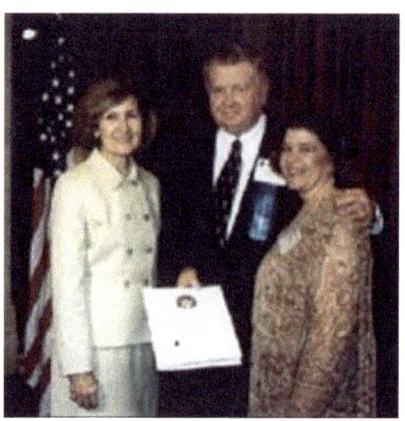

I have always been very appreciative of all the help I have been given over the years by nurses and ancillary medical personnel. So, one of the honors of which I am most proud is the Distinguished Surgeon Award, presented by the Association of Operating Room Nurses of Greater Houston at their first Triple Star Gala in 1998. As a bonus, my wife and I had the opportunity to meet President George H Walker Bush and have dinner with him at the River Oaks Country Club on that occasion. It was interesting observing his secret service escorts. He was very personable, friendly, and approachable, as indicated by the following story.

We all had a mushroom soup course, which was very good. President Bush really liked it because when almost finished, he put his spoon down and lifted the bowel to his mouth by its two small handles and finished it off. Well, you can guess what happened. Next, nine more people at that table did precisely the same thing, and everyone got a laugh about that. He was a very likable man. For a time, we frequented the same local grocery store, and my wife said he was going in the store at the same time as she was, and he stopped and said "after you little lady" and let her enter first. Another time she went to the frozen yogurt counter to get a treat, and the President happened to be there, and again, he invited her to go first.

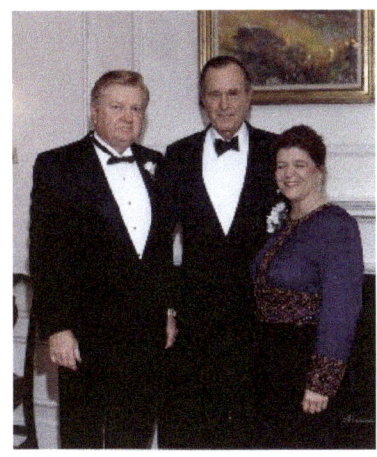

A famous television celebrity in Houston for decades was Marvin Zindler, who accompanied me on several Operation San Jose medical mission trips to Latin America. He had the opportunity to observe many operations that I performed on these trips. I had the chance to be one of "Marvin's Angels" by offering to take care of several needy patients whom he brought to my practice over the years. I was delighted when March 1st, 2000, on the KPRC TV channel in Houston, he said: "Dr. Cronin is one of the finest plastic surgeons in the country." I was pleased to serve as the Chief of Staff of St. Joseph Hospital 2002 to 2004. In 2003 I received The Dawn of Hope Award presented by the Helping Hands Medical Mission organization.

It was an honor to receive an award for the best member paper at the 2004 annual meeting of the Texas Society of plastic surgeons.

I was pleased to serve as President of the Texas Society of plastic surgeons 2009 – 2010. I was grateful to be recognized as Hometown Hero - Outstanding Volunteer by Halliburton at NRG Stadium at a Houston Texan game in 2011.

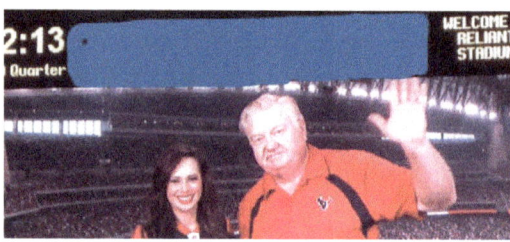 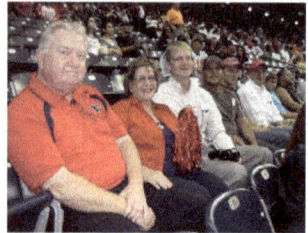

Another event for which I am grateful was the Board of my high school alma mater electing me to the St. Thomas High School Hall of Honor in 2012. I was especially pleased that, at that ceremony, a classmate of mine, Father Drew Wood, introduced me. He might have reminded me at that time that, as a high school student, he had dated my future wife years before I did. In 2013, my wife and I were Legacy Award recipients of the Christus Foundation for Healthcare. We had the pleasure of having a nice dinner the night before with Regis Philbin, who was the keynote speaker at the award luncheon. We both found him to be very skillful at getting to know a lot about everyone at our table, even those who were not particularly outgoing.

Although this section about the joys of plastic surgery may be quite short, it is because this entire book is a celebration of the pleasures of working in the field of plastic surgery. Indeed, I have also had many personal family blessings. All of my eight children are doing well; they are all married, productive members of society, and outstanding people. They have given my wife Candy and me 28 beautiful grandchildren, with one on the way at this time.

As I look back on my medical career and consider all the various awards which I have received, I am grateful for all my blessings. Although I believe I always tried to do my best for my patients, I feel bad for those patients under my care who did not get an optimum result. I am especially sorry for any patients who may have been harmed by my actions no matter how well-intended.

Chapter 14

The Place of Functional Plastic Surgery in the Healing Mission

Functional plastic surgery is surgery performed on abnormal structures of the body caused by congenital defects, trauma, infections, tumors to improve function, cure disease, or relieve symptoms.

Tumors benign and malignant

Various childhood vascular "birthmarks" are quite common. The most prevalent type, infantile hemangioma, usually appears in the first few weeks of life. Its natural history is to increase for a few months and then stabilize. I often leave them alone because many will spontaneously involute by age seven. Some hemangiomas leave almost no residual defect. However, most are reduced to an area of thin skin and subcutaneous tissue that will need a revision anyway. I recommended simple excision for "Caleb" below because I anticipated an excellent result that would obviate the potential issues of possible bleeding or infection in the lesion. More apropos excision would alleviate the parents' anxiety and worry over several years.

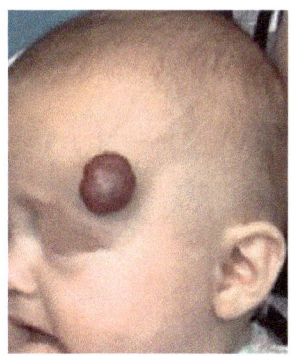 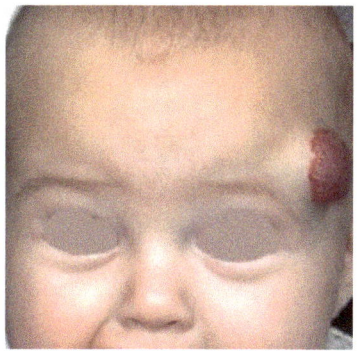

I did a simple elliptical excision and closure, as outlined below. The postoperative result is after a few months.

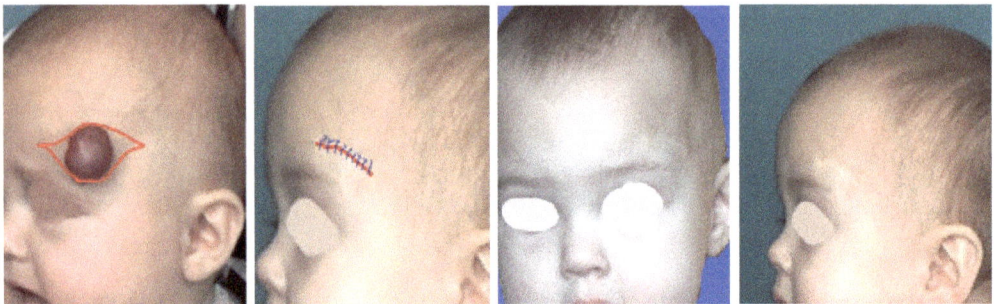

Baby "Markum" below demonstrates that sometimes this type of lesion will" outgrow its blood supply and spontaneously necrose and bleed. Of course, this can be a big nuisance and, on occasion, even life-threateningly dangerous.

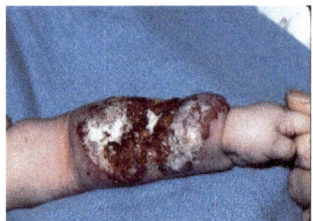

I treated another patient "Annie," below with simple elliptical excision and closure of the wound.

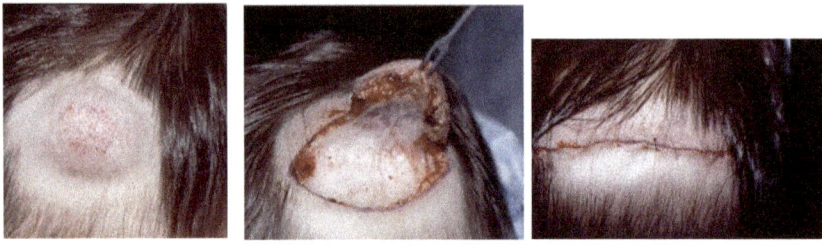

Another typical congenital lesion is a preauricular pit or sinus. Such sinuses are best left alone if asymptomatic. They can cause trouble if they get infected or enlarge, as shown in the three examples below.

The Healing Mission of Plastic Surgery

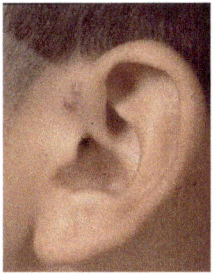 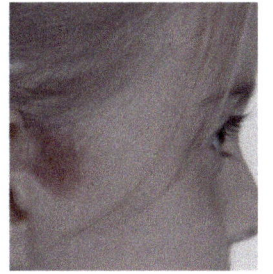 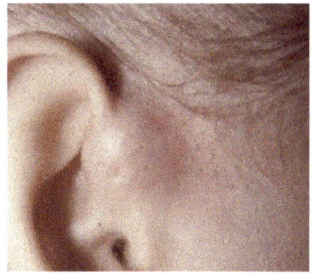

If they are symptomatic, I first rid them of infection and then excise the whole sinus. The pit typically goes deeper than is obvious, and I have found that one needs to remove some ear cartilage to cure the lesion. I have routinely used a mixture of methylene blue and hydrogen peroxide to instill into the sinus. The blue color lines the tract and marks any extensions, which ensures complete excision of the lesion, as demonstrated in the drawing below.

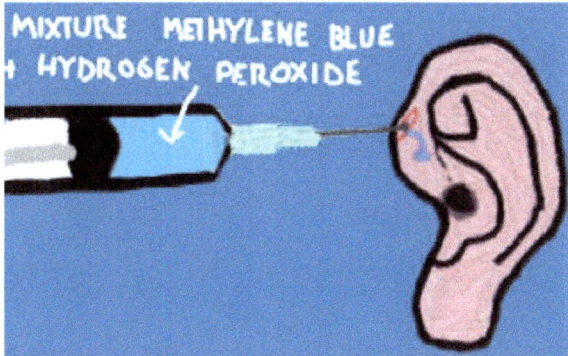

I delineate a sinus tract below left, and one can see the faint blue dye (also pointed out by the blue arrows) at the sinus skin surface held by the forceps and in the depth of the wound near the small retractor. In the middle photo, a flexible metal probe extends from the skin pit to the excised cartilage in the removed specimen.

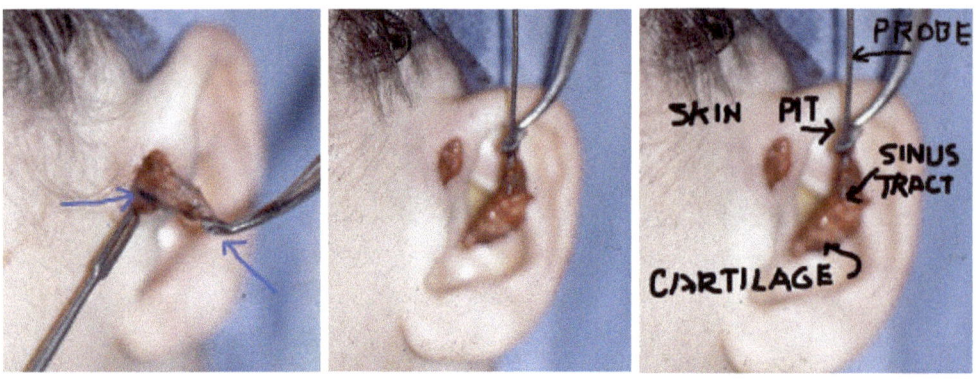

The drawing below illustrates the specimen includes the pit and the entire tract, including some ear cartilage. The post-op photo is on the right below.

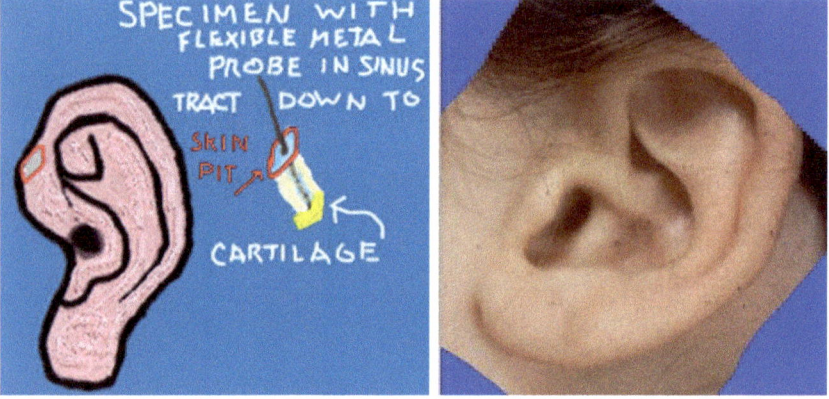

The patient below," Meg," came to see me at the insistence of her daughter. The patient was reluctant, because she was afraid she might have cancer and did not want to face that. Her lesion did not have any characteristics that made me suspect cancer. I removed a benign cystic lesion, and she was healing well on her return office visit. The preoperative forehead mass (left) and her early result (right) are below.

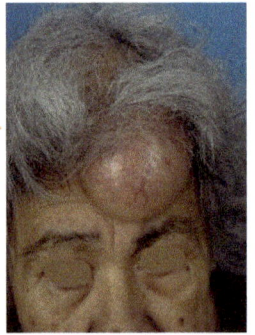 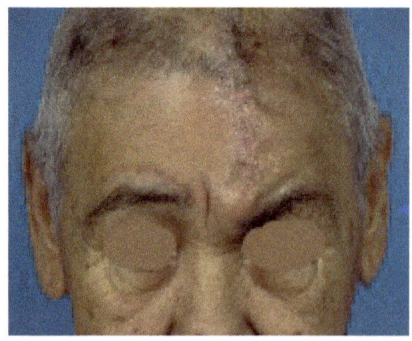

Salivary gland tumor

Salivary tumors can arise in the parotid gland in the cheek, in the submaxillary gland, just under the lower jaw, in sublingual and in tiny minor glands throughout the oral cavity. The drawing below shows the approximate location of these glands.

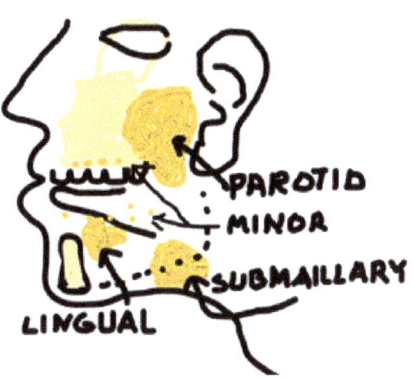

Parotid tumors are the most common, followed by submaxillary and sublingual gland tumors. Minor salivary gland tumors are much less common.

"Sean" had a painless, firm swelling develop in the left preauricular area over a few years. Fine needle biopsy indicated it to be the most common type of parotid salivary gland tumor, a benign mixed tumor or pleomorphic adenoma. These tumors consist of a mixture of cell types, hence the moniker. About 20% of parotid gland tumors are malignant.

The mainstay of treatment is excision with careful preservation of the facial nerve, which runs right through the gland, and separates it into a superficial and deep lobe. The first photo below shows the proposed incision outlined in blue ink. I marked the mass with blue dots. The second photo shows the skin flap elevated to expose the tumor, circled in blue. I use a standard method of protecting the vulnerable facial nerve while excising parotid tumors. I first identify the nerve (yellow), which is found deep just below the ear canal right after it exits the base of the skull.

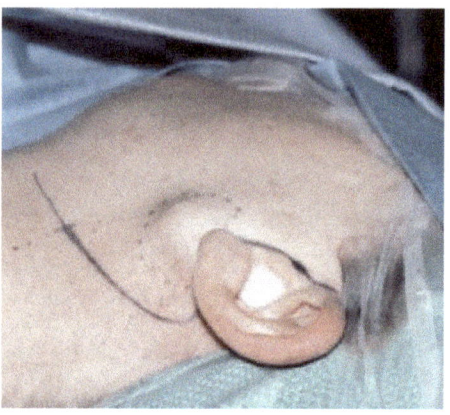
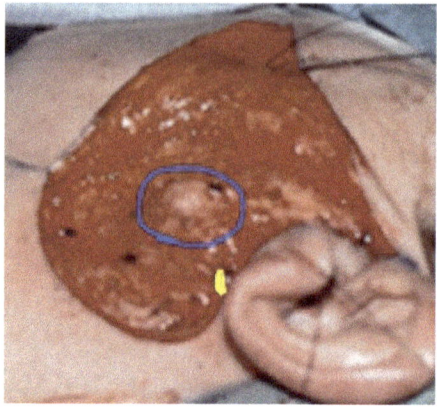

I can then follow the nerve distally, dissecting the superficial lobe while protecting the nerve, which bisects the outer and deep portions of the parotid gland. The necessity of careful dissection right on the surface of the nerve branches of the facial nerve makes this procedure rather intense. There always seem to be a lot of small obscuring "bleeders" all along the way! The first drawing below indicates the mass in the more shallow portion on top of the facial nerve. The second drawing represents the superficial lobe, including the tumor dissected off the nerve.

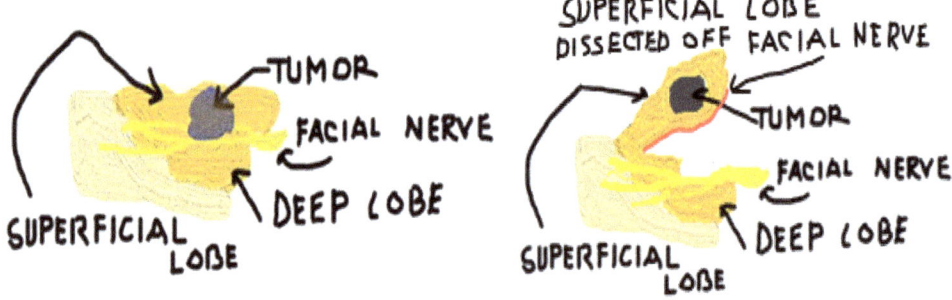

The photo drawing below illustrates the operation. I marked the tumor in dark blue and its previous location in light blue and the facial nerve in yellow. The photo shows I have almost wholly excised the superficial lobe and the tumor. The surgical specimen includes the external portion of the parotid gland and pleomorphic adenoma (mixed tumor).

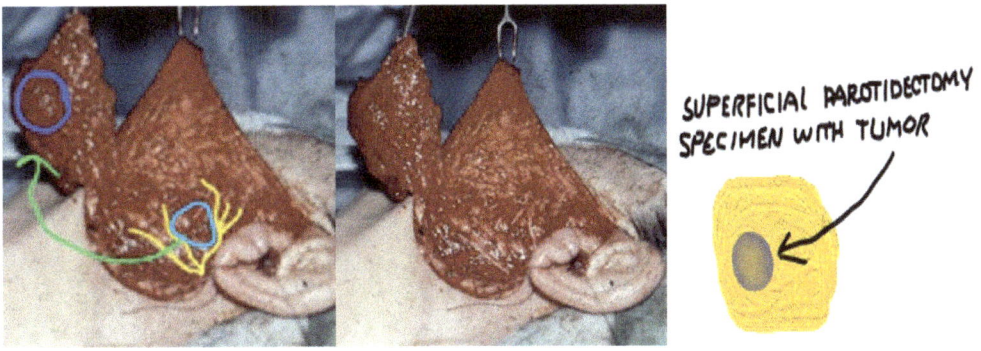

After superficial parotidectomy, the facial nerve is in the base of the wound. At the same time, the deep lobe remains in situ, as demonstrated below, unless it needs removal because of the tumor present there.

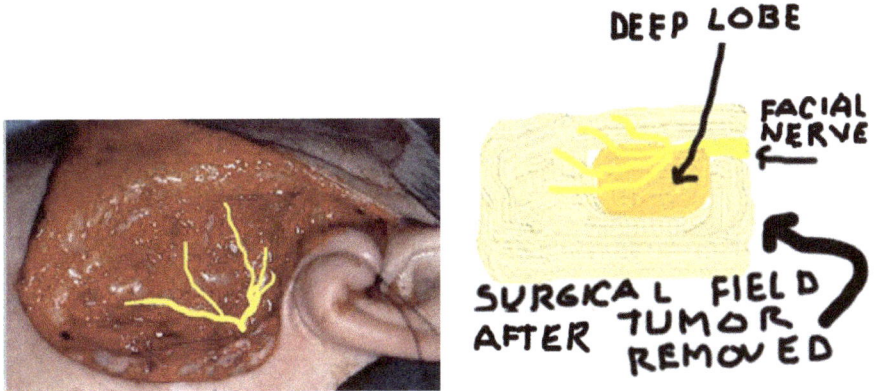

The post tumor excision photos and the immediate post-op photo are below.

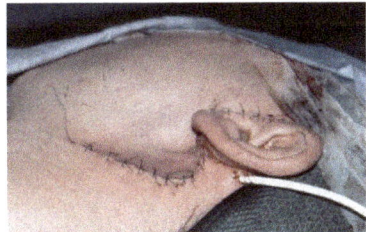

"Sean" did well postoperatively, with no facial nerve weakness.

Sub maxillary gland salivary tumor benign

The patient below was a very nice-looking administrator from another hospital. If I remember correctly, she was referred to me by a physician at our hospital. She had a rubbery swelling in the area of the left maxillary gland, which is a salivary gland, similar to the parotid gland in the cheeks. I approached this mass through an incision in the neck, in the regular crease lines, to leave a scar that eventually would be inconspicuous. I dissected the entire submaxillary gland with the tumor and sent it for pathological examination. The pathology report confirmed my suspicion that the mass was a benign tumor, even though a significant percentage of submaxillary gland tumors are malignant. She had an uneventful recovery.

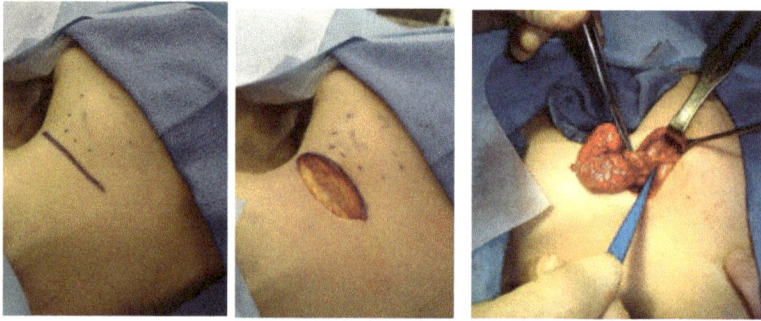

"Alicia" had the growth pictured below on her tongue. It had developed over just a few months.

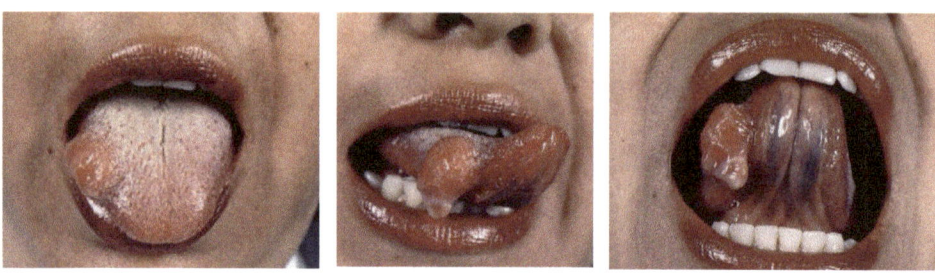

I performed a simple excision. The lesion was a benign neurilemmoma, a tumor that derives from nerve sheath Schwann cells. These cells line peripheral nerves: so neurilimmoma can originate from nerves almost anywhere on the body. Her postoperative result shows minimal tongue distortion and no functional impairment.

The Healing Mission of Plastic Surgery

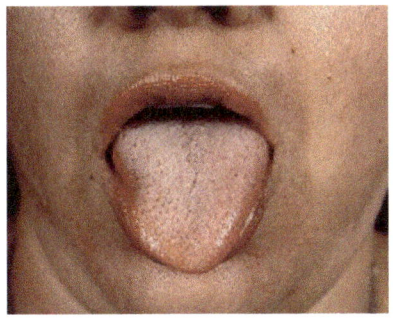
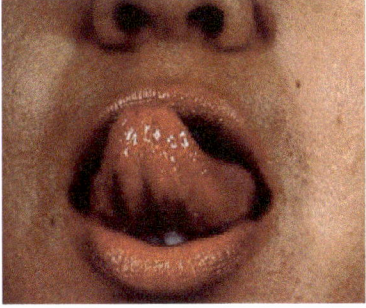

"Ginger" presented as a young adult with a mass in her left neck. However, this was a congenital second branchial cleft cyst that originated during embryonic development but only enlarged enough to be identified after she became an adult. It presented as a soft mass just anterior to the sternocleidomastoid muscle in the neck.

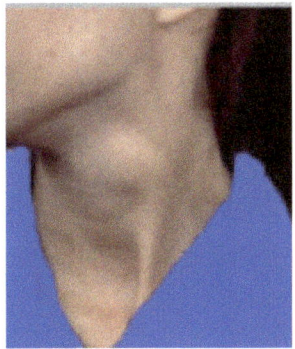
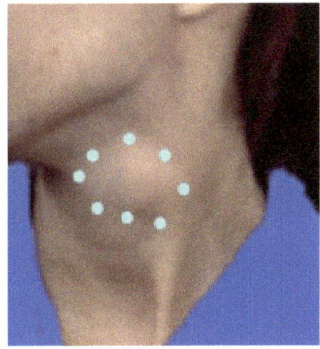

I excised this cyst through a small horizontal incision in the neck. The cyst was anterior and deep to the sternocleidomastoid muscle. It is essential to be knowledgeable of the complex anatomy of the neck to avoid large vessels and significant nerves when excising such a mass.

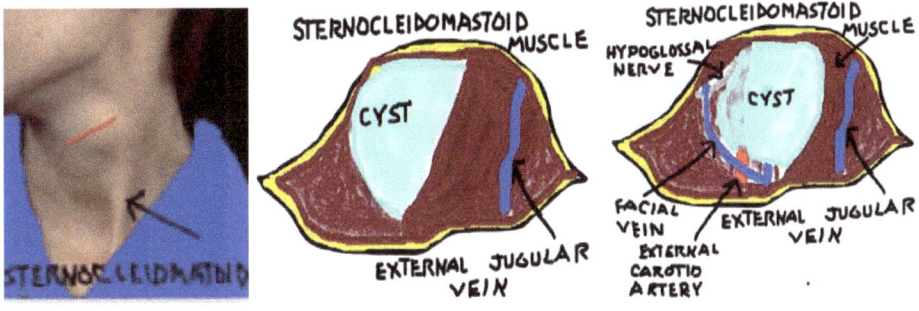

I dissected the branchial cyst, which was adjacent to the common carotid artery and internal jugular vein. There was a deep fibrous tract at the base

561

of the cyst, as illustrated below. I removed the entire cyst and amputated the fibrous tract.

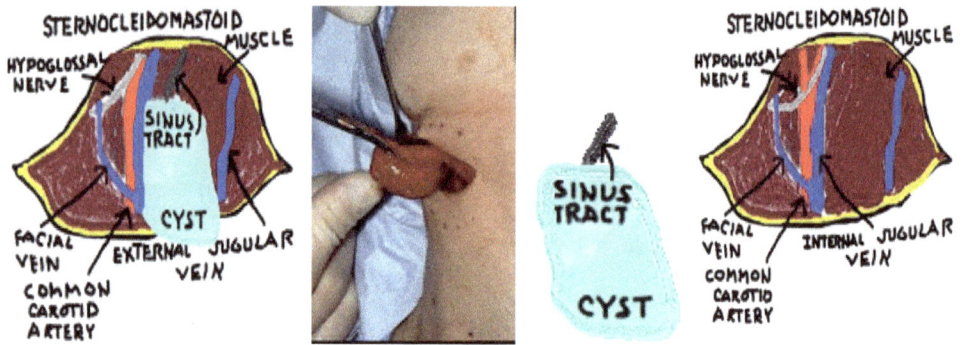

"Ginger" tolerated this procedure well and had an inconspicuous scar.

Recurrent skin cancer

The patient below "Dawn" was an elderly lady with recurrent squamous cell carcinoma of the lower lip. I did her case with the help of Dr. Michael Lypka, the senior resident at the time, and now medical director for Operation San Jose. Although the first view looks relatively innocuous, the second two photos show the area we needed to remove to assure clear margins around the tumor. Also, the third photo shows the extended incisions along the nasolabial fold, which we needed to get the movement of the tissue necessary for reconstruction with this Karapandzic technique.

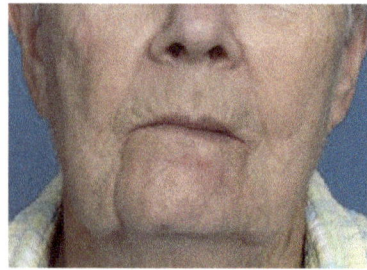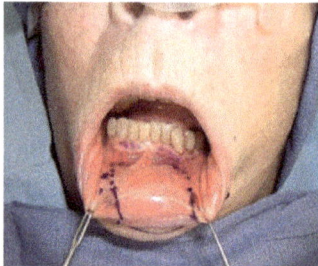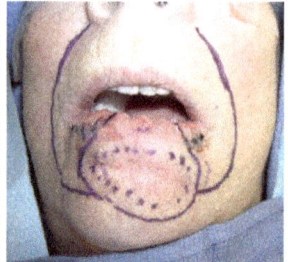

The intraoperative views below show an orange rubber loop around nerves and vessels which we preserved while freeing and then rotating the periolar tissue to repair the defect. We obtained the movement of the tissue flaps while safeguarding both the blood supply and the innervation. The immediate closure with the readjusted flaps is pictured on the right below.

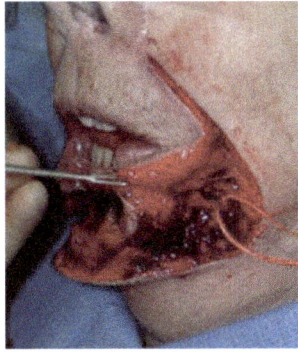 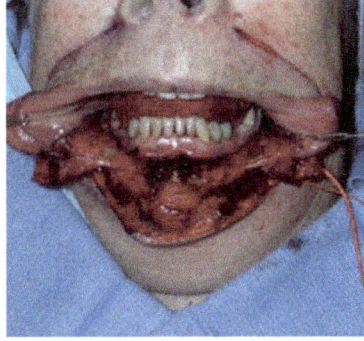 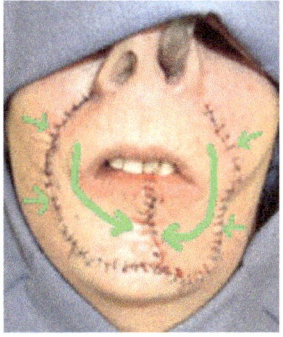

The two pictures below are both postoperative after about three months. I was pleased with "Dawn's" aesthetic and functional outcome.

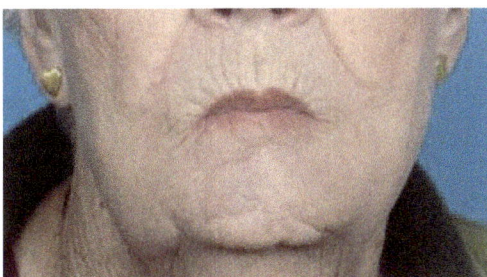 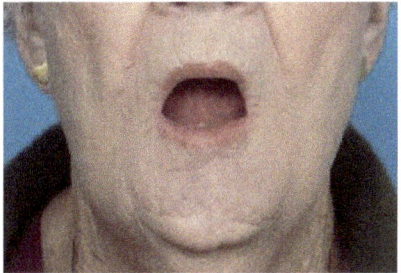

The drawing on the left represents the basal cell skin cancer on the helical rim of "Robert's" right ear. The first photo is after the excision of a basal cell carcinoma of the helical edge of a right ear and elevation of helical rim tissue on either side.

I reconstructed the helix by essentially stretching the lower helical tissue, which is without cartilage and advancing that, which also lifted the lobule a little. The upper portion of helix contained some cartilage, and I brought it inferiorly. Together these two flaps were enough to reconstruct the helical rim as shown on the right. The ear looks perfectly normal but is slightly smaller than pre-operatively

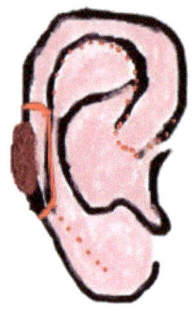 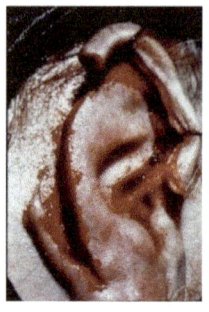 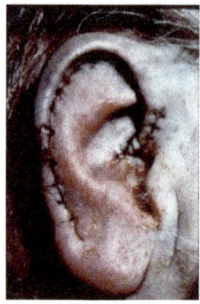

"Johnny" is shown with an extensive basal cell carcinoma of the left nasal ala. The pre-operative photos below show the lesion.

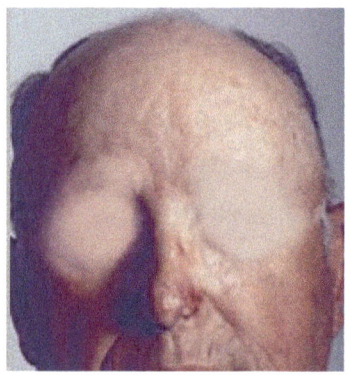 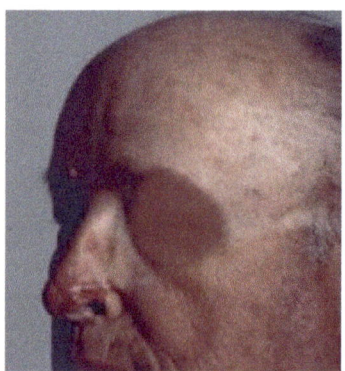

The close-up view on the left below shows the extent of the lesion and the proposed excision. On the right, I have drawn a midline forehead flap while awaiting frozen section clearance of the margins of the tumor.

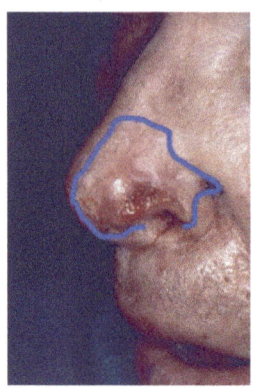 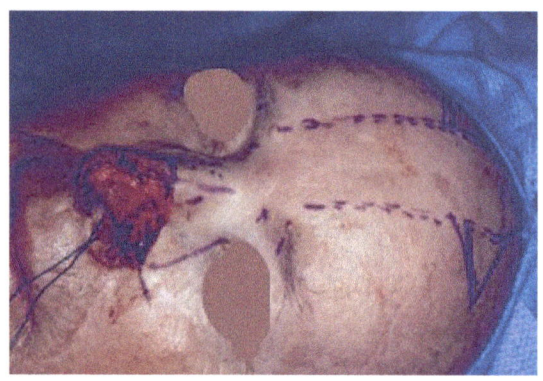

After getting clear pathology margins, the forehead flap was elevated and brought to the nasal tip, as demonstrated in the two photos below. Part of the donor site was left to heal by secondary intention.

The Healing Mission of Plastic Surgery

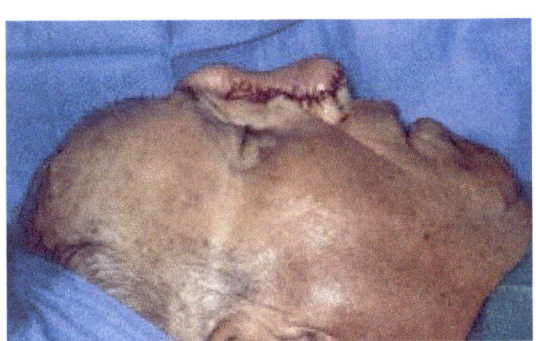
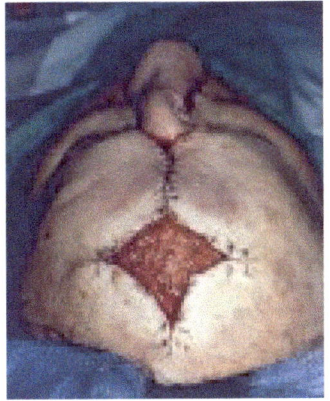

The final result below is several months later.

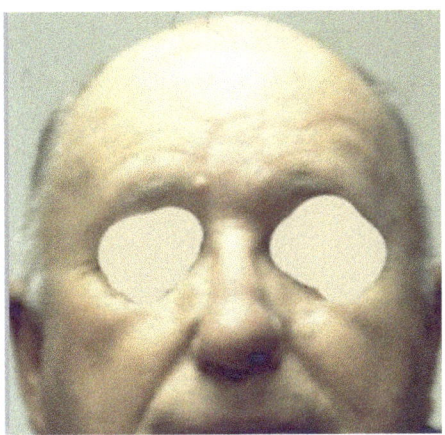
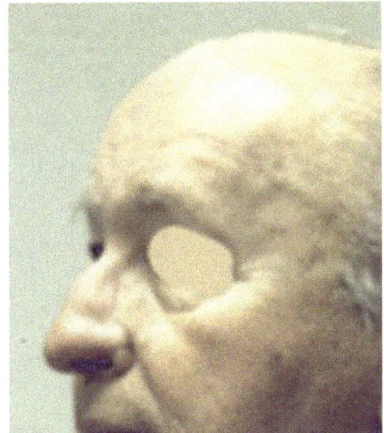

A head and neck surgeon colleague asked me to close the wound after he excised a squamous cell carcinoma of the lower lip in the patient "Mary" shown below. He also did an upper neck lymph node dissection as on the right.

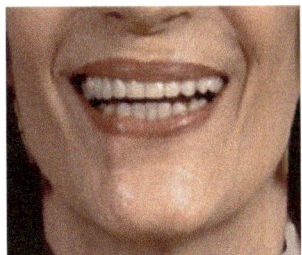
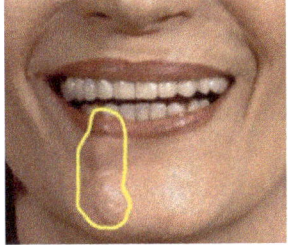
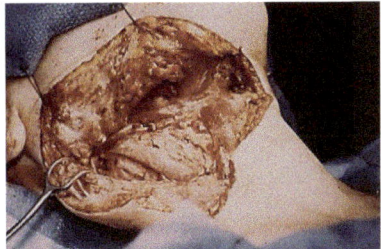

The photos below show the extent of lip excision. The last picture on the right indicates the mental nerve which the oncologic surgeon needed to clear of tumor.

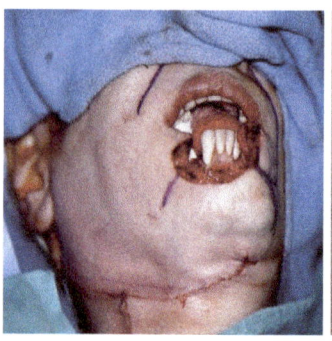 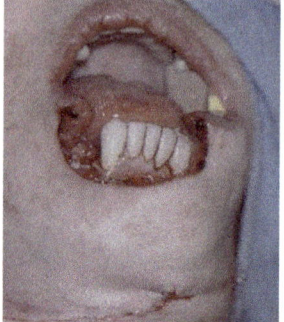 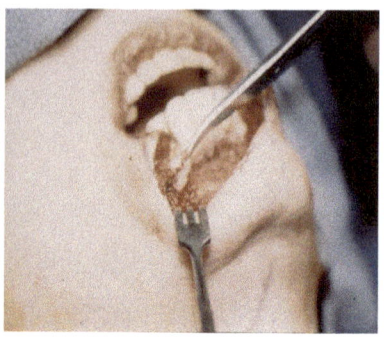

To close the defect, I advanced lip and cheek tissue from the right and rotated tissue from the left lower and upper lip. Her very early postoperative result is below. She continued to see her oncologic surgeon, but I lost her to follow up.

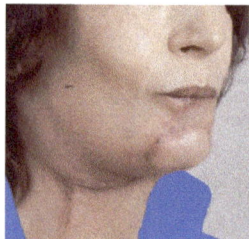 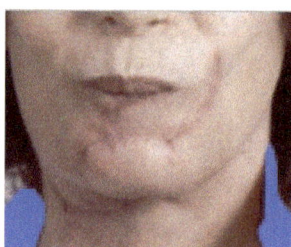 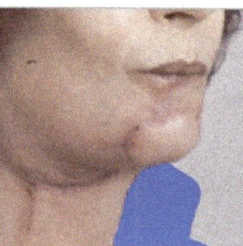 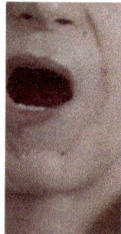

Decubitus ulcers or pressure sores

There is a great diversity in the way people handle adversity. On the one hand, we may have a person with paraplegia confined to a wheelchair who is unable to prevent a pressure sore because he will not lift himself for a few minutes every hour. On the other hand, we have amateur basketball teams, with all paraplegic players in wheelchairs who do not develop pressure sores. Such people are quite inspirational. I do not mean to say it is easy to prevent pressure sores; it's not.

The general public is somewhat aware that debilitated patients can develop pressure sores. These commonly occur in paralyzed patients who cannot move around to take the pressure off areas of their bodies frequently enough. Also, paralyzed patients usually suffer from numbness over significant areas and cannot tell when the pressure has been present too long. These ulcers can occur first on the skin surface. The weight of the patient presses their skin against a bed or a chair. Wounds also can occur internally from bony prominences crushing the tissue between it and the dependent skin surface. This internal tissue can also necrose from excess unrelieved pressure. Many of these cases are very sad.

What is not generally known is that plastic surgeons are routinely involved in the care of such patients if they develop more than superficial sores. It was interesting to me to note that the actor Christopher Reeves, who developed quadriplegia after a fall from a horse and did so much to publicize both the plight and the value of such patients, developed pressure sores that led to infection, sepsis and his death. It emphasized to me how easy it is to get pressure sores even in someone who had all the financial resources possible to prevent them. Over the years, I have seen several young male patients who had paraplegia because of gunshot wounds from gang activity. There are many impressive operations involving the movement of flaps of tissue, which plastic surgeons use to repair sizeable deep pressure bedsores. However, prevention is much preferred.

It can take only a few hours to cause enough damage to result in a deep pressure sore that might take a massive operation and weeks of recovery to repair. The psychological state of the patient is quite pertinent. An angry, uncooperative, or depressed patient is much more likely to have difficulty with the development or recurrence of pressure sores. They are also prone to problems in the recovery phase of such surgery. Occasionally it even seems appropriate to refuse to operate on a patient, whose physical condition might otherwise warrant or benefit from surgery. It may be that a patient's psychological state so predisposes him to recurrent pressure sores as to warrant intervention Sisyphean.

There are certainly cases where we do not perform surgery with flap closures for pressure sores. Senile debilitated patients who have reverted to a fetal position with stiffness and contractions of all the joints or a demented patient who is unable to cooperate or even a patient too malnourished to heal are not candidates for surgery.

If I believe I will have difficulty healing the wounds or that the patient will be back with recurrent pressure sores in short order, I recommend only debriding the dead tissue and treating the patient with dressing changes. I want to avoid futile surgery and discomfort, being more aggressive with treatment would not be beneficial to the patient.

Bedsores or pressure sores are a tremendous problem, both in hospitals, nursing homes, and bedridden homebound patients. It takes almost constant vigilance and outstanding nursing care to prevent these in predisposed patients. The cost of extended medical care and prolonged hospitalization is enormous. When a patient is unable to move and relieve the pressure from dependent areas of the body, tissue necrosis (death) can develop in as little as a few hours. Especially problematic are patients who lack sensation in dependent areas because of spinal injuries or strokes etc. These are not just nursing nuisances.

They can be very serious and often lead to infection, septicemia (infection in the bloodstream) and can result in patient death. Functional plastic surgery for bedsores gets relatively little attention because it is not at all glamorous. Avoidance is key. I believe this is an area where both nursing homes and hospitals need to put more emphasis on prevention rather than more costly treatment after the development of these problems. The topic "end of life issues" has gotten a fair amount of attention lately. One chapter in that discussion must be the prevention and treatment of pressure sores.

"Annamarie" developed paraplegia several years earlier after a cave-in at a site she was exploring. Pressure sores like the one below plagued her. She developed this ischial pressure sore from sitting too long in one position without relieving the pressure. The patient is face down on the operating table. The surgical hemostat demonstrates that there is a void beneath the skin, at least the size of the blue circle. The drawings represent the position of the bony ischium. The weight of the body, concentrated at the bony ischium (orange), causes necrosis of the soft tissue from within a relatively short period. It takes constant vigilance to avoid pressure sores. They can be made worse by maceration, contamination, and infection.

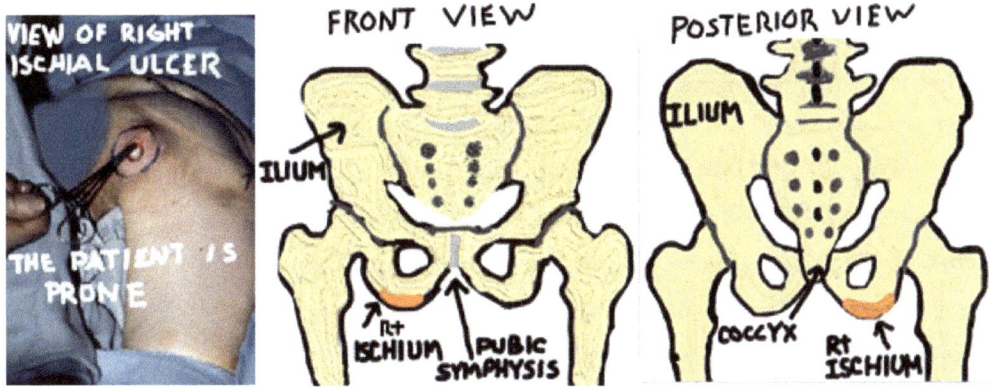

To better delineate the extent of "Annamarie's" pressure sore, I instilled a mixture of methylene blue ink and hydrogen peroxide into the wound to stain all the surface of the pressure sore. After I elevated a gluteal flap, one can see the extent of the injury is much greater than the original small opening. Because the surface of this type of wound is always contaminated, I next excised all of the tissue stained blue. The second photo below shows the large gluteal myo-cutaneous flap, which previously had been lifted out of the way, now being turned clockwise from lateral to medial, as shown by the blue arrow. I rotated the flap, of skin, subcutaneous fat, and gluteal muscle to fill in the void left after excising the pressure sore.

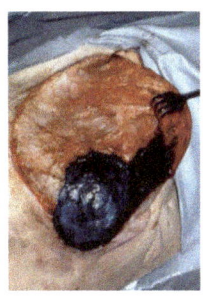 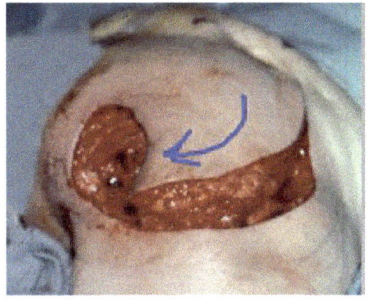

The first photo below shows the extent this bulky thick flap can be elevated and rotated. It also indicates that I have excised all the blue contaminated wound surfaces. The second photo shows the closure of the wound. Unlike many rotation flaps, for example, in the scalp, I closed both the pressure sore and the donor area. The last photo shows this right ischial area 10 months later.

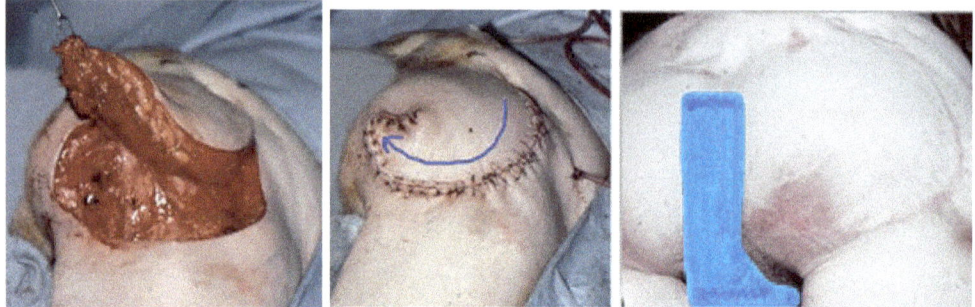

It is interesting, at least to me, that the only time I went to court to testify involved this patient. As I recall, she was suing the owners of the land where she suffered her paraplegic injury. I testified about her medical condition and susceptibility to pressure sores like the one demonstrated above. She was very grateful for the surgery we were able to do for her and was happy that I testified in court for her.

In another case shown below, "John," a paraplegic accountant, also developed an ischial pressure sore from unrelieved pressure while sitting in his wheelchair. As I recall, this was the first pressure sore "John" had developed although he had had paraplegia for several years.

In these intraoperative photographs below, the patient is face down on the operating table, and we are looking at the left posterior thigh. The left posterior knee is to the right, not visible. I closed the ulcer in a V to Y matter by moving tissue from the middle of the thigh to the upper leg over the ischium. The flap contains skin, subcutaneous fat, and underlying fascia. The blood supply comes from the inferior gluteal vessels which run beneath the wound and on the undersurface of the fascia of the posterior thigh. So even though I incised all around the flap, it still retains blood supply from underneath. I previously demonstrated this septocutaneous type of flap in chapter 4.

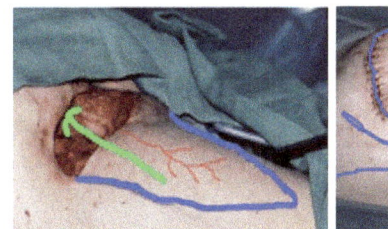 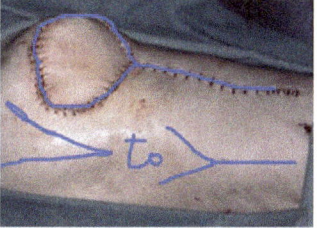 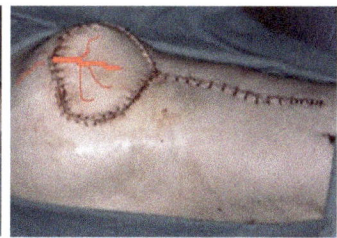

In the duplicate photos below, the dots help show the movement of the tissues.

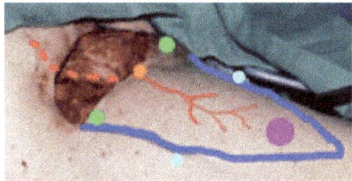 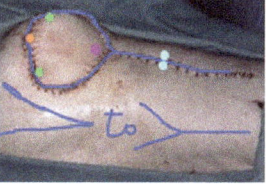 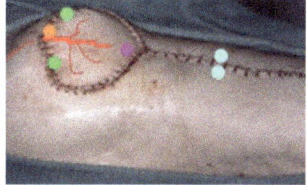

"Thaddeus" had paraplegia because of a gunshot to the back as a teenage gang member. He developed this pressure sore on the left trochanter from lying on his left side in bed without frequent enough relief of the pressure from his greater trochanter. The femur bone goes from the knee to the hip. The greater trochanter is a prominent part of the femur, which bears a lot of weight when one lies down on his side. The two drawings below illustrate the position of the greater trochanter relative to the femur and pelvis. In the left recumbent position, it is a bony point that pushes on the soft tissue with the weight of the entire trunk.

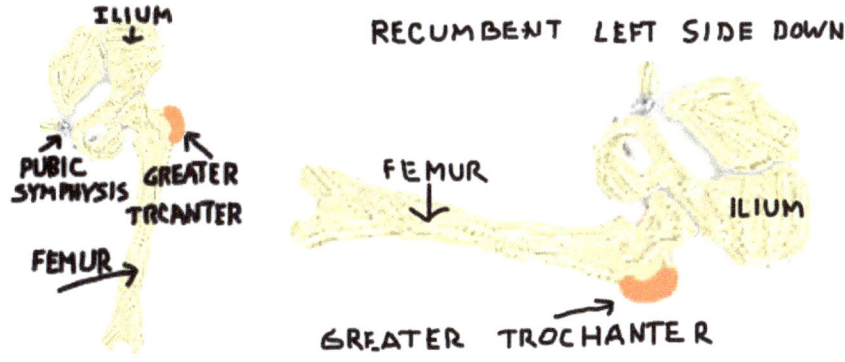

The drawing below shows a trochanteric pressure sore, which "Thadeus" developed at home. I have debrided the wound, and it is ready for closure. I performed a tensor fascia lata myocutaneous flap. This flap has good blood supply from a branch from the femoral artery, specifically the lateral circumflex artery, as demonstrated diagrammatically on the left below. The flap with skin, subcutaneous fat, fascia, and tensor muscle, is elevated and turned to cover the defect. The donor area is pulled together and repaired primarily. The completed reconstruction is on the right below. The colored dots help to understand the movement of the flap.

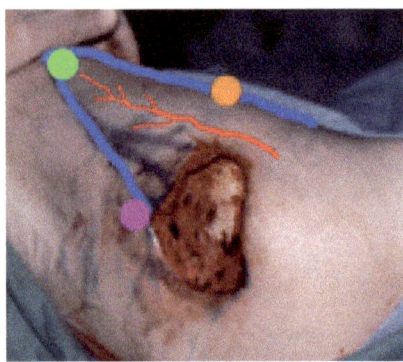 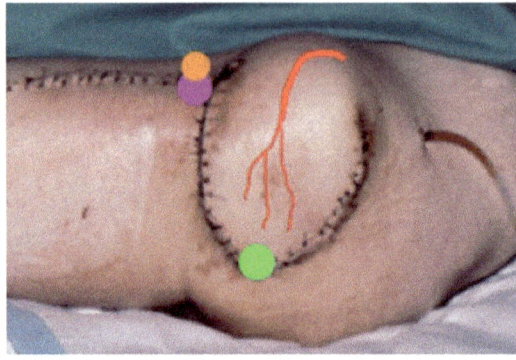

The paraplegic bedridden patient shown below "Chauncey" presented with multiple pressure sores, including the left trochanter and the sacrum. Multiple flaps were needed to close these wounds. "Chauncey" is likely to have recurrent pressure sores in the future.

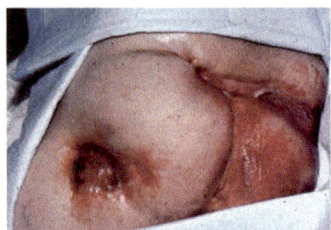 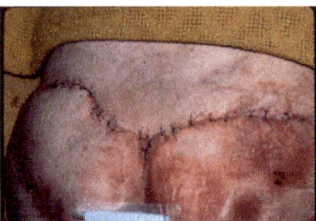 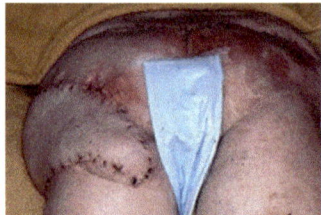

Flail thumb

An elderly gentleman, "V," had significant arthritis, which affected his hands. He suffered instability at the metacarpophalangeal joint of his right thumb. His thumb was almost useless. Since the thumb is responsible for about 40% of the function of the hand, it was a significant problem for him. The first two photos below show the preoperative flail condition of the thumb.

The Healing Mission of Plastic Surgery

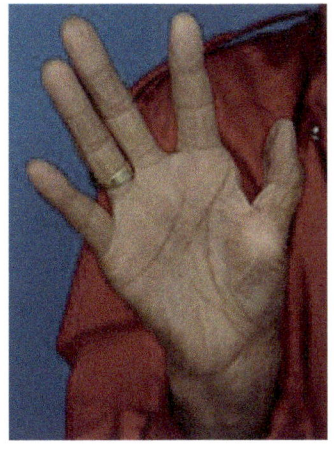
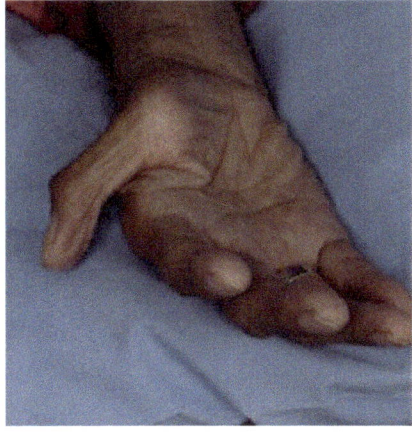

I fused the metacarpal phalangeal joint. I first removed all the residual cartilage and cut (red) the bony edges of the thumb metacarpal and proximal phalanx. The diagram below illustrates the procedure. I slightly flexed the proximal phalanx from the metacarpal then fixed the two bones with metal pins for several weeks.

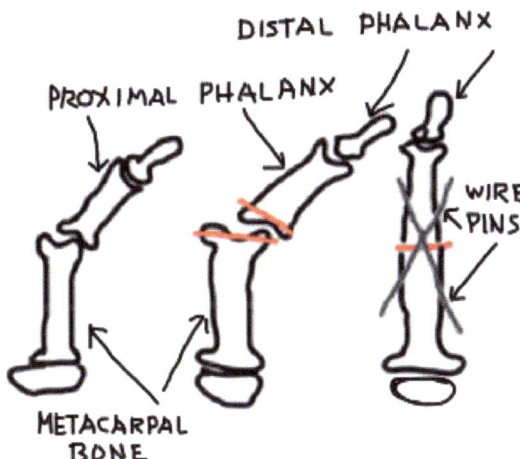

This procedure restored the function of the thumb almost to normal. The two postoperative photographs below illustrate the functional stability and near-normal mobility after surgery.

The Healing Mission of Plastic Surgery

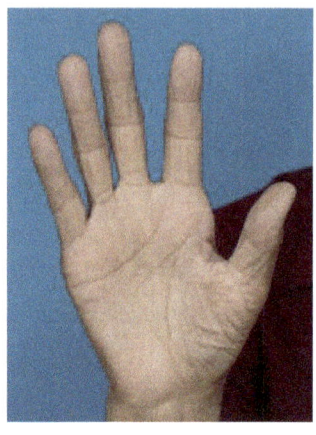
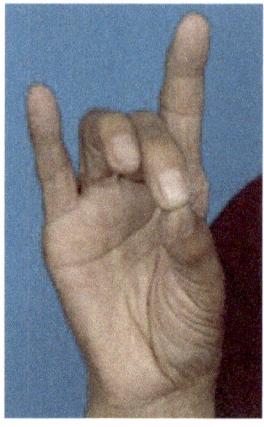

"V" was quite pleased with his improvement. He said that he was better able to do practical maneuvers of daily living such as buttoning and unbuttoning his clothes because of the surgery.

"Francine" burned both forearms in a steam press work injury. When I first saw her, she had bilateral extension contractures and was unable to extend her hands to a neutral position, as shown in the two photos below.

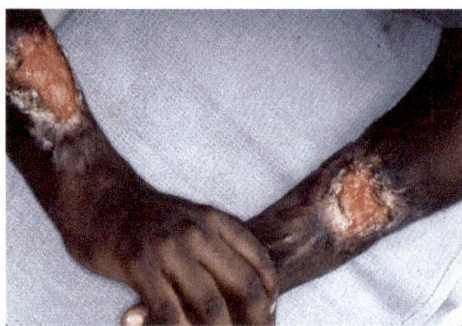
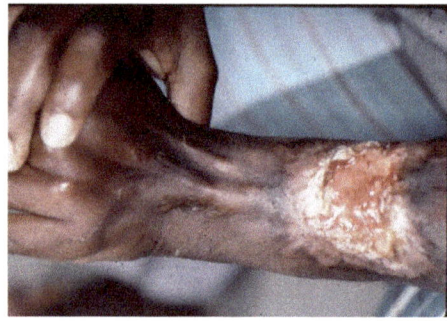

In the operating room, I debrided both wounds and released the contractures, as shown in the first photo below. The resultant wounds were unsuitable for skin grafting because of exposed tendons. Therefore, I prepared an abdominal pedicle flap for coverage of the injured areas. The picture on the right below shows the donor site ready to receive the forearm.

The Healing Mission of Plastic Surgery

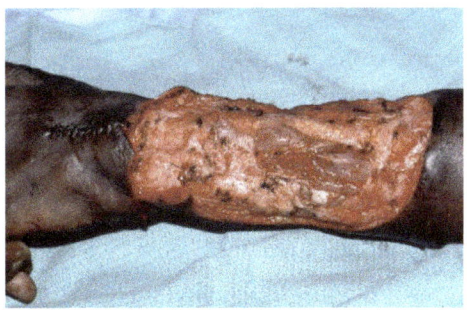
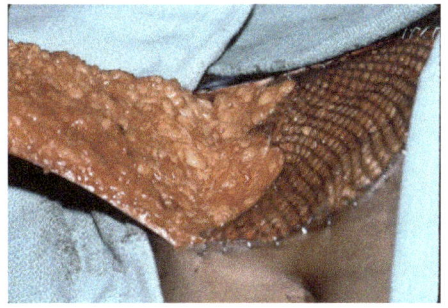

I placed the forearm so the flap would cover the raw surface, as demonstrated in the two photos below.

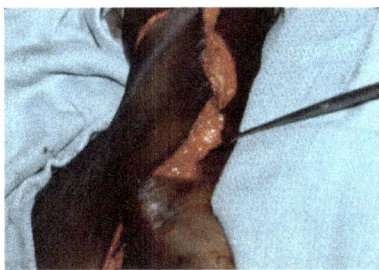
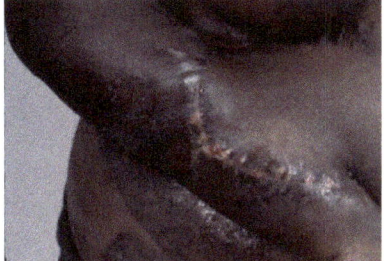

I left the forearm in place for two weeks and then cut the base of the flap with the abdominal flap tissue remaining on the forearm. I did the two forearms sequentially so that she would have only one arm restrained at a time. The excellent function with the final result is evident below, but also the considerable donor site cosmetic cost.

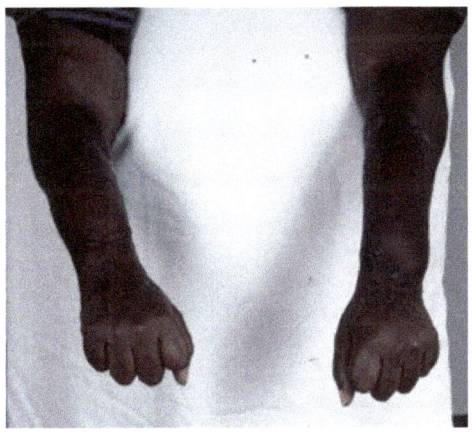
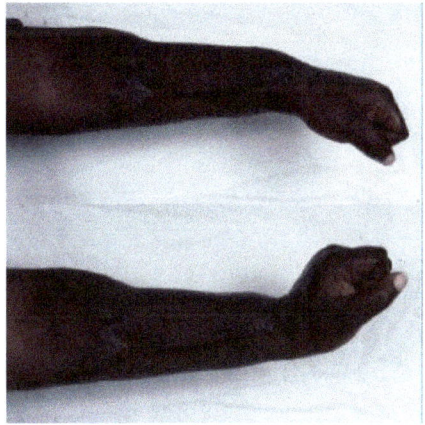

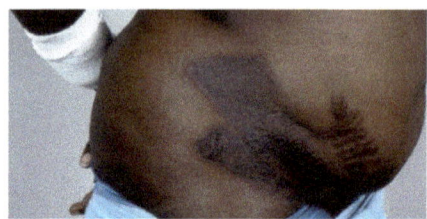

I performed this case many years ago. Today an alternative would likely be a free tissue microvascular flap transfer, which would not require the arm to be fettered, and would have less severe cosmetic ramifications.

Dupuytren's contracture

Dupuytren's contracture is an acquired functional deformity of the hands, which causes the fingers to contract towards the palm preventing straightening of the fingers. It can be very debilitating in severe cases. It is most common in Celtic and northern European people. The ring finger is involved more than any other digit, but all can be affected. It is often correctable if not too advanced. However, the recurrence of deformity does happen frequently.

There is a severe form of the disease called the Dupuytren's Diathesis, which affects other areas of the body, such as the sole of the foot and the penis. Surgery involves the removal of the scar-like bands of tissue that form in some of the natural fiber structures of the palm and fingers. Sometimes these scar bands will wrap around the small digital nerves that supply sensation to the fingertips. Therefore, dissection of this scar tissue can be tedious and is routinely done with magnification to help avoid injury to these small nerves and the small blood vessels of the fingers.

A moderate case is demonstrated by "John" below. The first drawing shows the ring finger drawn up because of the contracted tissue of the palm outlined in yellow dots. The red line is the proposed incision to expose the subcutaneous scar tissue. Simply closing such a straight-line scar would promote contracture of the wound at the skin level, which would be antithetical to the purpose of the operation. When I use such a straight-line incision, I make Z-plastys at closure to break up the straight-line. Alternatively, I would make a zigzag incision. The third photo below shows the involved scar tissue exposed and outlined with yellow dots.

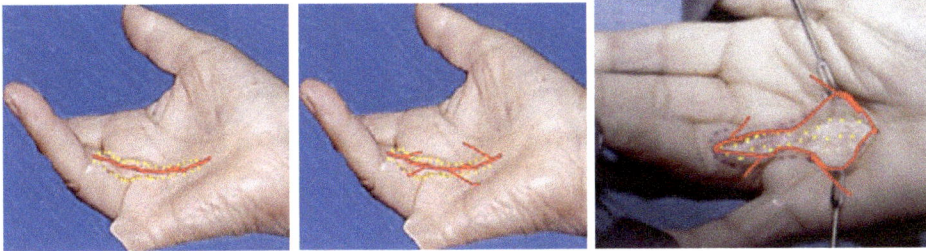

The next photo below shows that scar tissue accentuated by the yellow marker. The following two photos show the Duyputrens tissue dissected and lifted, ready for removal.

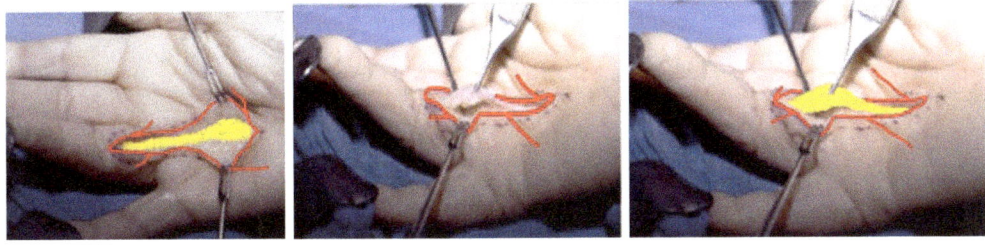

The photo on th left below shows the excised Dupuytren's scar tissue. On the right, the yellow marker accentuates the scar.

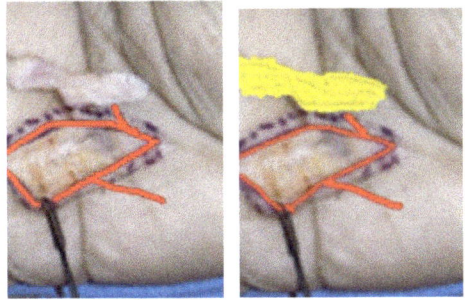

As demonstrated by the photos below, I broke up "John"s" original straight-line incision with two z-plastys, one in the palm and one on the proximal finger. Transposing the z flaps transforms the straight- line to a zigzag scar pattern. The colored dots indicate the movement of the flap tips from their original to their final position. "John " obtained an excellent functional result, as shown in the last two pictures.

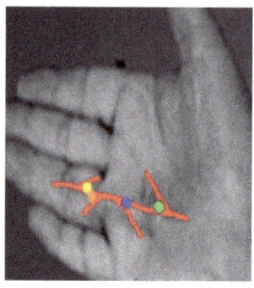 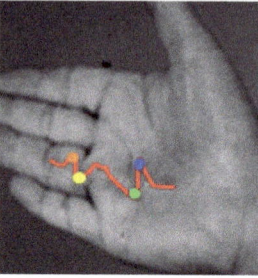 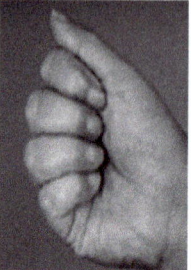 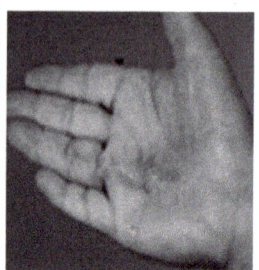

Giant Cell Tumor of finger

This patient "Gloria" presented with a painless swelling of the index finger. The enlarged area was somewhat firm and rubbery; I suspected it was a giant cell tumor. This idea was reinforced at the surgery when the mass had the typical appearance of a giant cell tumor. The growth incased the ulnar neurovascular bundle in the finger.

This tumor was benign but could recur if I did not remove it entirely. In "Gloria's" case, I had to carefully dissect the mass from the neurovascular bundle so that the finger would survive the removal without loss of the blood supply or sensation to the fingertip. On the left below, one can see the tumor surrounding the ulnar neurovascular bundle; on the right, I have excised the mass and preserved the neurovascular bundle. The pathological examination confirmed the diagnosis. The patient did well postoperatively.

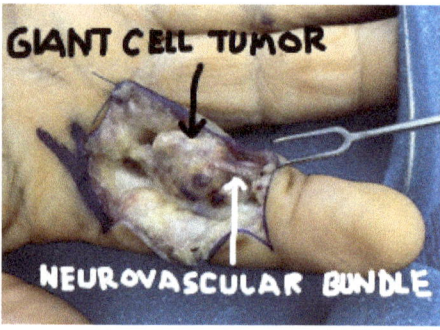 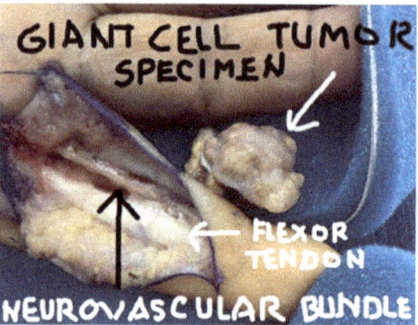

Polydactyly

Polydactyly is a frequent congenital deformity that may affect the ulnar side, the thumb side, or the central hand. The manifestations can be very complex or quite simple, as in the case below of baby "Mark." The most common expression is a small reduplication on the ulnar side of the hand, as demonstrated by the bilateral example below.

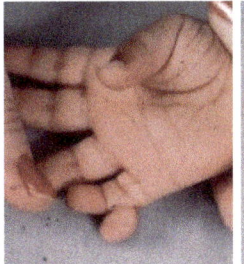
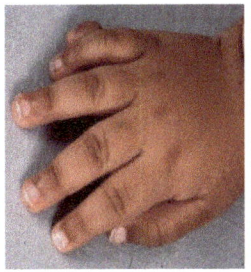
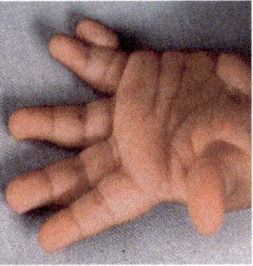
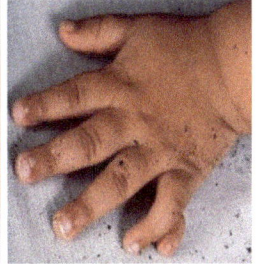

Treatment was a simple excision of the extra digit. The postoperative photos are below.

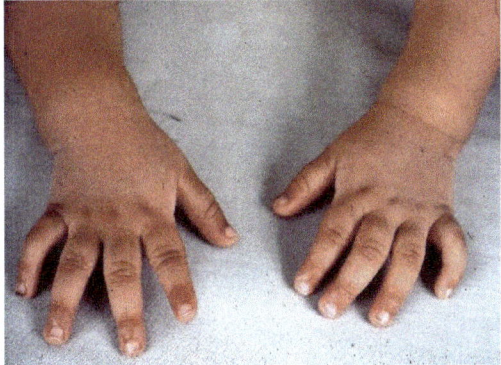

Orbital region

Eyelid ptosis

Sleepy eye is a colloquial term for eyelid ptosis. It can be a congenital or acquired problem.

The young boy "Johnny" demonstrates congenital ptosis or droopiness of his left upper eyelid, partially blocking his vision. His ptosis is both a functional and cosmetic issue. I corrected his ptosis by an operation in which I harvested fascia from his lateral thigh. I made strips of fascia to connect the upper lid to the frontalis muscle of the forehead, which ordinarily raises the brow. See the middle photo below. This frontalis muscle's tension and activity produced a better functioning left upper eyelid. I used this method when the levator muscle in the eyelid is too weak to shorten, as is usually done in acquired ptosis. The third photo shows the postoperative result.

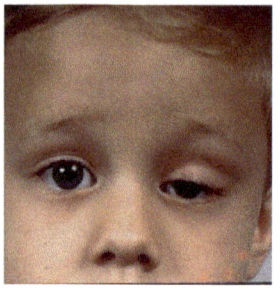 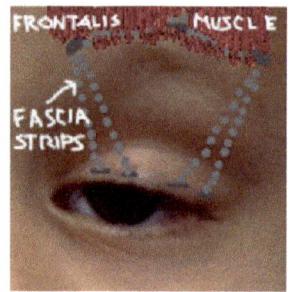 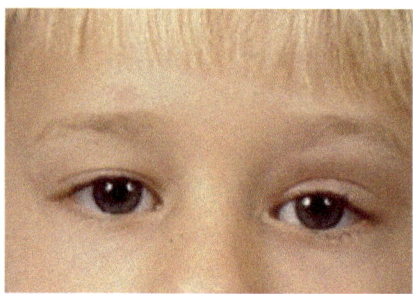

"Roberto" shown below is a 60-ish man with bilateral acquired or senile ptosis of his upper eyelids. The upper lids are partially blocking his line of vision.

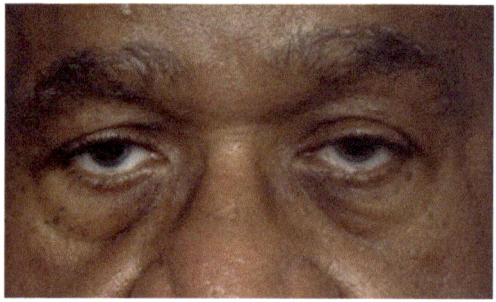

Ptosis may result from trauma to the upper eyelid, but most cases are senile ptosis, which is a degenerative problem common and with aging. Unlike congenital ptosis, there is usually some residual activity of the levator muscle, which lifts the lid. The preoperative physical examination can ascertain the excursion of the lid with active use of the levator muscle. If there is not enough activity, then a procedure like the one done for the child above is needed. However, usually shortening the levator mechanism is sufficient.

The traditional method of repair was actually to cut out a segment of the levator muscle. However, various suture techniques to shorten the levator mechanism seem more natural to execute and just as effective. The first upper eyelid drawing below shows a method that connects the fibrous tarsal plate of the upper eyelid to the levator muscle just above the aponeurosis with a blue suture. The tarsal plate is the dark gray structure. A blue suture has been placed in the tarsal plate and brought out in the levator muscle just above the aponeurosis drawn in white.

In the second drawing, the upper edge of the gray tarsal plate is pointed out by the green arrow. The levator muscle is pointed out by the purple arrow. In this lateral view, one can see that pulling the tarsal plate up to the levator muscle shortens the levator mechanism, which had been elongated by stretching of the levator aponeurosis.

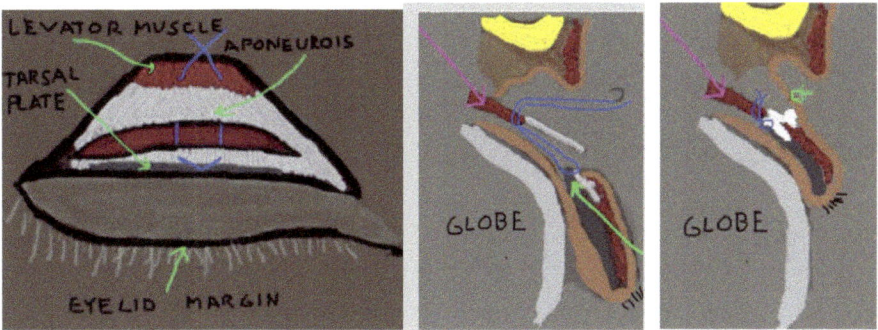

"Roberto's" postoperative result is below, showing correction of the bilateral upper eyelid ptosis.

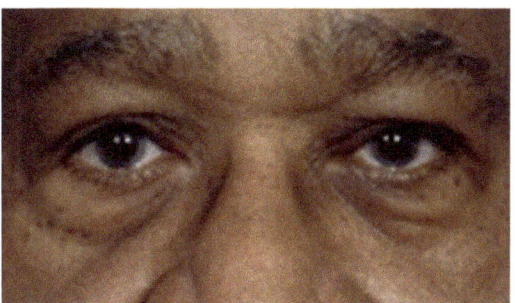

The above procedure, known as the three-step technique, is described in much more detail for surgeons by doctors Mark Codner and Clinton McCord and popularized by them.

The traditional technique of cutting out a segment of the levator muscle is usually done under local anesthesia so that the surgeon can get feedback from the patients by asking them to look up and down, etc.. An advantage of this three-step technique does not require the patient's active participation. So it can be done with the patient asleep if more convenient. The surgeon can get feedback himself with close observation and minimal physical testing of the eyelid tension. "Roberto" was treated with this technique, as were the additional adult patients below.

"Jan" had acquired ptosis the right being more severe than the left, partially blocking her visual field. As is usually the case, I operated on both the right and left upper eyelids. I used the three-step technique. Pre- and postoperative photos are below.

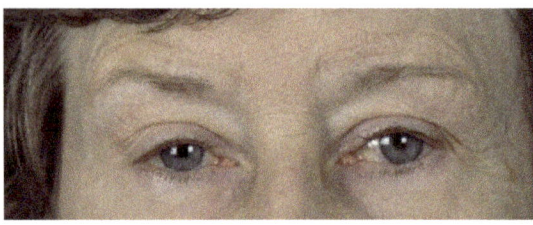
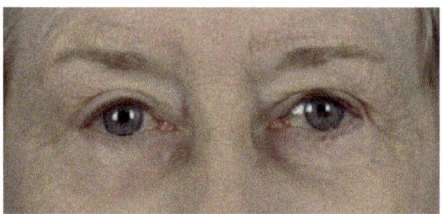

"Raymond," below, was bothered with restriction of his upward and lateral gaze. I performed an upper eyelid ptosis procedure for him with the result below. I did nothing to the lower eyelids.

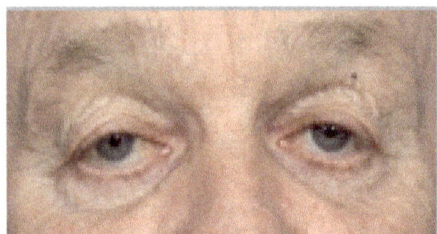
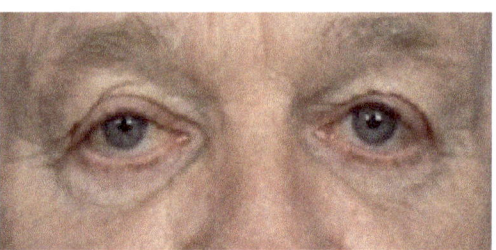

"Shirley" shown below had severe ptosis with a visual field abnormality. She obtained the result below after I performed a three-step procedure.

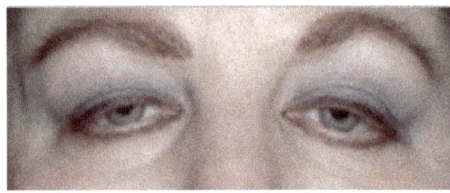
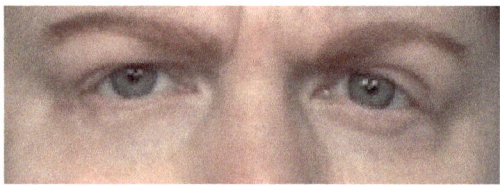

"Fernando" shown below had ptosis worse on his left. I did a bilateral ptosis three-step procedure for him. I did not operate on the lower eyelids.

The Healing Mission of Plastic Surgery

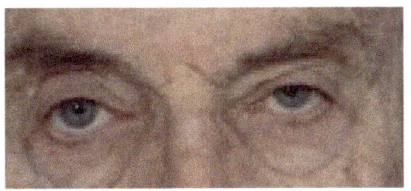
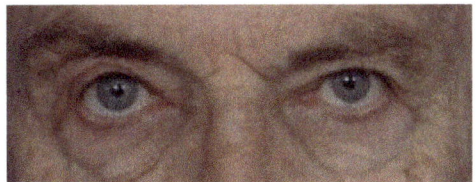

"Abby" had significant bilateral ptosis. I performed a three-step ptosis procedure for her. I slightly overcorrected the left eye. I had her pull down on that lid frequently for several days postoperatively, which helped some. Such action is standard practice when there is an overcorrection. Interestingly, although I believed she obtained a good result from the operation, she was not pleased and was never satisfied.

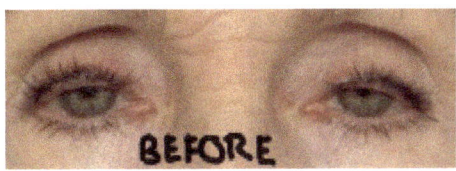
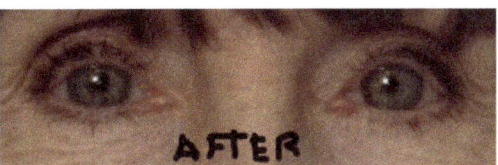

The patient below "Ronnie" had severe left upper eyelid ptosis and the mild right upper eyelid ptosis. I performed a bilateral levator shortening procedure upon her. Her pre-and postoperative photos are below.

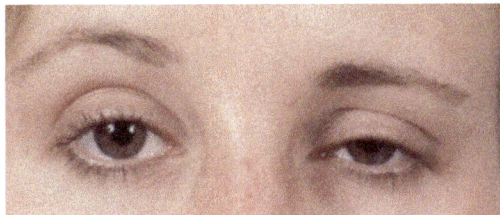
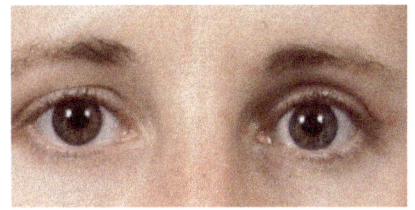

Lower eyelid ectropion

"Truman," pictured below, had a bilateral senile ectropion, which was quite irritating for his eyes. He also had considerable excess fatty tissue of the lower eyelids.

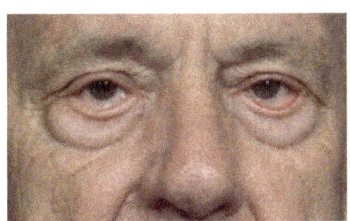
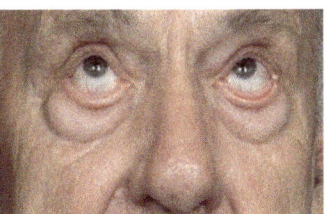
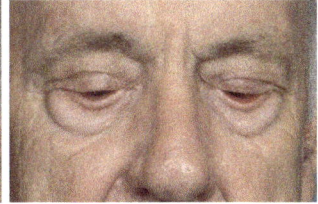

I recommended a tarsal strip procedure for him. This procedure shortens the horizontal length of the lower eyelid, thereby tightening the eyelid. I did this by removing the skin and mucosa from a segment of the tarsal plate. The tarsal plate is a fibrous structure in the superior portion of the lower eyelid. In the photo below, I have already "stripped" the lower eyelid tarsal plate, which I am holding with forceps.

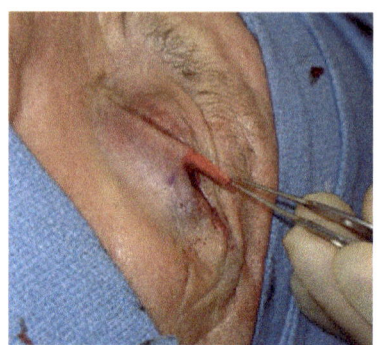

I then moved that portion of the tarsal plate superiorly and laterally sutured it to the periosteum at the lateral orbital rim. In the drawings below, the area denuded is outlined in red. The denuded tarsal strip is inserted superiorly and laterally and secured to the lateral orbital rim. This maneuver horizontally shortens the lower eyelid and corrects the ectropion. The last photo below shows "Truman's postoperative result after this tarsal strip procedure. I also removed excess fatty tissue from the lower eyelids.

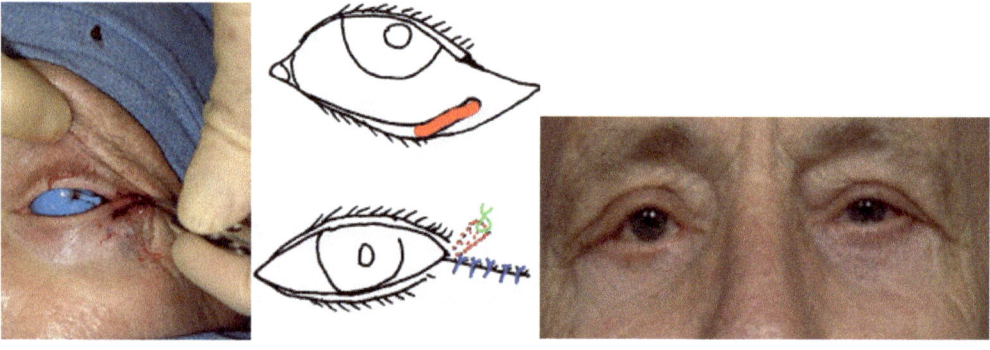

Below is another severe case of ectropion. In this case, "Chad" had suffered a stroke with paralysis of the right side of the face. He has not only right lower eyelid ectropion but also significant brow ptosis on the right. "Chad" presented with a watery and irritated right eye. He was quite debilitated because of interference with visual acuity. I shortened the horizontal length of the eyelid by removal of some tissue and then tightly fastening the remaining lateral edge of eyelid at that lateral aspect of the orbit similar to the previous case above.

I also lifted his right brow with direct excision of forehead tissue and removed some upper eyelid skin. I performed these procedures on this elderly gentleman under mild sedation and local anesthesia as an outpatient. The process was quite successful in restoring the function of his right upper and lower eyelids. His early postoperative result is on the right below.

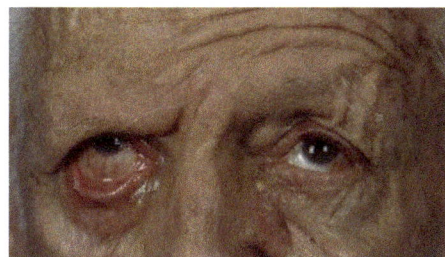 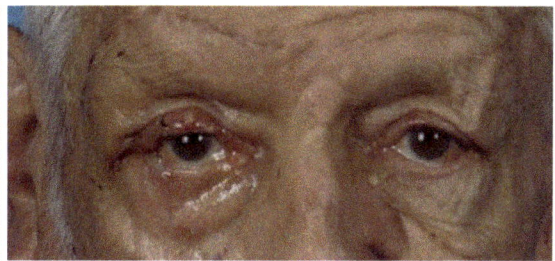

Facial skin cancers

Basal cell and squamous cell carcinoma are the most common types of skin cancers. Melanoma is more dangerous but less common, although it is on the increase in areas like Texas, where I practiced. They are usually associated with excess sun exposure. Plastic surgeons routinely take care of patients with these lesions, both excising them and reconstructing the defects created by their removal. Also, dermatologists or other practitioners may send patients to plastic surgeons, post excision for complex reconstructions. Care of skin cancer patients can be a significant part of many Plastic surgeon's practices. The following are several examples of flap closures, many with some flap designs already presented in chapter 4.

The patient below "Hank" had a basal cell carcinoma of the left lower eyelid outlined in blue on the left. The middle photo indicates the full-thickness lower eyelid excision that I planned. I excised the lesion and obtained frozen section checks of the margins from the pathologist. After getting a wound free of tumor, I proceeded with a two-stage type reconstruction.

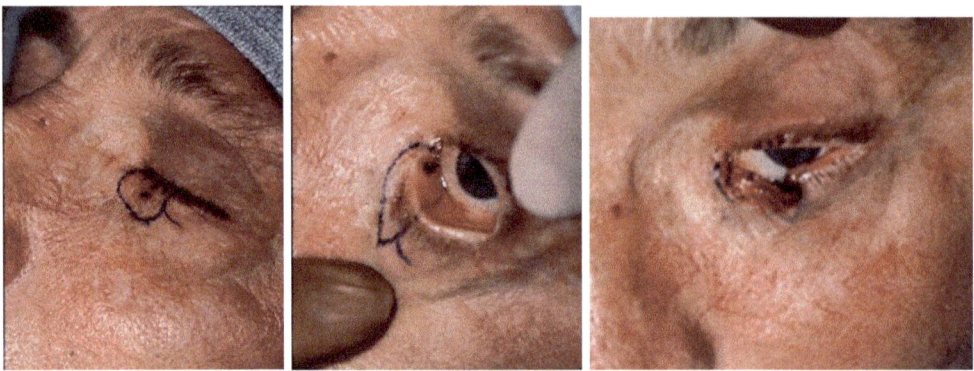

I made an incision under the upper eyelid and brought tissue from the upper eyelid into the lower eyelid and sutured it in place temporarily, as shown in the left photo below. Several days later, the bridge was separated, leaving the donated tissue from the upper eyelid in the lower eyelid for reconstruction. This post-separation result is on the right below.

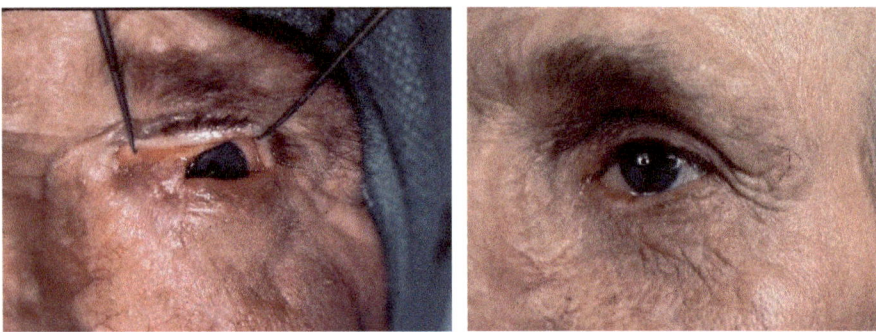

Eyelid and Nose Basal Cell Carcinoma

"Bart" had extensive sun-damaged skin and a history of multiple skin cancers. He had a distinct right lower eyelid lesion and a sizable but less visible nasal lesion.

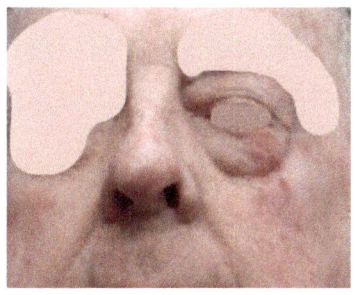 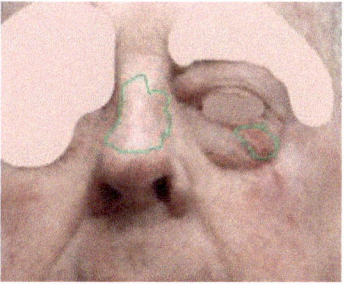

I excised the eyelid lesion and obtained a free margins report from the pathologist with frozen sections. I raised a skin and muscle flap from the upper eyelid, which was based laterally. I rotated it about 50 degrees and placed it to cover the lower eyelid defect created by the skin cancer excision. I sutured the donor defect of the upper eyelid in a straight line. w The diagrams below depict this procedure

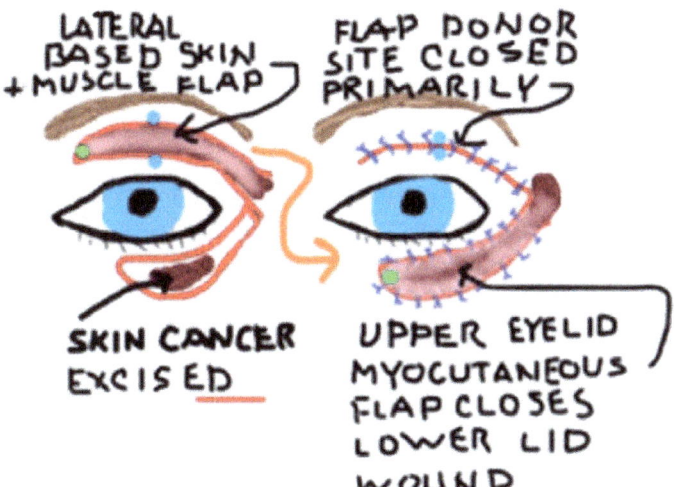

The photos below show the extensive nasal defect. I have sutured the lower eyelid reconstructed from the upper eyelid flap, as well as the donor site from the upper eyelid primarily.

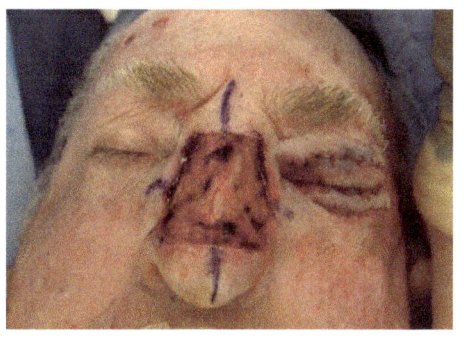 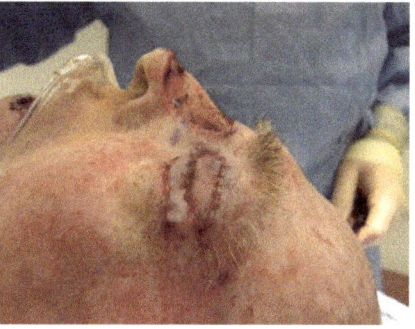

I treated the large skin deficit left on the nose after removal of the extensive skin cancer with a full-thickness skin graft taken from the neck just above the clavicle.

The first picture below shows the full-thickness skin graft donor site already closed in the neck. The second photo shows a stabilizing bolster dressing tied over the nasal full-thickness skin graft.

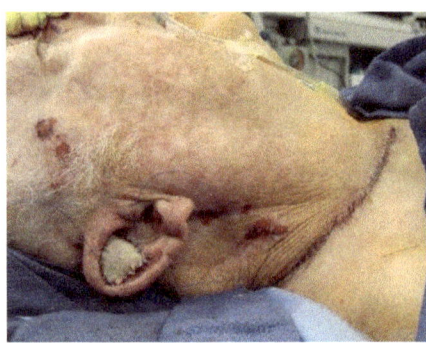 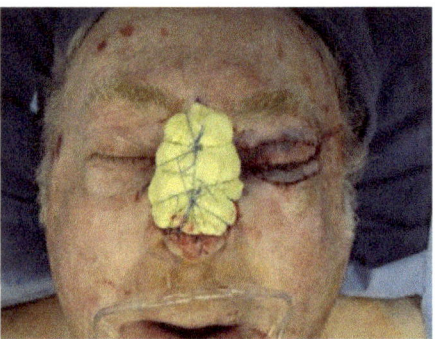

Postoperative photos of "Bart" show his final result.

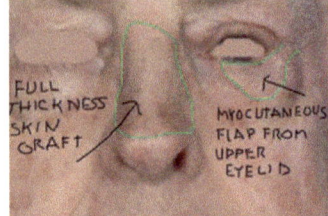 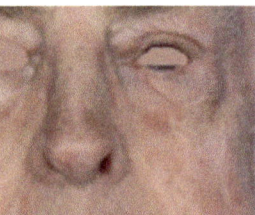 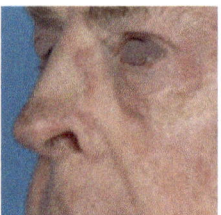 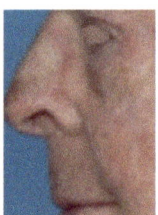

Nasal Tumor

"Emma" below had a lesion of the nose that would bleed periodically. I recognized it as a basal cell carcinoma.

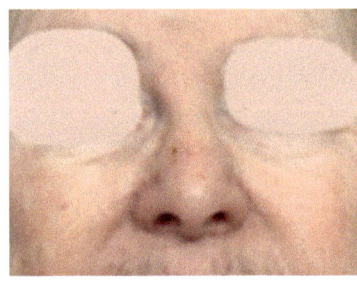 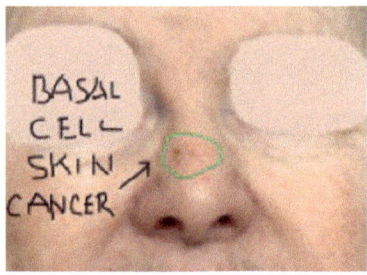

I took her to the operating room and under IV sedation, surgically removed the lesion, and oriented it for the pathologist. He performed fresh frozen section checks of the margins. When clear, I designed a dorsal nasal V-Y advancement flap as diagramed on the patient below. The dots will help show the movement of the nasal flap.

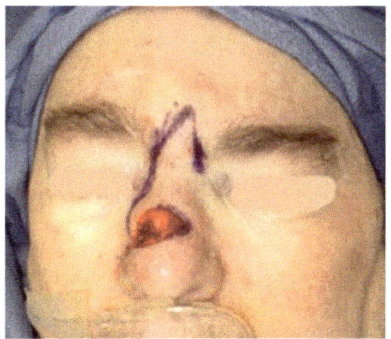 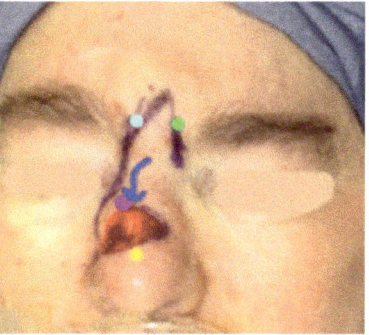

The immediate on the table result is below.

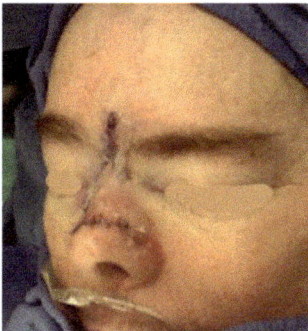 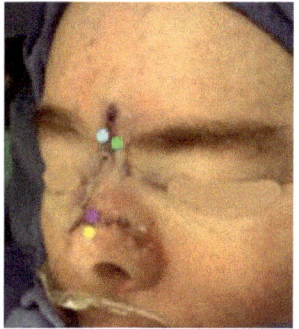

I outline the final scar placement on the left below. The post-op results are on the right.

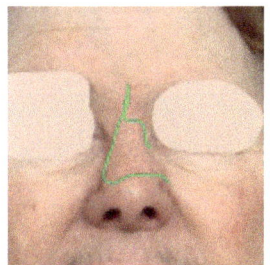 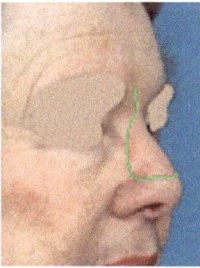 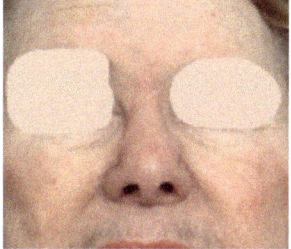 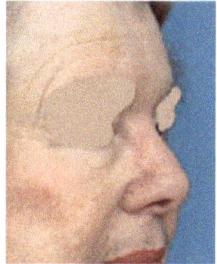

"Alexander" below had a squamous cell carcinoma of the lip. The blue line marks the excision of the cancer. The margins were free on fresh frozen sections. I reconstructed the lower lip with tissue, including skin muscle and mucosa, advanced from lateral to the lesion. Next, I excised redundant triangles of cheek tissue and adjusted, as shown in this "Bernard" procedure.

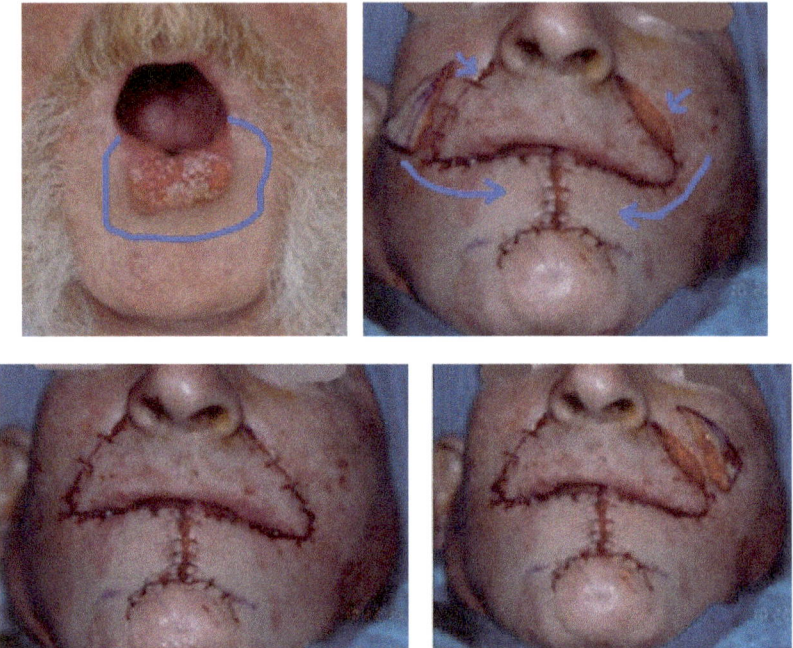

His postoperative result is below.

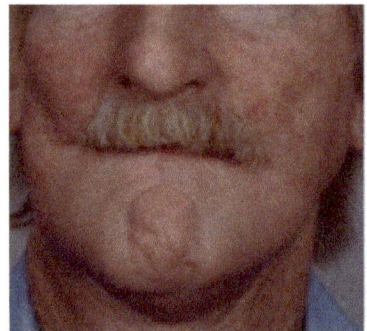

"Charlotte" had a pigmented basal cell removed. The surgical specimen was divided and oriented so the pathologist could obtain Complete Circumferential Peripheral and Deep Margin Assessment (CCPDMA) with reconstruction with a random rhomboid flap as below. The colored dots show the rearrangement of the tissue.

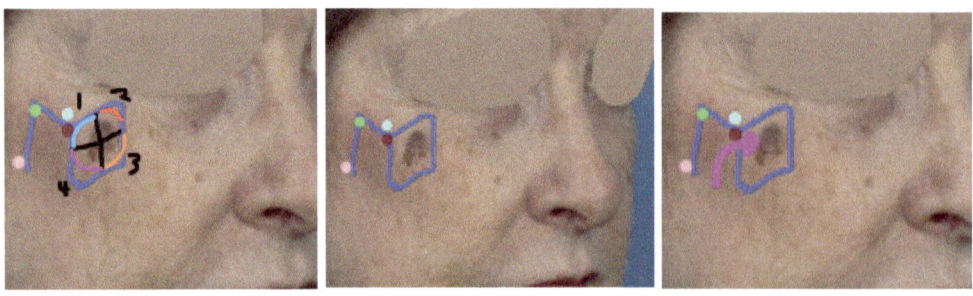

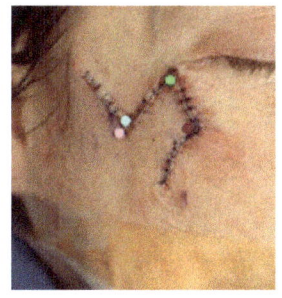 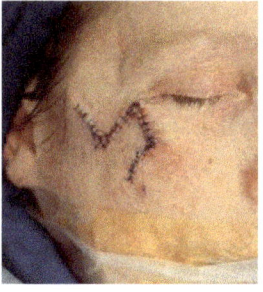

"James" had a discrete basal cell carcinoma of the nose. I excised it as indicated by the blue circle. The margins were clear on fresh frozen sections. I used a tiny muscle-based V-Y flap, shown in red, to close the defect. I sutured the donor site primarily

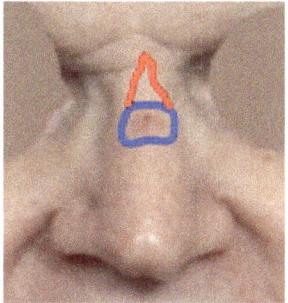 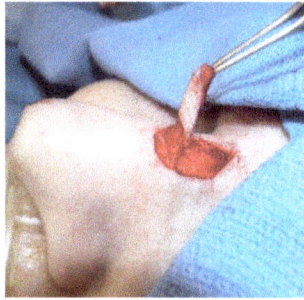 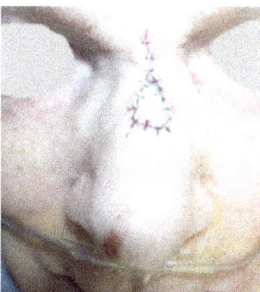

"Mark" had a basal cell carcinoma removed. The resection margins shown in the first photo below were not clear. After additional resection, I had free margins on frozen sections, as in the second photo. I planned a bilobed random flap for closure, as outlined in blue below.

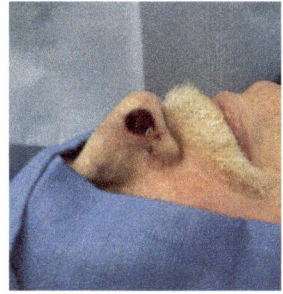 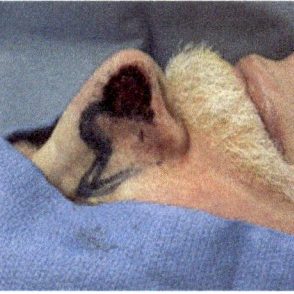 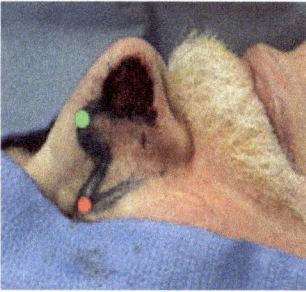

I elevated the random bilobed flap and transferred it, as shown below.

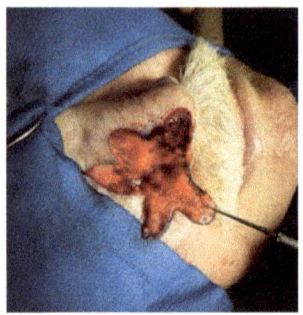 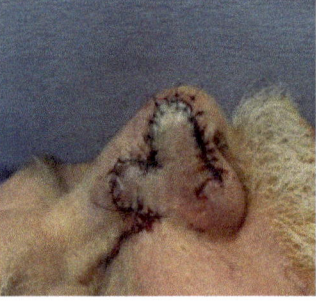 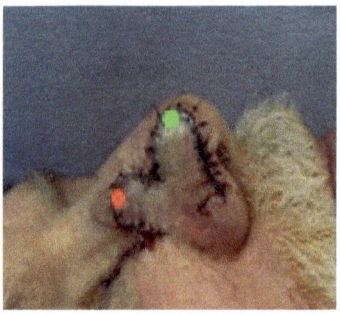

Below is the postoperative result.

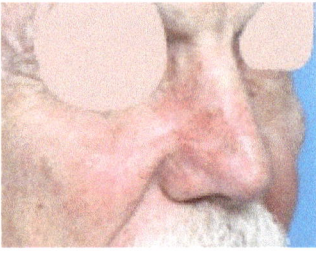 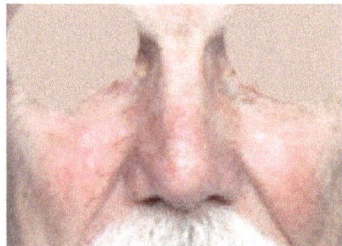

Mohs micrographic surgery

As a plastic surgeon, I often worked in concert with other physicians; in this case, I was asked by a dermatology colleague to reconstruct a defect after removal of a tumor. The patient below "Mia" was sent from the dermatologist office to mine the day following a Mohs procedure for an extensive basal cell carcinoma. The photos below show the complex defect.

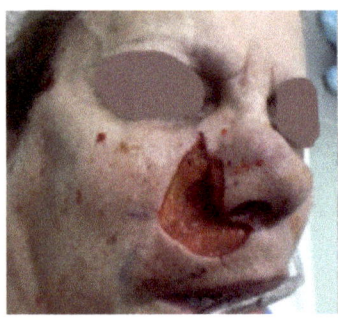 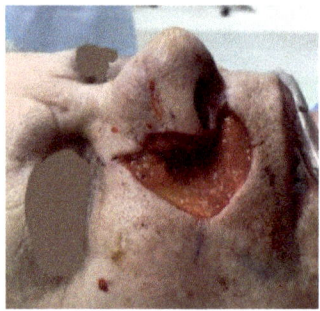

Below I reconstructed the defect with a random advancement flap from the cheek and a rotation flap of the lip as outlined. The photos are only about two weeks later. The scars had not yet matured or faded, but because her form and structure were excellent, I forecasted an excellent result.

The Healing Mission of Plastic Surgery

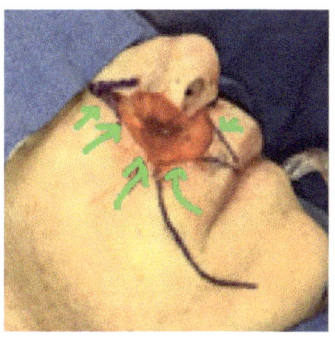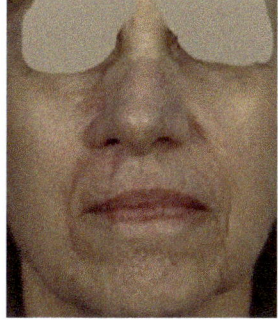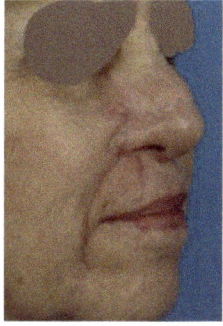

Also referred by her dermatologist for reconstruction after removal of a basal cell carcinoma of the nasal tip was "Victoria" below. She presented to me the day after her Mohs procedure.

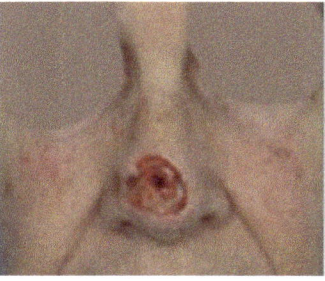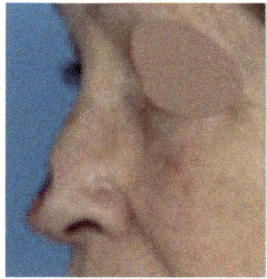

I designed a full-thickness skin and muscle dorsal nasal/glabella flap was with the help of a sterile cloth pattern to predict the movement of the flap tissue. This maneuver can help prevent a flap from failing to reach the full extent of the defect. Measure twice and cut once.

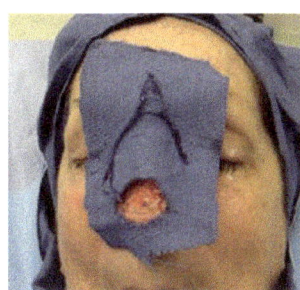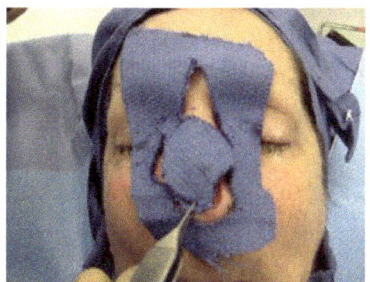

Below the actual flap is rotated and enables closure of both the Mohs wound and the donor area. The dorsal nasal flap is very reliable and useful.

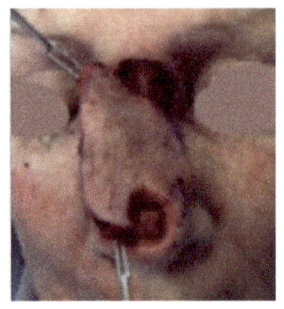 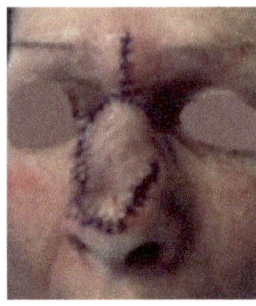

Her postoperative result is a few several weeks later. Over time the flap will continue to blend in.

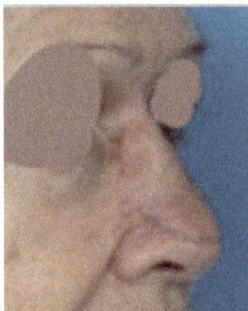 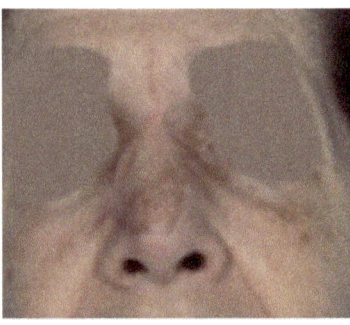 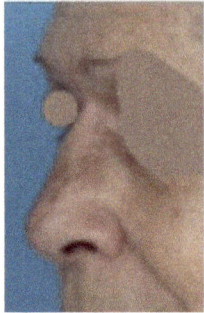

"Liam" was a gentleman with a small basal cell carcinoma in a sensitive location. If I did a primary closure, it would have distorted the nasal ala on the right side. The rotation flap I performed gave him a proper reconstruction without distortion, as shown below.

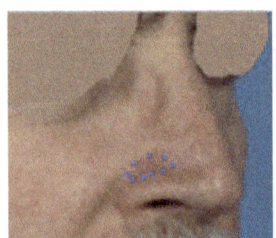 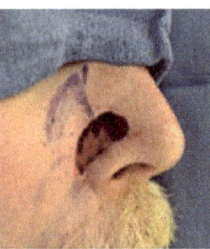 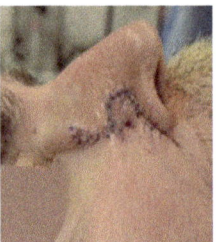 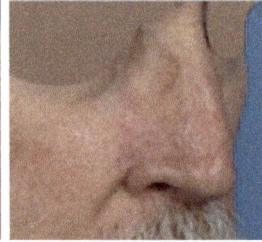

"Marivel," below, was sent to me from her dermatologist, who removed a small basal cell carcinoma. The defect was minor but in a delicate area. I treated this with a superiorly based nasolabial flap, as shown below.

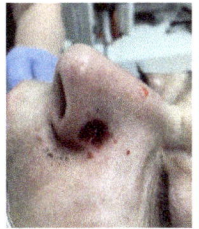 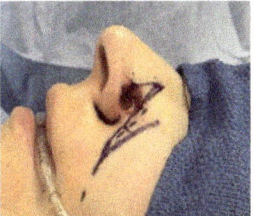 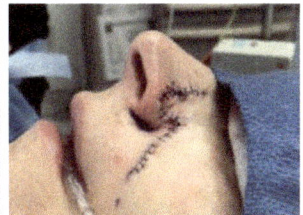 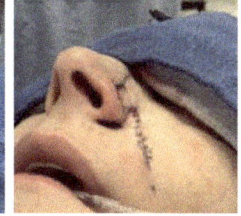

Below the next patient, "Glenda" had an inconspicuous basal cell carcinoma of the nose but needed an excision a little larger than the yellow circle below. She was a businesswoman who was in the public eye and was keenly concerned about her appearance. I excised the lesion and obtained fresh frozen sections of the margins from the pathologist. I performed a nasolabial flap procedure like the one I did above on "Marivel." The last three pictures below show "Glenda's" result after several weeks.

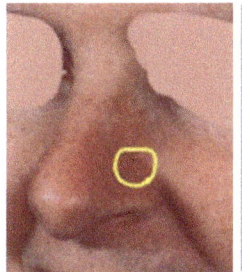 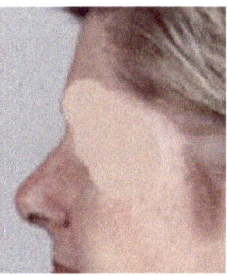 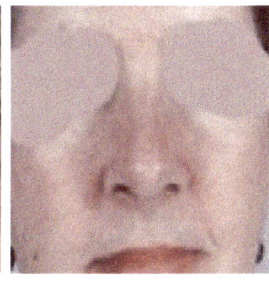 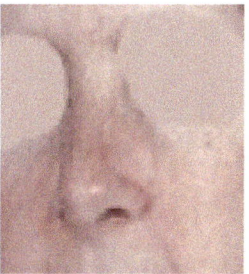

"Frederica" is another patient whom I treated a basal cell nasal defect with a dorsal nasal flap. The first photo below demonstrates the wound. The second and third photos show the deep level from which I lifted the flap and then rotated it to repair the defect. The last picture shows the post-op result several weeks later.

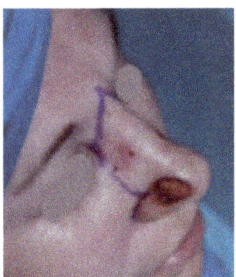 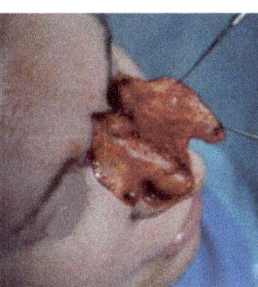 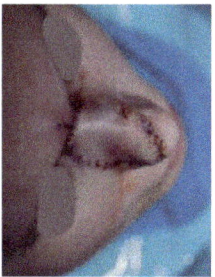 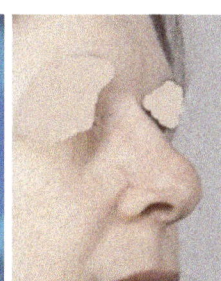

"John has a basal cell carcinoma outlined in blue ink in the first photo below. The defect after frozen section checks of the margins is in the center photo. I have illustrated my plan of repair in the photo drawing.

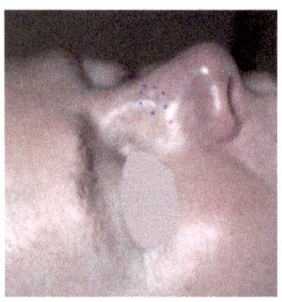 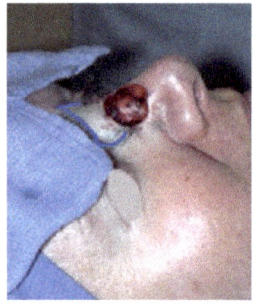 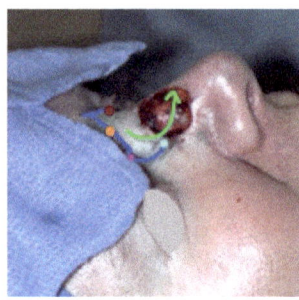

The dots help one see the movement of the flap. The immediate result on the operating table and the result after a few months are below.

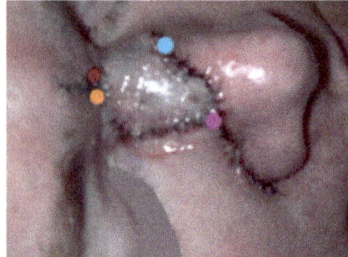 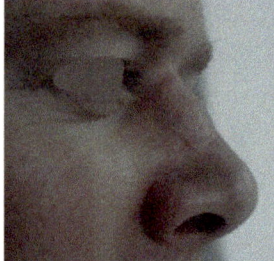 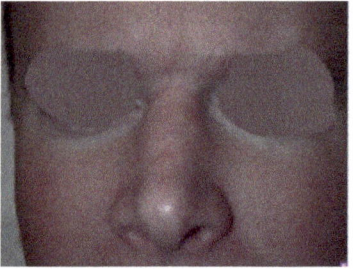

"Clark" had a basal cell carcinoma, as shown in the first photo below. He had a wide nose with loose skin, so I did an elliptical excision. The frozen section margins were clear. Therefore, I elected a simple straight -line closure. The last photo on the right is a few months post-op

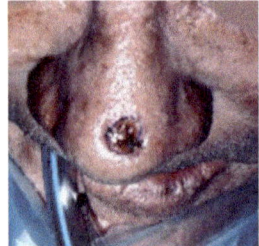 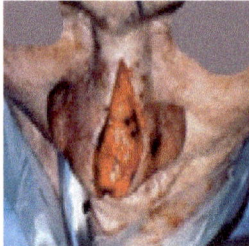 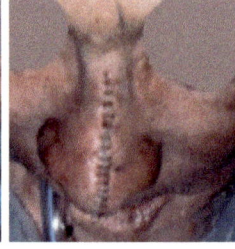 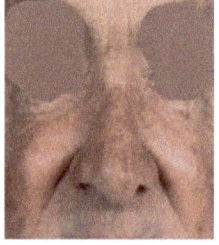

"Marcuse" had a basal cell carcinoma, as shown below, outlined in ink. To facilitate frozen section checks of the margins, I divided the lesion into smaller sections 1-4. The pathologist checked the perimeter and depth of each with frozen sections.

The Healing Mission of Plastic Surgery

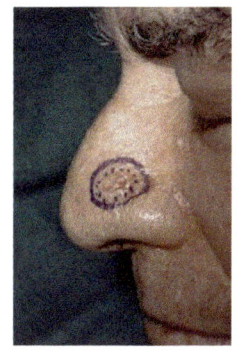
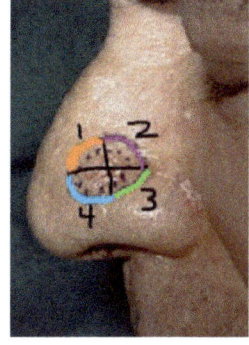

After obtaining clear margins, I repaired the resultant defect with a bilobed flap, as outlined below.

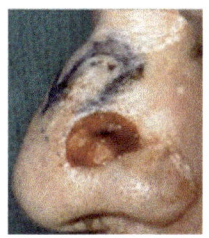
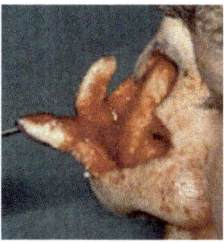
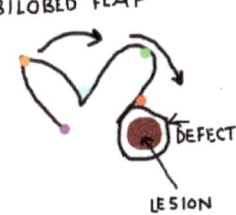
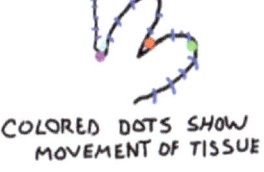

Below are the results on the table and after a few weeks.

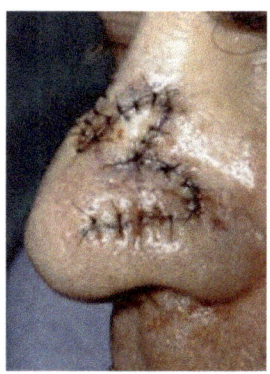
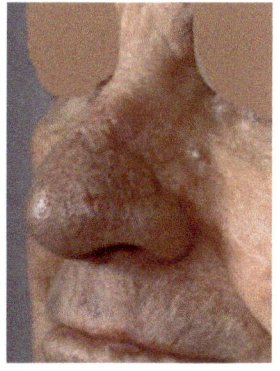

"Alexander" has a basal cell carcinoma of the nasal dorsum. I turned a glabella flap down to repair the defect.

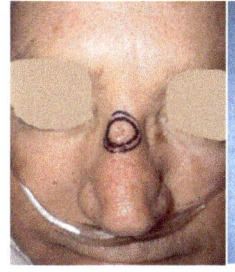
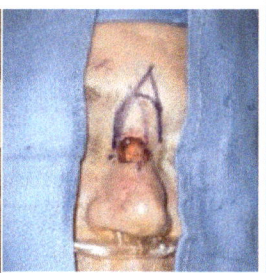
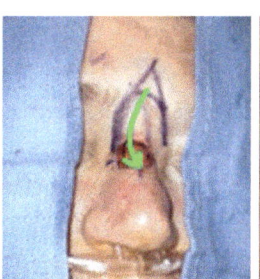
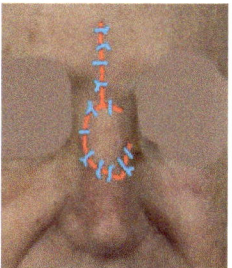

His early postoperative result is below.

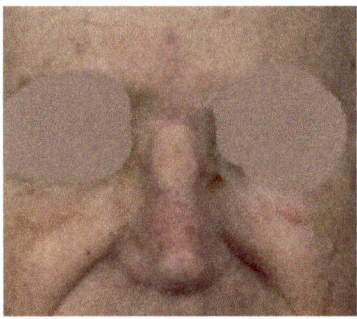
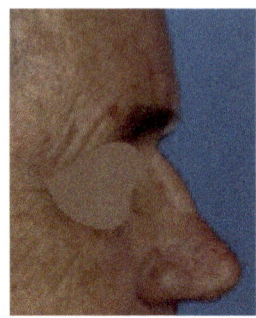

I repaired a skin cancer defect for "Margarette" with a nasolabial flap, as shown below with her, on the table result.

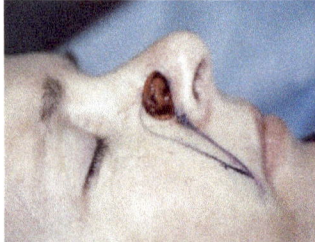
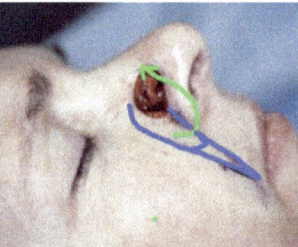
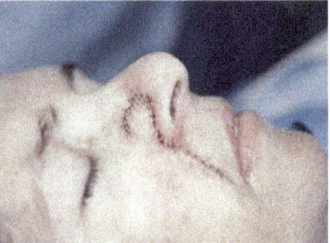

I performed a similar nasolabial flap for "John" who had a small basal cell skin cancer. The flap is blending in nicely.

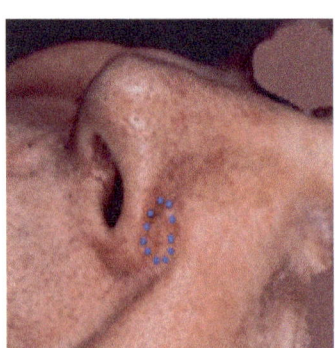
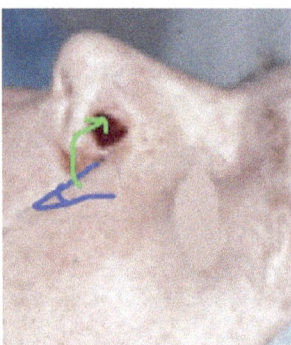
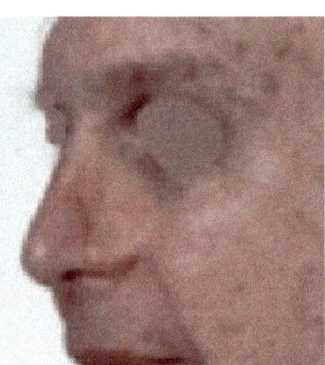

Melanoma

"Juanita" was referred to me by a surgical oncologist. He had diagnosed melanoma of the upper lip and was planning an excision and sentinel node biopsy. The oncologist injected a radioisotope near the tumor two hours before the procedure. At the start of the operation, he also injected blue dye near the tumor. Both the stain and the isotope migrate to the draining lymph nodes.

At the time of the excision, the surgeon explored the area of the draining lymph nodes, with the aid of a Geiger counter and the visual inspection for blue dye. The first or sentinel node is identified and removed for pathological examination. The status of the nodes will help in staging the tumor and selecting any adjuvant therapy. The first picture below shows the innocuous appearing lesion. The second is after the oncologic surgeon has removed the cancer. The third is after I have begun to mobilize adjacent tissue to reconstruct the defect.

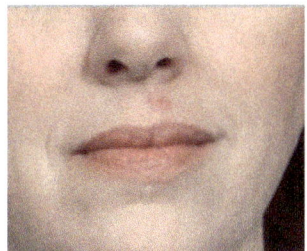 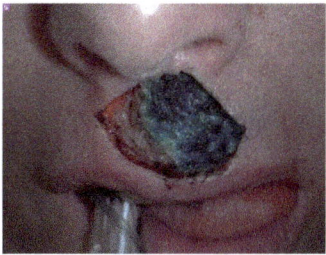 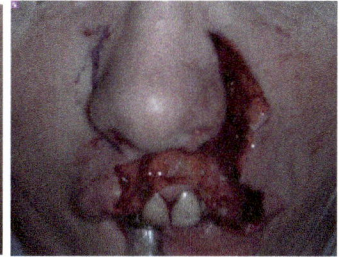

The first photo below is on the table result, and the others are very early post-op photos. The oncologic surgeon followed her, and I believe she did well.

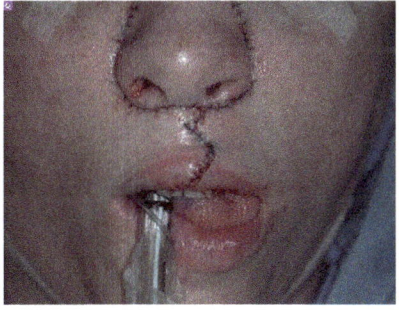 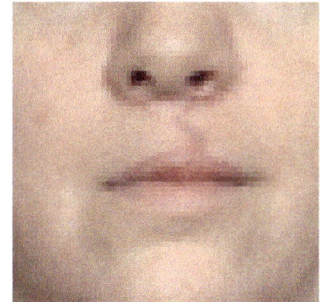

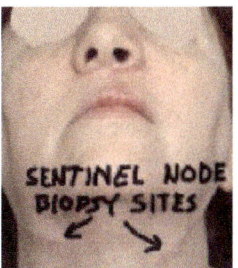 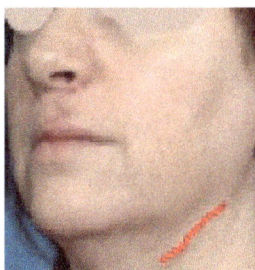 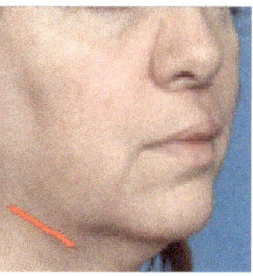

Benign eyelid tumor

The young girl "Annie" shown below had a benign upper eyelid tumor, which I removed. The center photo shows the tumor better exposed for excision. There is a white corneal protector in place. Her post-op result is on the right.

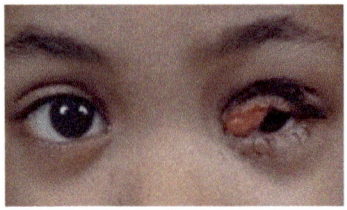 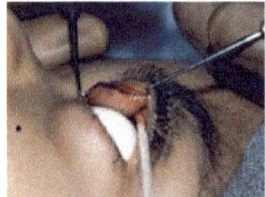 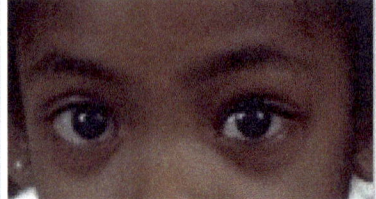

Macrostomia or large mouth

This macrostomia patient, "Bobby," has bilateral # 7 rare Tessier clefts. I repaired these clefts with the same technique as the patient with bilateral # 7 clefts in chapter 4. His before photo and a five-year post-op photo are below.

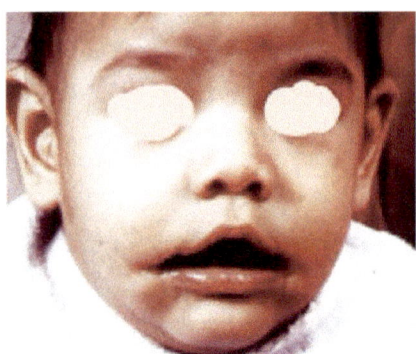 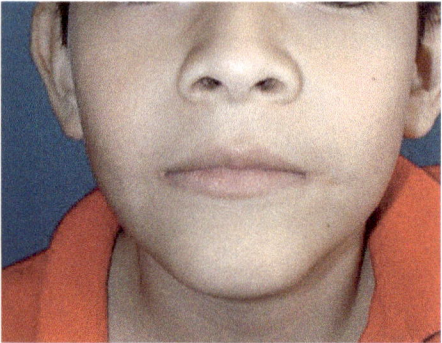

Below "Karl" has a unilateral # 7 cleft on the right. His preoperative and a few weeks post-repair photo are below.

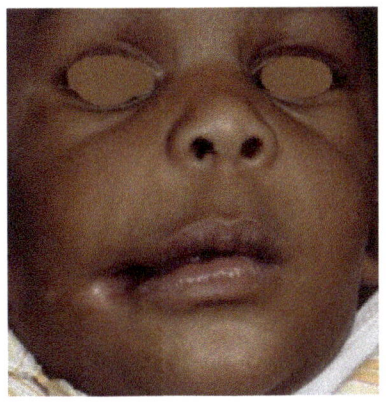
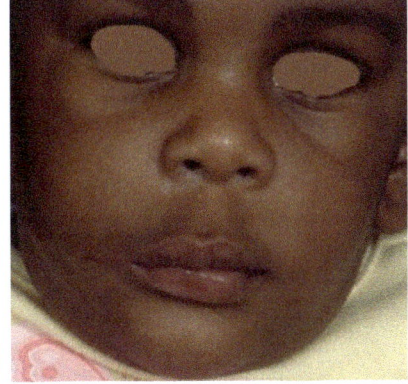

Free flap heel reconstruction.

The octogenarian patient "Horace," below, had a chronic nonhealing ulcer of his right heel. I treated him by excising this ulcer entirely down to the bone. The wound was not suitable for a skin graft closure, so I elected to perform a free tissue transfer of vascularized temporoparietal fascia to the wound. The posterior tibial vessels were convenient for an anastomosis, as in the drawing.

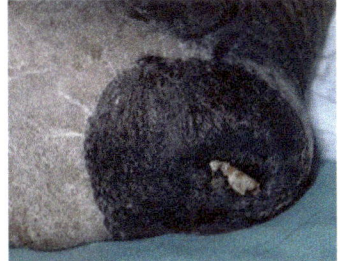
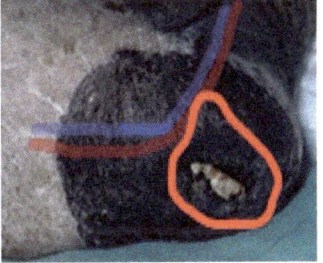
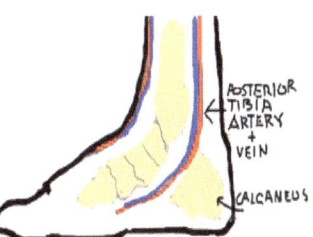

In the first photo below, recipient posterior tibial vessels in the foot were isolated and prepared to receive donor vessels. The second photo shows the temporoparietal fascia flap dissected from the side of the head and the supplying vessels isolated with a small orange rubber strap.

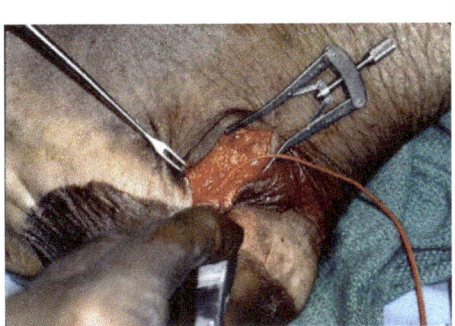
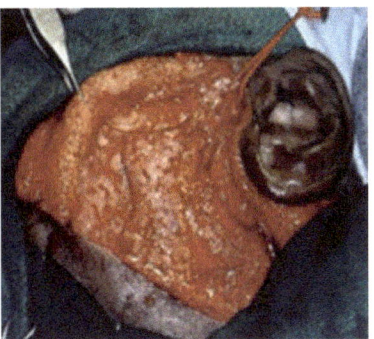

The next photo drawing below shows the facial donor vessels, which are the blood supply to the flap, isolated before being severed. The final picture below shows the temporoparietal flap elevated before being separated from the patient.

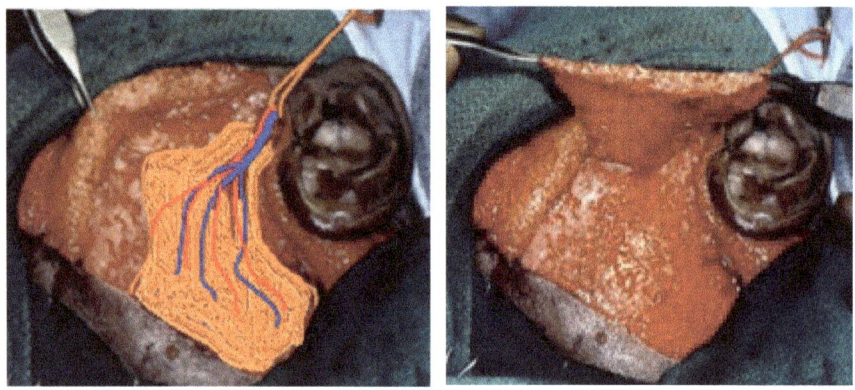

I transferred This thin flap was, and the flap vessels were sutured to the recipient vessels in the foot to re-establish the blood supply. I anastomosed the flap vein to the severed end of the posterior tibial vein. In contrast, the flap artery was anastomosed into the side of the tibial artery so as not to interrupt blood flow to the foot. I placed the flap into the defect created from the excision of the ulcerated wound of the heel. I then covered the flap was with a split-thickness skin graft.

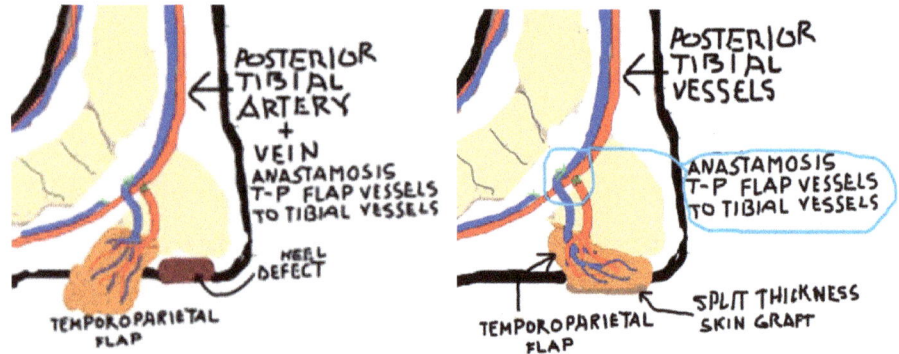

The postoperative results are below. He was able to resume walking without difficulty.

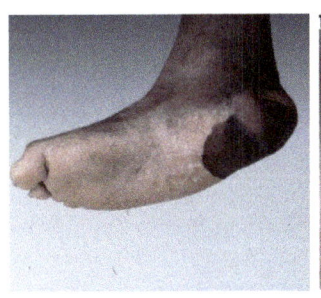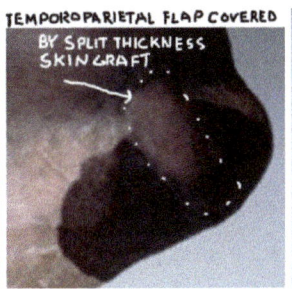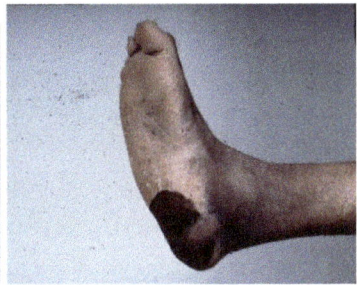

Obesity

Body contouring surgery and Liposuction

We're supposed to be in an epidemic of obesity in the United States, with more than 30% of the public significantly overweight. Primarily because of the success of various bypass surgery procedures aimed at the morbidly obese patient, we began seeing more and more patients who had lost massive amounts of weight.

In many of these patients, the skin will not correspondingly shrink to their new size; therefore, they will have considerable hanging excess skin for which the only solution is surgical removal and tailoring. Some predict such body contouring as a new growth area in plastic surgery. We must keep in mind that this is significant surgery prone to various complications and must be considered only after genuinely informed consent.

Sometimes surgery done on obese patients can be considered functional because the excess weight makes it difficult for them to do tasks of ordinary living.

Big boy bed

A huge man, "Ignatius," came into the office one day. He said that he had already lost about 150 pounds, having had a stomach stapling procedure a year earlier. He complained of a large pannus of abdominal tissue, which hung down and lapped down below the knees. He wanted to have this large apron surgically removed so that he would be more mobile, more comfortable, and would be able to continue losing weight and get into better shape. Except for his obesity, the gentleman was in good medical condition. I agreed that the removal of this abdominal apron would be advantageous for him. His preoperative photo is below.

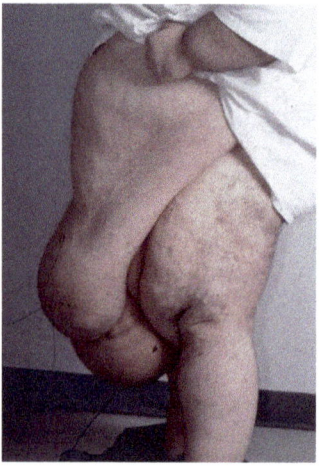

I remember a few things about him that were unusual. On the day of his surgery, because of the heaviness and the abundant, thick nature of the abdominal apron, I arranged to do his operation with a large hoist available. After induction, we preliminarily prepped the patient and placed large clamps into the pannus. We fasten the clamps to the hoist so that it could lift the pannus to facilitate the surgery. Otherwise, it would be difficult to push the large, heavy, abdominal tissue out-of-the-way to make the incisions and to remove the tissue. The two photos below (from another patient "B" with a smaller abdominal pannus) illustrate a pannus lifted by clamps tied a hoist.

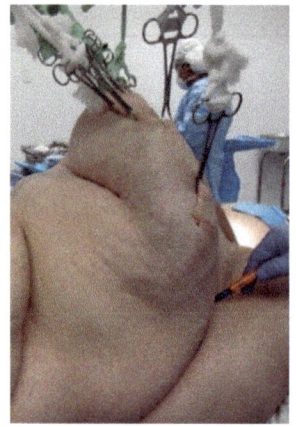 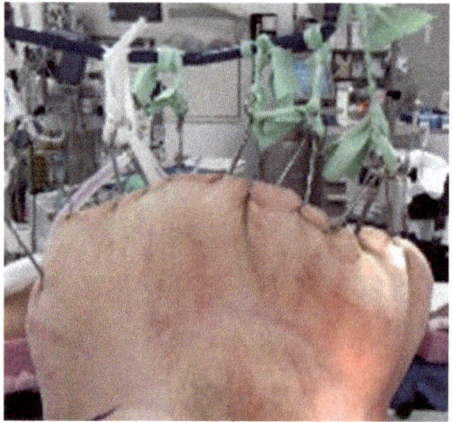

During the surgery for "Ignatius," I removed approximately 45 pounds of skin and fat from his abdomen. The operation is somewhat more complicated than one might think because it is hard to stay oriented in this sea of fatty tissue. I have heard of instances where a surgeon trying to cut into the abdomen on massive patients instead angled off somewhat and cut down until he cut through the skin again and saw the operating table, never having been in the patient's abdomen! The slightly gross picture below is of a pannus weighing 36 pounds, which I removed from patient "B."

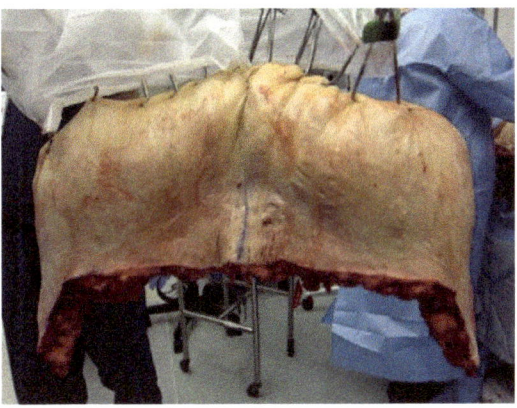

The two pictures below are intraoperative photos from Ignatius's surgery. The first view shows the thickness of the subcutaneous fat of the residual abdominal tissue. The second view shows the closed abdominal wound after the removal of the pannus.

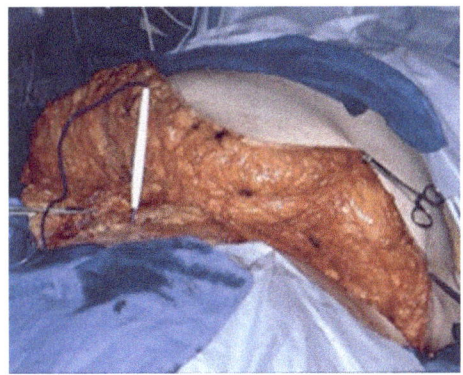 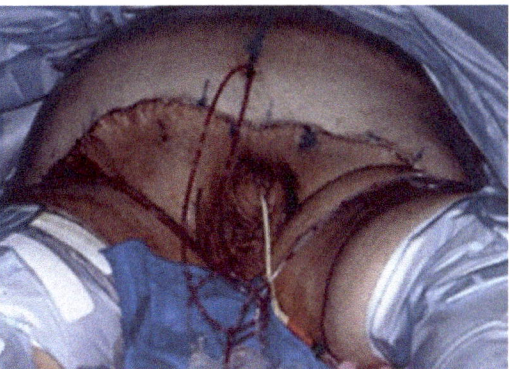

Because of the extensive nature of this operation and the man's obesity, he spent the night of surgery in the intensive care unit. We had a unique bed for him called a big boy bed, which could facilitate bringing the patient to a standing position. It worked somewhat like a dump truck that could be tilted, allowing the patient to put his feet on the ground and then stand up. In my first experience with this bed, we began leaning the bed up so that the patient could stand up. Mind you; this is still a 400 - pound man. As I was standing in front of him, seeing the bed keep coming up and the patient becoming more upright suddenly, I realized that if he was not steady enough on his feet, he might fall forward on top of me. It was a very unpleasant sensation for a few moments. He did well, healed satisfactorily, and improved his activity level after the removal of 45 pounds of tissue. He also said that his ability to maintain personal hygiene was much improved.

Although one can see his very fatty thighs in the first two postoperative photos below, he no longer had abdominal tissue hanging below his knees. He was now in a much better position to lose additional weight.

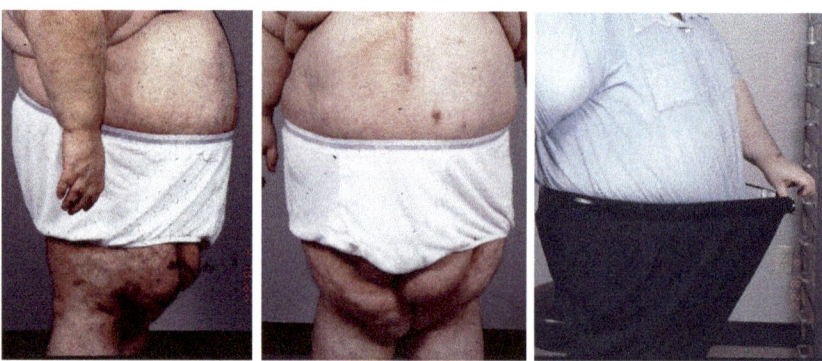

Long Palate Case

A middle-aged man, "Zavier," was referred to me by a physician colleague who thought he might need a nasal septoplasty. "Zavier" had sleep difficulty with loud snoring, which was interrupted by the sensation that he could not breathe. He said he would sometimes sleep in an upright, easy chair and have less frequent interruptions.

On examination, I found that he could breathe well through his nose when he was in an upright position; however, when I placed him supine with his head back at the same level, he would immediately have trouble breathing. When I carefully looked in his mouth with him supine, the problem was obvious. His palate was so long and relaxed that I observed his uvula and posterior soft palate resting on the posterior pharynx. He had a form of obstructive sleep apnea. Some other causes are severe nasal septal deviation or a large tongue that falls back and obstructs the airway etc.

The first photo on the left below illustrates normal breathing through the nose in the supine position. The second photo shows obstruction of the pharyngeal airway when the palate is too long and floppy and therefore rests on the posterior pharyngeal wall in the back of the throat. I observed this problem on "Zavier's" physical exam.

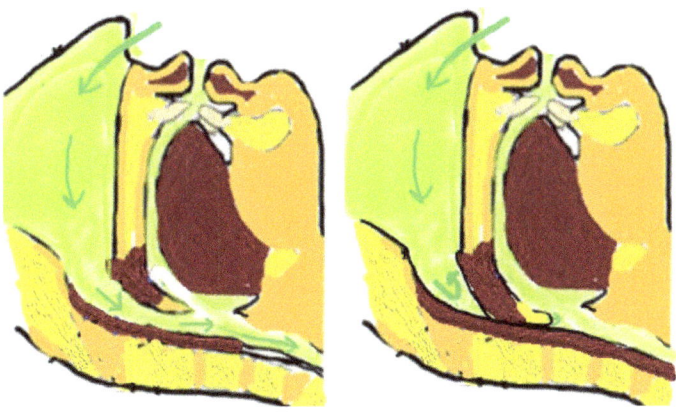

After discussing this with him, I found out that he had had a sleep study and was already using a CPAP machine. CPAP machines are often beneficial for patients with obstructive sleep apnea. However, he had trouble using it. He would usually remove it after trying to sleep with it for an hour or so. I presented an alternative treatment that I thought might be helpful for his circumstance.

I proposed shortening his palate surgically so that it would be less obstructive. He was ready to try something new as the CPAP was not working for him. A few weeks later, I took him to the operating room and performed a shortening of his soft palate, which removed his uvula and about an additional 1.5 centimeters of his soft palate. The drawing below on the left represents the trimming of the soft palate and uvula. The illustration on the right shows the relief of the obstruction.

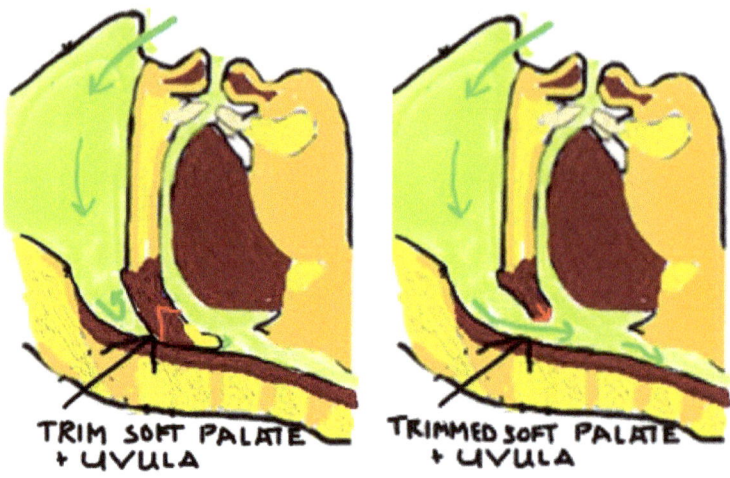

After allowing a couple of weeks for the swelling to subside, we were both happy that his sleep apnea greatly improved. A potential complication of this surgery is hyper-nasal speech because of nasal air escape from the oral cavity into the nasal cavity. Fortunately, he did not have that issue.

Functional Abdomen

Recurrent Abdominal Hernia

Recurrent abdominal hernias are a more common problem than one might think. Because plastic surgeons are so concerned with wound closures, they are sometimes called upon by our general surgery or gynecology colleagues to help with closures of recurrent hernias. Such consultations have increased since the development of the component separation technique of closure.

Mid-drift over bulge

This lady, "Elesia," had previous abdominal surgery but developed a large incisional hernia with an abnormal bulge in the lower abdomen. This condition was not only unsightly but was also quite uncomfortable when she had to strain for any reason. Through a tummy tuck approach, I repaired the abdominal wall hernia and removed the excess abdominal skin. Although she did have some cosmetic improvement, this was fundamentally a functional surgery, which made her more comfortable and better able to do strenuous activities. I did this procedure before the component separation technique was available.

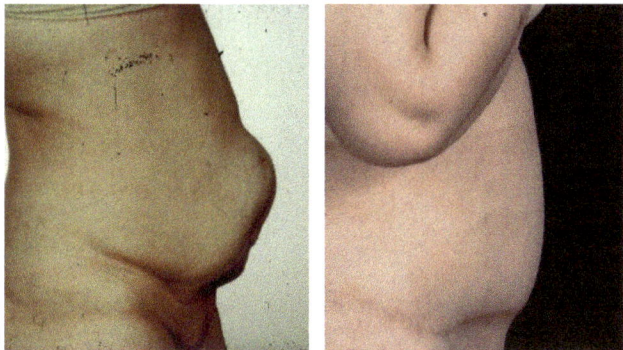

I did the following severe hernia case was done with a general surgeon colleague. This patient had a large ventral abdominal hernia with loss of muscle domain or control.

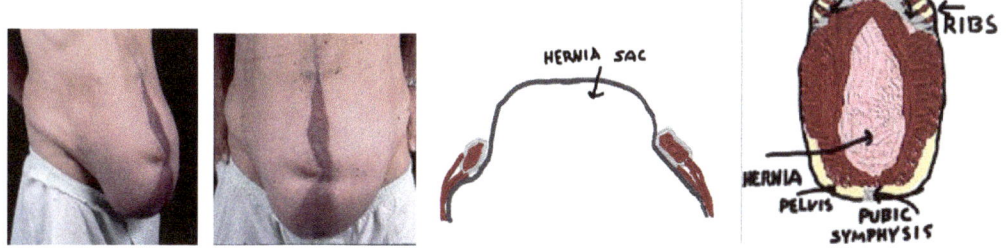

In his case, we used a large mesh to support the entire abdominal wall, as we were unable to obtain good muscle repair with the rectus fascia. We sutured the mesh to fixed structures, the pubis and ilium below, and ribs above. We also fastened it to the muscles laterally. I also excised redundant skin leaving an inverted T shaped scar.

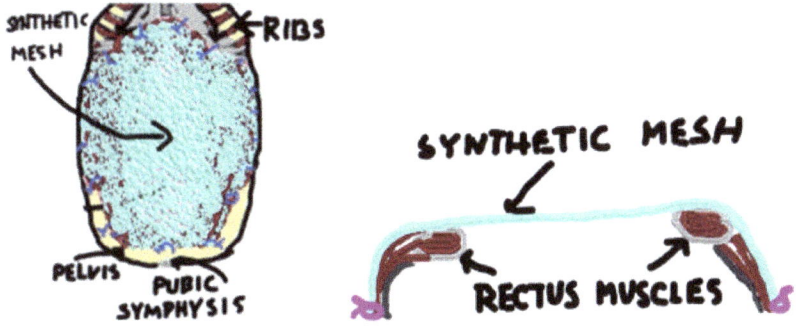

His postoperative result is below

The Healing Mission of Plastic Surgery

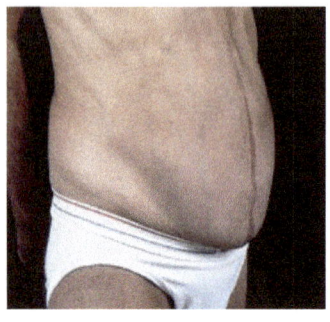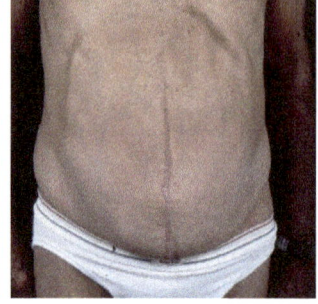

Recurrent Abdominal Hernia

Component Separation Technique and dermal matrix

The patient represented below "Gregory" was sent to me for consultation by a general surgeon colleague of mine. This patient had previously had a large hernia develop after abdominal surgery. He also had already had two procedures attempting to repair his abdominal hernia. Both had failed. Surgical colleagues often request plastic surgeons to help close difficult or complicated wounds all over the body. "Gregory's" preoperative pictures are below.

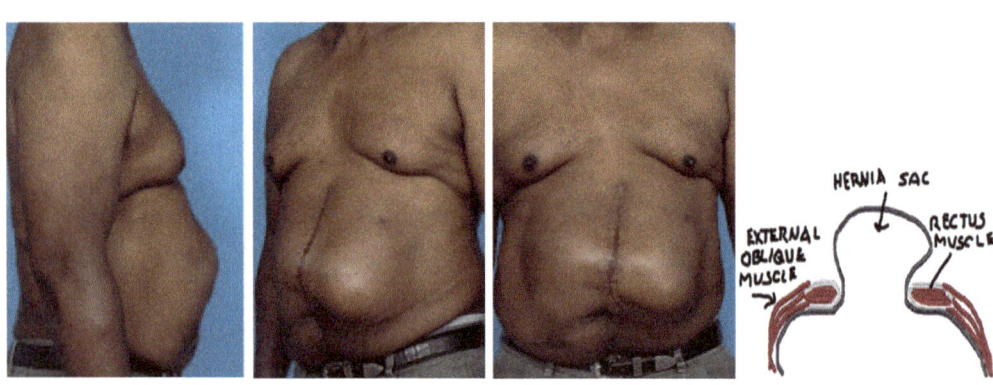

In his case, I recommended a components separation method introduced by doctor Oscar Ramirez. In this case, the general surgeon began the operation and identified the hernia, remove the hernia sac, and place the abdominal contents which had herniated through the abdominal wall back into the abdominal cavity. The first photo below shows the situation after he removed the hernia sac, and the intestines are back where they belong. The yellow dots indicate the edge of the fascia of the abdominal wall and show the size of the hole or hernia defect in the abdominal wall.

The Healing Mission of Plastic Surgery

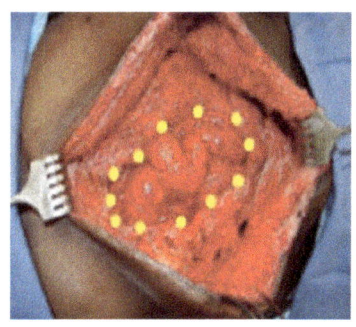

I then took over the operation to repair the abdominal wall to prevent the recurrence of the hernia. I combine several techniques to obtain a robust abdominal wall closure. First of all, I cut the external oblique muscle on either side laterally in the abdomen to allow better mobilization of the rectus muscles as in the second intraoperative photo. The two blue lines show the amount of stretching that has been accomplished by the release of the external oblique muscle and fascia laterally. The rectus muscle (held by forceps) and fascial edge (yellow dots) can now stretch beyond the midline. I repeated the same maneuvers on the opposite side so that I could close the midline fascia without any tension.

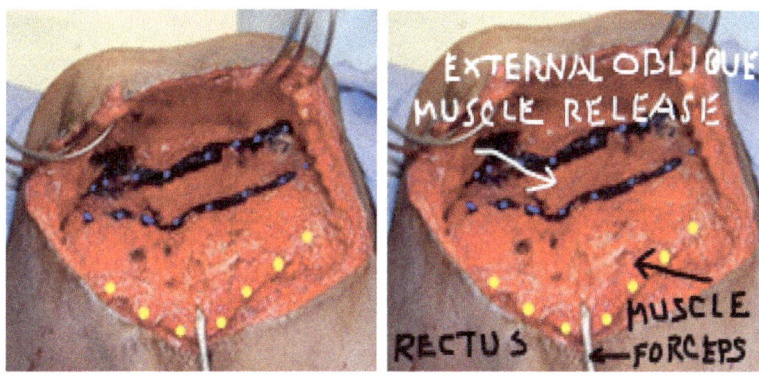

Before repairing the fascia, I first sutured a layer of dermal matrix between the abdominal contents and the inside of the abdominal wall against the fascia and rectus abdominus muscle as an internal reinforcement. The purple dots in the intraoperative photo below are on the dermal matrix underlay. The pink sheet in the drawing represents the dermal matrix.

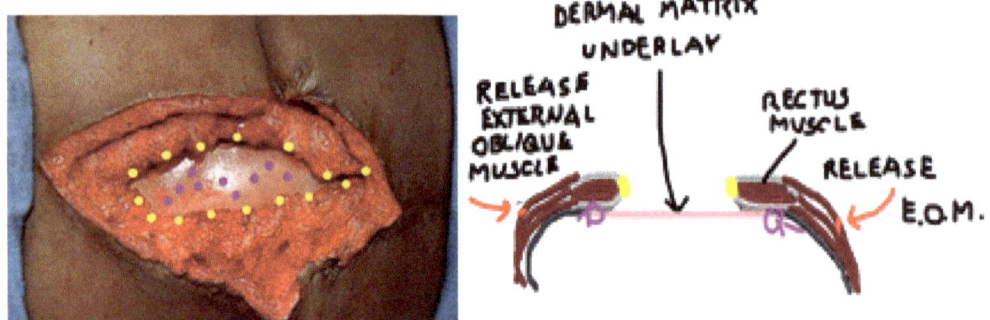

I then sutured the rectus fascia in the midline, as shown in the drawing below. The lateral muscle release made this possible.

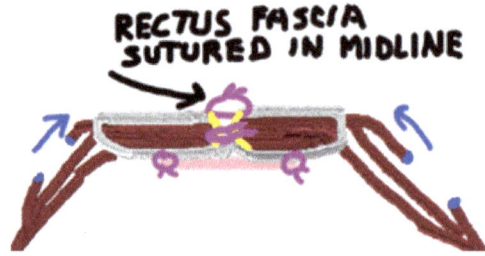

Following the closure of the rectus fascia in the midline, represented by the two rows of yellow dots, I reinforced the repair with a synthetic mesh overlay as in the intraoperative photo and drawing below. I overlayed the fascia repair by a couple of inches on either side. I sutured it to the abdominal wall represented by the gray dots. This repair was like a belt and suspenders. Because of this recalcitrant problem, I wanted to do as much as I could to prevent another recurrence. Underlays are much more reliable than overlays. The drawing also illustrates the release of the external oblique, which allowed the rectus muscles to move more readily to the midline.

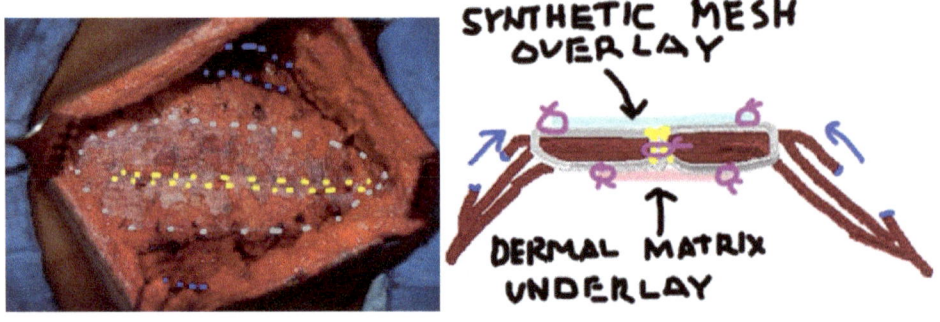

The postoperative photos below show the functional and cosmetic results. This three-layer closure of this multi recurrent hernia was successful.

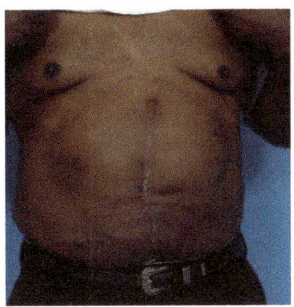 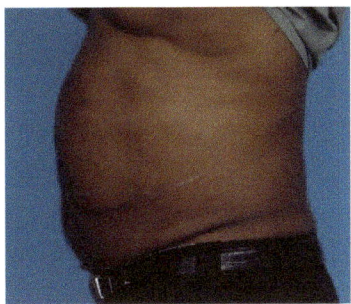

Pelvic Issues

Vaginal Fistula Repair

A 54-year-old lady, "Gloria," had cancer of the rectum and underwent chemotherapy and radiation therapy. An ultrasound revealed a recurrent tumor. Therefore, her oncologic surgeon performed a partial rectal resection. However, after that surgery, she developed a rectovaginal fistula, which is an abnormal connection or passageway between the rectum and the vagina. This fistula allowed fecal matter to leak into the vagina. She, therefore, needed a diverting colostomy.

Then her oncologic surgeon took her back to surgery for closure of this fistula between the rectum and vagina. However, this attempt to directly close the connection was not successful. Her surgeon then referred her to me for the closure of this fistula. Because she had previously undergone radiation therapy, the local tissues were damaged and had a subpar capacity for healing. She was very distraught by this situation, although she was happy that she had no residual evidence of cancer. My two drawings below are representations of normal anatomy, showing the vagina and the rectum separated by a relatively small amount of tissue.

The Healing Mission of Plastic Surgery

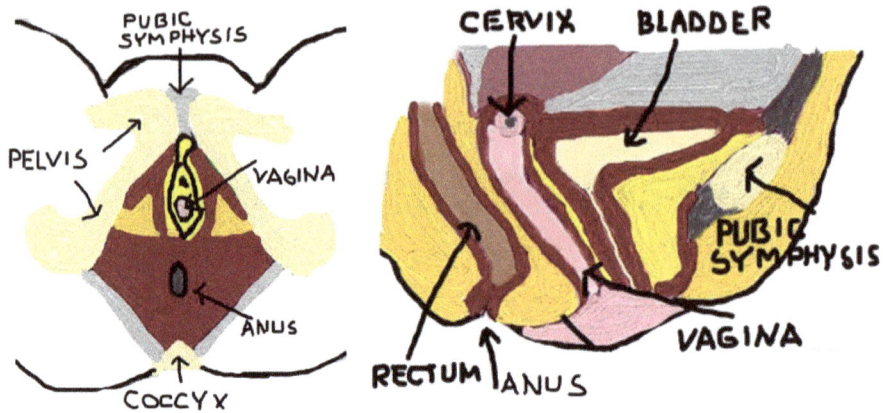

My drawing below shows the location of the fistula circled in light blue. I devise a plan for closure, which would entail surgery to separate the walls of the vagina from the rectum and, if possible, close each layer independently to separate one from the other.

However, knowing the poor condition of these tissues and the likelihood that there would be a breakdown of these closures, I decided that interposing a muscle flap would be advantageous. I planned to take the gracilis muscle from the medial thigh and turn it upward so that it could be placed between the rectum and the vagina to offer healthy with better blood supply to help with the healing.

Hence the need for the diverting colostomy she already had. My surgery intended to restore normal function by re-separating the rectum from the vagina.

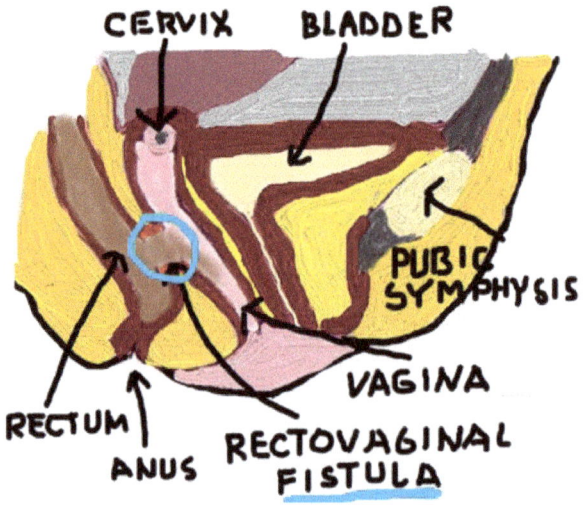

The Healing Mission of Plastic Surgery

I did the surgery from below with the patient in the lithotomy position (feet up in stirrups). With the patient asleep, the examination of the vagina and rectum revealed a large opening about 2cm x 4cm connecting the two. As I palpated, around its edge, I felt multiple staples from the previous surgery. I first removal more than a dozen of these metallic staples through the vagina. Following this, I made an incision through the skin between the vagina and the anus, sparing the sphincter muscles. I then dissected between the vaginal and rectal layers and soon reached the fistula. I sharply freshened the edges of the fistula, and then I continued the dissection well past the fistula. I was able to do separate direct closures of the vagina (green sutures) and the rectum (dark blue stitches), both circled in light blue in my drawing below. The previously dissected space (white void) separated these two closures.

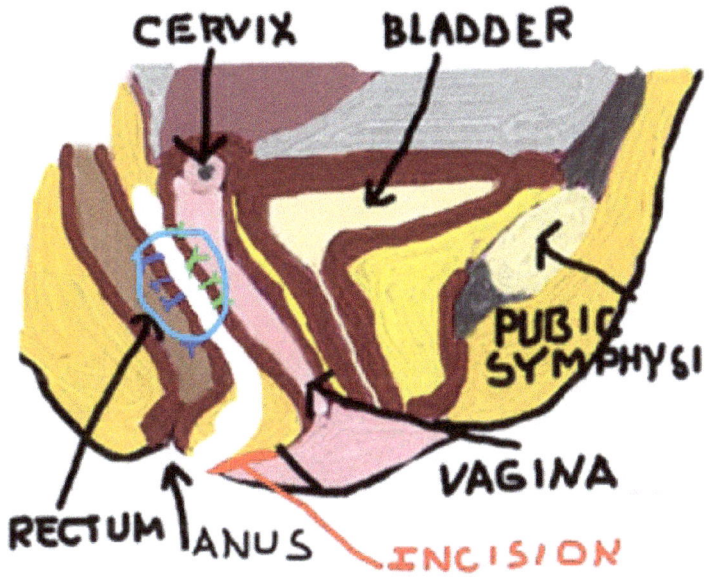

Next, I made an incision in the upper thigh and dissected the gracilis muscle from its insertion and freed it toward its pubic origin.

The Healing Mission of Plastic Surgery

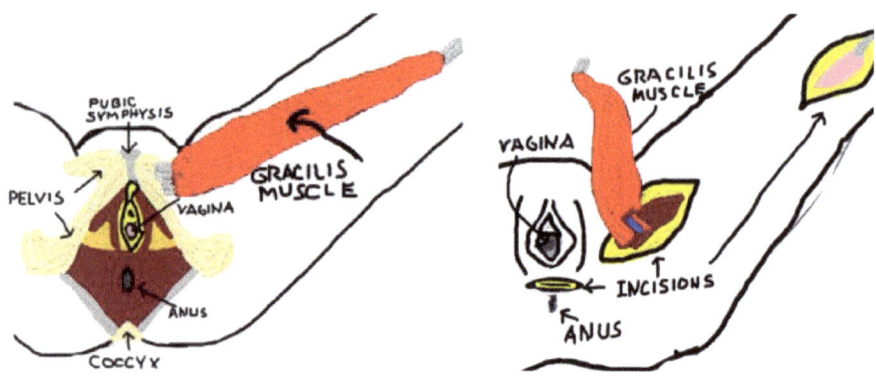

I tunneled this long thin muscle under the skin and then turned it upward into the space between the vagina and the rectum and sutured it as high as possible. The drawings below show, from two different views, the gracilis muscle between the two preliminary closures of the rectum and vagina. Its purpose was two-fold. First, to offer new blood supply and, therefore, better healing capacity into the area that received so much previous radiation therapy, secondly, to provide a somewhat thick tissue barrier between the closures on the two sides of the previous fistula. Even if there was a small breakdown on either the rectal or the vaginal side, the interposed muscle provided a barrier of healthy tissue for healing.

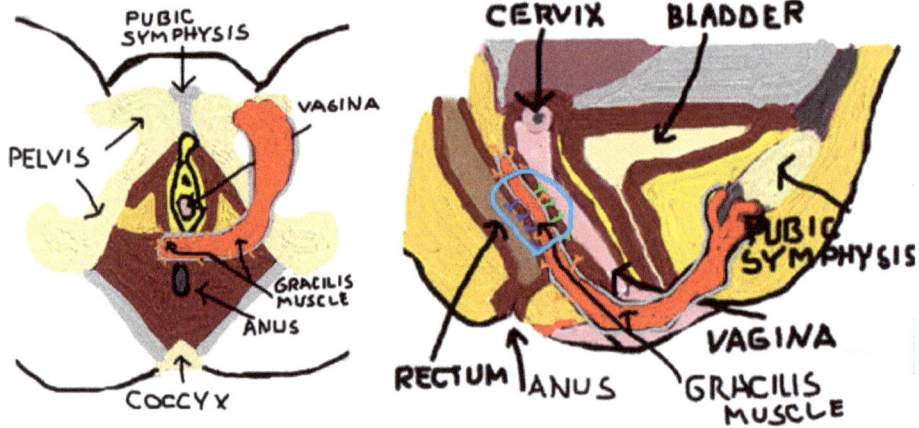

The surgery was a success, so her general surgeon took down the colostomy several weeks later. "Gloria" was able to resume normal bowel function and again have near-normal vaginal anatomy. She became a much happier camper and was very grateful for the care I was able to give her.

Colorectal surgeons often need to deal with patients who have developed such rectovaginal fistulae. I recall a patient "Maggie" with inflammatory bowel disease I saw at the request of a colorectal surgeon. She had developed a rectovaginal fistula because of inflammation and infection. She was treated with a diverting colostomy for several months to see if the fistula would heal on its own. When this did not happen, the colorectal surgeon decided to explore the area in the operating room and asked me to help with the repair. She had persistence of the fistula.

The colorectal surgeon separated the rectal and vaginal walls and repaired the rectal side of the fistula. I then sutured the vaginal side of the defect and placed a gracilis flap into the wound to separate the vagina from the rectum, just like "Gloria's" case above. "Maggie" did well and had the colostomy reversed later.

Vaginal reconstruction with gracilis flaps

The following patient, "Rosanne," illustrates the difficulty of perineal cases as she suffered complications in her healing that necessitated additional surgery. She had cancer of the rectum near the anus. Her surgical oncologist treated her with an abdominal perineal resection (A-P resection) of the rectum. In that procedure, the surgeon uses both an intraabdominal approach and one from the perineum. She needed a permanent colostomy with an opening in the abdomen because of the extent of the rectal resection. The first drawing below shows the perineal incision in red for the A-P resection. My second drawing is a sagittal view of the carcinoma and its resection, which included wide excision of the anus and resection of a large segment of colon and a part of the posterior wall of the vagina.

The Healing Mission of Plastic Surgery

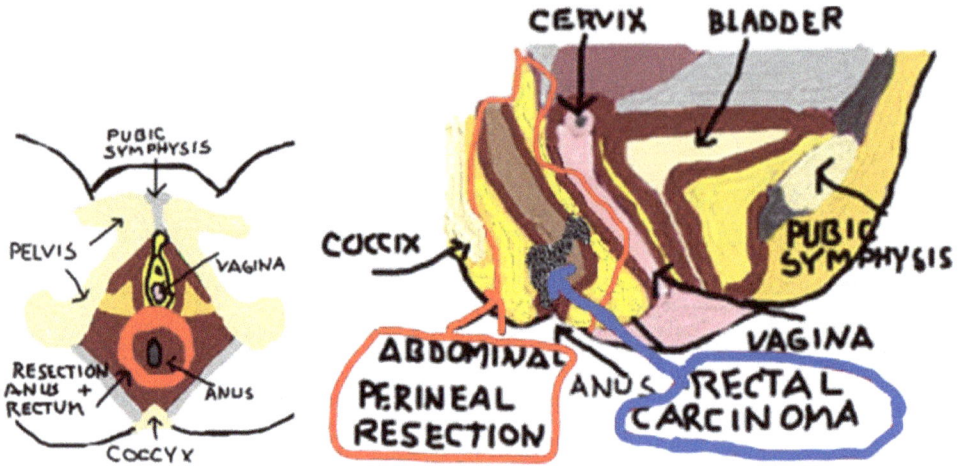

My first drawing below shows that a void exists from the removal of the perineal tissue, rectum, and colon. The second drawing also shows that part of the posterior wall of the vagina is missing. The void created by an A P resection can be quite capacious.

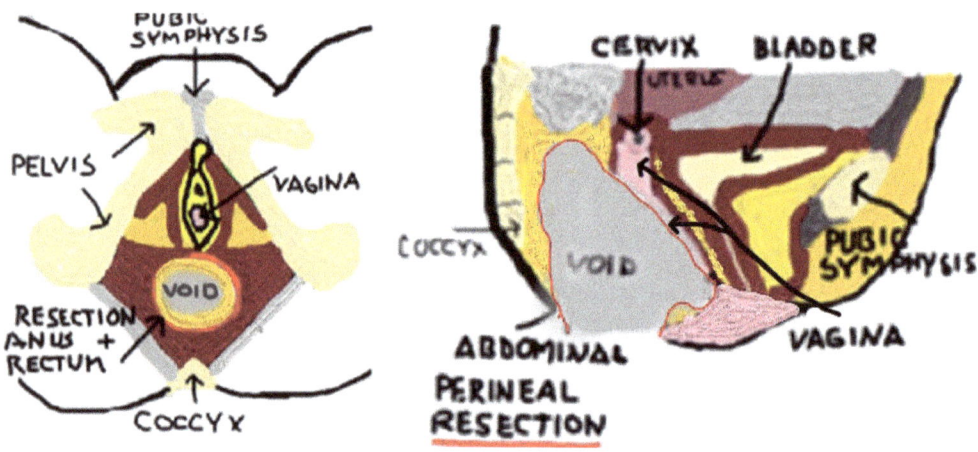

The intraoperative photo below, with the patient in the lithotomy position (in stirrups), shows the significant perineal/sacral surface defect. The deeper void is not seen well, because of the collapse of adjacent tissue into the wound. The photo also shows bilateral gracilis myocutaneous flaps. The drawing on the right shows the proximal portion of the skin island has been partially de-epithelialized so that I can bury that section for the deep reconstruction. The green dot is at the proximal end, and the purple dot is at the distal end of the flap.

The Healing Mission of Plastic Surgery

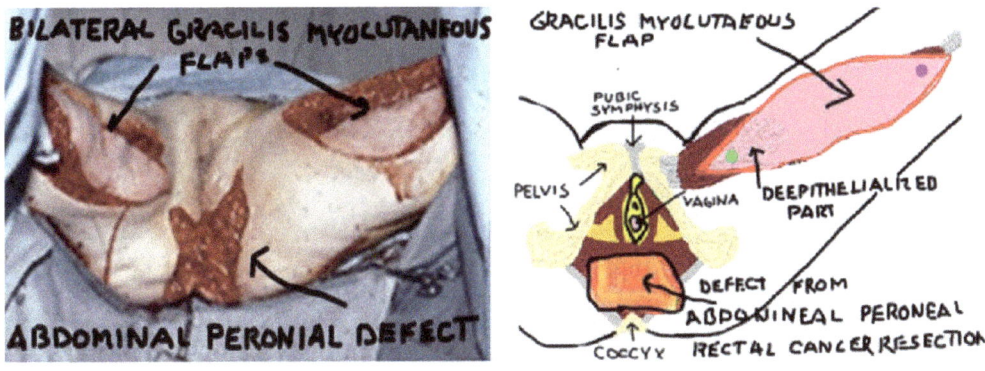

The drawings below show how I filled in the deep void with the de-epithelialized portions of the gracilis myocutaneous flaps, which I tunneled to the perineum. I used part of one flap to reconstruct the posterior vaginal wall.

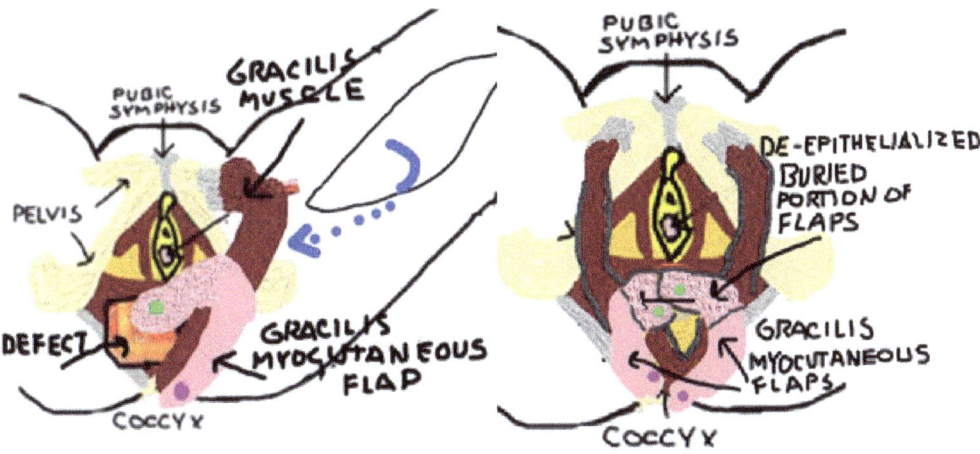

The drawing below shows the proximal skin island (green Dot) buried deep in the void and part used to restore the posterior vaginal wall (orange line). I utilized the distal portion of the flap (purple dot) to reconstruct the large perineal/ sacral surface defect. The intraoperative photo on the right (the patient is in the lithotomy position) shows the flaps in place at the end of the procedure. At this point, everything looks successful.

The Healing Mission of Plastic Surgery

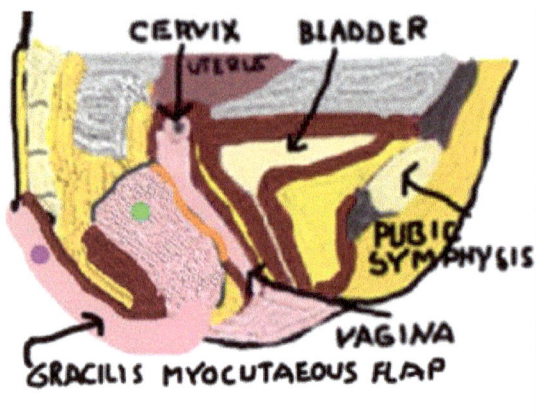
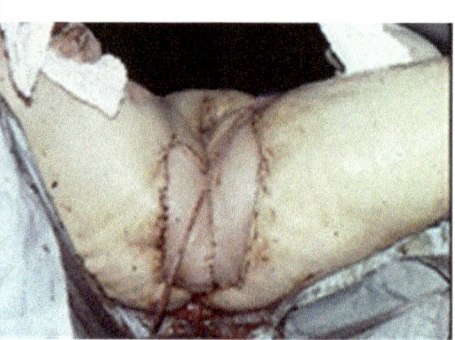

T

The drawing below is a key to the previous photo showing the orientation of the proximal and distal skin islands.

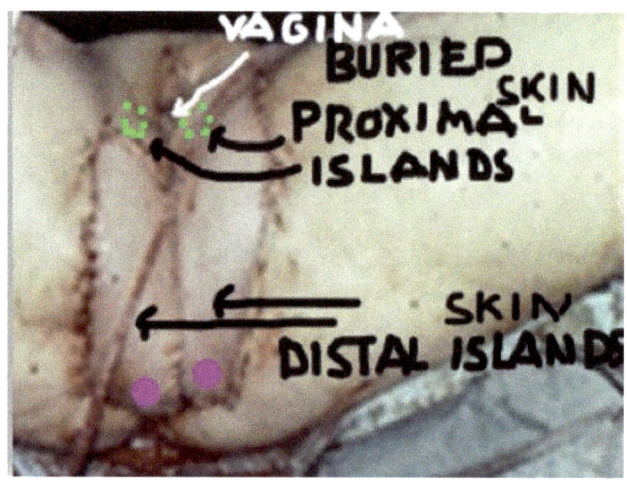

However, everything was not ok. Although the vaginal reconstruction and the perineal reconstruction were healing well, some of the lateral skin islands toward the sacrum necrosed. This failure may have been because this part of the skin island was not well center over the muscle to receive perforating blood supply. The photo on the left below was taken several days after surgery. The patient is in a prone position rather than the lithotomy position. I took her to the operating room for debridement of the necrotic tissue. The photo on the right is after the excision of the dead tissue. The rubber bands are around the gracilis muscles, which are still viable.

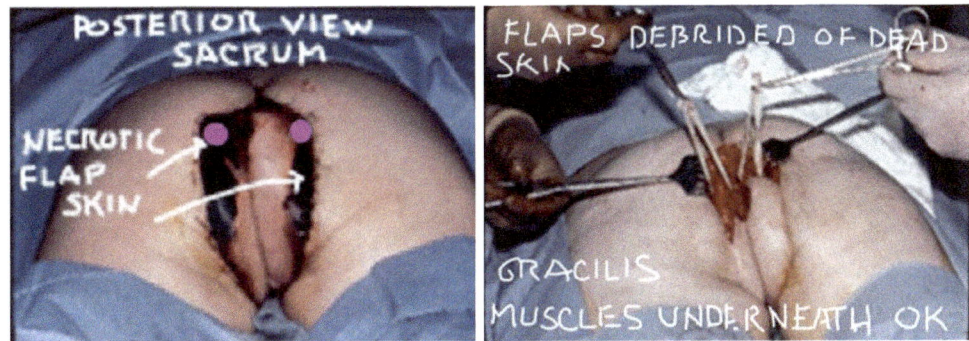

The intraoperative photo on the left below is the immediate result after debridement and closure at the revision surgery. The post revision photo on the right, taken a few months later, shows that the patient has completely healed the troubled area.

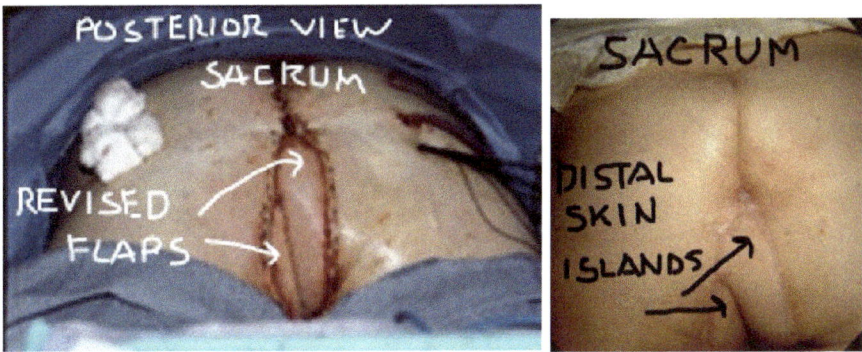

So, she had an extensive abdominal perineal resection of the rectal/anal carcinoma, a permanent colostomy, a reconstruction of the vagina, and perineal/sacral defect. These are examples of functional plastic surgery. "Rosanne" did well for many years after these procedures

Chest Wall

As a plastic surgeon, I would occasionally be called by cardiovascular surgeons to close dehisced sternal chest wounds. Coronary artery bypass surgery was even more prevalent before stent placement, and balloon angioplasty procedures became popular. Occasionally an infection would develop, and wound dehiscence would result. Three different examples are below.

The Healing Mission of Plastic Surgery

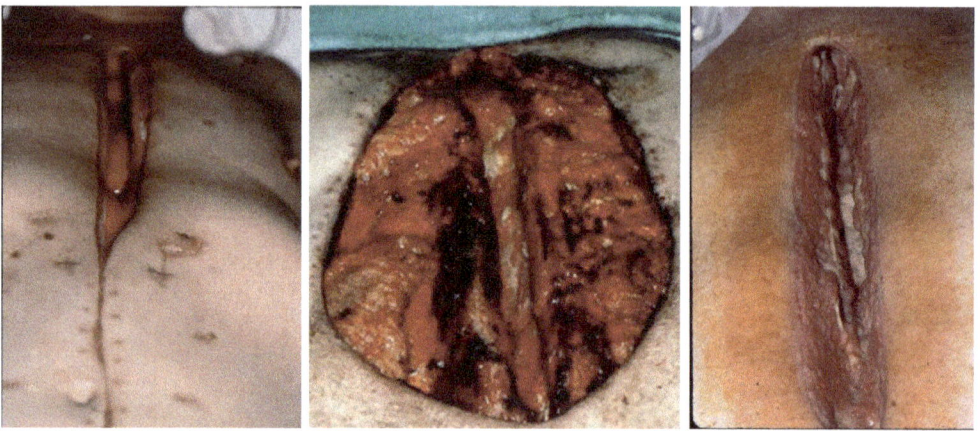

The last patient, "George," was repaired by first debriding the wound of any nonviable tissue. In his case, I used three muscle flaps to bring in new, well-vascularized tissue and closed the extensive wound. The pectoralis major muscles maintained blood supply from the thoracoacromial vessels, and the left rectus abdominis muscle kept blood supply from the superior epigastric vessels. The first photo drawing below shows the blood supply to the two pectoralis major muscles and the left rectus muscle. The second picture is a photo drawing showing both pectoralis major muscles released from their insertion on the humerus and rotated to close the upper portion of the wound. At the same time, I transferred the left rectus abdominis muscle to the lower part of the defect for full closure.

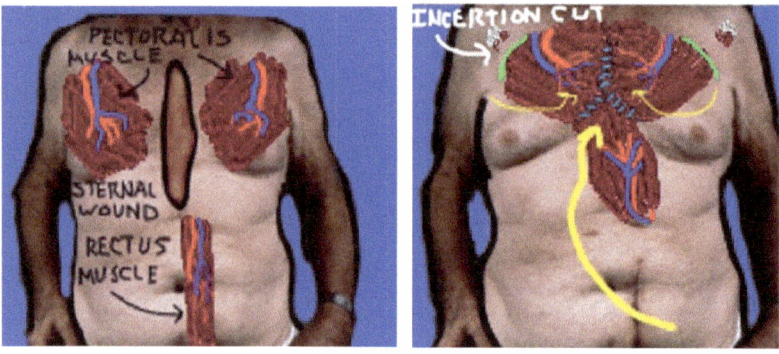

Below left and center show the muscle flaps have fully closed the sternal wound defect. The final result is on the right. I closed the surface wounds primarily because there was no skin loss.

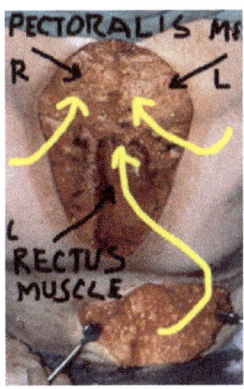 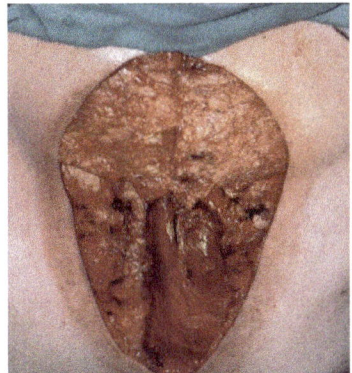 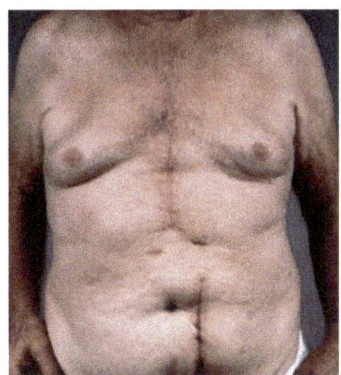

Functional Breast

I cover breast reconstructions in chapter 9.

Breast Reduction

Breast reduction surgery is a prevalent surgery that is usually considered functional. Many patients have pain in the back, neck, and shoulders because of large, heavy, and pendulous breasts. They often have intense shoulder grooves from bra straps pressing into the flesh. Sometimes they have rashes in the intertriginous areas where the breast skin rests on the abdominal skin and causes maceration. There have been studies that validate the benefit of breast reduction in decreasing discomfort and improving maneuverability and quality of life. As a result, medical insurance commonly covers breast reduction, although it is not unusual for there to be a specific exclusion in some policies.

There are only a few basic concepts needed to understand breast reduction. First, the procedure removes excess breast tissue and some overlying skin. The operation preserves the nipple either by leaving it on a de-epithelialized buried pedicle of underlying breast tissue or by removing it and transferring it as a free composite graft to a new de-epithelialized position on the breast. A breast lift is integral to breast reduction. The surgeon must take into account both the blood and nerve supply for sensation to the nipple in the creation of a pedicle flap.

A severe complication of breast reduction is necrosis of the nipple because of inadequate blood flow. If a nipple dies occurs, it may require debridement and secondary reconstruction. A much more common but usually insignificant healing complication is minor necrosis at the inverted T junction in the inframammary crease area. The vast majority of breast reductions utilize one of the myriad pedicle techniques because the nipple maintained on a pedicle is usually better preserved than with a free graft. I will present a few examples of commonly used breast reduction techniques.

Free nipple technique

The free nipple technique uses the nipple and areola as a full-thickness skin graft. The surgeon removes the nipples, amputates the appropriate amount of breast, and then reshapes the remainder. Only after that, he grafts the nipple and areola on de-epithelialized skin at its new location. I performed this amputation and free nipple graft technique occasionally on large breasts, usually in older patients. There is usually some loss of sensation to the nipple with this technique, although in patients with quite large breasts, often there is already diminished sensation. Another issue is there may be some pigment loss with the nipple graft, especially in dark-skinned patients.

"Lory" was a middle-aged lady who wanted relief from discomfort caused by her large pendulous breasts shown below.

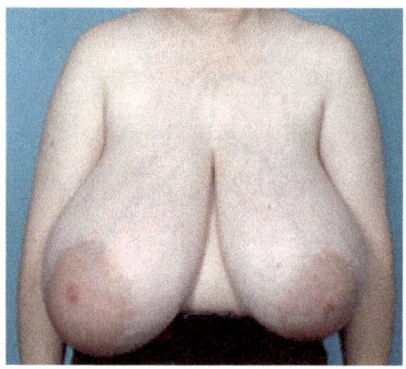
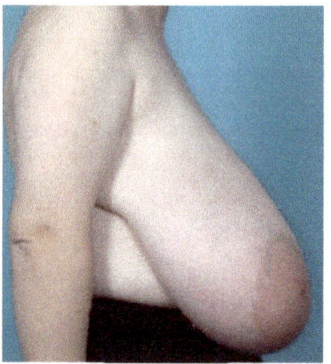

In the photo drawing below, I have drawn an elliptical incision in red, taking into account the desired new position of the nipple (purple). First, I excised the nipples from the breasts and set them aside as shown below right, to be later replaced on the breasts as full-thickness/composite grafts.

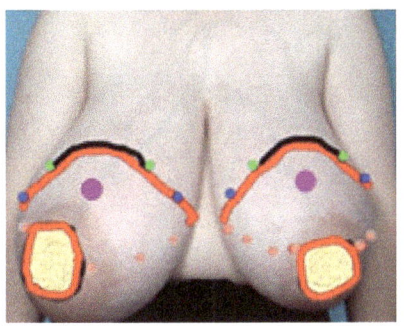 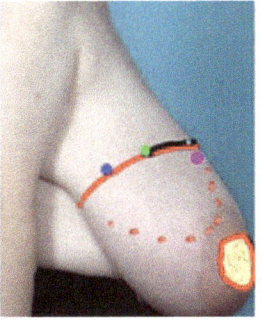 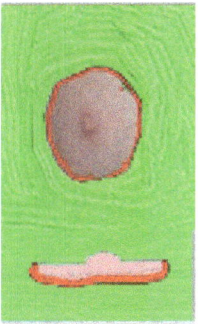

Next, a large portion of each breast was amputated through a horizontal elliptical incision (red) and then oriented and sent for pathological examination.

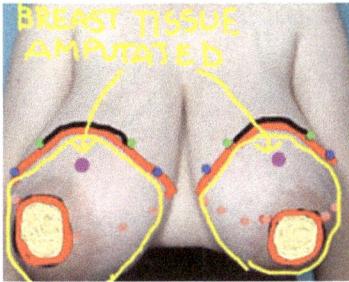 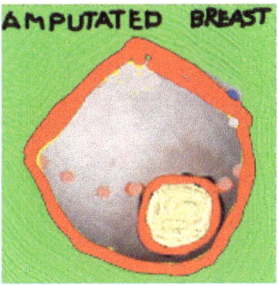 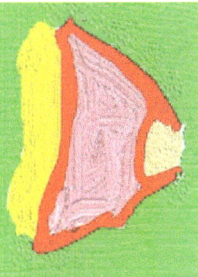

As the photo drawings below indicate, to shape the remaining tissue, I closed the elliptical incisions beginning in the midline of the breast from superiorly in an inverted T fashion, which gave shape and projection to the breast. I placed the sutures first firmly in the deep breast tissue and then in the skin. The colored dots illustrate this closing movement. The yellow circle and purple dot indicate the new areola and nipple position.

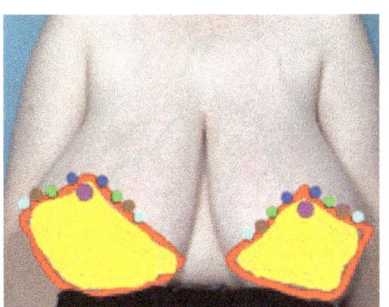 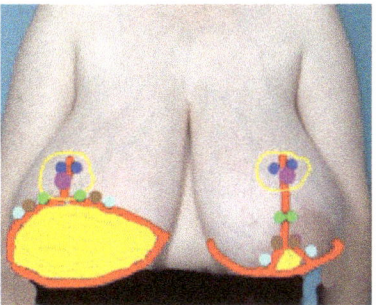

Upon completion, the final incision shape was that of an anchor, as shown below.

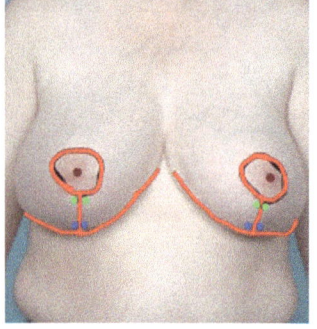 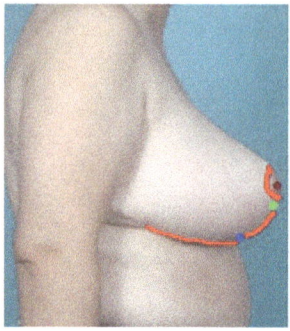

The final result below for "Lory" is after the amputation and free nipple graft technique. Compare with her pre-operative photos previously shown.

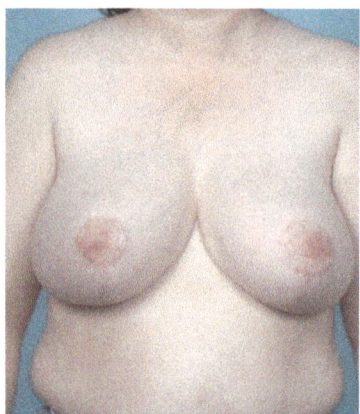 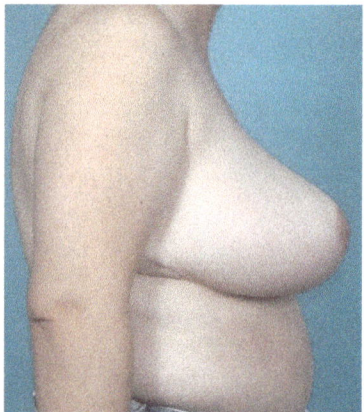

Another amputation and free nipple graft case like the one above of Lory is that of "Victoria." She has excellent shape for such a large reduction but does also have some loss of pigment in the nipple-areola area.

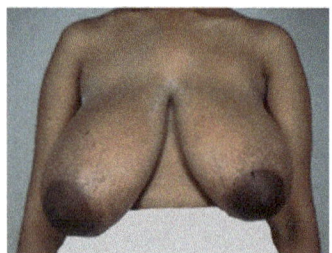 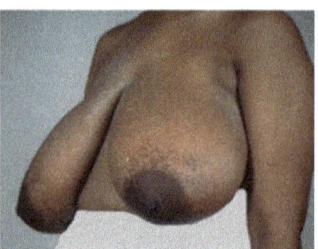 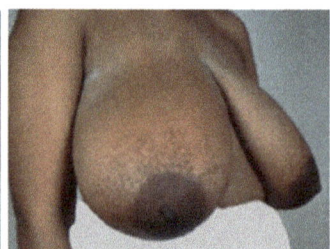

The Healing Mission of Plastic Surgery

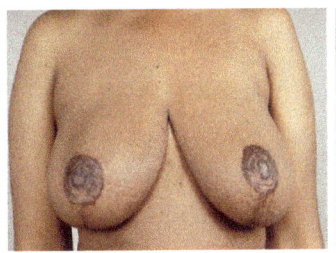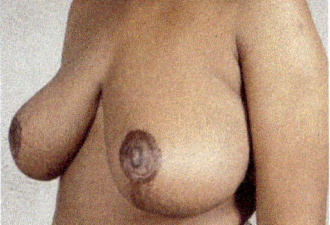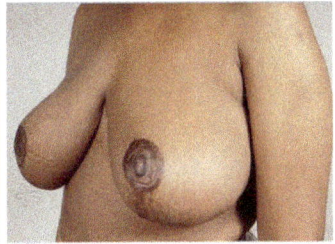

Pedicle techniques and the Wise pattern

In contradistinction to the above cases, I performed most breast reductions with techniques that leave the nipple attached to a de-epithelialized pedicle. Because I have de-epithelialized the flap, I can bury it under other breast tissue and skin. If the flap were not de-epithelialized, the epidermis would shed skin cells and create large cysts of epithelium on top of the flap. I use the wise pattern for most breast reductions.

Dr. Robert Wise, one of my mentors who I introduced in chapter 3, developed the "Wise" design. He developed this by studying brassiere patterns from Frederick's of Hollywood. These patterns could be made from X-ray film so that they were sturdy but flexible enough to bend a little, and the surgeon could sterilize it if he wanted it after the surgery began. I show an example of the pattern below. It is placed on the breast as in the second picture and oriented to correspond to the proposed new location of the nipple (pink dot).

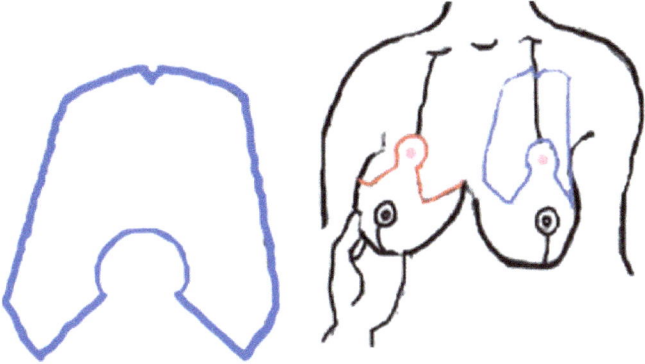

After making cuts along the red lines and removing breast tissue, the surgeon brings together the limbs of the pattern as shown to produce the conical shape desired for the new breast. The nipple, maintained on a pedicle, is lifted beneath this new position and sutured in place.

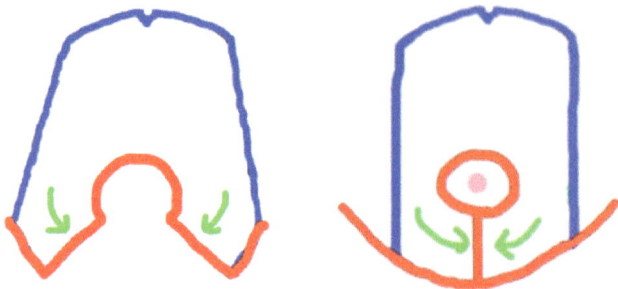

I thought it was fascinating that Dr. Wise told me the amputation and free nipple technique was his favorite breast reduction procedure.

The three most common pedicle methods for breast reduction are the vertical bipedicle, inferior pedicle, and superior-medial pedicle. They all use the Wise pattern and end with an anchor-shaped scar pattern.

Vertical Bipedicle

The first reduction mammaplasty technique my mentors taught me as a plastic surgery resident was the vertical bipedicle operation of McKissock described below. I deployed this technique many times. The first diagram below shows breast tissue removal is from either side of the de-epithelialized vertical bipedicle (pink) and from beneath the flap and the nipple, as shown in the second diagram, which is a lateral view.

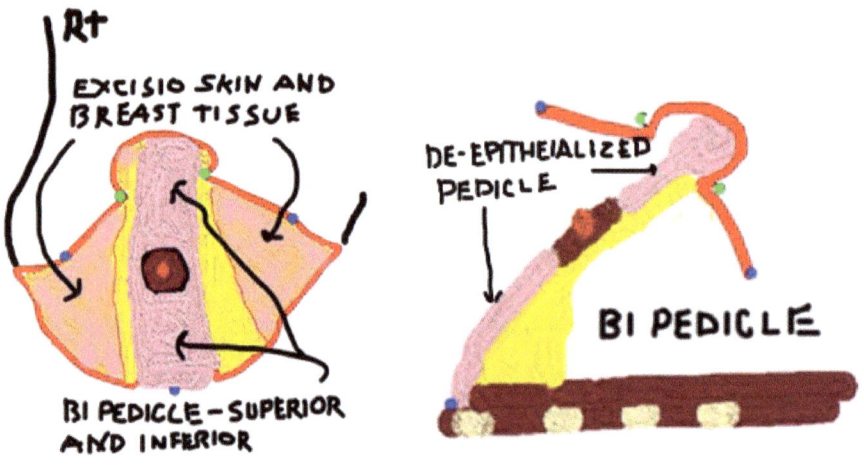

The area under the nipple must be thin enough to fold upon itself both above and below the nipple, as in the diagram below. The remaining breast and skin flaps of the Wise pattern are brought together as usual in an anchor-shaped scar pattern, as shown below.

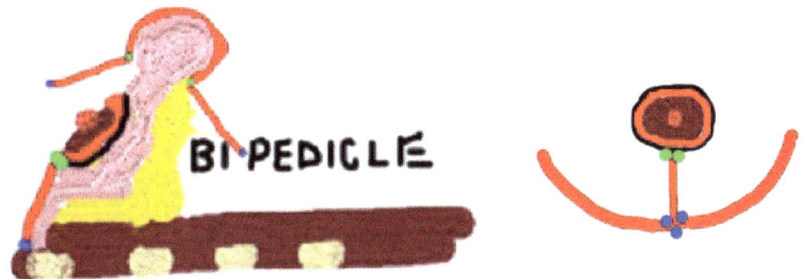

"Angelina" below complained of discomfort because of her large pendulous breasts.

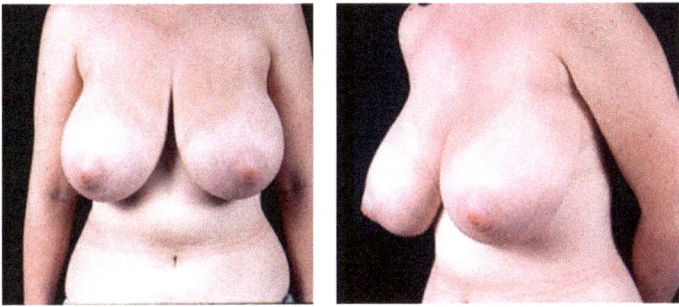

I used a standard Wise pattern as drawn on her breasts below.

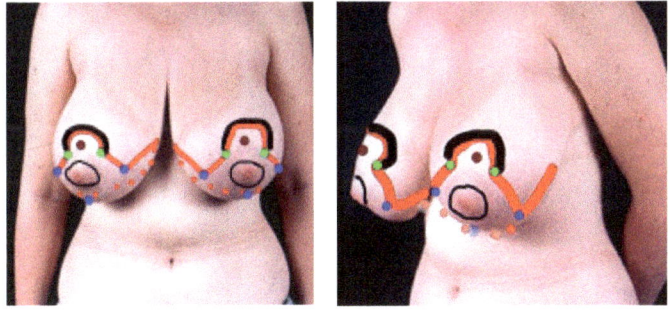

I show the vertical de-epithelialized bipedicle flap in orange below.

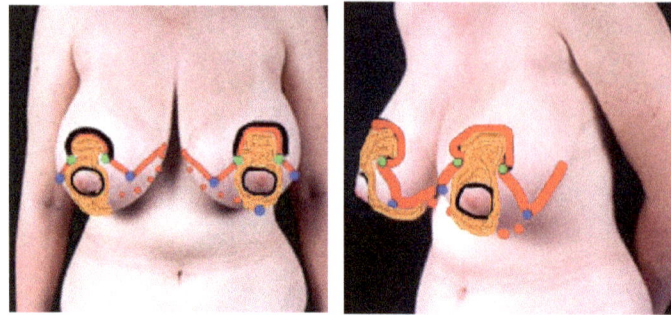

I illustrate the anchor-shaped closure below.

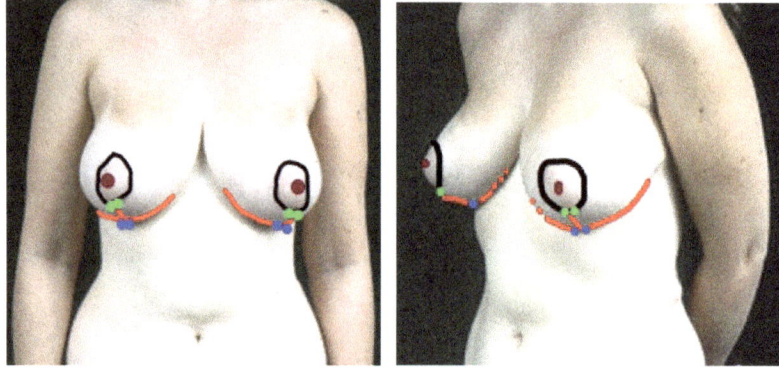

The final result for "Angelina" is below.

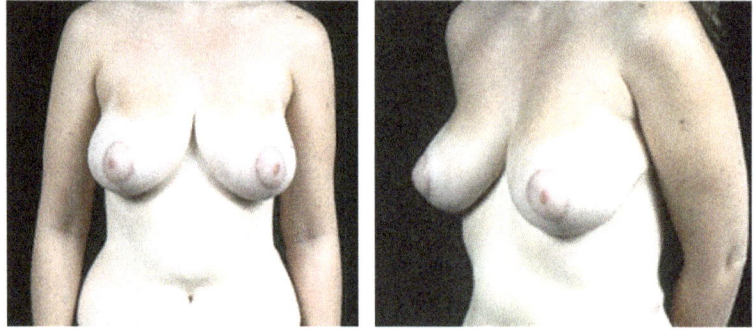

"Margery" complained of large, dense breasts that were too ptotic. I performed a verticle bipedicle reduction mammaplasty procedure for her. Her postoperative results are on the right below.

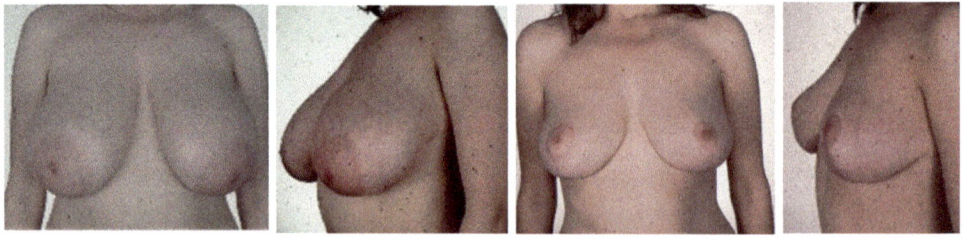

I also performed a verticle bipedicle for "Julia." She wanted a considerable reduction to try to relieve her back and shoulder discomfort. Both she and I were pleased with the results. Her before and after pictures are below.

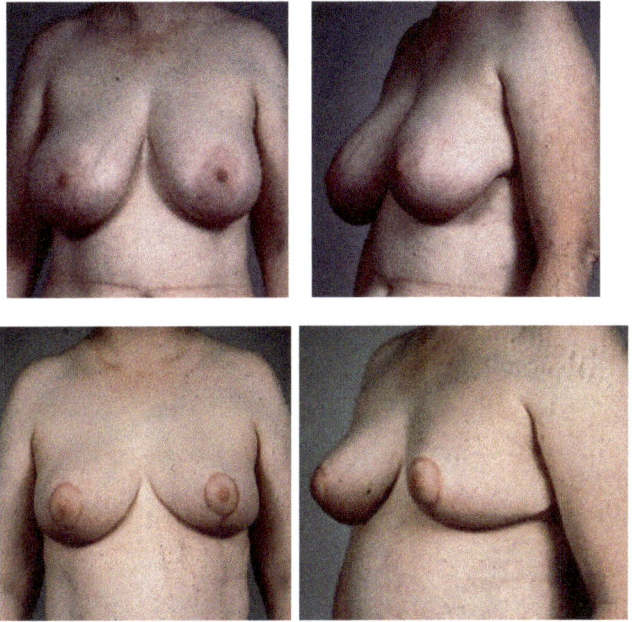

Inferior pedicle

The inferior pedicle technique, popularized by Courtiss and Goldwyn, became common near the completion of my residency training. I found it more versatile and applicable in more significant breast reduction cases. This inferior pedicle has a thicker base than the inferior portion of the bipedicle flap technique. My drawings below illustrate this method.

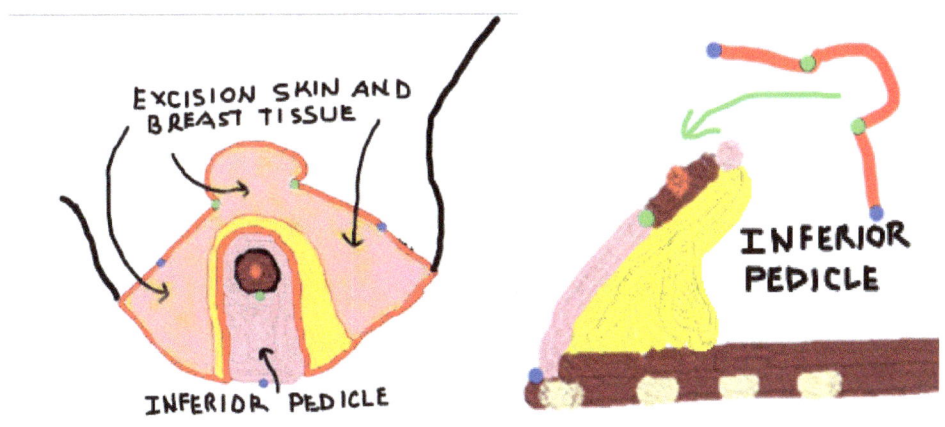

This flap is also folded on itself as below to fit the anchor-shaped Wise pattern closure.

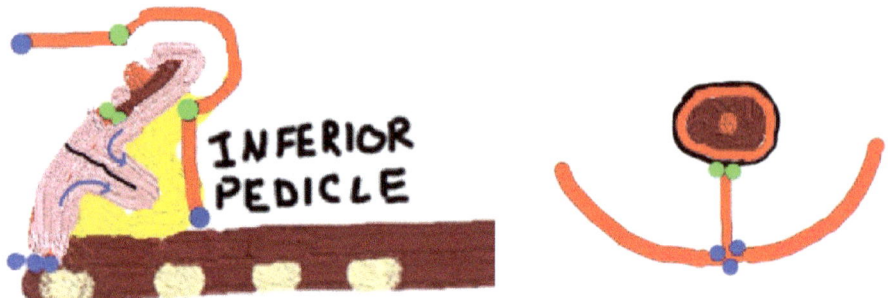

"Alice" was plagued with back and shoulder pain from her large, dense breasts and came to me seeking relief. The amount I planned to remove would be more than I would have been comfortable doing with a bipedicle procedure; I recommended the inferior pedicle technique. I show her preoperative condition below.

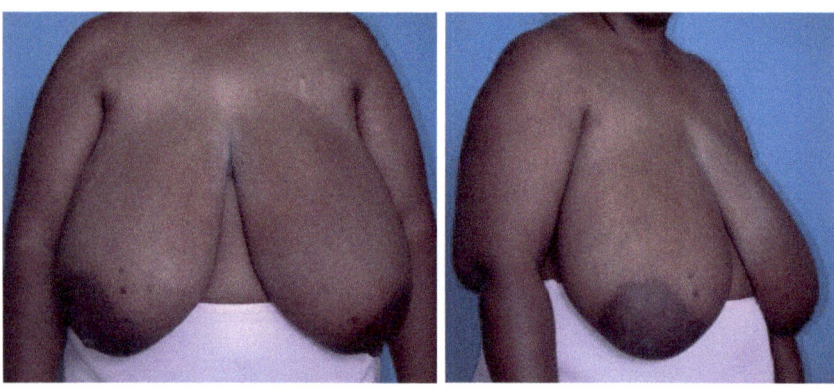

Again the Wise pattern plan is illustrated below.

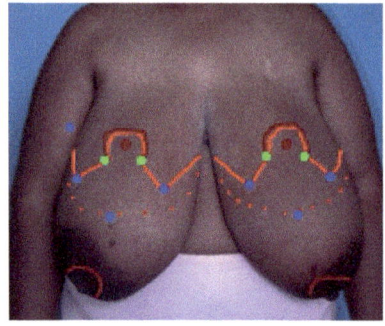
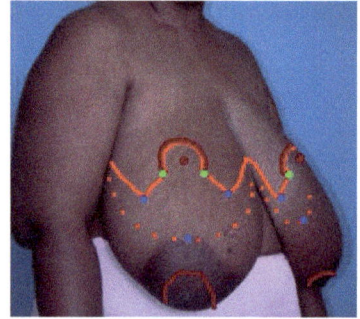

The de-epithelialized inferior pedicle, which is mostly on the deep underside of the breasts below in this view, is indicated in orange.

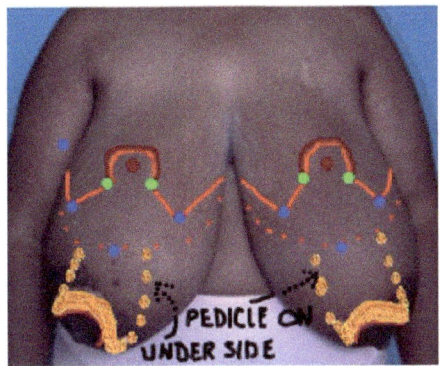
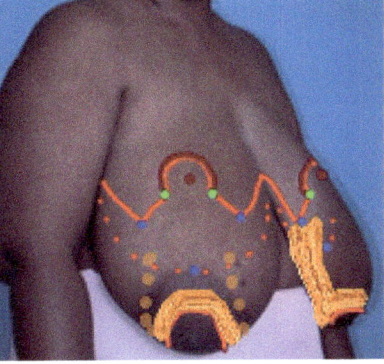

The photo drawings below show the anchor-shaped closure of the Wise pattern after removal of the indicated breast tissue.

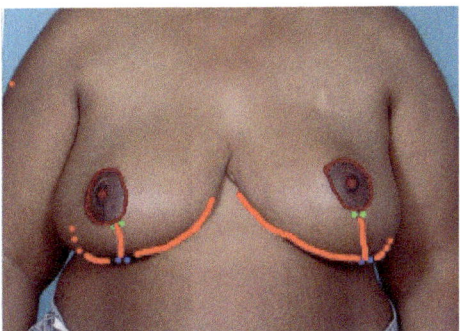
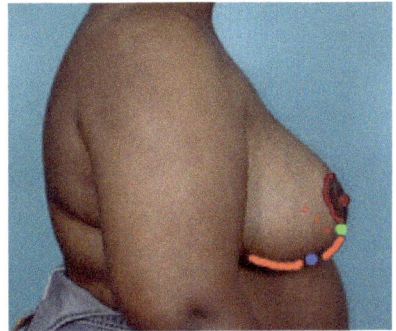

As one might imagine from "Alice"'s postoperative photos below, she was much more comfortable after the procedure without the massive pendulous breasts.

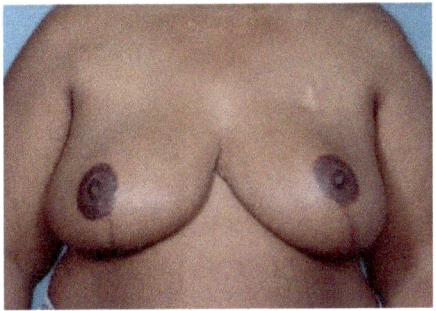
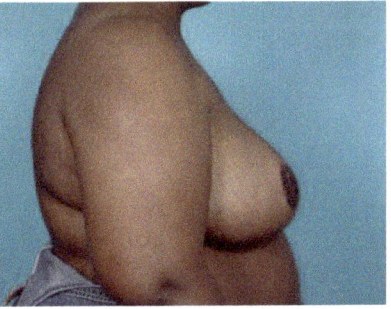

Another patient upon whom I performed an inferior pedicle reduction mammaplasty was "Josephina" whose pre and postoperative photos are below. She had postoperative relief of pain and discomfort and was additionally very pleased with her new appearance.

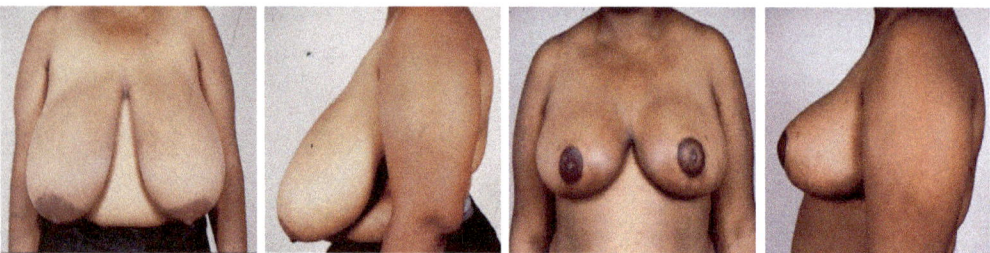

"Clarice" was another patient who sought relief from discomfort caused by large pendulous breasts. I did an inferior pedicle reduction technique. She experienced significant improvement in her symptoms. Her before and after pictures are below.

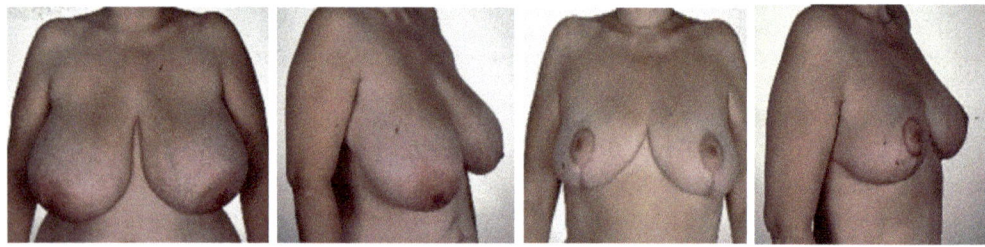

"Monique" was uncomfortable with pain in the back and shoulders from large pendulous breasts and sought relief. I recommended a reduction mammaplasty with an inferior pedicle technique. She did well and had improvement in her symptoms and was pleased with her new breast size and shape. Her before and after photos are below.

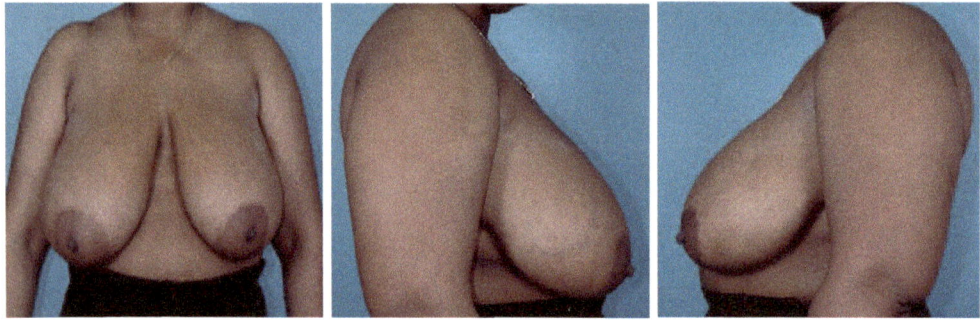

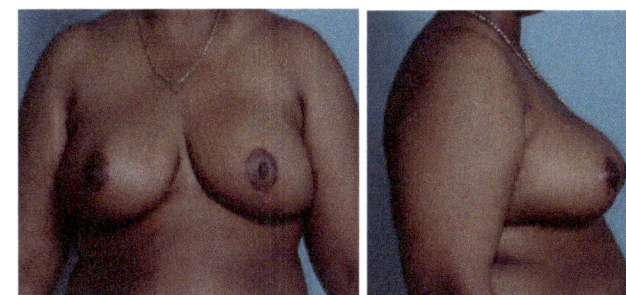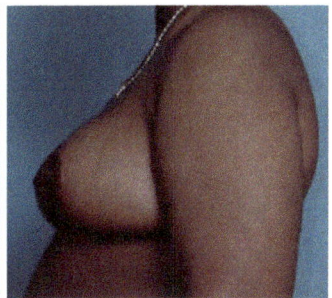

Superior Medial Pedicle

The superior medial pedicle technique evolved from various superior pedicle operations. I found this to be reliable and usually a little more rapid than the inferior pedicle technique. I found it perhaps easier to obtain a pleasing shape with less maneuvering of the flaps. I diagramed the superior- medial flap technique below.

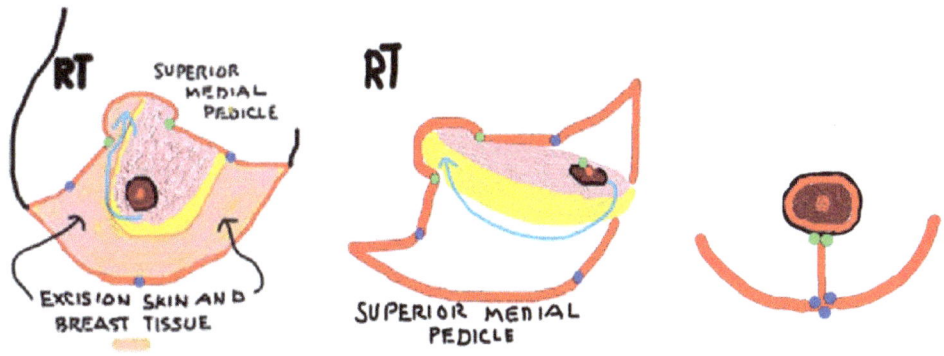

"Abigail," who had moderately large breasts, requested reduction. She sought relief of back discomfort and also just wanted smaller breasts. Her pre-operative photos are below.

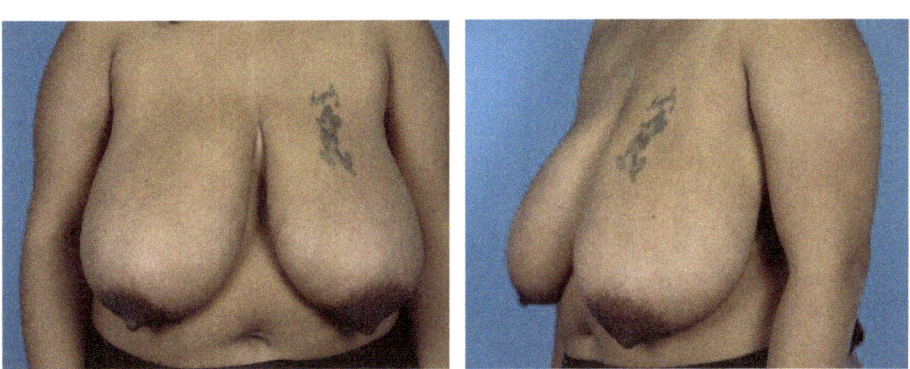

I again used the Wise pattern.

The Healing Mission of Plastic Surgery

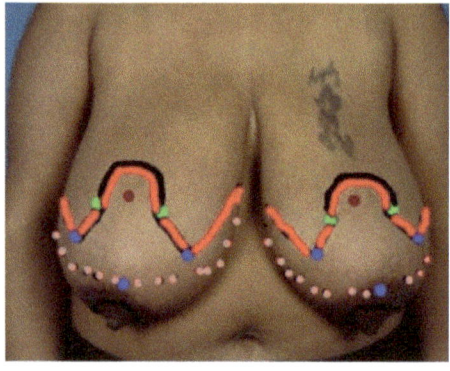
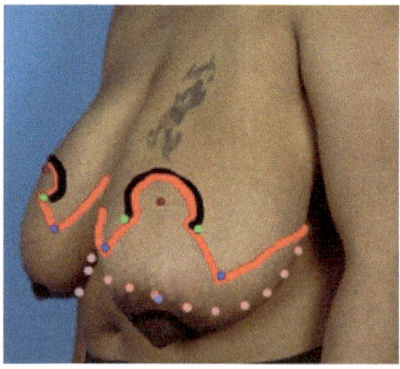

I used a de-epithelialized superior-medial pedicle, as outlined below.

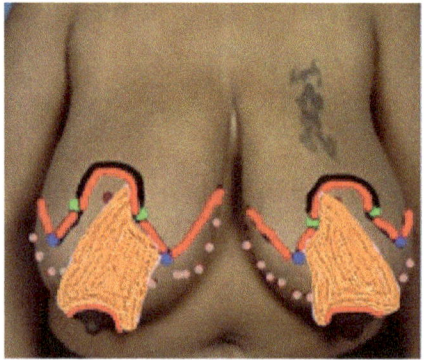
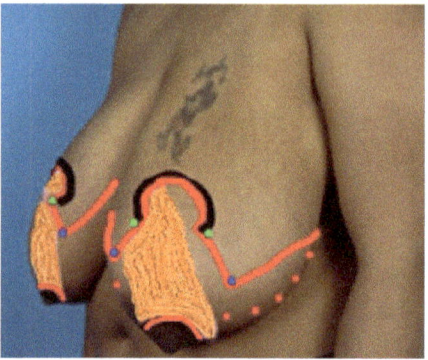

The Wise pattern closure is below.

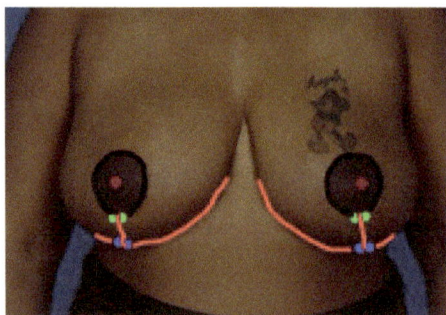
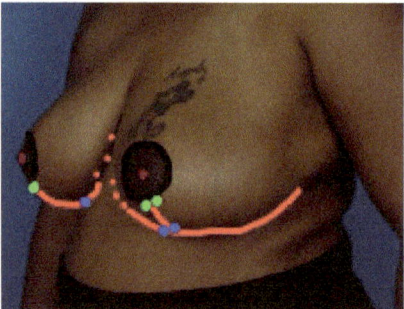

Both she and I were pleased with her result shown below. Because of the tattoo, it is easier to appreciate the improvement when comparing her preoperative condition with these postoperative photos. She has an excellent breast shape post-reduction.

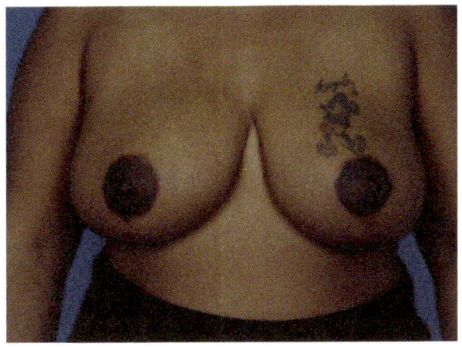 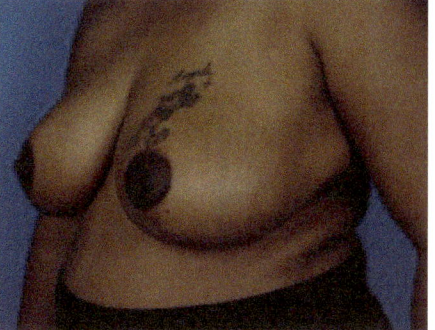

Another patient, "Ruth," not only complained of discomfort from large breasts but that they affected her posture.

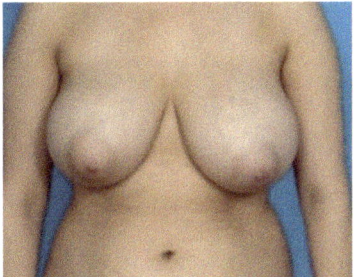 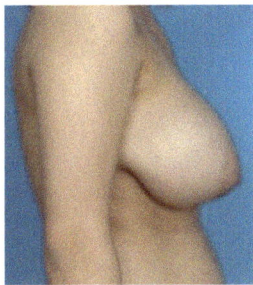

Below is after I performed a superior-medial pedicle breast reduction.

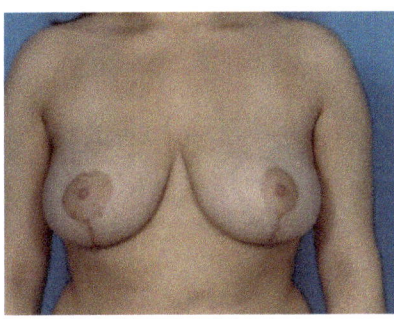 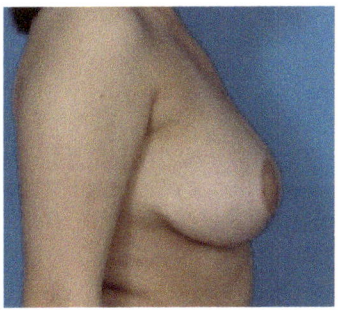

She seemed to have an improvement in her posture as well as getting some relief from back pain. Aditional pre and then postoperative views are below.

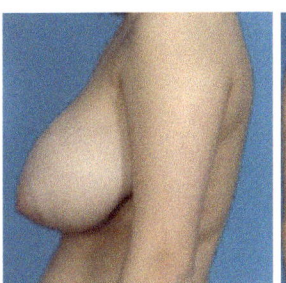 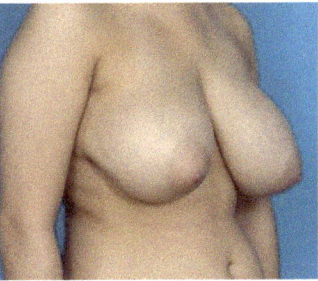 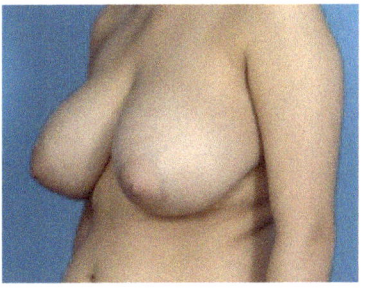

The Healing Mission of Plastic Surgery

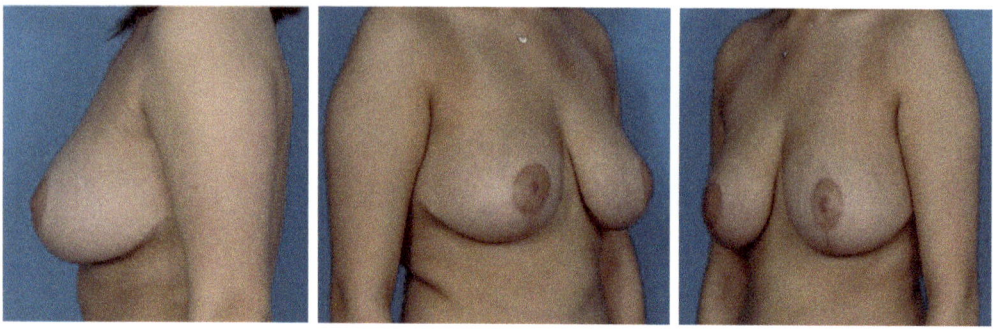

I was pleased with the result in "Barbara's" superior-medial pedicle reduction mammaplasty case. She had both relief of physical discomfort and was happy with her size and shape. Her before and after photos are below.

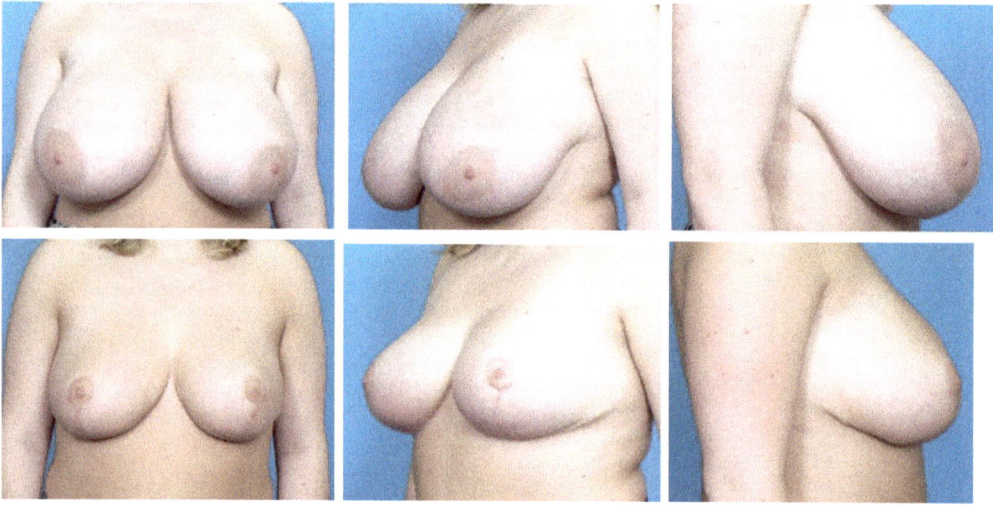

"Grace" also benefited from a superior-medial reduction mammaplasty. Her pre-op and post-op photos are below.

The Healing Mission of Plastic Surgery

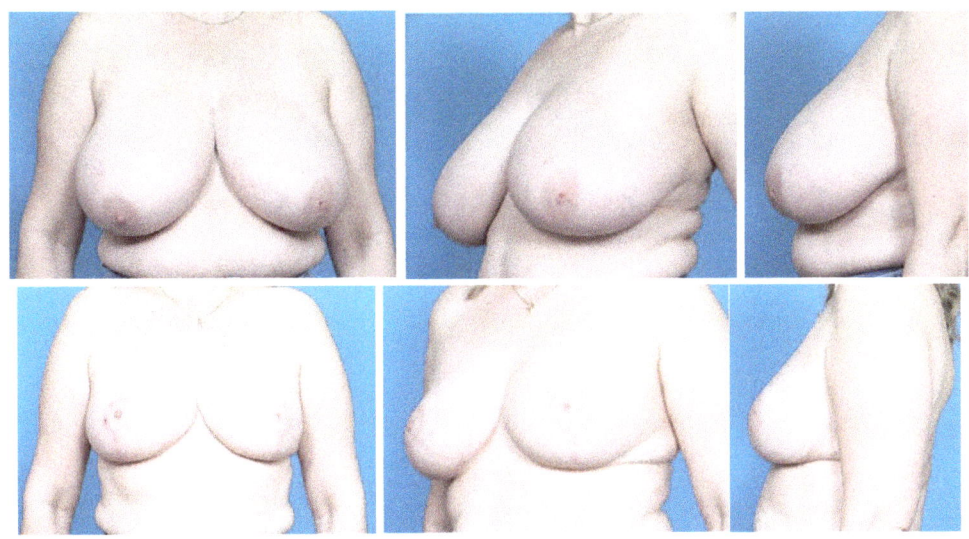

"Kathaleen" wanted smaller and less sagging breasts. I performed a superior-medial pedicle reduction mammaplasty for her. She was pleased that she received the results that she wanted. Her before and after pictures are below.

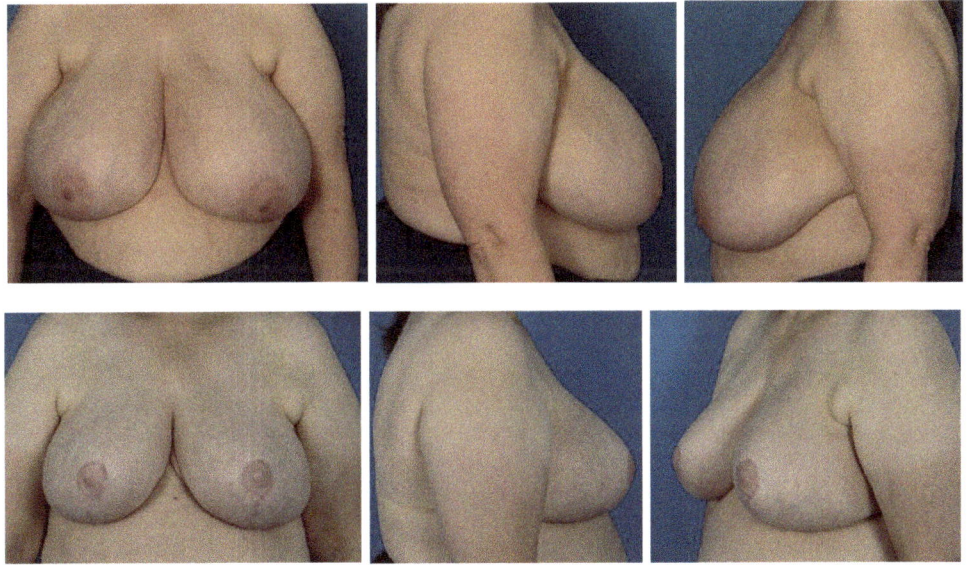

"Dede," said she was tired of large breasts and wanted them smaller so that she could wear better fitting clothes. I did a superior-medial reduction mammaplasty for her that satisfied her wants. The pre-op and post-op photos are below.

The Healing Mission of Plastic Surgery

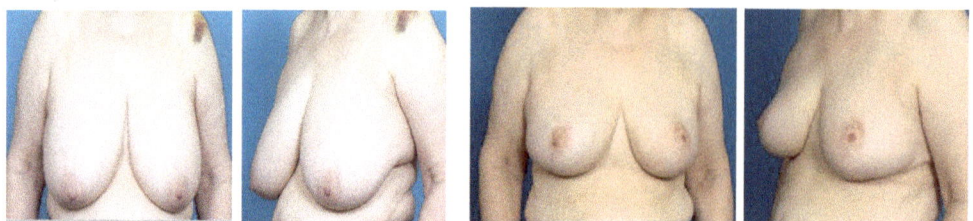

Another patient for whom I performed a superior-medial pedicle reduction mammaplasty was "Donna." In her case, the amount of reduction was relatively small. Insurance companies usually do not cover reductions of less than 500-600 grams. She may have had to cover the expense of her surgery herself.

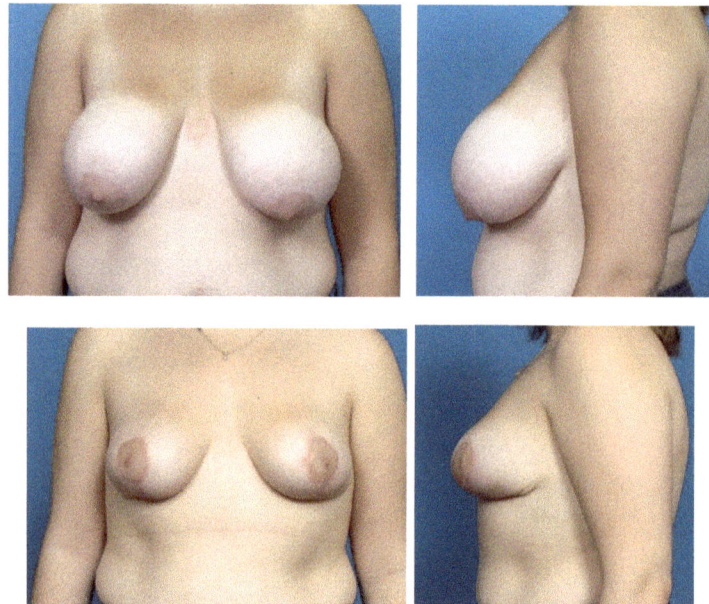

Burns

"Thelma" had a thermal burn of the face and developed scar contracture of the mouth with significant limitation of opening. The second photo shows the patient after the Z-plasty of the oral commissures. The third photo shows an acrylic splint with projections coming out of the mouth at each lateral commissure. It was necessary to maintain this splint for several months until the scar matured enough that contracture would not recur. The fourth photo shows the mouth after the maturation of the scar. She was now able to open her mouth to eat more comfortably.

The Healing Mission of Plastic Surgery

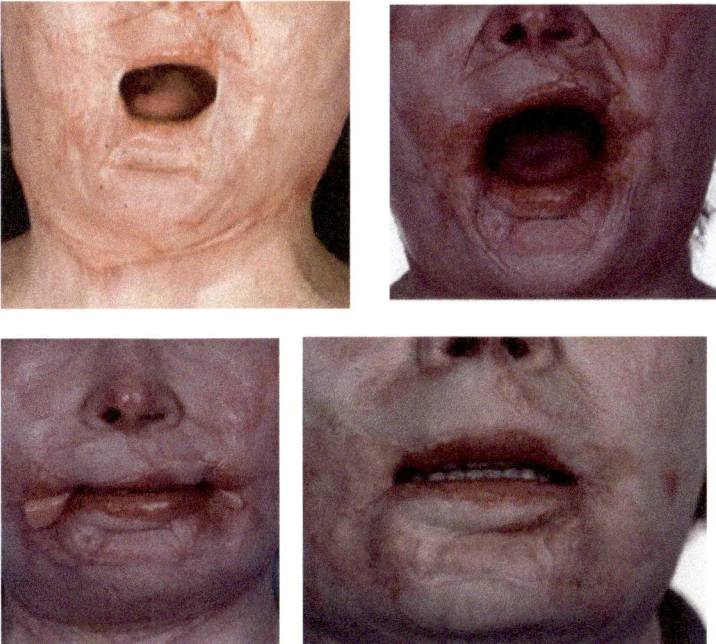

Malocclusion & facial distortion

This 19-year-old "Bob" had a severe open bite class III malocclusion, a narrow upper arch, a long face, and vertically long chin. The first preoperative picture below shows the severe malocclusion; the second and third photos show the excess vertical dimension of the chin and lack of projection of the chin.

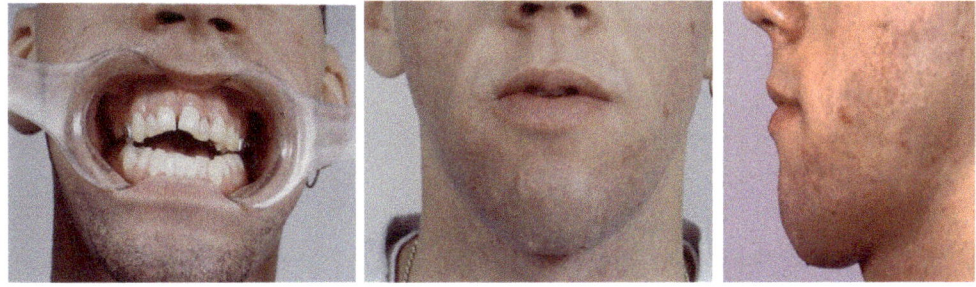

The first procedure I did for him was a modified Le Fort I osteotomy and midline palate osteotomy(cut) with rapid palatal expansion. That is, I mobilized the midface, split the palate in two, and made it wider. I had a cooperative orthodontist's input to help me with this case.

At the second operation, I performed bilateral mandibular osteotomies and setback, genioplasty, and hydroxyapatite implant augmentation of the maxilla. That is, I repositioned the lower jaw and separately advanced the chin and augmented the cheeks with an implant. The postoperative photo below shows the new occlusion. His surgery improved his ability to chew correctly. The second and third photos show a better projection of the chin after the jumping genioplasty procedure.

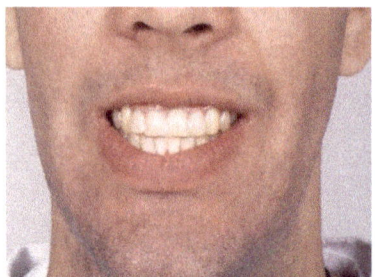 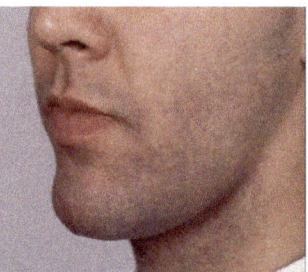 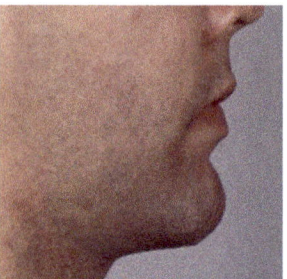

Chapter 15

The Place of Reconstructive Plastic Surgery in the Healing Mission

Reconstructive plastic surgery is surgery performed on abnormal structures of the body caused by congenital defects, developmental abnormalities, trauma, infections, tumors, or disease to approximate a more normal appearance, not specifically to improve function.

I had to look closely to appreciate some of the deformities "Anita" was pointing out. It was apparent she did have ptosis (drooping) of her right eyelid but not enough to hinder her visual field. That and a subtle depression of the right side of her face were now unbearable deformities that "Anita" related to abuse by her mother when growing up. She forgave neither her mother for the abuse nor her father, who looked the other way and buried himself in his work as a professor. I was certainly concerned that perhaps she was making too much objection to the actual deformities.

We discussed everything in great detail and at great length. "Anita" focused on the deformities because they were a constant reminder of the abuse. She hoped that improving the stigmata of the prior abuse would improve her self-esteem, body image, and make her feel better. I believed we had an excellent chance of making a substantial improvement in the eyelid symmetry. I was much less sure we could make her feel better about the remaining facial balance. I planned a ptosis procedure to lift the right eyelid to match the left. Fat grafting to the right cheek would add contour to help correct the facial asymmetry. It was with some hesitation that I took her to the operating room. I marked the contour changes I planned on her cheek with a medical marking pen.

The Healing Mission of Plastic Surgery

It is an awesome feeling to take a knife from the scrub tech and bring it to the patient's eyelid and then cut through the skin to begin the correction. I dissected through the orbicularis muscle, cleaned the fat off the levator muscle that lifts the lid. I took a fine electrical cautery to zap small bleeding blood vessels. I then placed sutures in the levator muscle to shorten it and thereby reposition the lid to a higher level. I did her procedure under local anesthesia, one stitch at a time asking Ms. Jones to look up and down so I could titrate the amount of muscle shortening. (Later in my career, I preferred a technique that did not require the patient to be awake and cooperate. Examples are in chapter 14.) After the position seemed just right, I closed the wound with fine sutures.

I aspirated fat from her abdomen, prepared it by centrifuging it gently for a short period, then decanting it to remove most of the blood and oils, leaving a concentrate of fat cells. Then using a small syringe and fine needle, I injected the thick fat concentrate into the pre-marked areas of the face to attempt to correct the contour deformity.

She had an uneventful recovery. It was a little hard to read her assessment of her result. She did seem to appreciate she had some improvement by the corrective procedures. A few months later, she returned inquiring about facial rejuvenation surgery. At this point, she was complaining that as she was aging, she looked more and more like her mother, and this was disconcerting. I was not very encouraging regarding her requested surgery. I didn't do any further surgery for her; I think she probably went to another surgeon.

Ear Reconstruction

Left Ear Deformity

The little girl below, "Mary," has a congenital deformity of the left ear with duplication and extra tissue in front of the ear. The left ear is also much more prominent than her normal right ear. We can well imagine the child asking her mother, "why is my ear different from everybody else's? I removed some and rearranged some of the extra tissue in front of the ear. I folded and fixed in position with sutures the cartilage of the ear to bring it closer to the side of the head. With her better-matched ears from this reconstructive effort, she should be able to avoid body image problems. The first two photos are pre-op, and the second two are post-op.

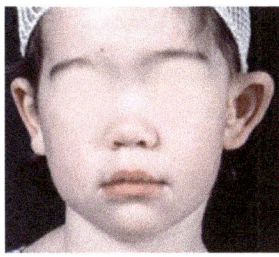 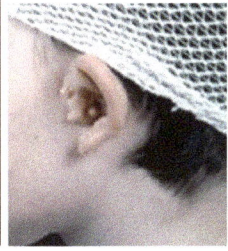 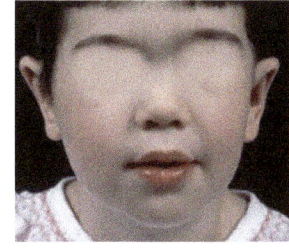 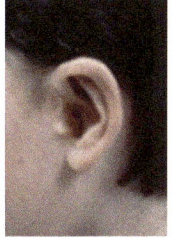

"Zelda" displays a lop ear deformity in the first photo below with a vertically shortened ear because of the crimping of the upper pole of the ear. I corrected her lop ear by molding the cartilage with sutures I placed on the back of the ear cartilage, similar to that previously described in chapter 4 under otoplasty. The second and third photos below are postoperative.

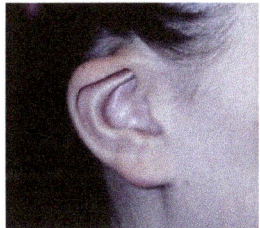 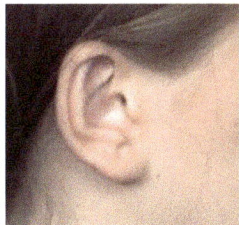 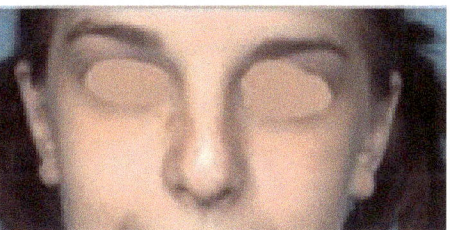

The patient below "Alexander" has a typical microtia (small ear) deformity with an underdeveloped ear with gnarled cartilage shown in the first two photos below.

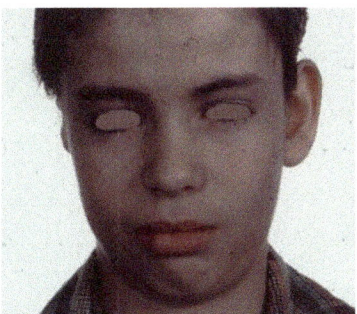 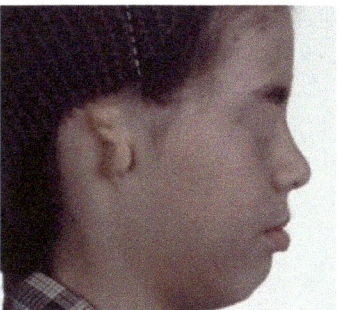

The first photo below shows the residual skin after the removal of the original snarled diminutive cartilage to make room for the rib cartilage construct. The second photo shows the cartilage ear framework I made from the rib. Thirdly, the cartilage is being placed into the vacated space.

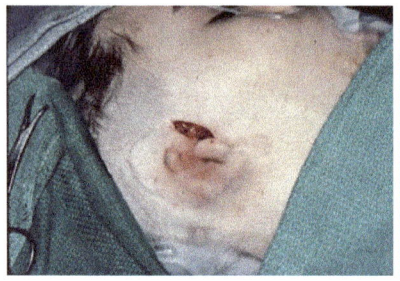 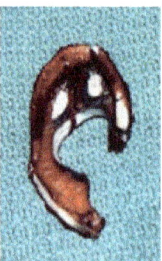 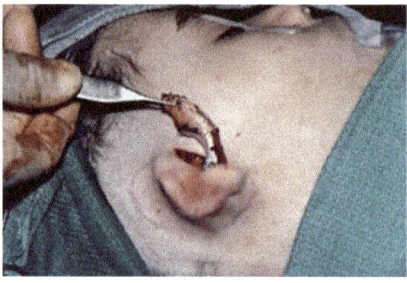

The first photo shows the cartilage construct in place during the first operation. The second photo is at the next procedure, where I revised the tragus and elevated the ear is from the side of the head.

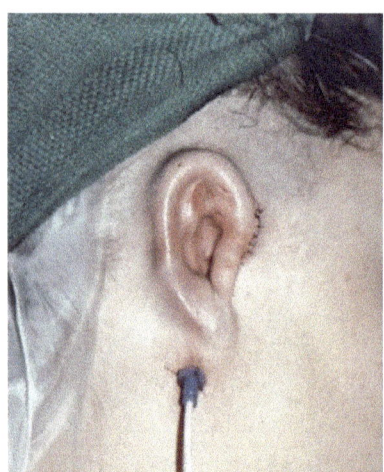 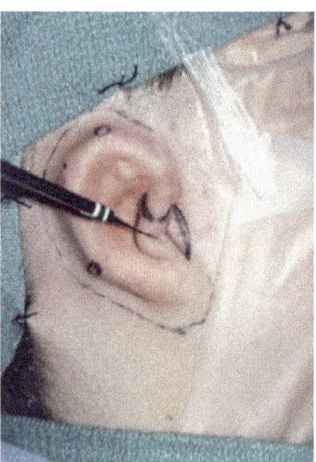 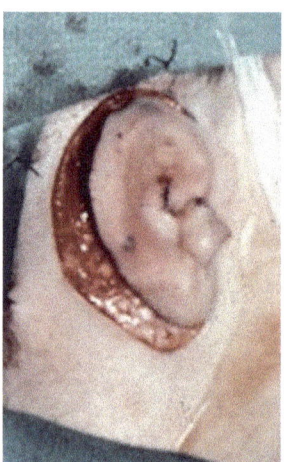

The final result is below.

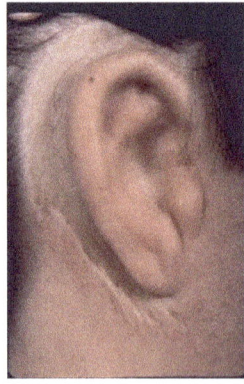 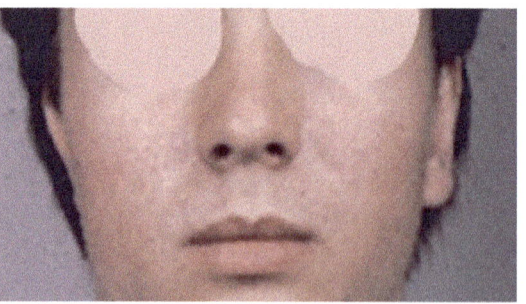

"Carolina" has microtia, as in the first photo below. The second and third photos are after the placement of a synthetic ear framework implant.

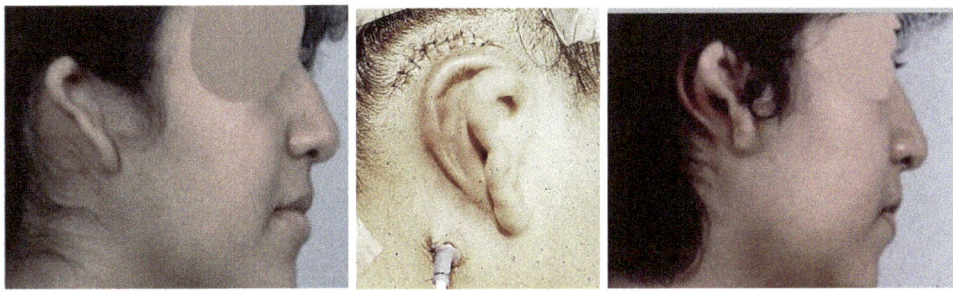

Carolina's post-op result after rearrangement of the soft tissue around the implant is below.

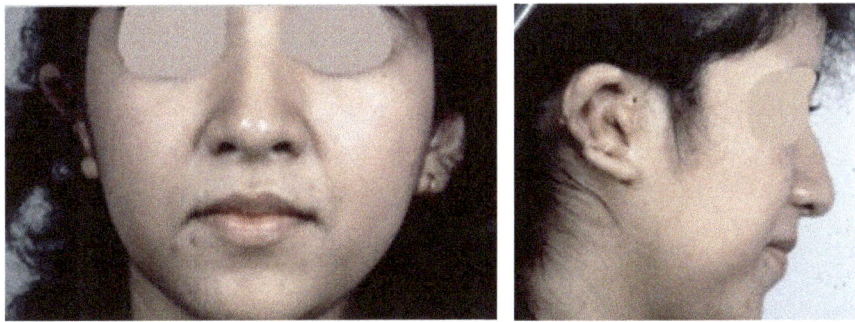

Below "Margo" was a 10-year-old girl born with a congenital microtia on the right and a healthy ear on the left. I harvested cartilage from the rib cage on the left side.

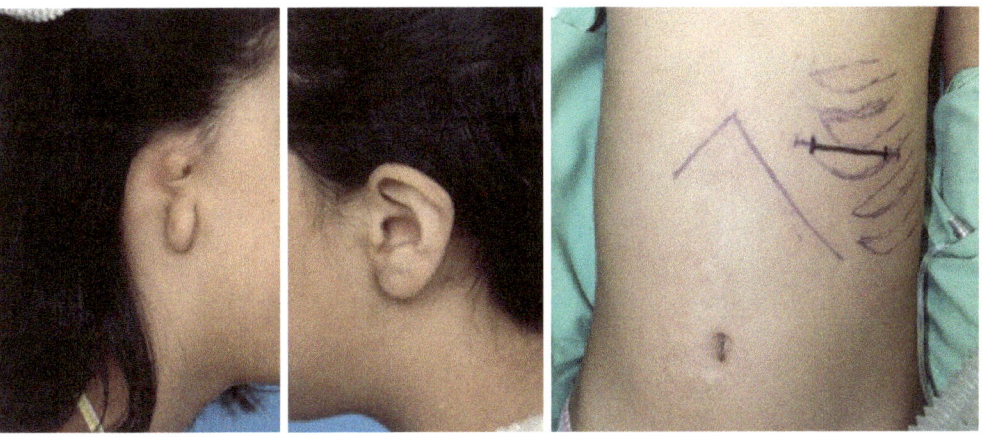

I used a plastic template of the opposite left ear as a model to help construct a cartilage framework from the rib, as shown below. Th next photo shows the frame implanted after removal of the preexisting cartilage. Her intermediate result is on the right.

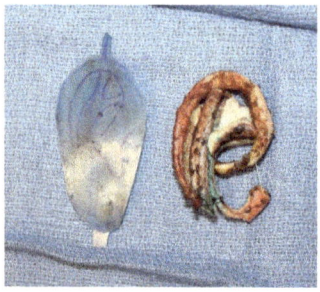 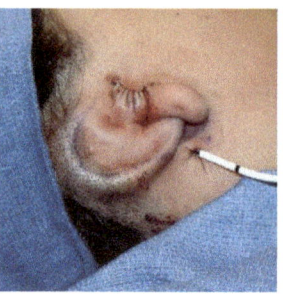 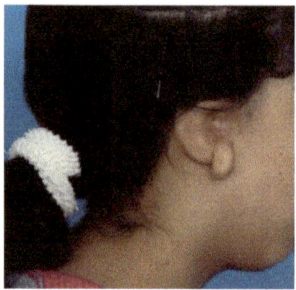

After elevation of the ear, she lost some definition of the helical rim. So, I brought a three-staged cigarette flap from the neck to the helical edge to give a better representation of an ear. The second and third photos below show her result.

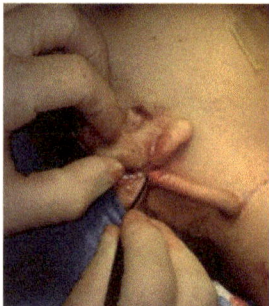 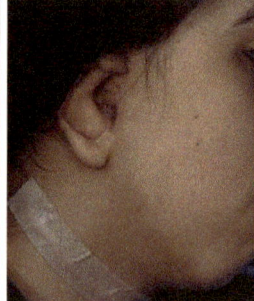 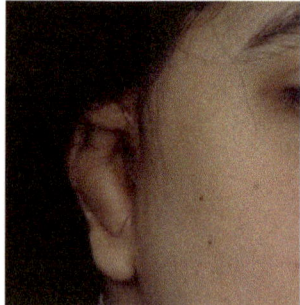

Forehead reconstruction after trauma

"Clint" suffered trauma to the left forehead area losing bone, thereby causing the contour defect shown in the preoperative pictures below. I decided, after consultation with the patient, to use cranial bone for the reconstruction of this forehead defect. I made an incision from ear to ear across the scalp and turned the anterior scalp forward over the face to gain access to the depressed area. In the third picture below, I outlined the defect in blue.

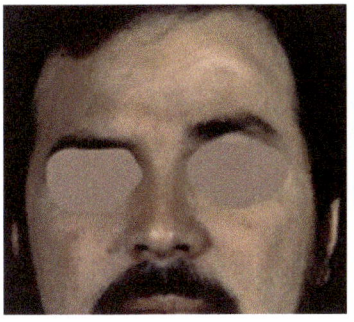 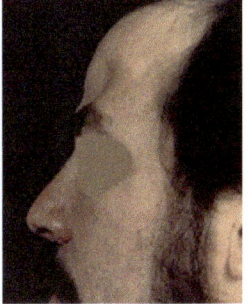 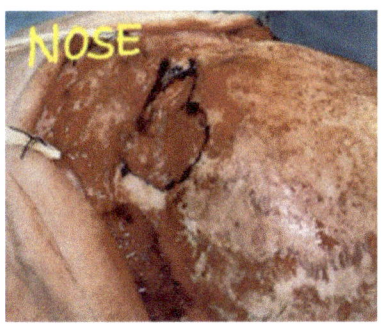

Below a blue template of the defect was placed over the parietal bone. The neurosurgeon harvested a full-thickness piece of the parietal bone, as shown in the second photo below.

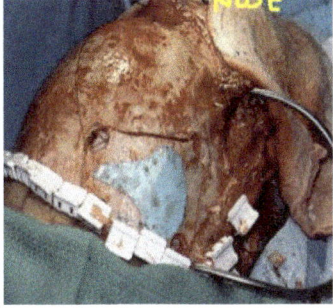 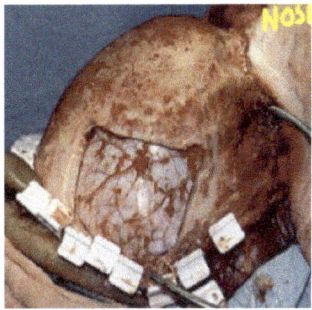

I then split this bone into two. I returned half to close the donor area. I shaped the other half to repair the original traumatic defect and also used bone dust to fill in the cracks between the bones.

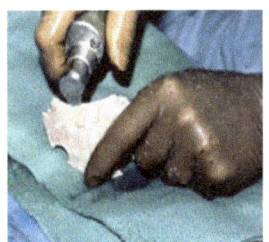 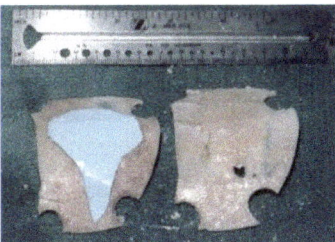 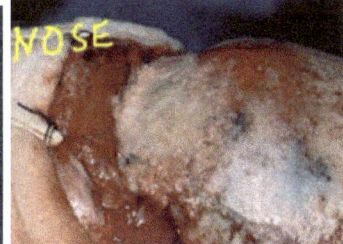

The postoperative result a few months later is below.

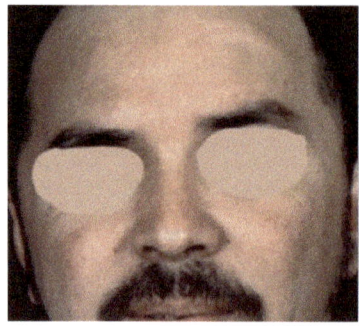
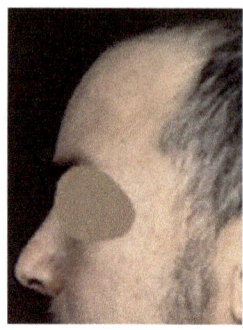

I used a different method of forehead reconstruction in "Doreen," the elderly patient below. The first two photos show the extent of the forehead defect with extensive loss of bone. The third photo is an intraoperative view after I turned the scalp flap forward. I have placed wires across the area of absent bone, ready to receive a viscus acrylic reconstruction material.

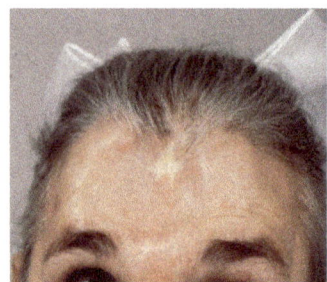
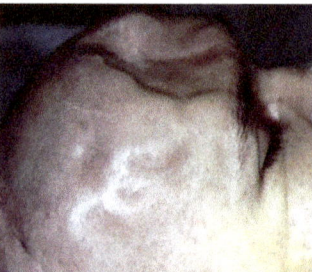
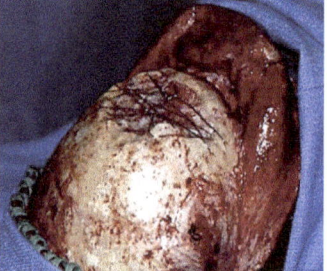

Below I have shaped the acrylic in place and allowed it to harden. The last photo is the postoperative result.

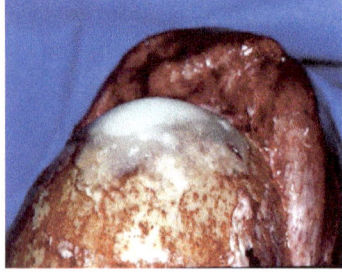
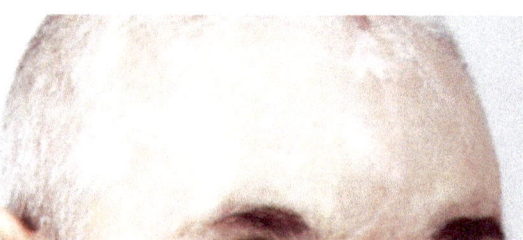

Another forehead reconstruction for trauma is represented by "Roberta," shown on the left below. She has a depressed defect that has also distorted the brow. In the intraoperative photo, I have turned forward a scalp flap that temporarily covers the nose and face.

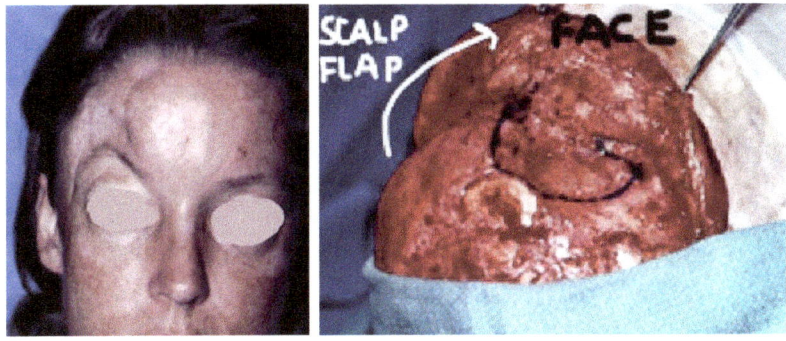

I harvested iliac bone graft from the pelvic girdle and shaped it to the dimensions of the defect. I wired this graft in place. I did her case before we had micro plating systems.

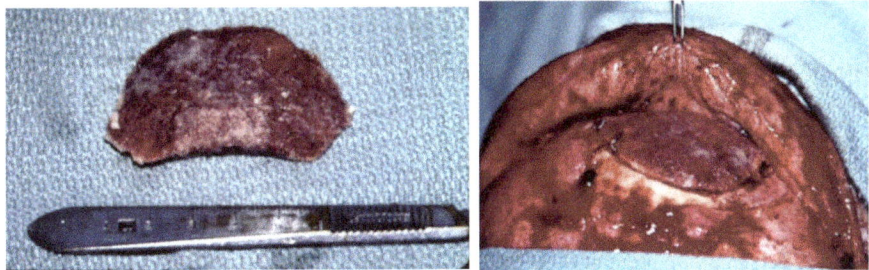

Her early postoperative result is below. She has a better contour of the bone, and her brow position is improved.

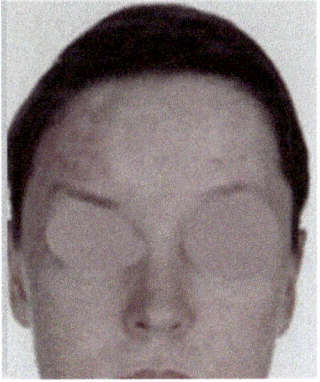

The patient below, "Margo," had a benign parotid tumor removed. However, this left her with a depression in the left cheek, as shown in the first two photos below. She wanted to have something done to improve this depression on the left side of her face.

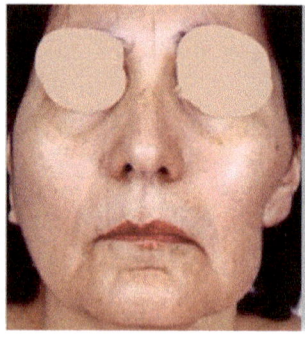 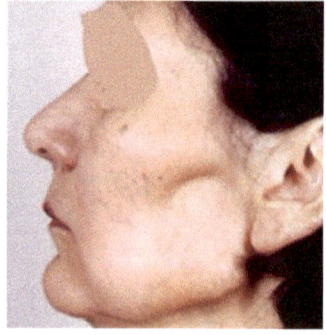

To reconstruct this defect, I made an incision in the scalp and turned temporoparietal fascia down to repair the defect. The photo-drawing shows the origin of the fascia. The second picture below is from another patient that shows the elevation of a temporoparietal fascial flap pointed out by a blue arrow. The orange arrow points out the temporalis muscle. The use of temporoparietal fascia leaves no functional issues. The last two photos show the postoperative result.

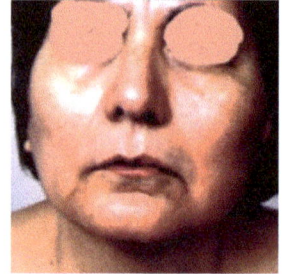 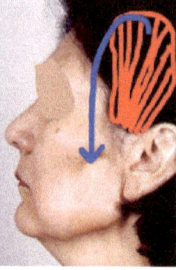 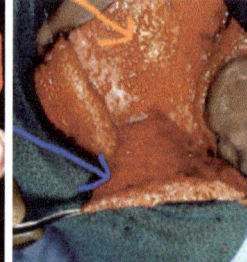 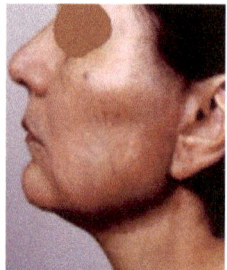

"George" suffered a tibial fracture in a motorcycle accident. The orthopedic surgeon consulted with me. The first photo below shows the bones were pinned with an external fixator to hold them in place. The loss of skin and soft tissue exposed the bones, which needed soft tissue coverage to heal. I elected to take a latissimus dorsi myo-cutaneous flap from the patient's left lateral and posterior chest as in the second and third pictures. The last picture on the right shows the free flap ready to be transferred to the leg. The thoracodorsal blood vessels are pointed out by the small purple arrow.

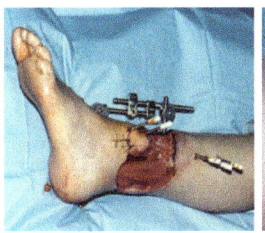 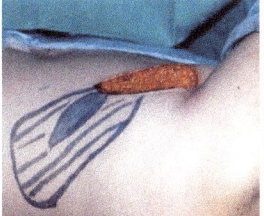 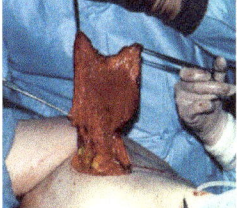 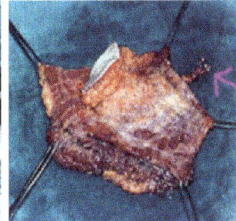

I then anastomosed the flap thoracodorsal blood vessels to the anterior tibial blood vessels in the lower leg. I then wrapped the muscle around the bone to cover it and promote healing. I then placed a skin graft on the muscle. The patient did well and was able to have the external fixation device removed several weeks later.

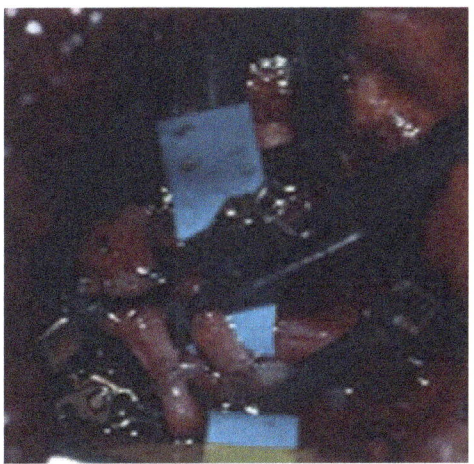 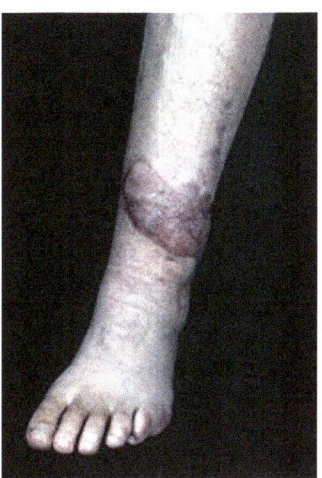

Gynecomastia

Gynecomastia is the enlargement of the male breast. Adolescent males often develop minor gynecomastia, which spontaneously resolves in two or three years. It can be bilateral or unilateral. The possibility of a cancerous lesion must be ruled out, especially in unilateral cases. Persistent cases may be caused by some endocrine system physiologic disorder or from medications.

Many cases are idiopathic. (of unknown cause). An endocrinologist usually evaluates these patients to rule out any treatable cause. I have treated gynecomastia surgically, often with small incisions around the areola and piecemeal removal with direct excision and liposuction as needed to smooth out the affected areas. Treatment for gynecomastia can sometimes be a gray area between reconstructive versus cosmetic. Medical insurance companies refused to cover many of the procedures I did for affected patients.

"Freddy" was a young man who is embarrassed by this breast enlargement, which was predominantly on the left side. I treated him with a small incision at the areola for a direct excision of breast tissue and feathered the surrounding tissue with liposuction. He was pleased with his results, as shown in the last two photos below.

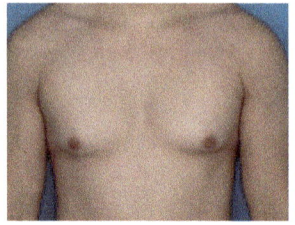 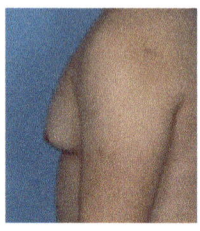 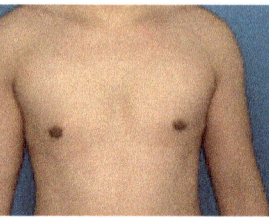 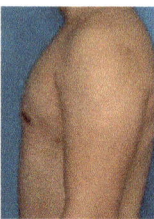

"Mark," below, was a 20 something-year-old with persistent gynecomastia. He was treated with a small incision at the inferior aspect of the areola and liposuction or feathering the edges. His pre-and postoperative photographs are below.

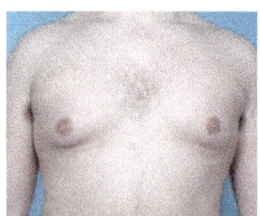 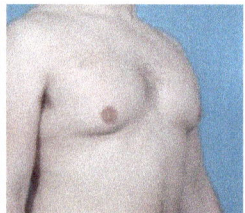 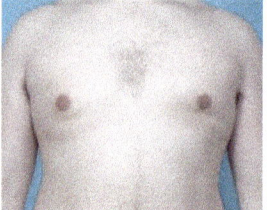 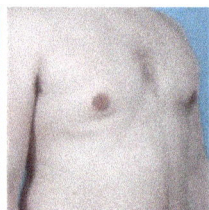

"Jason" was a young man with left unilateral gynecomastia. The biopsy was negative for cancer. He underwent direct excision of the gynecomastia through an inferior areolar incision. I used liposuction to feather the edges of the resection. His pre-and postoperative photographs are below.

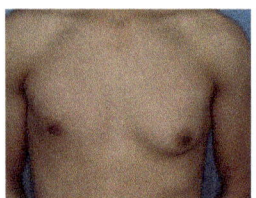 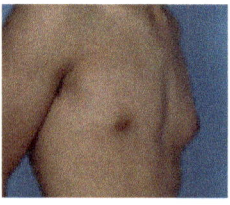 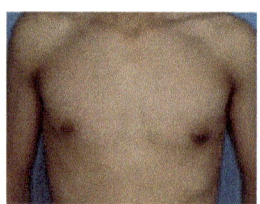 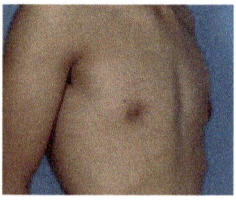

The Healing Mission of Plastic Surgery

"Clyde" below was in his 30s when he presented with bilateral gynecomastia. I excised the breast tissue through an areolar incision. I performed liposuction through tiny incisions at the inframammary crease. These incisions have not yet faded in th early postoperative photographs, which show improved contour.

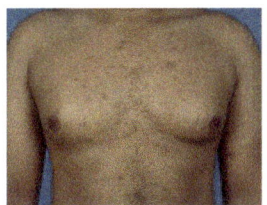 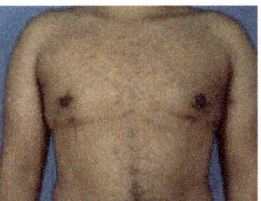 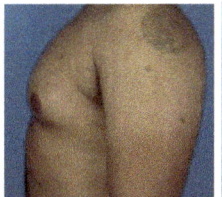 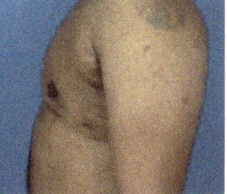

"Alberto" below was on the borderline of having to excise the skin as well as remove breast tissue directly. We approached him with a small incision, excision of the breast tissue, liposuction to feather out the removal. Although he still has some excess skin, he's probably better off than having a large scar from skin removal.

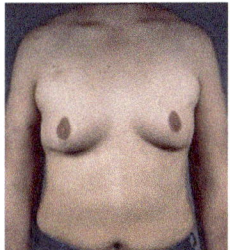 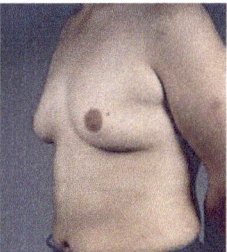 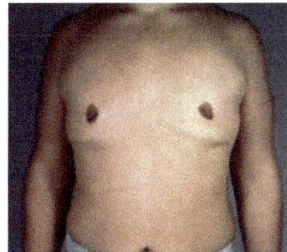 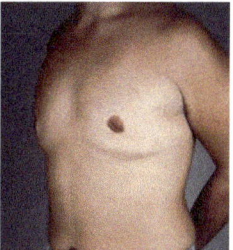

Breast Asymmetry

"Angelina" shown below demonstrated more significant breast asymmetry. I treated her breast asymmetry with an inferior pedicle Wise pattern technique. I performed a breast lift on the left and a reduction on the right.

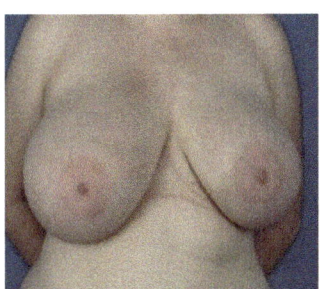 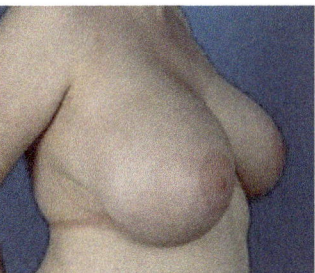 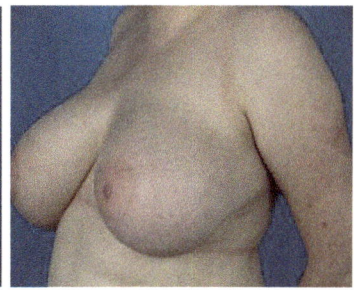

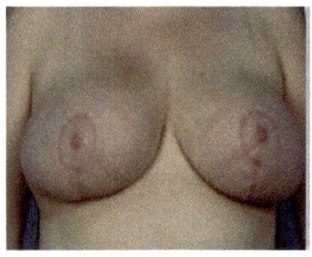 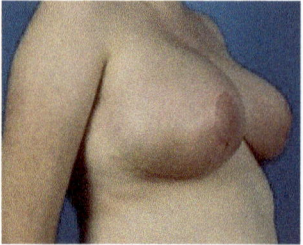 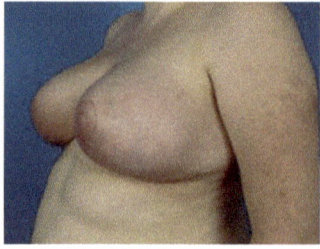

"Gina" below had significant breast asymmetry. I performed a medial pedicle Wise pattern technique with a minimal reduction on the left and a more substantial decrease on the right.

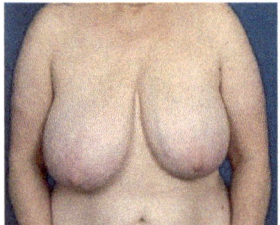 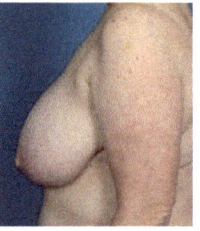 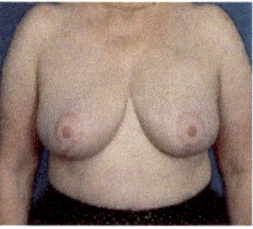 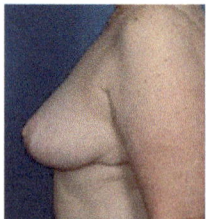

"Moire," below, had significant asymmetry; I treated her by doing a superior pedicle reduction mammaplasty on the right and a breast augmentation with a silicone gel implant on the left side. This surgery gave her much-improved symmetry, as shown in the post-op photograph, also below.

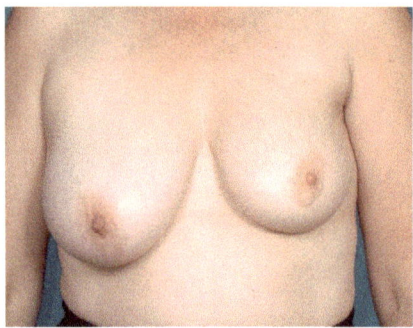 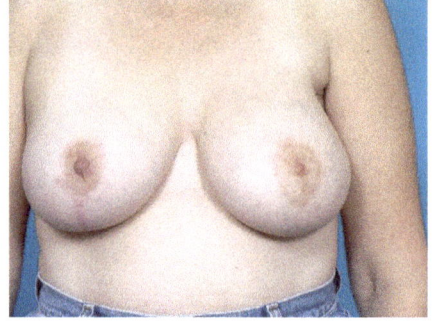

Facial Reconstruction

Facial Paralysis

"Sue" shone below had a long-standing left-sided facial paralysis. She was concerned with her sagging mouth. After discussing options, we decided to address her concern with a cheek suspension flap. I de-epithelialized the area in blue in the second picture.

The Healing Mission of Plastic Surgery

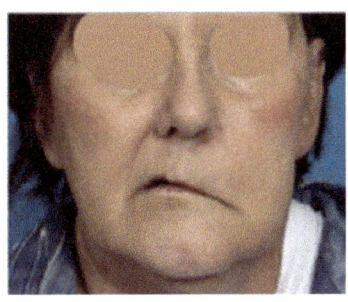 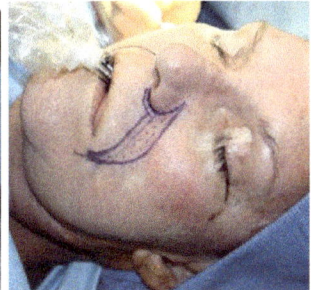 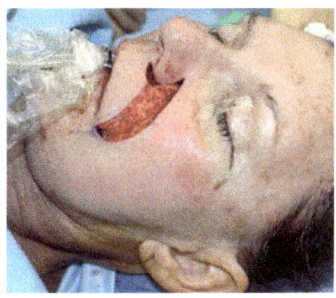

The de-epithelialized flap was elevated, advanced, and sutured to the periosteum of the cheekbone. The result is on the right below.

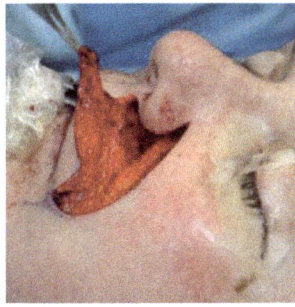 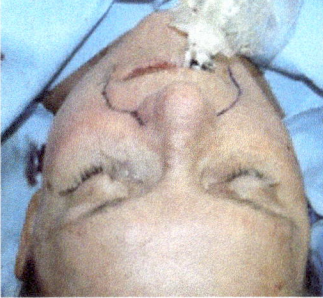 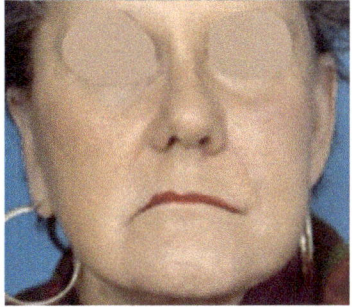

I treated another facial paralysis patient, "Deborah," whose pre-operative relaxed and smiling photos are below in a similar way.

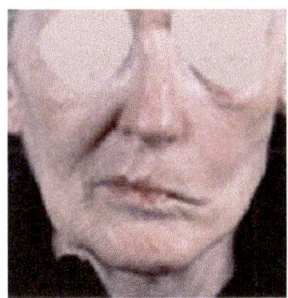 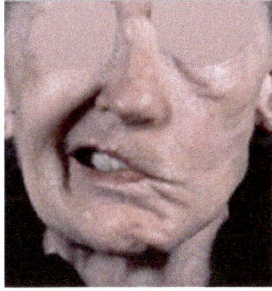 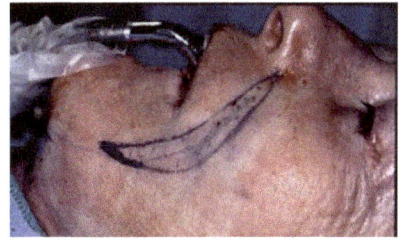

Her postoperative relaxed and smiling photos are below.

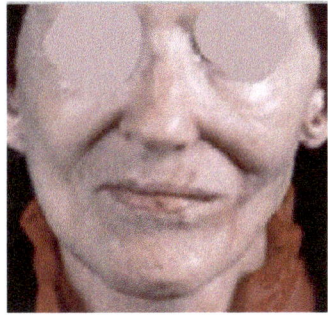 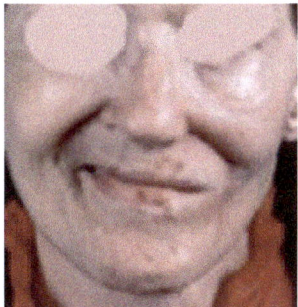

Free Flap Facial Reconstructions

"Loretta" had a defect from the removal of an eye tumor and subsequent radiation therapy. She had a resultant relative lack of growth on the right side of the face. She had a prosthetic eye. Her preoperative pictures are below. One of my partners at the time, Dr. Brauer, referred her because he thought she needed a free flap. I agreed, and together we planned a free tissue transfer.

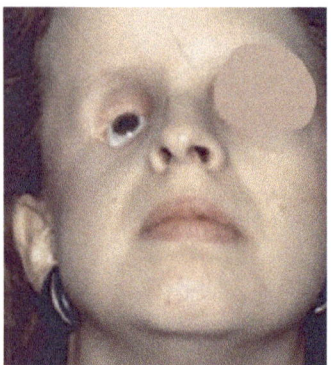
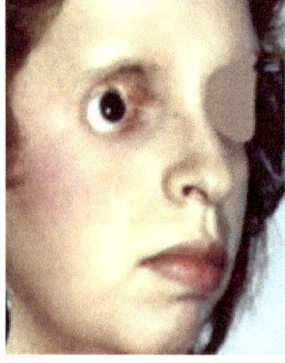
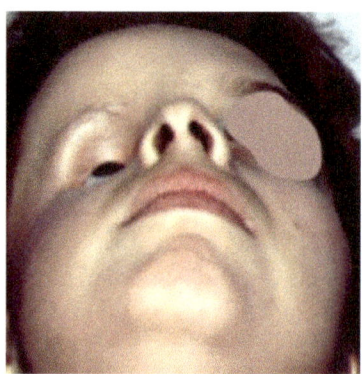

The paper template on the patient's right back helped to design, orient, and shape the flap. The scapular flap of skin, subcutaneous fat, and fascia are shown in the second intraoperative photo below partially dissected. In the photo-drawing, the flap remains essentially connected only by the blood vessels supplying the flap, otherwise ready for transfer.

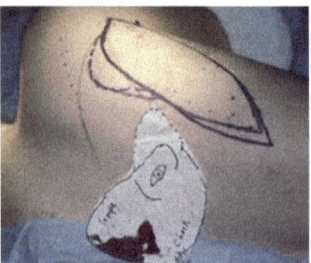
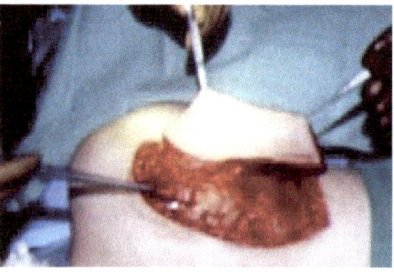
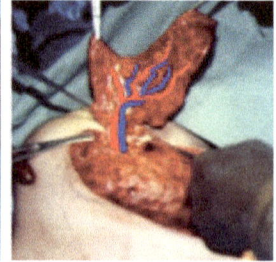

I identified the recipient facial vessels in the neck and undermined the facial skin to make room for the scapular flap, which I planned to place beneath it. I then cut the supplying vessels to the scapular free flap. I transferred the flap to the face, anastomosing the flap, and recipient neck vessels to re-establish the blood supply to the flap. I trimmed and shaped the flap to produce as much symmetry of the face as possible.

The Healing Mission of Plastic Surgery

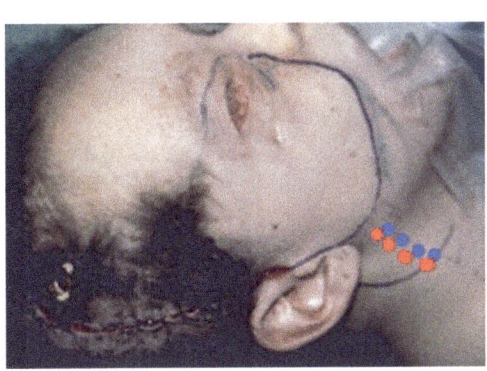
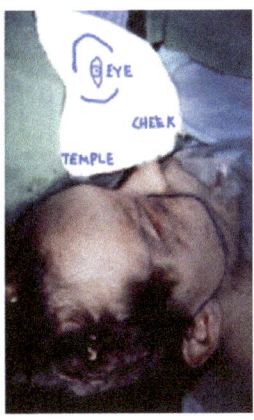

The first two photos below are early post-op views. The last picture, after several months, shows both better contour and better fitting of her ocular prosthesis. The glasses helped to camouflage her residual asymmetry.

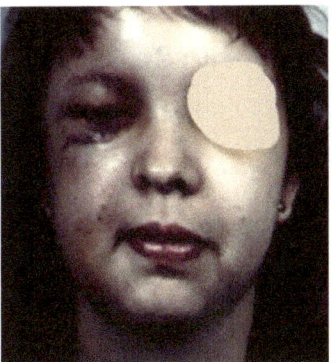
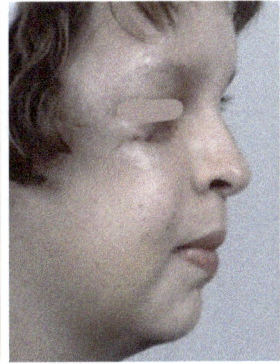
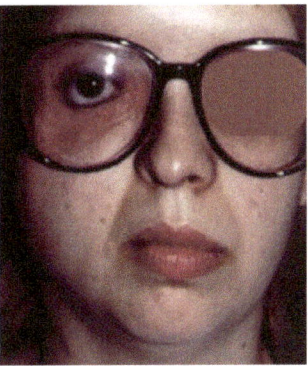

"Joseph" below was a patient I inherited from Dr. Tessier when he stopped coming to Houston. He previously had several operations for left hemifacial microsomia, including upper and lower jaw surgery and bone grafts. He had proper occlusion but was still deficient in left facial contour.

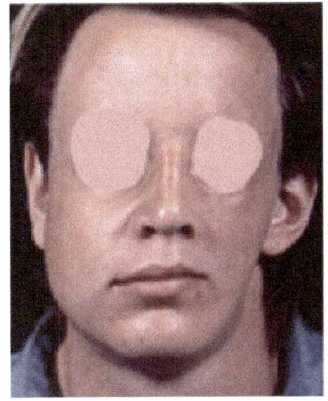
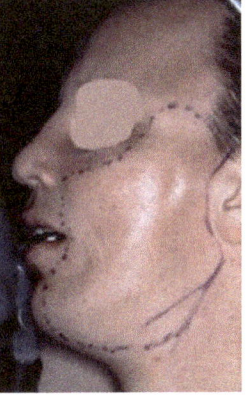

Like the previous case, I used a scapular free flap to add bulk to the face. His postoperative results are below.

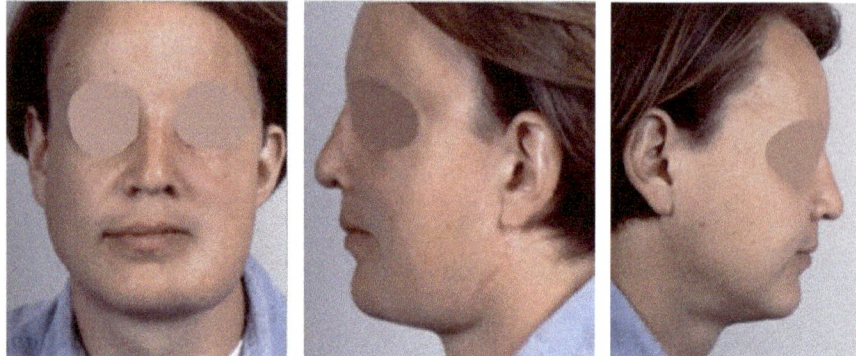

"Victoria" had a severely short columella with a stubbed nose after previous cleft lip surgery done elsewhere.

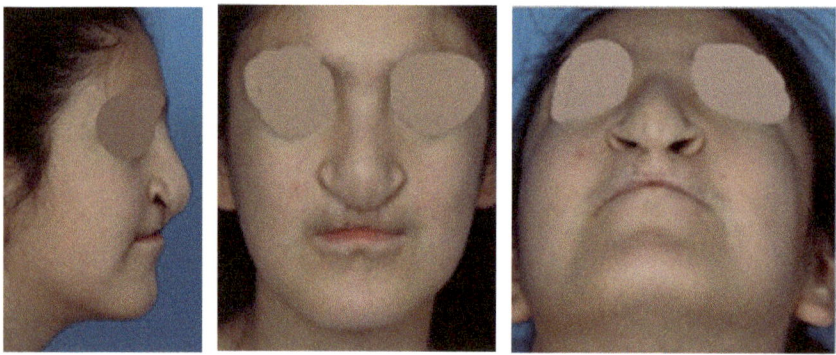

I performed a two-stage Abbe flap lip switch procedure, like that done for "Jim" in chapter1. I released the central lip prolabium upward to become the nasal columella, which allowed the nasal tip to be freed and project more normally. The upper lip was made fuller by augmentation from the transferred lower lip tissue. Below are her early postoperative views after the separation of the Abbe flap.

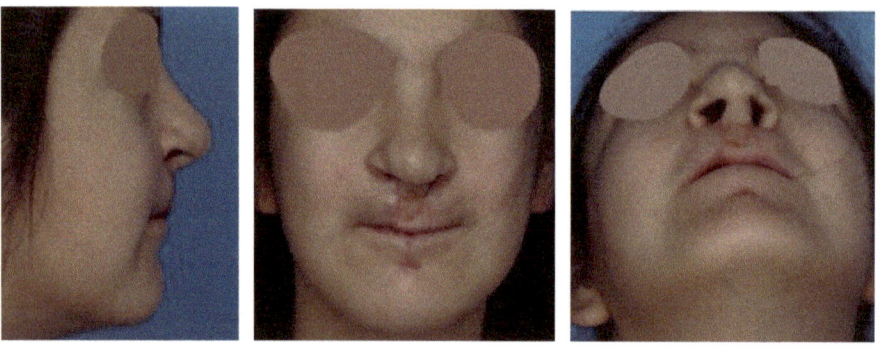

"Reginald" also presented many years after having a cleft lip and palate procedures. He was desirous of cosmetic improvement even though he had lived with this condition for many years. His deformity was similar to the above patient's, but not as severe. I treated him with a different technique. I performed a local columella lengthening procedure and a lip revision.

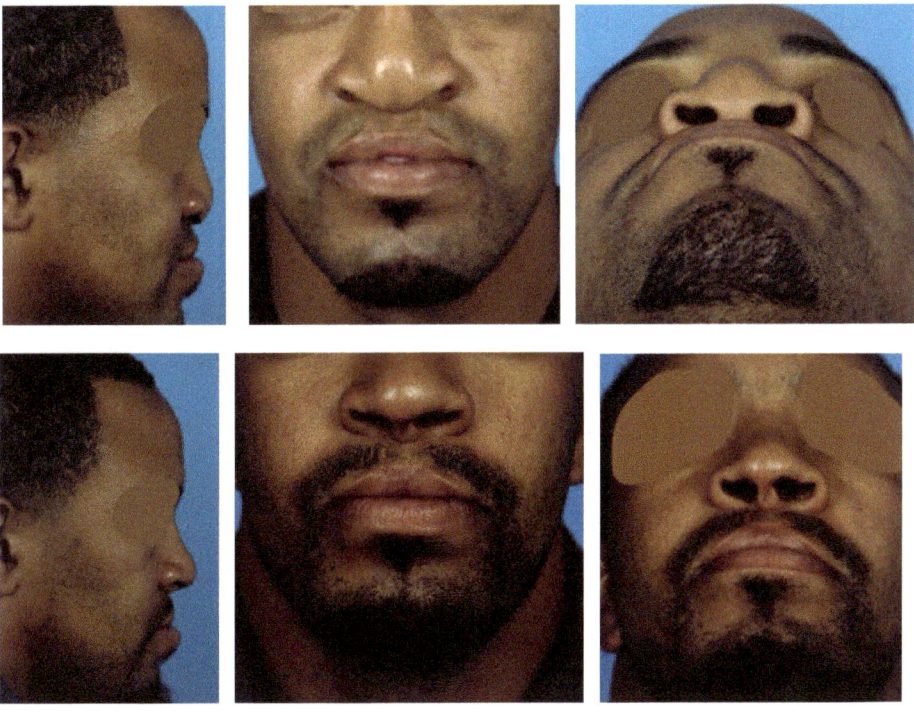

This child "Victoria" shown below was born with an intensely pigmented congenital giant nevus of the scalp. Large darkly pigmented nevi have a propensity to degenerate into malignant melanoma; this is probably proportional to the size and how dark the pigment is. Recalling the patient discussed in chapter13 who eventually died from melanoma, I was anxious to remove this nevus in its entirety. I planned to remove the lesion and replace it with a split-thickness skin graft. The graft was located both on the forehead and frontal scalp. The STSG would constitute forehead reconstruction. The plan would be to later move hair-bearing scalp to the location needed for anterior scalp hair with tissue expansion like "Suzzy" in chapter 2.

The Healing Mission of Plastic Surgery

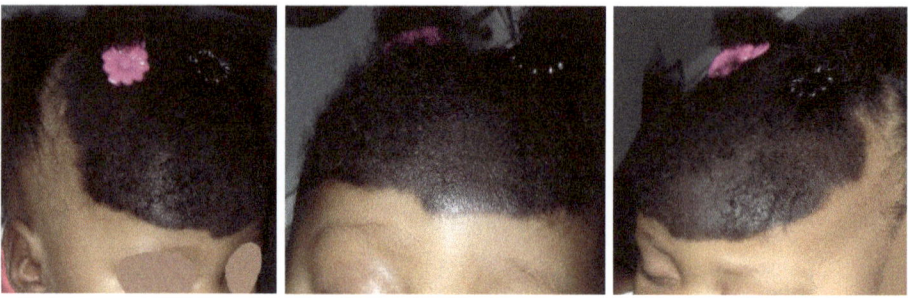

The child is shown below after STSG to the forehead and scalp.

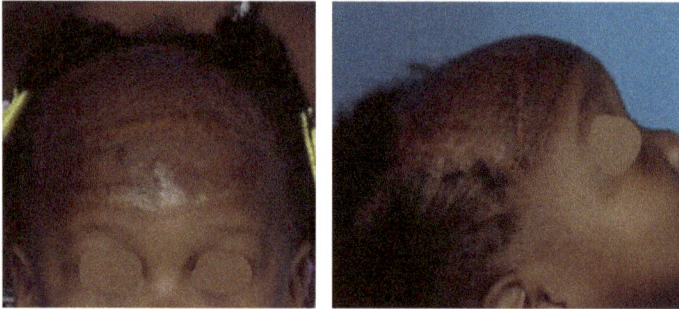

I anticipated the scalp reconstruction to take a few stages. In the photo-drawings below, the orange dotted line represents the expected eventual anterior hairline. Several months after the excision and skin grafting, I removed a strip of the STSG posteriorly and undermined and advanced hair-bearing scalp forward. I did not yet use tissue expander balloons to stretch the scalp.

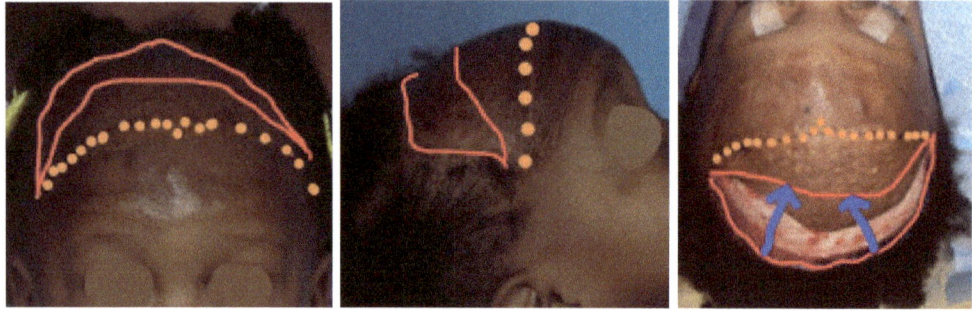

As you can see in the photos below, she still needs a significant segment of STSG replaced with the hair-bearing scalp. I anticipated I would utilize a tissue expander balloon technique to finish the reconstruction. I regret that, because of my retirement, I was unable to finish her case.

The Healing Mission of Plastic Surgery

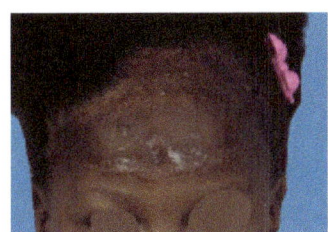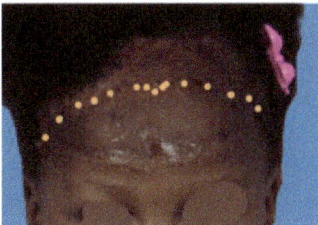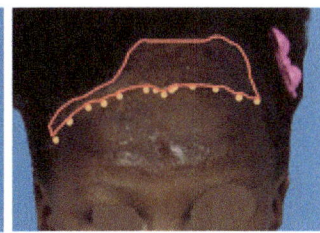

Chapter 16

The Place of Cosmetic Surgery in the Healing Mission

Cosmetic plastic surgery, also known as aesthetic surgery, is surgery performed to reshape normal structures of the body to enhance appearance. It often improves body image and increases self-esteem. Cosmetic surgery now holds a mainstream place in the field of plastic surgery. As alluded to in the first chapter, there is a quite tangled relationship between functional, reconstructive, and aesthetic surgery. Although plastic surgery has become very prevalent, a large percentage of the general population thinks plastic surgery is synonymous with cosmetic surgery. If you read the preceding chapters, you know differently already. There is also a significant portion of the general public, which frowns upon cosmetic surgery as being vain and extravagant.

Such a reading of the aesthetic part of the field of plastic surgery, I think, is inaccurate and shortsighted. It is true that occasionally I have seen a patient requesting cosmetic surgery who comes across to me as extraordinarily narcissistic and interested in extremely subtle signs of aging or such minor imperfections and that I have difficulty engaging in their requests.

Such neurotic patients are quite unusual. Most of the patients who come seeking cosmetic surgery are entirely reasonable with either realistic expectations or can be informed to have realistic expectations. It may be true that cosmetic patients may be somewhat more demanding and expect something closer to perfection than the average functional or reconstructive patient. However, this is not universal. Some cosmetic patients are quite happy with anything you might do to improve their situation. Some reconstructive patients are quite fastidious and nitpick results.

As mentioned before, when I was a teenager, I had a mole grow in the center of my forehead. At first, I didn't mind this until one of my friends began teasing me by calling me Cyclopes. After that, it concerned me enough that I went to see my plastic surgeon uncle so that he could remove this for me. He cured me with a simple office procedure, under local anesthesia, that took only a few minutes. I remember leaving the office a happier young man. Because of that experience, I understand little things can be concerning to anyone at particular times in our lives.

After I had been in the practice of plastic surgery for a few years, I developed some puffiness under my lower eyelids from some excess fatty tissue. I looked tired all the time, even when I was not. I knew a lower blepharoplasty could correct this. Therefore, I consulted with my partner Benjamin Cohen who graciously obliged me. My lower eyelid surgery alleviated the problem, and I was able to go about my business more contentedly. Again, this type of experience helped me to understand how people can look upon some cosmetic imperfection as something they would like to improve upon to feel better about themselves. When this type of problem is approached in an orderly and reasonable fashion, looking for realistic solutions from professionals, most people have no problem with it.

Every plastic surgeon has many extremely grateful patients after helping them with functional problems or with reconstructive issues. What might not seem as obvious is that some of the most appreciative patients a plastic surgeon has are cosmetic surgery patients.

Before I get into specifics about cosmetic surgery with multiple examples of actual patients, I want to briefly discuss the phenomenon of shoppers that all plastic surgeons, especially those in private practice witnesses. Of course, we all recognize and welcome that patients often need a second opinion before they are ready to proceed with any significant surgical procedure.

Shoppers

It was not uncommon to have potential patients call our office to price shop for frequently performed cosmetic procedures. I have never wanted to be either the highest priced nor the lowest-priced surgeon. Such telephone shoppers rarely come in even if they make an appointment. It was most comfortable for our office manager to go ahead and give some general prices, though we might prefer to have the patient come in for a visit to assess their need and get accurate costs for them.

Another variation on shoppers is the patient who has a specific issue, such as a large nose. He may begin by rattling off a litany of names of plastic surgeons and, in this case, also ENT surgeons with whom he has already consulted. Often these patients are very time-consuming and unable to make any decision.

One particular patient that comes to mind was a young South Asian man with a large nose. I saw him on three different occasions for consultations. We went over his exam and looked at numerous views of his pictures. I made some prediction drawings, and he showed me pictures that he thought demonstrated the nose he desired. After all that, he then sent me several e-mails with additional images, together with multiple questions about them. I finally tired of the whole process after answering a couple of such e-mails. I told him he needed to come back to the office if he was interested in scheduling surgery. He never returned.

Another type of shopper is one who has no intention of scheduling cosmetic surgery with me but wants to have an in-depth consultation going over all the risks, benefits, and alternatives of their desired procedures. They have already seen the surgeon they want to perform their operation, but they want to clarify a few things and are hesitant to "bother" the other surgeon with questions.

Still, another sort of shopper is the patient who is sent by his attorney because of some scars. Sometimes these are minimal scars that are not a functional problem. Also, they may be such that it is debatable whether or not any surgery, such as scar revision or dermabrasion (sanding), would be helpful. After I explain the pros and cons of any revision surgery, they say they need an estimated cost for those possible procedures even if I do not recommend them in their case. The reason is, although they may have no intention of having surgery to improve the scars, they do want to make an insurance settlement that will be greater if it includes funds for potential intervention.

I had a lady come to see me in the office who had been injured by a dog several months previously. She had well-healed scrapes of the upper and lower lip on the left side, which were. She had very slight vertical scars that mimicked her pre-existing smoker's lines. The smoker's lines on the uninjured right side of her lips were more prominent than the small scars left from the accident. Also, she complained that her cupid's bow on the left was not as distinct as before the dog bite, even though the trauma had not extended fully to that area. There is a lot of normal variability in the prominence and distinctiveness of the cupid's bow. Also, with aging, the bow often becomes less distinct. I was so under impressed with the cause and effect relationship in her list of complaints that I lost my cool momentarily and said: "give me a break." Although with further discussion and explanation of her situation, our rapport improved, she never did schedule a procedure to enhance the scars.

Another shopper presentation is two ladies who come together and want to have their consultations simultaneously. They usually inquire about a facelift, but sometimes, it may be for augmentation mammaplasty or something else. They may be out on a lark shopping, or they may genuinely be serious about having surgery. It is hard to tell sometimes. One will usually schedule first as the less bold one wants to wait and see how her friend turns out from the surgery.

I have never subscribed to the marketing tool for having free consultations. As a professional, I expect to give my opinion about the patient's situation and not try to talk the patient into surgery. Often, I found myself telling the patient I do not recommend surgery.

I remember a young lady who came to see me in consultation regarding her lips. She thought fuller lips would enhance her attractiveness. Of course, there are various injectable fillers available for this purpose. Occasionally there are situations where I recommend surgical procedures with or without some implant or autograph such as fat or fascia from the patient. What was remarkable in her case is that she had already had multiple injections with fillers and had an exaggerated fish lip appearance, the" trout pout" look. I told her I did not think additional injections, or any other procedure would presently be a good idea and declined to intervene. I thought of the famous line from Robert Burns's poem To a Louse, translated as, "Oh, would some power the gift to give us to see ourselves as others see us."

Cosmetic body contouring surgery

Aesthetic body contouring surgery has been an expanding field in plastic surgery, partly because of the obesity epidemic in the U.S and the successful weight loss operations meant to counteract it. But also because there are new effective contouring procedures to help not only those overweight patients but others as well. Abdominoplasty, circumferential body lift, thigh lifts, arm lifts (brachioplasty), as well as traditional breast lifts, have all become more fashionable. Certainly, liposuction has gained a significant role in contemporary body contouring.

Circumferential body lift

A young lady, "Ida," presented with complaints of back neck and shoulder discomfort from large pendulous breasts. She was moderately obese. She thought, if she had a reduction mammaplasty, it would also incentivize her to lose weight. I performed a reduction mammaplasty procedure for her, and she did well. Subsequently, she shed a considerable amount of weight over a year or so without any bypass surgery.

However, by then, she felt needed another boost. She consulted with me again. I decided that liposuction of her abdomen, hips, and thighs would be beneficial, especially if followed later by skin tightening surgery. She acceded to my recommendations. So, I lipo-suctioned a significant amount of fat from the abdomen, hips, and thighs with excellent benefit and no complications.

About two years later, after she had lost additional weight with dieting, I performed an extensive operation consisting of abdominoplasty with a circumferential body lift and an inner thigh lifting procedure. Her transformation made a huge difference in her attitude toward life as well as her appearance. I was impressed even though I was the surgeon. She also appreciated that she received a very copacetic result. Below left are her preoperative photos, and on the right are her postoperative pictures after this three-year process.

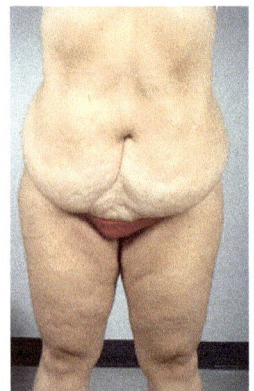 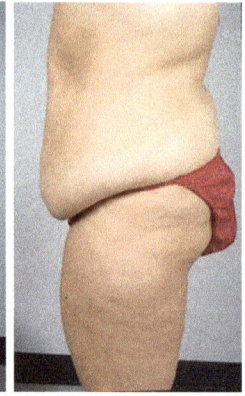 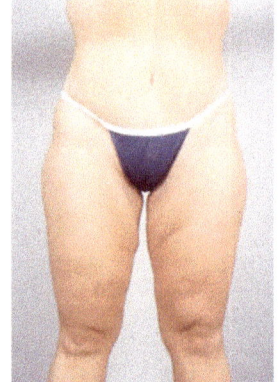 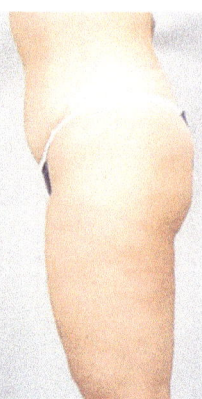

"Harper" had lost a lot of weight dieting. She complained of excess abdominal skin and loose skin of the buttock and hips. She also had a dark birthmark that I advised her to remove. I performed an extended abdominoplasty with a circumferential incision. The operation tightened the hip and buttock, removed the birthmark, and reshaped the abdomen. Below is the preoperative view, the proposed amount of skin excision, and the postoperative result.

The Healing Mission of Plastic Surgery

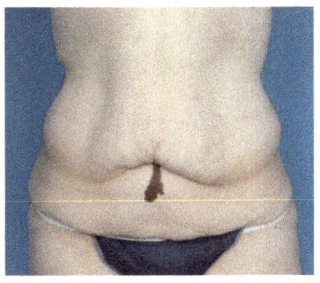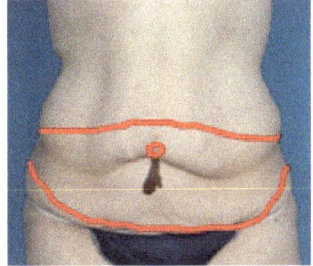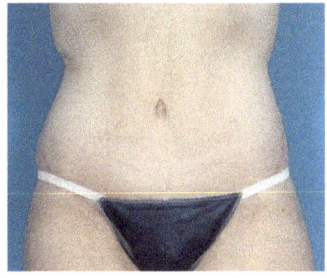

Below the lateral preoperative view, the proposed amount of excision, and the lateral postoperative result.

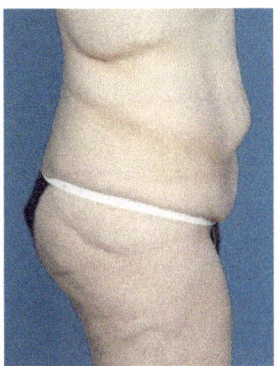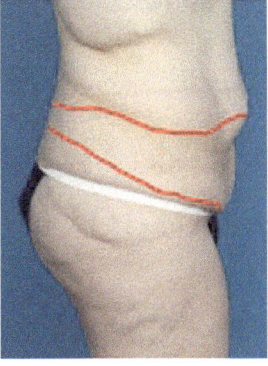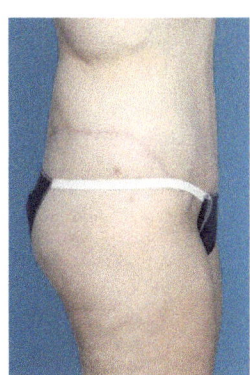

Abdominoplasty

One of the most common body contouring operations is abdominoplasty, popularly known as a tummy tuck. Ordinarily, this operation not only removes excess skin but also tightens the abdominal wall its musculature. In the case below, "Sandra," I performed an abdominoplasty, which tightened the skin and muscle fascia, and reduced the protuberance of the abdomen. Her before and after photos (before scar maturation) are below.

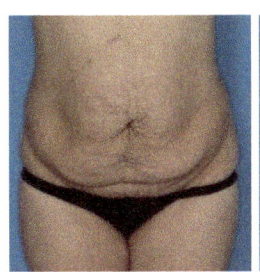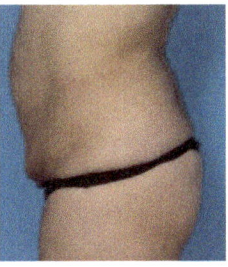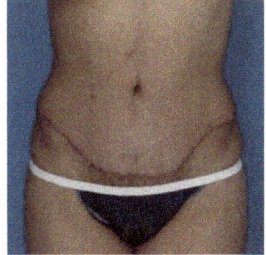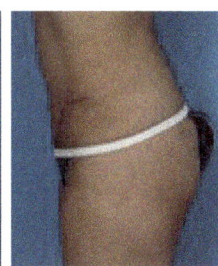

"Amelia" was displeased with the loose skin of her abdomen, which no amount of exercise would eliminate. I performed an abdominoplasty, tightening her muscles and removing the excess skin. This procedure relieved her displeasure with the excess skin and improved her body image.

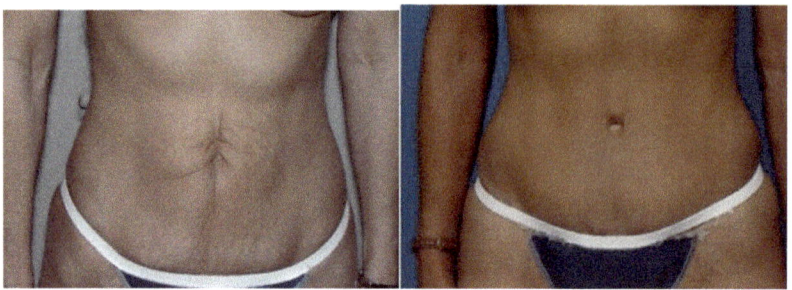

"Roberta" below complained of her protuberant and wavy abdomen. An abdominoplasty with plication of the rectus muscles, removal of excess skin, together with liposuction of the stomach and thighs, gave her a healthier appearance.

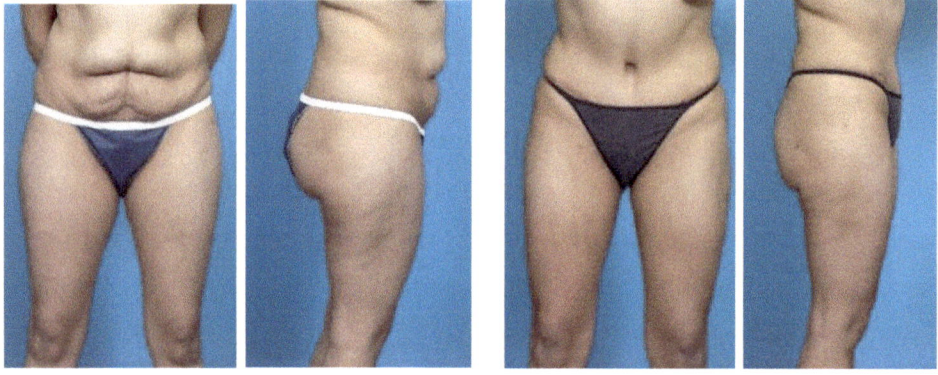

"Blyth" below had loose excess skin of the abdomen and a weak protuberant abdominal wall. She sought improvement and was willing to undergo an abdominoplasty (tummy tuck), which included extensive tightening of the abdominal wall fascia and musculature. Her preoperative and postoperative photos are below.

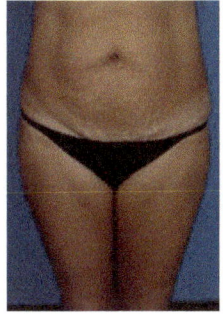 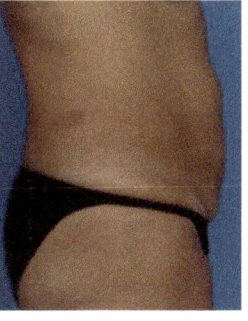 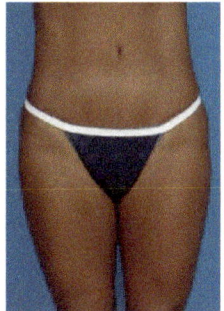 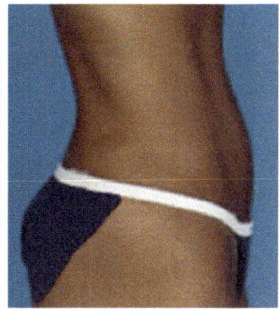

The lady below "Charlotte" was overweight and sought improvement with liposuction and abdominoplasty. Of course, I encouraged her to lose weight. She needed a boost to get her on track to obtain a better physique. Pictures of her preoperative condition are below.

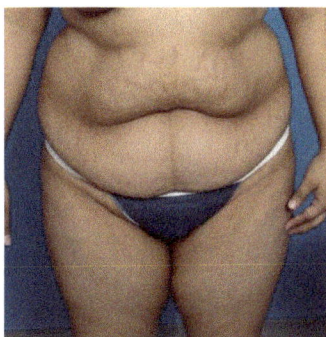 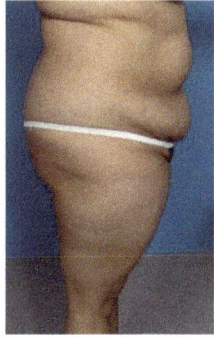 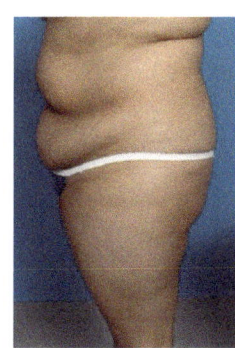

I performed circumferential liposuction of her thighs and liposuction of her hips and abdomen. Also, I performed an abdominoplasty removing excess skin and abdominal fat. I think she obtained a lot of improvement from this plastic surgery intervention. I hope she took advantage of this "boost" and continued with her weight loss and physical fitness program.

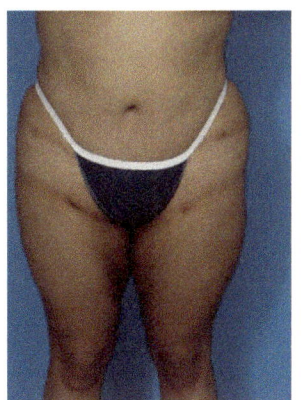 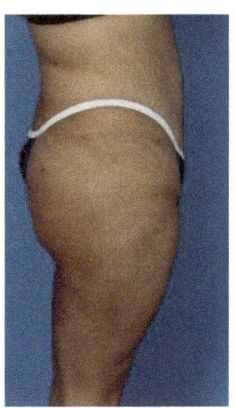 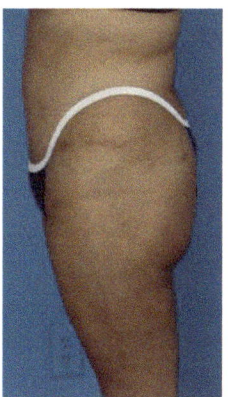

Additionally, "Charlotte" sought to improve the appearance of her breasts and, at the same time, reduce them a moderate amount. Her preoperative photos are below. I blotted out a distinctive chest marking.

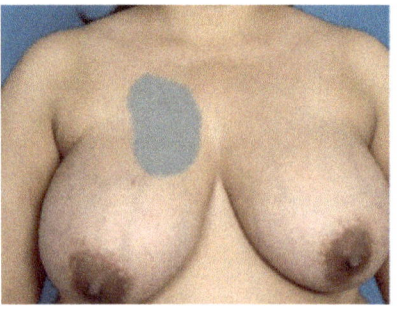 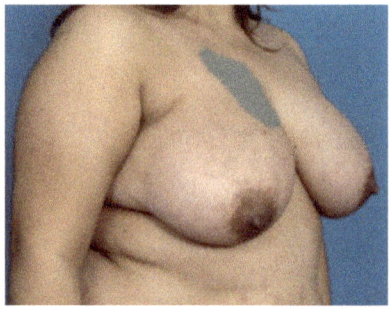

I performed a modest reduction with a superior-medial pedicle flap and Wise pattern closure. Chapter 14 has more details on breast reduction techniques. Her postoperative result is below.

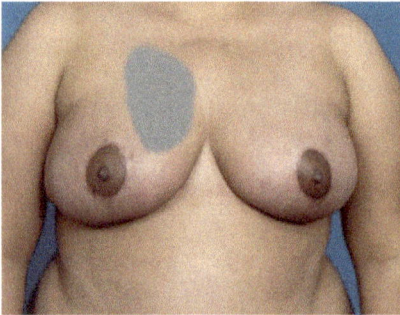 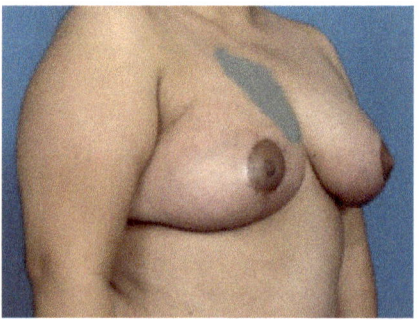

"Dallas," shown below, had had surgery on her abdomen as a young child. She presented with two complaints. She objected to the weakness and prominent bulging of her stomach, and additionally, to the residual depressed scar adjacent to her umbilicus.

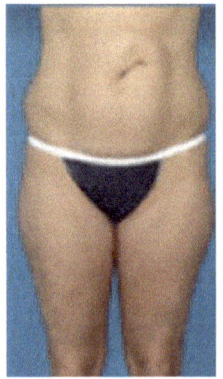 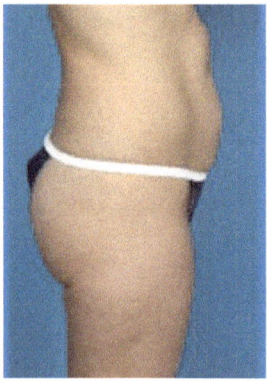 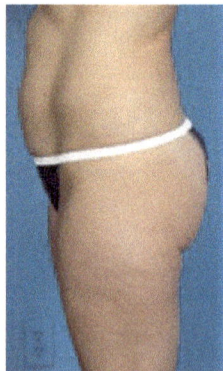

Through a lower abdominal incision, I plicated the fascia of the abdominal wall, making it stronger and less protuberant. I directly revised the old scar making it less depressed.

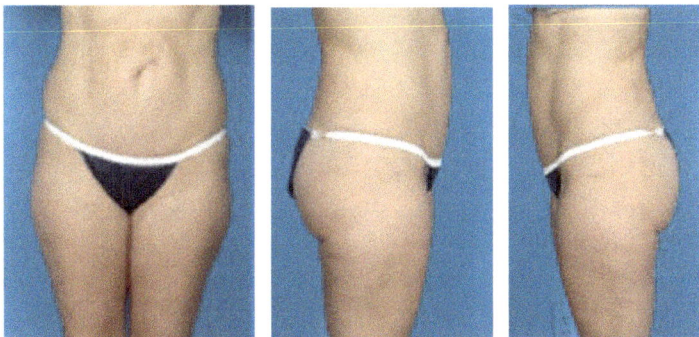

"Graciella" shown below was displeased by excess and wrinkled abdominal skin. I did an extended abdominoplasty for her (outlined in red), which substantially tightened and smoothed the abdomen. In the post-operative photo, she has special tape over the healing incisions to promote less scar tissue

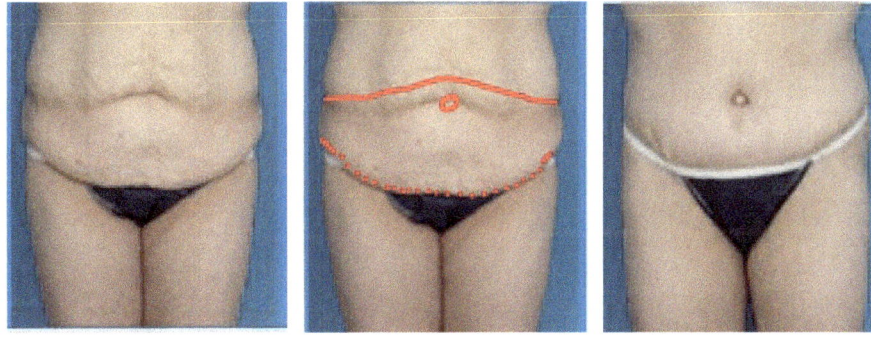

"Amber" sought body contouring rejuvenation. She disliked her excess abdominal skin and the upper thigh and buttock fulness. She also desired fuller breasts. Her preoperative pictures are below.

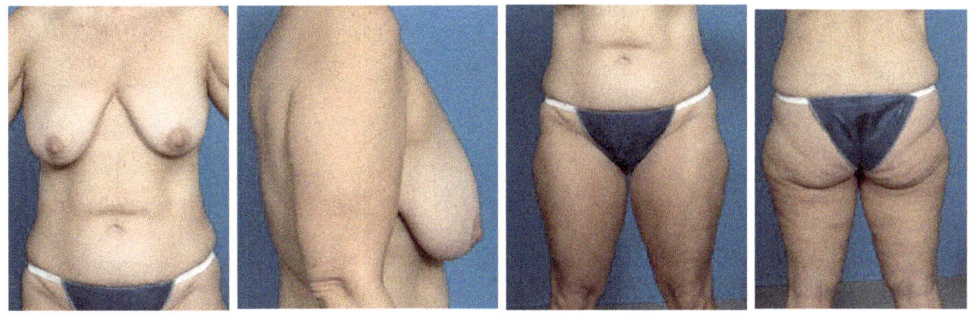

The intraoperative photos below illustrate the extent of circumferential abdominal and buttock/ upper thigh excision. The picture on the left is prone, and the image on the right is supine.

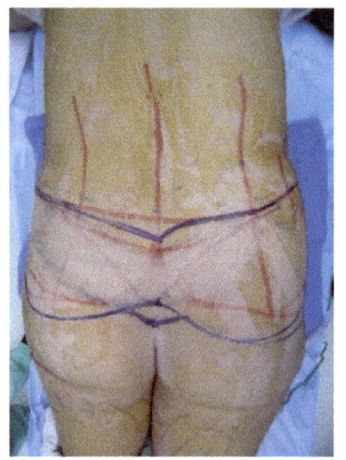 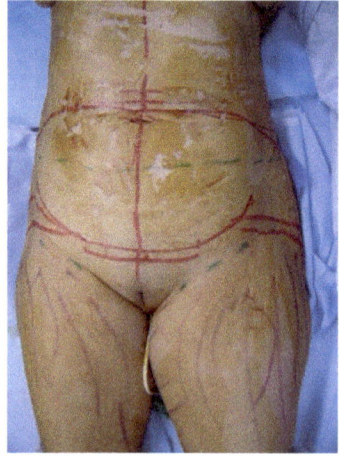

The photos below show the posterior view after the skin and fat excision and before closure.

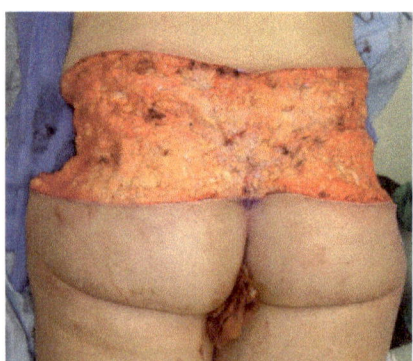 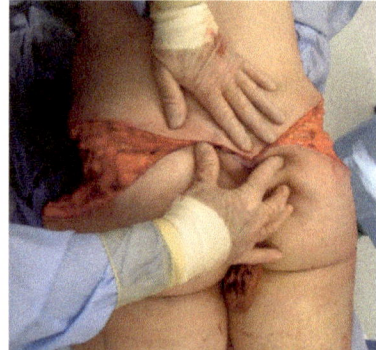

The intraoperative views below show freeing the lateral thigh with a distinctive long dissector that loosens the thigh skin. I then pulled up the skin and subcutaneous tissue to tighten the thigh, as shown in the immediate on the table closure on the right.

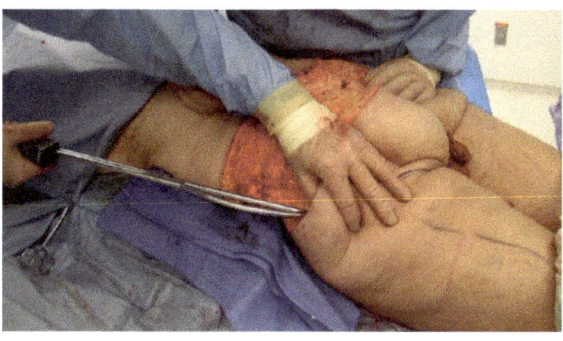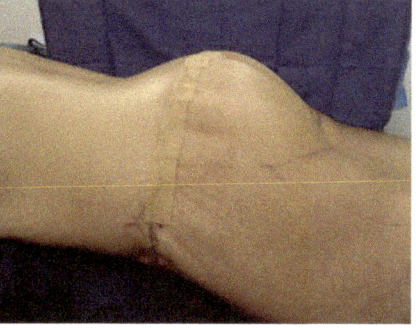

Another posterior and an anterior view, on the operating table, after a circumferential body and thigh lift and augmentation mammaplasty are below

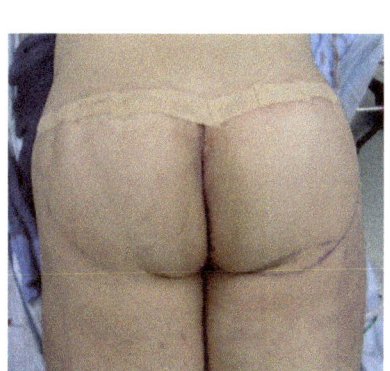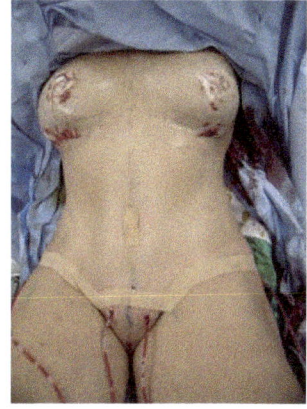

Compare postoperative views below with the above preoperative views.

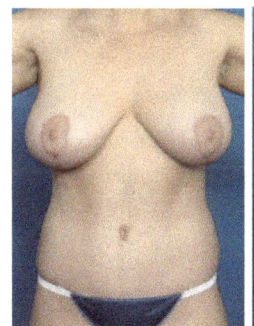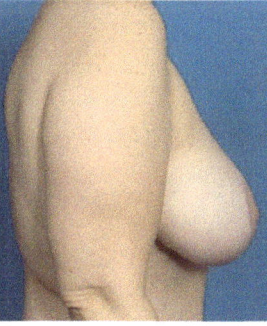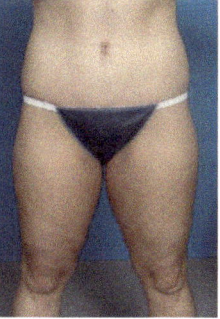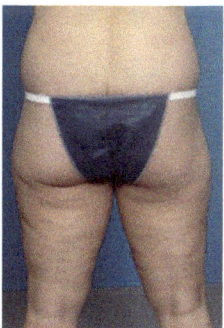

"Monica" complained of weak abdominal muscles and excess lower abdominal skin. She had separation (diastasis) of her rectus abdominis muscles from childbirth. I plicated her rectus muscles and removed excess skin and fat tissue. Her pre and postoperative photos are below.

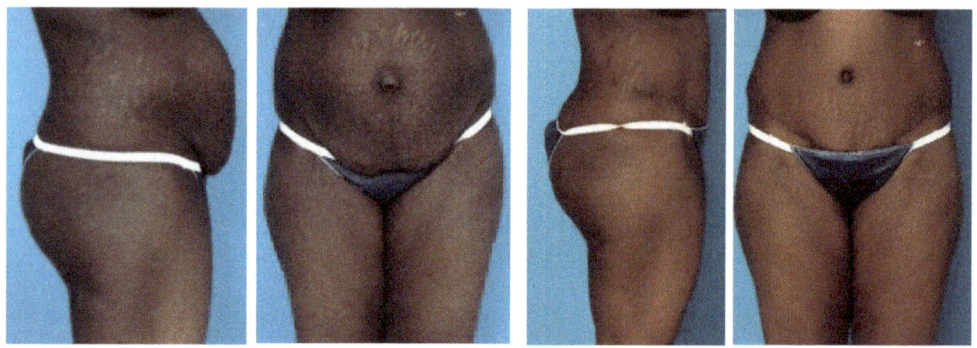

"Dido" had not only excess skin of the lower abdomen, but she had a bulge of the upper stomach from diastasis and week muscles. I plicated her rectus abdominis muscles to correct the fullness. I excised the redundant skin and fat with the incision outlined in red below.

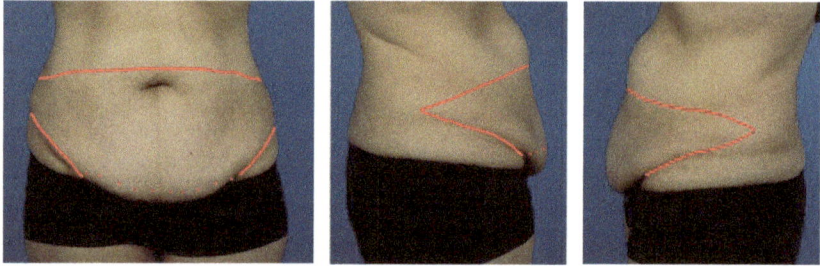

Her before and early after pictures are below.

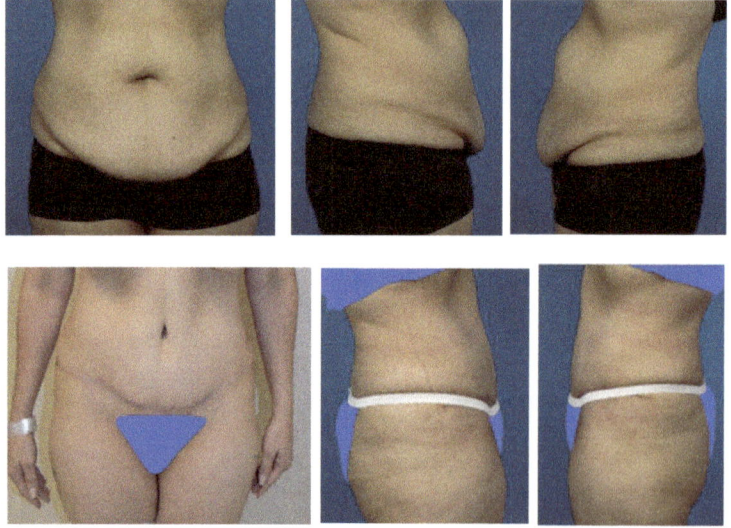

"Evelyn" wanted to do something for herself. She was unhappy with her excess abdominal skin. She always wanted fuller breasts as well.

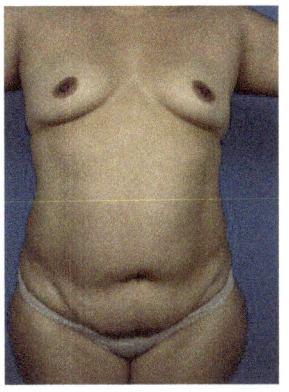 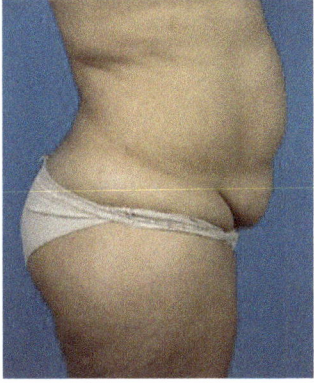

So, I performed an abdominoplasty and an augmentation with a silicone breast implant for her. Her results are below. She was pleased that she finally decided on these procedures. Her Considerable intra-abdominal fat limited her abdominal effect. She must address that fat with dietary weight loss.

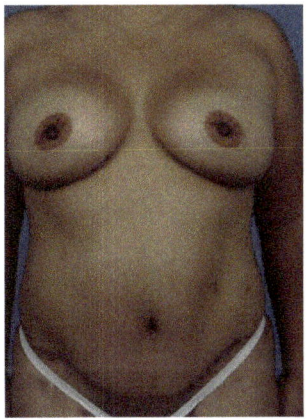 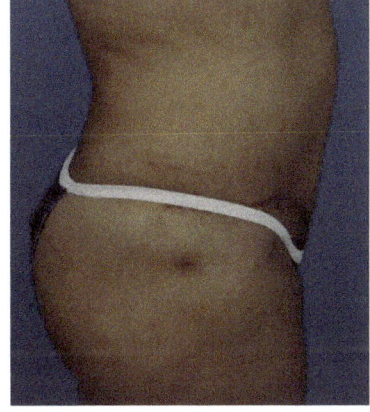

I performed two large volume liposuction sessions about two years apart for "Alexia." Large volume liposuction is usually considered anything over 5 liters of aspirate. I think she got an excellent result. The photos on the left are preoperative. Those in the center are after the first session. Those on the right are final results

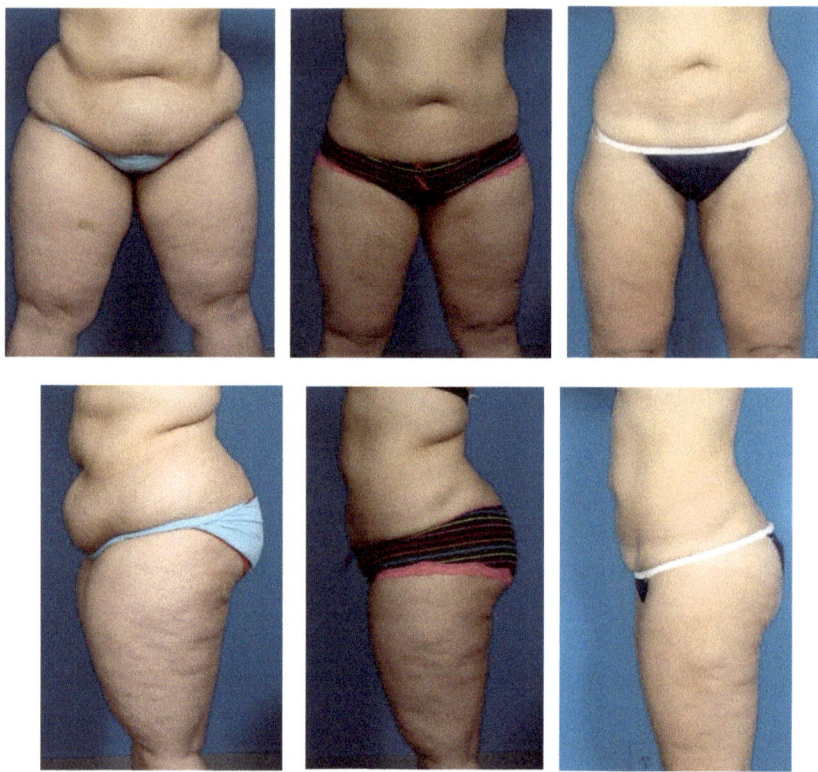

The patient below "Antonia" is typical of the patients seeking a "mommy makeover." That is, she has some flabby excess abdominal skin and somewhat deflated breasts after having children. I did an abdominoplasty and an augmentation with silicone gel implants. She found this was a rejuvenating experience. Her preoperative pictures are on the left and postoperative on the right below.

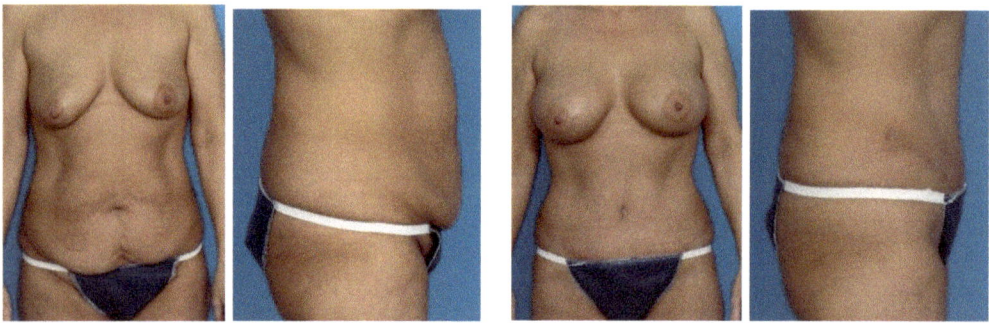

"Roberta," below, wanted to tighten her whole abdomen and get rid of excess skin. Her before photos show excess loose skin and a protuberant upper abdomen. I planned to plicate the fascia of the abdominal wall. But before doing that, I needed to repair the two small hernias that I incidentally found and marked in the photo below. I performed an abdominoplasty for her in which I plicated the abdominal wall fascia and removed excess skin.

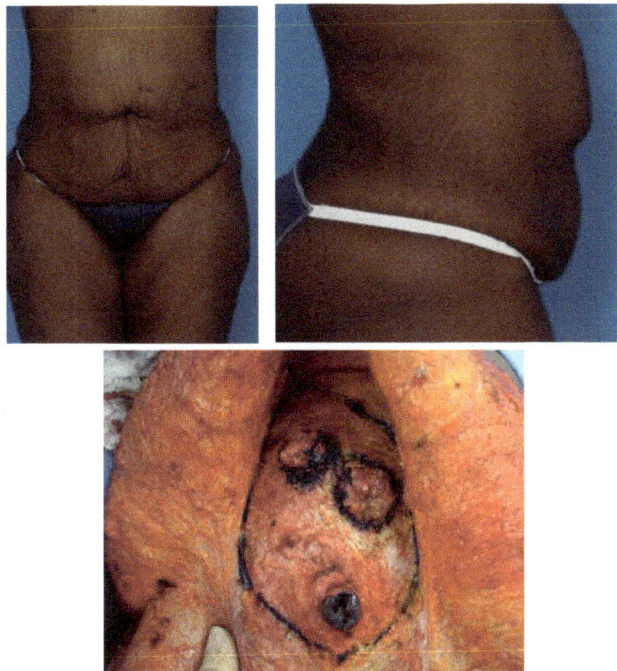

Her result shown below is distorted a little by the strap of the privacy briefs.

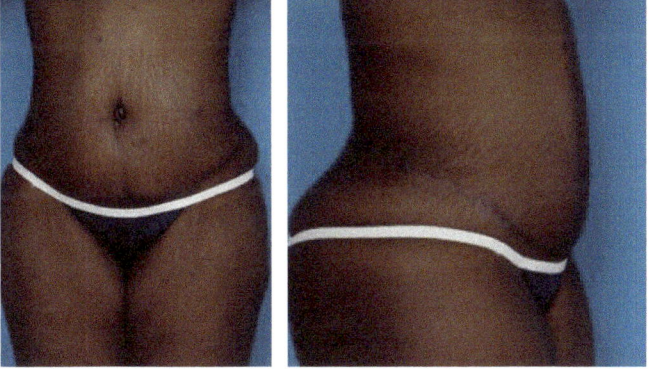

"Evangeline" felt her breasts "deflated" after having her children. She wanted to restore their former fullness. She also sought to tighten her abdomen.

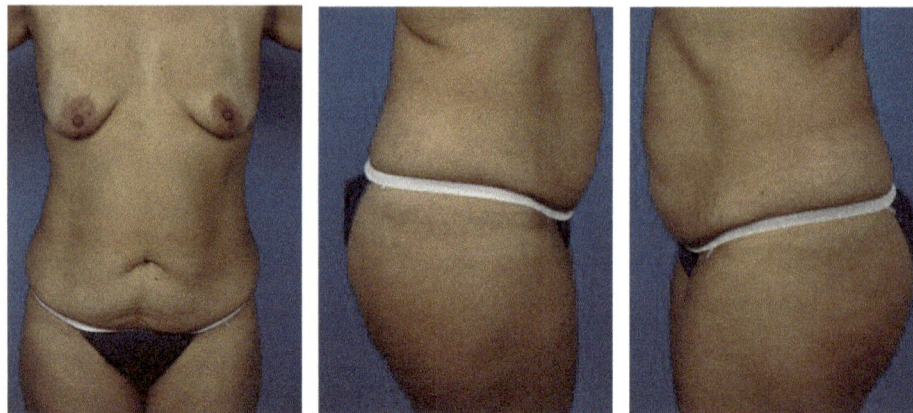

I performed an augmentation mammaplasty and abdominoplasty for her. Her result is below.

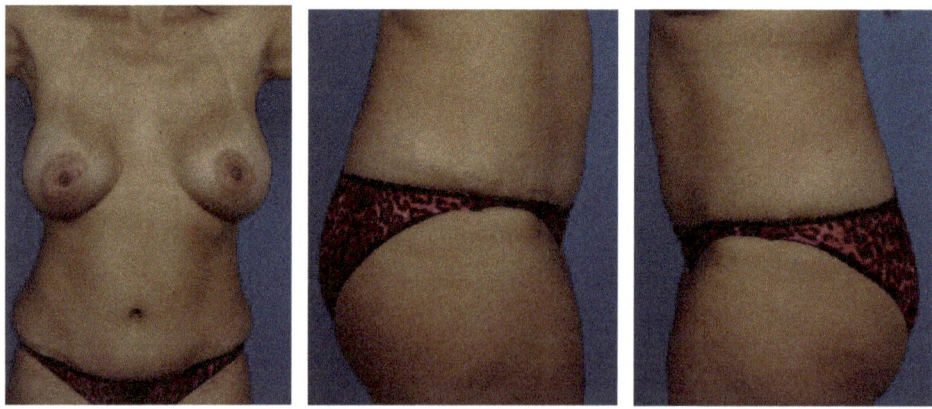

"Carolina" had lost a lot of weight with dieting. She wanted to get rid of the considerable wrinkled and sagging skin of her abdomen. She also wanted to restore some firmness in her breasts, which had become loose and smaller with weight loss. Her preoperative pictures are below

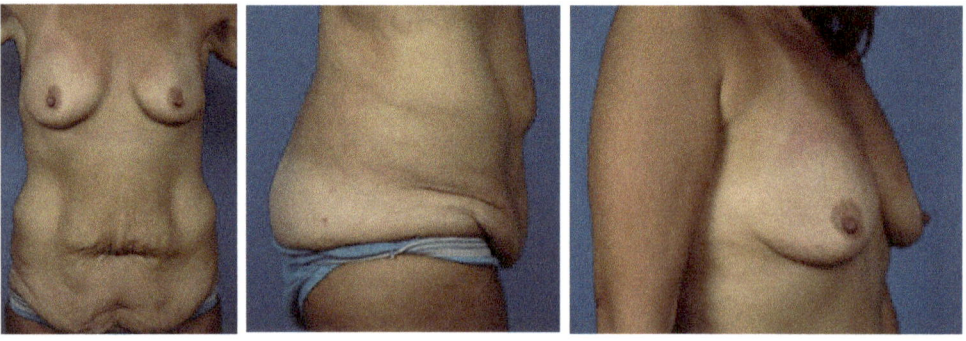

I did a circumferential abdominoplasty and augmentation mammaplasty for her. I drew the extent of the trunk incisions on her photos below.

The Healing Mission of Plastic Surgery

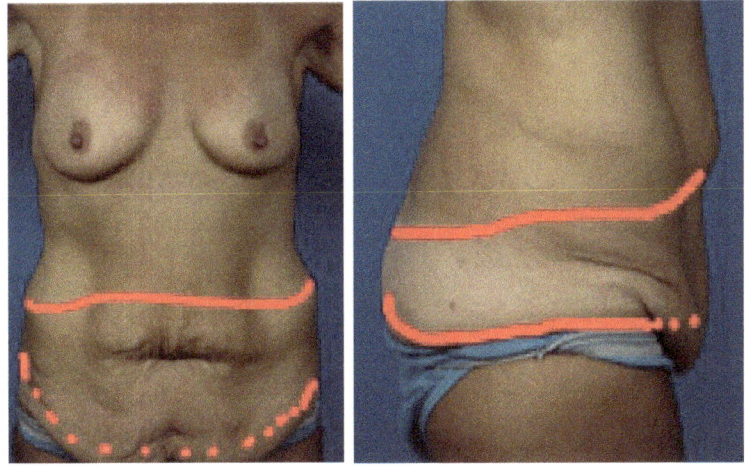

Her early postoperative results are below. The scars have not yet matured.

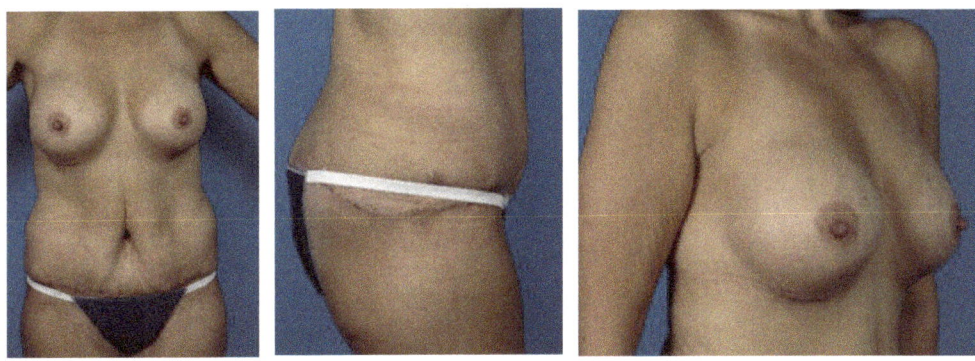

Lower extremity lipodystrophy

"Angel" had lipodystrophy(disproportionate fat) of the lower extremities with excess fatty tissue of her thighs, especially on the left, as shown in the preoperative photos. The intraoperative pictures below show the outline of the skin and subcutaneous fat I am in the process of removing from her thighs.

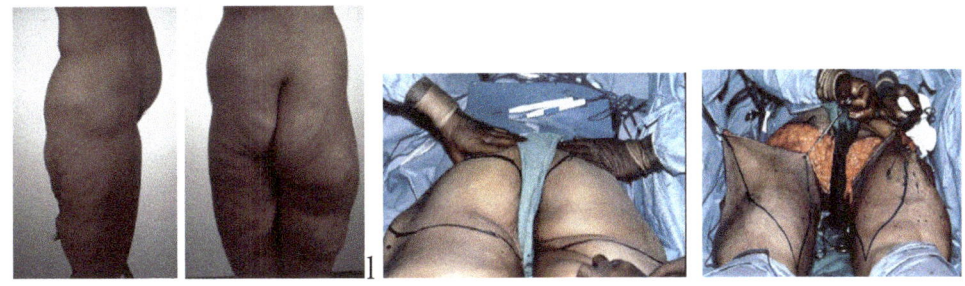

Her postoperative photos are below. This thigh reduction was quite helpful to her finding clothes that fit better, but it also gave her more agility. The improved shape more than compensated for the necessary scars, which will continue to fade.

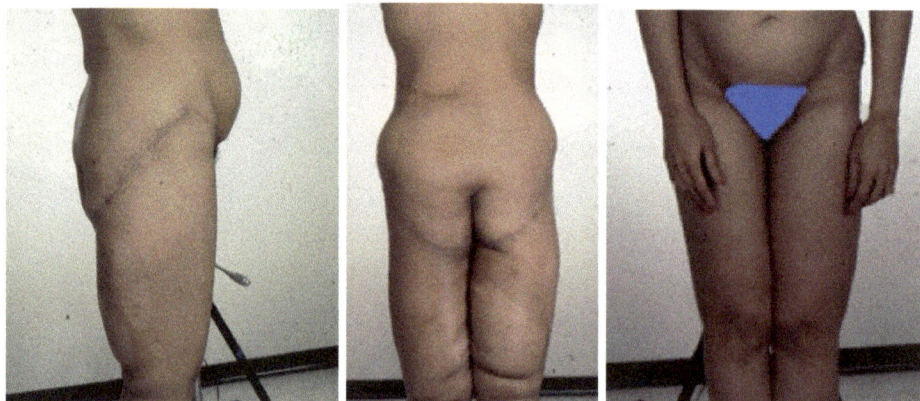

Brachioplasty

Brachioplasty is an arm lift procedure that is often beneficial after massive weight loss. It removes excess loose skin or excess fatty tissue. Its main drawback is the scar that results.

"Roberta" lost more than one hundred pounds. One of her concerns was the excess skin of her upper arms (batwing deformity), as shown below.

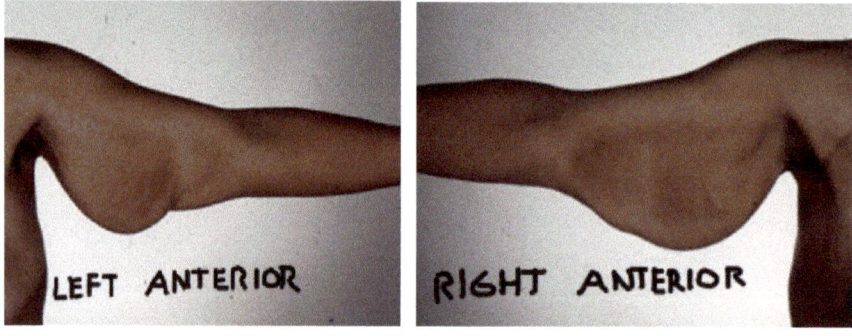

I have drawn the proposed incision on the left arm below. I made the upper incision and undermined the tissue I planned to remove. Next, the flap of skin and fat was brought forward and excised (red) at the appropriate level to allow closure with only mild tension.

The Healing Mission of Plastic Surgery

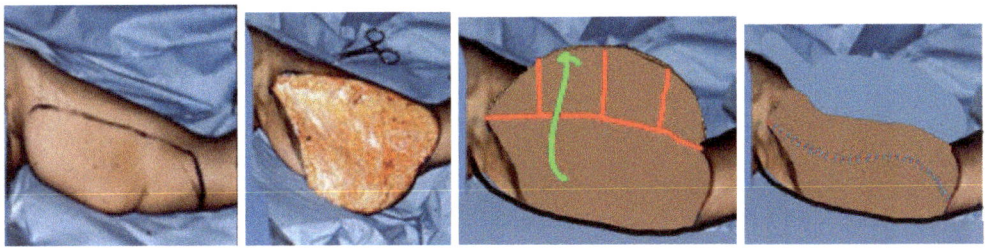

Below is an early postoperative photo.

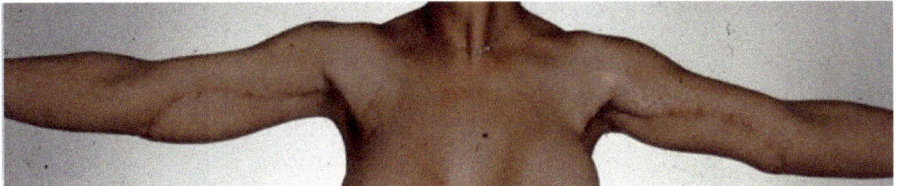

Below "Alexandria" demonstrates a moderate amount of excess skin and fat of the upper arms after losing weight with dieting and exercise. I have drawn the proposed incisions. I cut on one side and undermine the skin and fat. After checking to be sure I can close the wound without undue tension, I then cut the second side of the incision.

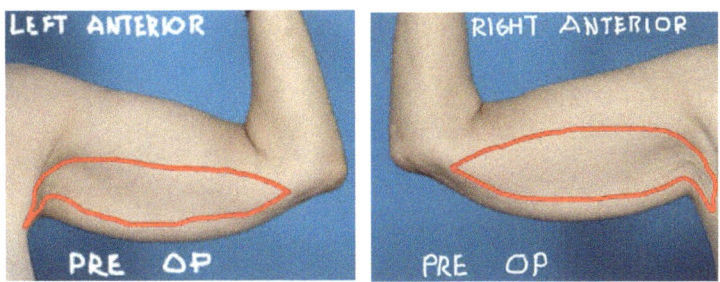

The left photo is of typical excised specimens. The right side pictures are immediate on the table results.

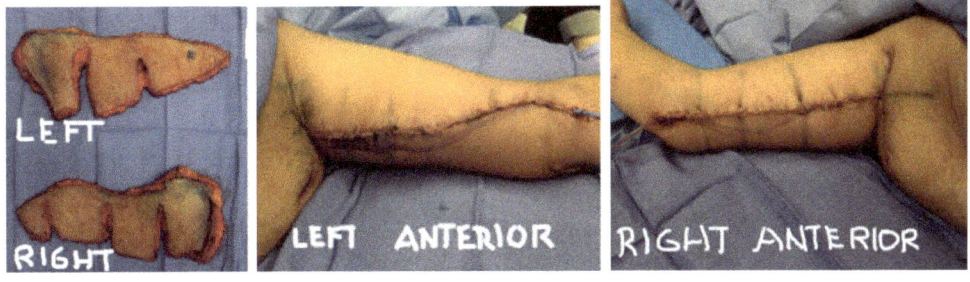

The Healing Mission of Plastic Surgery

Below are the preoperative and postoperative results for "Alexandria" several months after surgery.

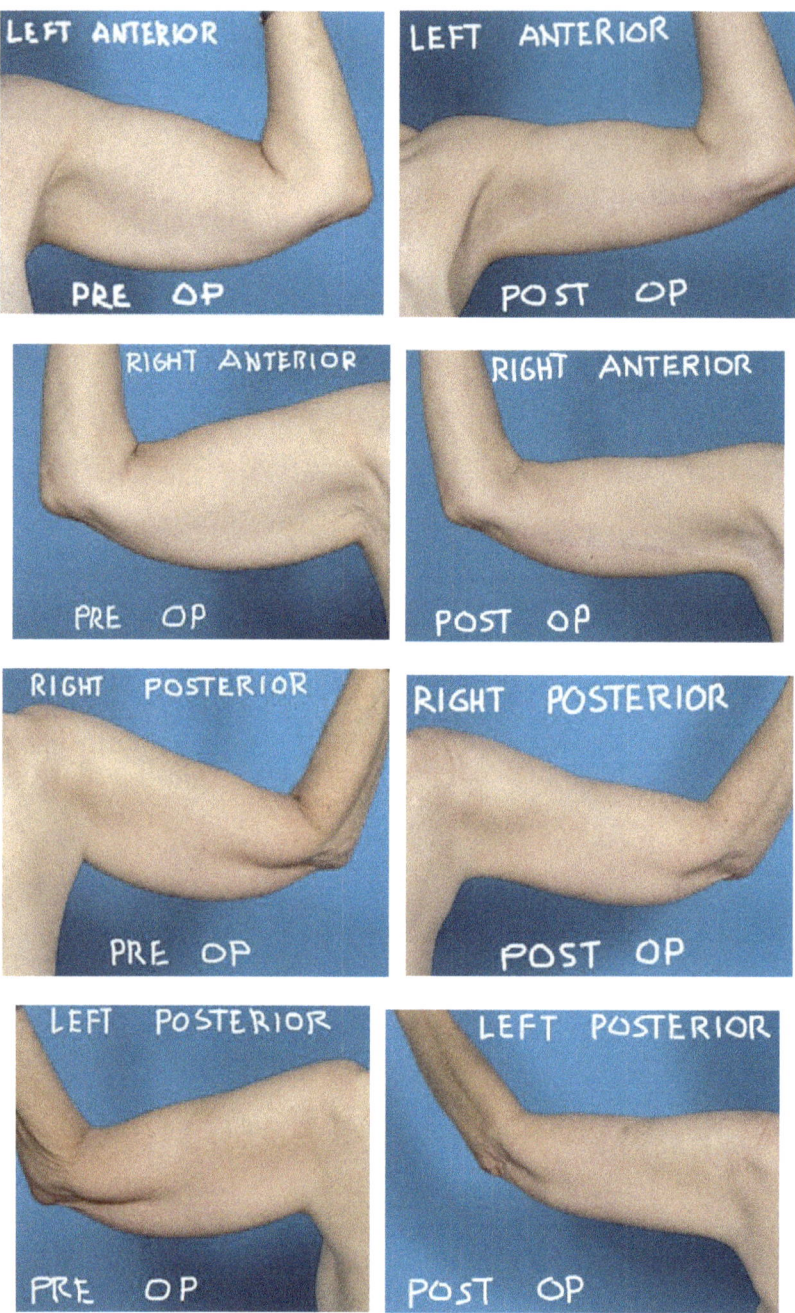

Face Lift

Facelift surgery involves incising the skin in relatively inconspicuous areas, then dissecting beneath the skin and sometimes deeper, beneath the superficial muscular aponeurotic system (SMAS). Tightening portions of this deeper tissue, such as the platysma muscle, helps counteract the sagging tissues of aging. Also, when the deeper tissue is tight, the skin incisions can be closed with less tension after excess skin removal. The chart below shows one example of facelift skin incision placement and skin removal in red. The gray line represents the incision of the deeper tissues. Usually, I tighten and secure the deep tissue (SMAS) with sutures in a more vertical direction than the skin tightening and excision.

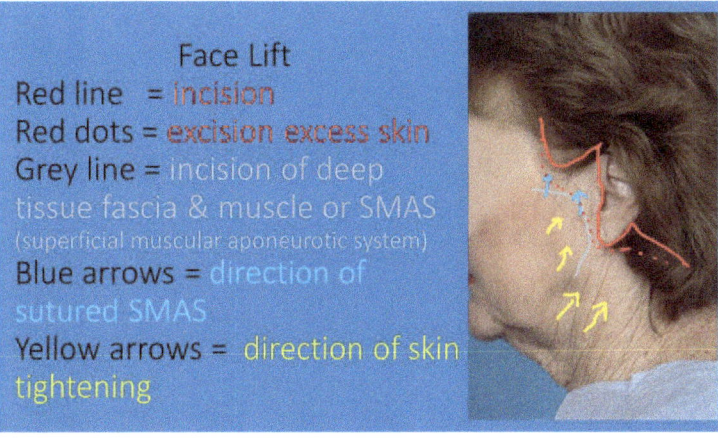

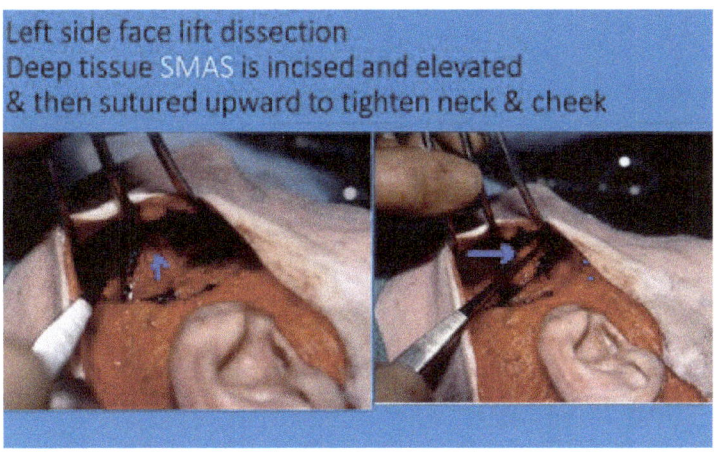

Facelift surgery has become very common. Considerable improvement can occur in these patients, especially when there are excess skin and fat of the neck. Some examples of facelift surgery follow.

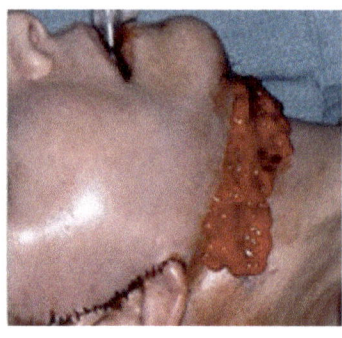

I not only tightened the neck skin but also directly removed fatty tissue for "Margaret" below. As in the above example, I tightened the platysma muscle in the neck too. The postoperative photographs show a significantly improved profile. This type of improvement can be very favorable for the patient's self- image.

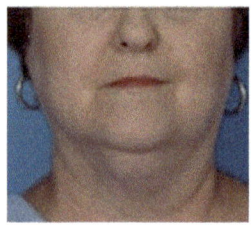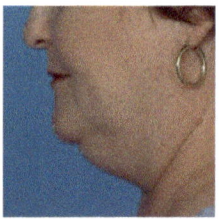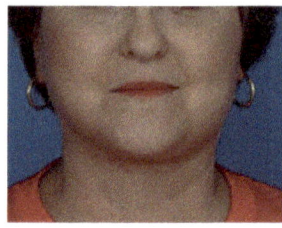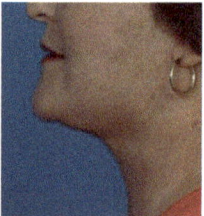

"Caroline" had fullness in the neck and jowls, as demonstrated in her preoperative photos on the left below. She shows improvement in the neck, jawline, and cheeks in the postoperative images on the right below. I directly removed fatty tissue and plicated the platysma muscle in the midline of the neck. I also plicated the SMAS (deep tissue) in the cheeks.

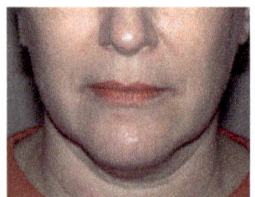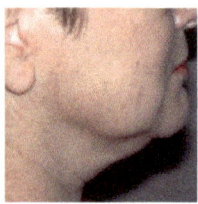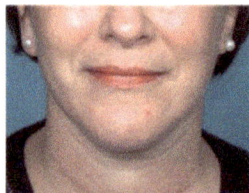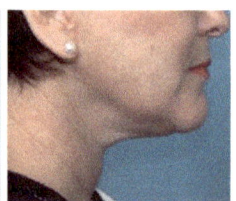

"Sharon" had early jowl formation and considerable excess skin in the midline of the neck. I performed a facelift with tightening and the removal of excess skin, producing the result below.

The Healing Mission of Plastic Surgery

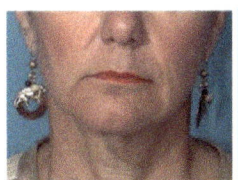 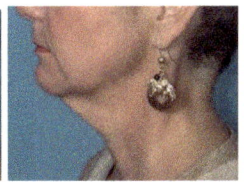 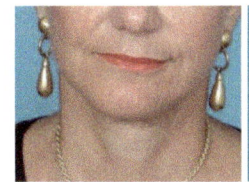 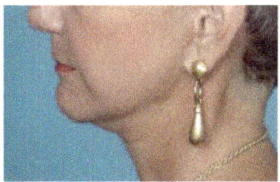

This gentleman below "Sami" had a facelift partly to help improve acne scarring. I remove some fatty tissue in the neck directly and with liposuction. The skin tightening can dampen the appearance of acne scars as in this patient. The skin tightening and fat removal is to improve the neck in both frontal and profile view.

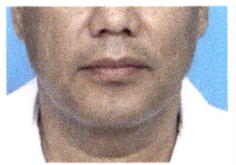 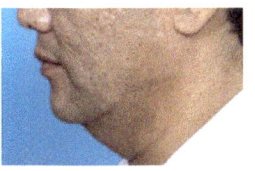 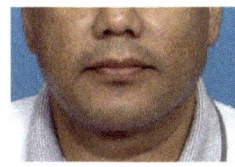 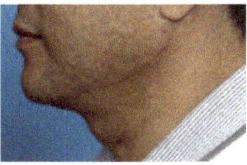

Another interesting phenomenon is that some reconstructive patients decide to undergo cosmetic procedures to improve their overall appearance. For example, it might be that a point of diminishing return has occurred in the reconstruction of their defect, and the most expeditious way to further improve their appearance might be to work on adjacent typical structures to improve their overall appearance. They may be able to accomplish their goal of looking better and feeling better about themselves by combining reconstructive and cosmetic surgery.

Below is an adult patient "Elizabeth" who was born with cleft lip and palate. She came to me for a consultation about some minor revision of the cleft lip. She decided to do not only that but also a facelift and facial fat grafting for cosmetic purposes. I did a facelift and fat injections of the peri-oral area. The photographs below demonstrate improvement in the jowls, neck, and periroal region.

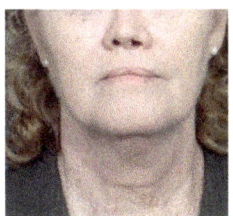 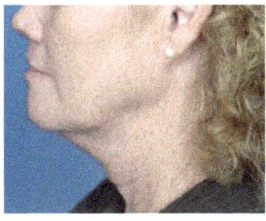 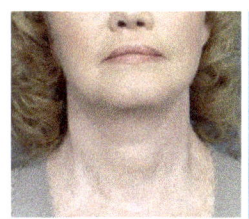 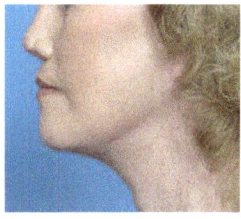

"Marguerite" below had fat grafting to the nasolabial fold area as well as a facelift with tightening of the platysma muscle in the midline.

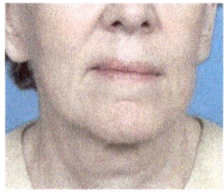 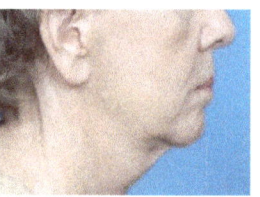 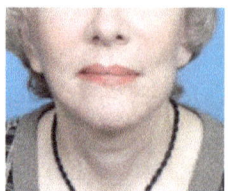 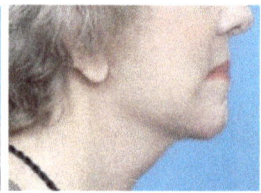

The patient below, "Francine," was especially unhappy with the excess skin of her neck. I performed the facelift by removal of excess skin and tightening of the SMAS in the cheeks.

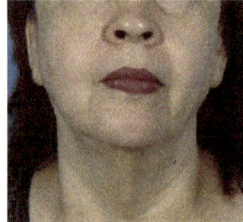 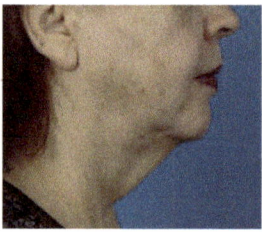 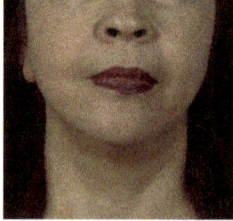 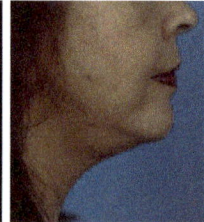

"Kathleen," shown below, objected to her jowl formation and excess skin in the neck. She also wanted improvement in the wrinkles around her mouth. She underwent a facelift with the removal of excess skin and tightening of the SMAS with plication sutures. At the same time, I did a perioral chemical peel. The postoperative photos show her improvement

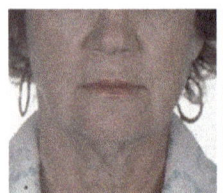 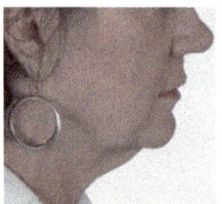 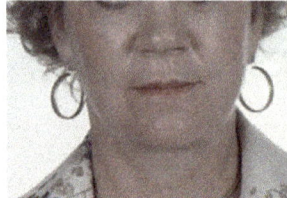 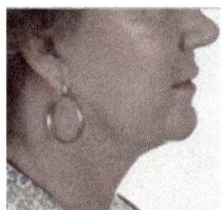

The patient below, "Marianne," especially objected to her profile view. She underwent a facelift with the removal of fat in the neck, removal of excess skin, and placement of a moderate-sized chin implant. The combination of fat removal skin tightening an augmentation of the chin has given her an improved profile in the neck and lower face.

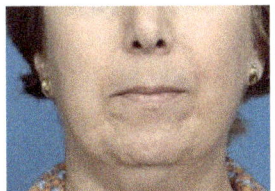 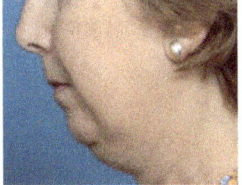 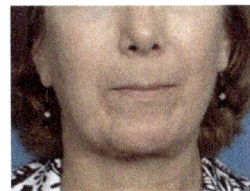 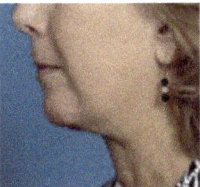

"Juanita" did not like the "turkey gobbler" type deformity in her neck. I performed a skin tightening facelift for her, which provided her considerable improvement, as shown in the photos below right.

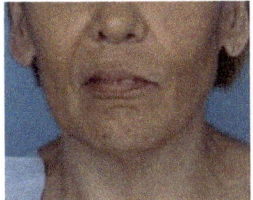 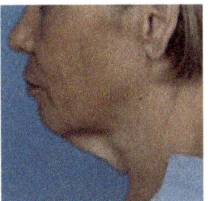 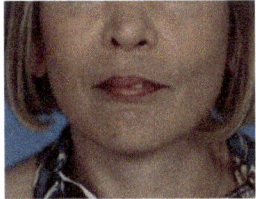 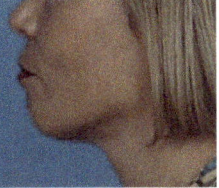

"Betty" wanted improvement in her neck, which she felt was too full. Fat removal in the neck directly and with liposuction combined with skin tightening and SMAS tightening was helpful. She also had a perioral skin peel to reduce rhytids of the upper and lower lip.

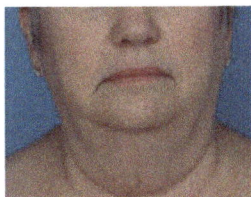 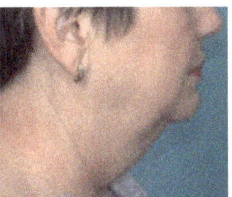 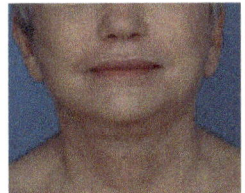 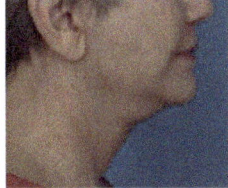

T - Z Plasty

The T - Z plasty is an operation developed by my uncle Thomas Cronin and his partner Dr. Tom Biggs. They designed it for improvement of the male neck in patients who did not want to have a facelift. It can be great for the patient who has a turkey gobbler type neck and does not mind a relatively inconspicuous scar directly on the neck. The surgeon pinches together excess skin from side to side to estimate the amount of removal. The desired amount is removed in a vertical elliptical manner, as shown below. The underlying platysma muscle can also be trimmed and tightened with plication. The surgeon tacks together the incision vertically, which produces bunching of skin (dog ears) on either end of the incision. This bunching is smooth out with horizontal excisions of the excess tissue. Then, a Z – plasty is performed in the center of the vertical closure, which lengthens the scar and prevents scar contracture.

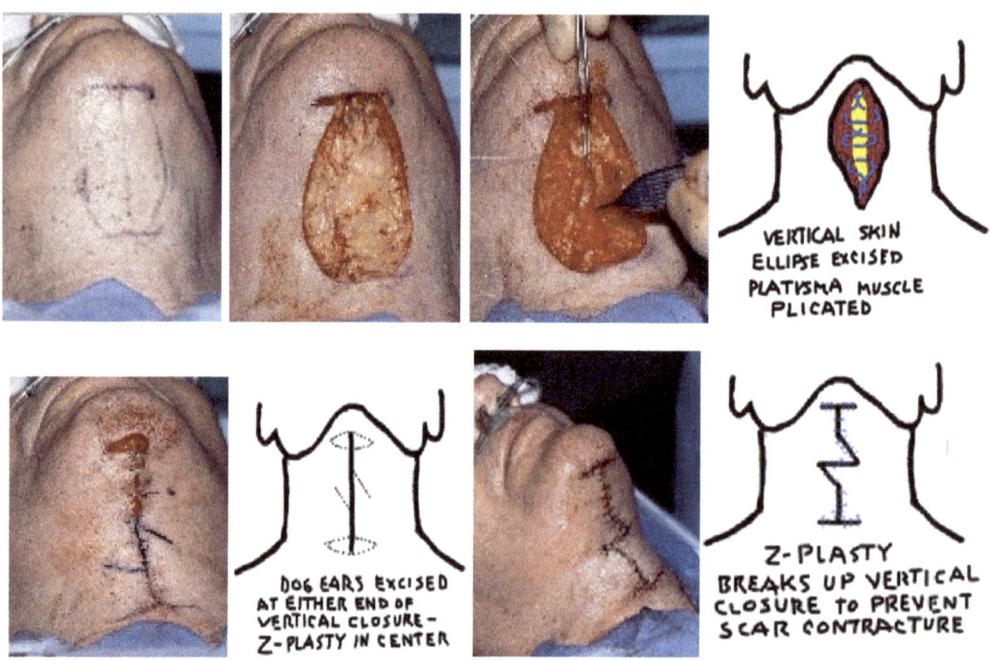

"Robert" was referred by his physician son because of just such a complaint. He did not like the excess skin of his neck nor the fact that he could no longer see his Adam's apple. His preoperative photos are on the left below. When presented with the option of a facelift versus a T- Z-plasty, he did not hesitate to choose this direct approach to the neck, which would correct what he perceived as his main problem. He was pleased with the result shown below on the right.

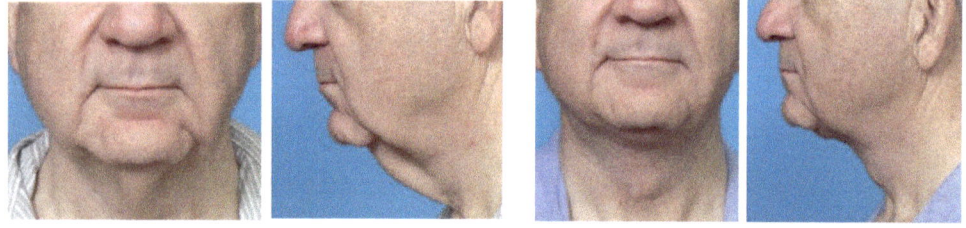

Another patient below also complained that the "turkey gobbler neck" bothered him, but he was confident that he did not want a facelift. As long as the patient can understand that this neck procedure will not give improvements in the face but only the neck and that there will be some scar, he may be an appropriate candidate for this operation.

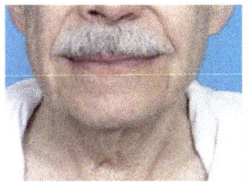 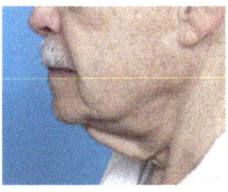 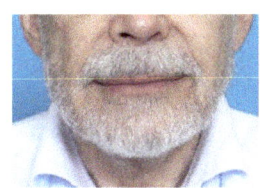 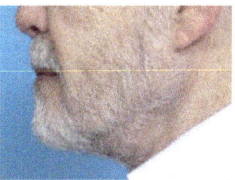

The T - Z - plasty is ordinarily reserved for male patients. However, in the following patient, a T - Z- plasty was used to help correct a problem that developed after a facelift by another surgeon. "Mary" came to see me several months after having a facelift. She had an unsightly scar contracture in the submental region below the chin. She was quite unhappy with this somewhat unusual complication from a facelift. There was a significant and persistent firm scar ball in the area, recalcitrant to steroid, and pressure therapy. I felt the only solution was to remove that affected skin and scar tissue even though it would necessitate putting some new scar in the area.

After discussing her options and considering my opinion, she decided to proceed with a T - Z - plasty. Pre-revision facelift photos(left) and post revision with T - Z - plasty photos(right) are below. I believe this procedure substantially solved her problem.

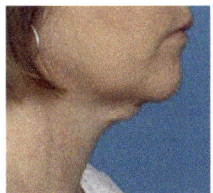 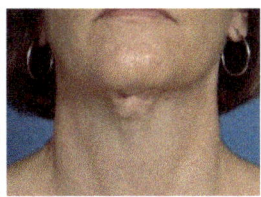 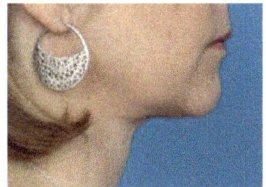 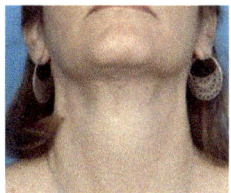

Blepharoplasty

The photograph below schematically shows the two upper and three lower fat pads that I often reduce by direct removal in cosmetic blepharoplasty. The red lines schematically represent common lies of excision of skin and sometimes underlying muscle in routine cosmetic blepharoplasty.

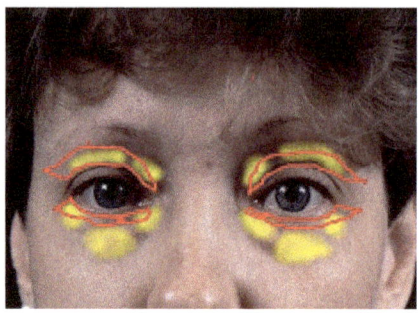

The patient below, "Janet," complained of excess skin, especially of the right upper eyelid. She also was happy unhappy because of the asymmetry of the upper eyelids. She had removal of more upper eyelid skin on the right side than on the left and minimal fat excision. I also removed and a small amount of skin from the lower eyelids. Her postoperative result(right) shows improved symmetry as well as the elimination of excess upper eyelid skin, especially on her right.

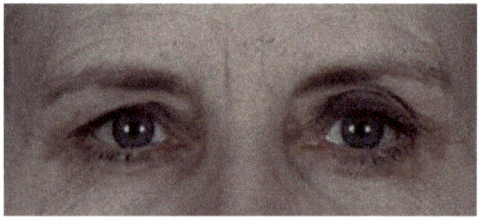 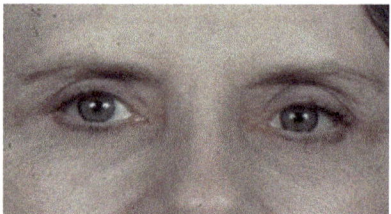

"Clara" did not like the appearance of her upper eyelids. She wished to have a fold visible. I performed a standard blepharoplasty with the removal of excess skin and a small amount of fat from the two upper lid fat pads. She obtained the improvement demonstrated in the post-op photo below right.

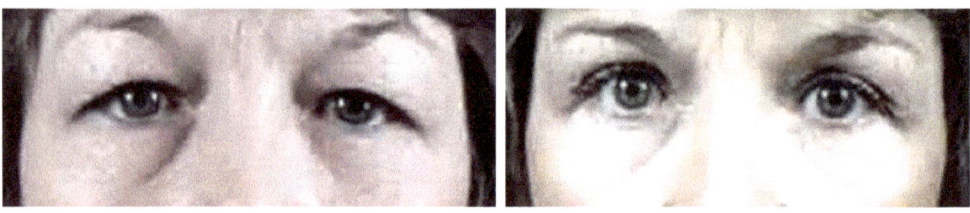

"Gladys" below complained of drooping upper eyelid skin. I addressed her problem with an upper eyelid blepharoplasty excising a moderate amount of skin and a small amount of fat; preop is on the left, postop on the right.

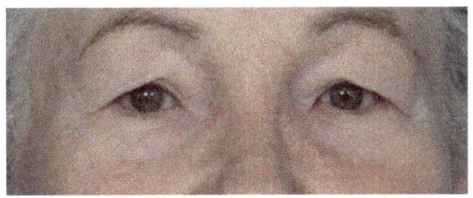 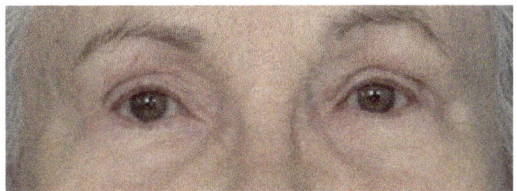

"Alan," below complained of excess and droopy upper eyelid skin and excess fat in the lower eyelids. He had excision of skin and fat from both upper-fat pads. I removed a lot of fat from all three lower eyelid fat pads, and I only re-draped the skin of the lower eyelids. I did not remove any skin from his lower eyelids.

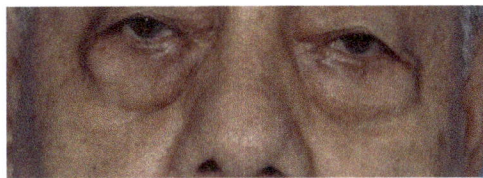 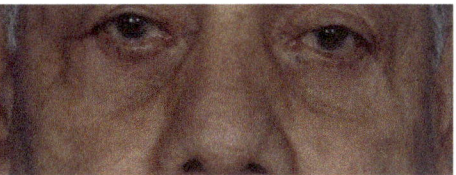

Cosmetic rejuvenation was the aim of "Helene" below. She had excess upper eyelid skin removed and a small amount of fat from the medial fat pad of the upper eyelid. In the lower eyelids, she had a small amount of fat removal from the three fat pads, some skin removal, and tightening of the muscle. She received considerable improvement and has a more youthful and rested appearance, as well as better symmetry of the upper eyelids.

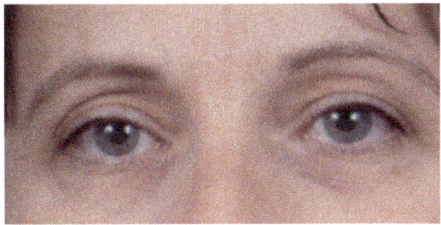 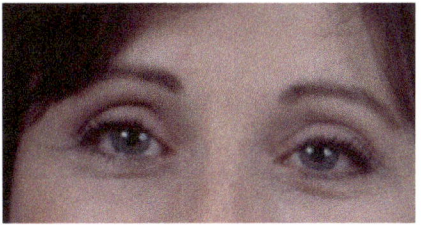

"Bobbie" above had moderate upper eyelid skin removal and minimal fat removal from the two fat pads. She was pleased with this result.

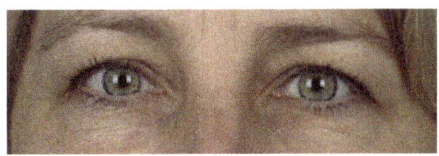 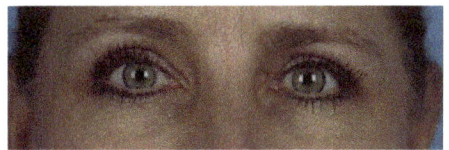

I obtained a nice regenerative improvement for "Stacy" below, who had a moderate amount of excess upper lid skin removed together with a small amount of fat from both fat pads. In the lower eyelids, I excised a small amount of fat from all three fat pads and got rid of a tiny amount of skin together with some tightening of the orbicularis muscle.

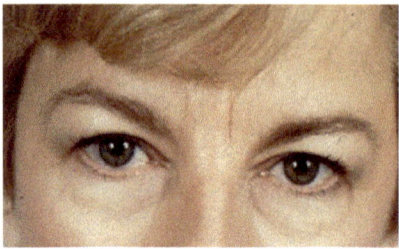 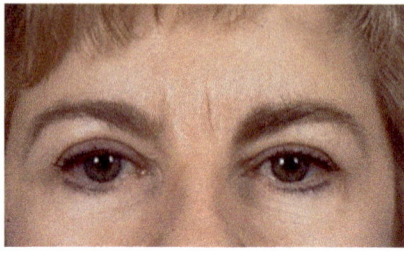

The elderly patient below "Thomas" had so much excess tissue of the upper eyelids that the upper blepharoplasty was covered by medicare as functional. Preoperative visual field testing confirmed the visual field partial obstruction. Additionally, I removed excess fat from the lower eyelids.

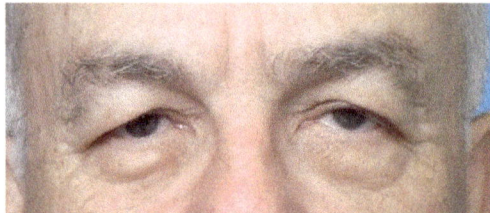 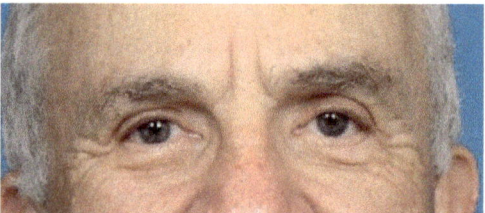

The patient below" Pearl" wanted to have a fold in the upper eyelids. I sutured skin and muscle to form a new relationship with the tarsal plate of the upper eyelid. This method was a "so-called" westernizing blepharoplasty. In my 38 years of practice in Houston, I only had a handful of such cases.

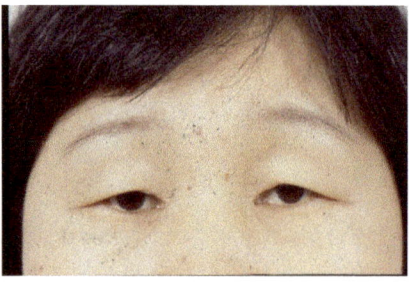 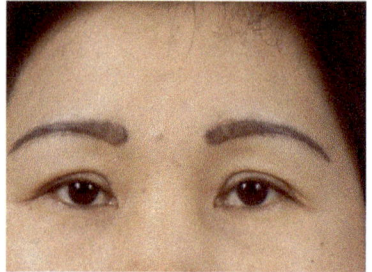

The Healing Mission of Plastic Surgery

Brow Lift

There are various methods of performing brow lifts. Some involve long incision from ear to ear within the scalp, undermining of the scalp and forehead, removal of a strip of the scalp, which pulls up the brow and forehead as indicated in the first drawing below.

Other techniques involve an incision at the hairline, undermining of the forehead, and removal of some forehead skin, thus lifting the brow. Still, other different methods include the use of the endoscope with wide-undermining not only of the forehead but posteriorly over broad areas of the scalp. Then the brow is lifted and pulled up in secured in place with a temporary screw or other fixation.

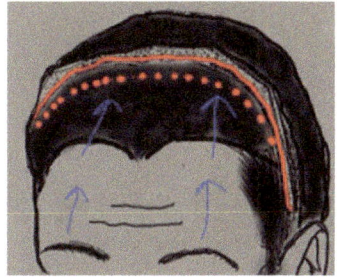 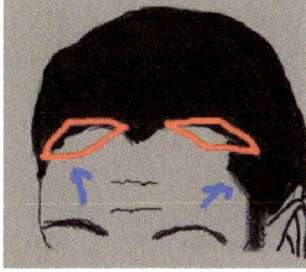 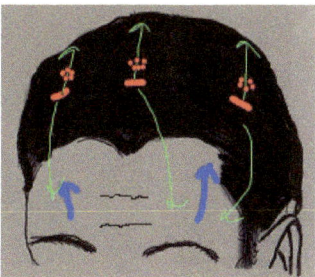

I did an endoscopic brow lift for "Jimmy" shown below. At the same time, I performed an upper and lower blepharoplasty. Note improved eyebrow symmetry.

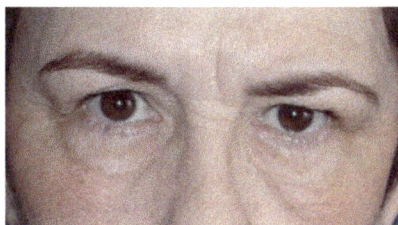 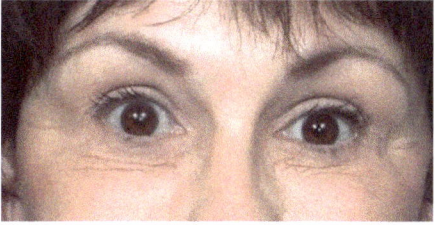

"Roberta" below had a lateral brow elevation procedure by taking an ellipse of skin out at the hairline on either side. Her pre-and postoperative photos are below.

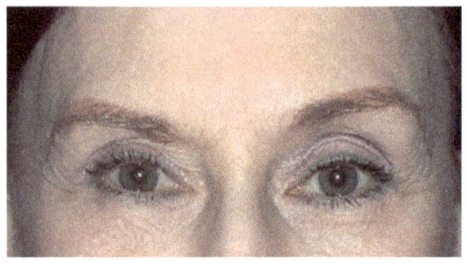 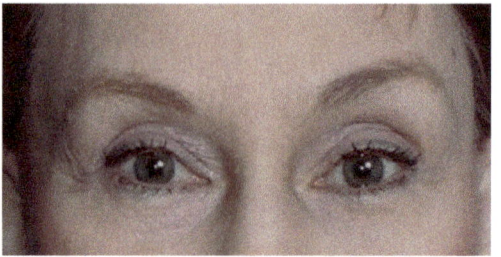

Below "Jacqueline" had lateral brow lift with forehead excision at the hairline. Her pre-and post-op photos are below.

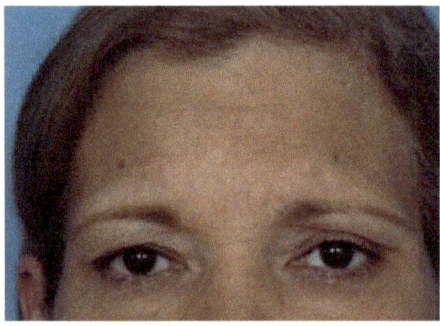 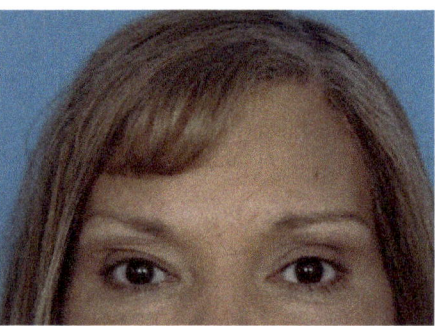

"Margaret" shown below had upper and lower blepharoplasty and, at the same time, a brow lift procedure with the endoscopic technique.

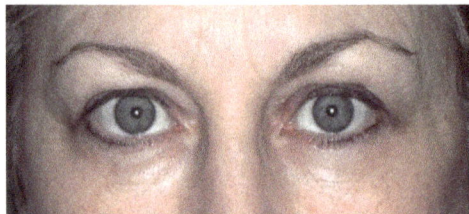 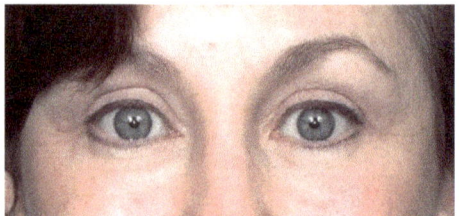

Perioral skin resurfacing

There are many methods for skin resurfacing. All of them destroy the surface layers of skin and then rely on the skin to re- epithelialize and heal. Lasers burn the skin, thus destroying the outer layers. Chemical peels coagulate or chemically burn the outer layer of skin. Dermabrasion destroys the epithelium by mechanical abrading or sanding the surface. I'm not sure the body knows the difference between these different ways of killing the outer layer of skin.

So, lasers, chemical peels, or dermabrasion can resurface perioral skin with similar results. These different modalities ablate or destroy outer layers of skin. The body then regenerates a new epithelial surface to replace the previous sun-damaged surface. These procedures dampen the wrinkles, thereby improving the appearance.

The elderly patient below, "Clair," had a deep chemical peel with phenol of the perioral area with significant improvement.

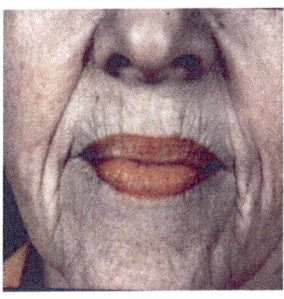
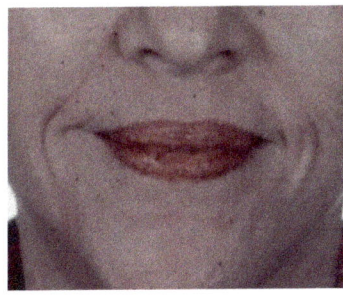

I performed dermabrasion of the perioral area for "Brittany" below. She got substantial softening in skin texture and the diminishment of vertical wrinkles.

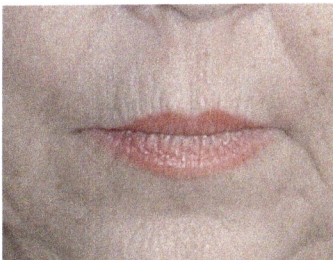
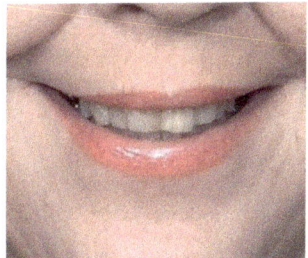

This patient below "Suzy" had a combination of trichloroacetic acid peel (medium depth) and dermabrasion. Her before and after photos are below.

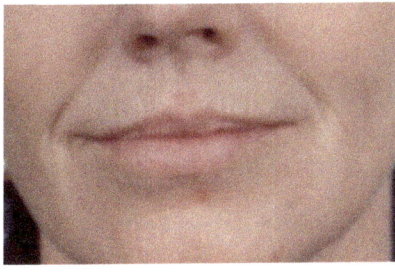
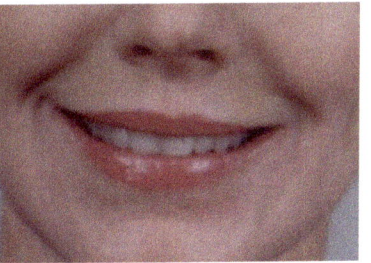

The patient below "Tayna" had a trichloroacetic acid peel with some smoothing of the perioral skin.

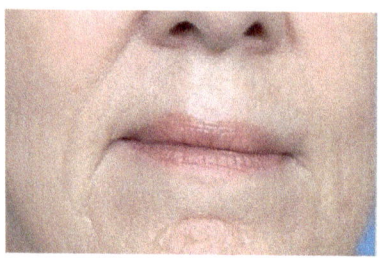 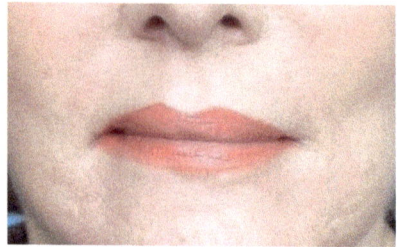

Breast surgery

I deal with augmentation mammaplasty in more detail in chapter 8. It is interesting to note that it has become a more prevalent surgery again as we have gotten further from the silicone scare of the 1990s. The reapproval of gel implants again for primary augmentation mammaplasty in 2007 has contributed to increased demand for this surgery. It can be a very satisfying surgery for many patients. On many occasions, I have had patients, like the one below, "Janine," tell me they are "proud "of their surgery.

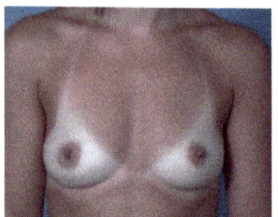 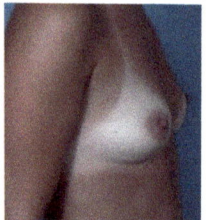 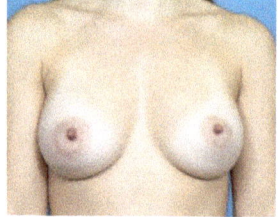 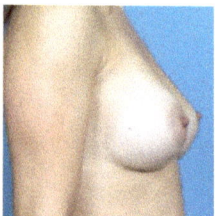

I discuss breast reduction surgery in detail in chapter # 14

Mastopexy

Mastopexy is breast lift surgery performed to make the breast more youthful and aesthetically pleasing. The surgical method is repositioning the existing tissue. Ordinarily, the surgeon only removes some skin and no glandular breast tissue. Sutures hold the breast parenchyma in the new position.

There is a trade-off between improving the shape of the breast and necessarily leaving some scars on the skin surface. The amount and location of the scar vary with the particular technique of mastopexy. Most mastopexies utilize the Wise pattern and leave an anchor-shaped scar pattern. The maximum incision is anchor-shaped. It has a circle around the nipple-areola complex, with a vertical component down to the crease and a horizontal segment in the crease under the breast. Some procedures leave only part of the anchor-shaped scars.

The patient below "Keyna" is happy with the size of her breasts, but she is unhappy with the sagging nature of the breasts. She was willing to accept some scars to have more shapely breasts.

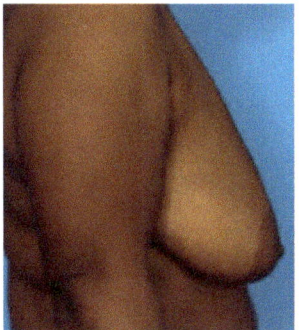
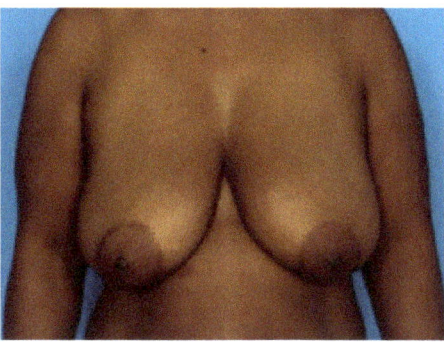

I de-epithelialized the outer layers of the skin of a superior pedicle to reposition the nipple. (de-epithelialized skin can be buried under other tissue and heal). Also, to uplift and give more projection, I developed a de-epithelialized inferior pedicle and tucked it under the remaining breast tissue, as shown in the intraoperative photos below.

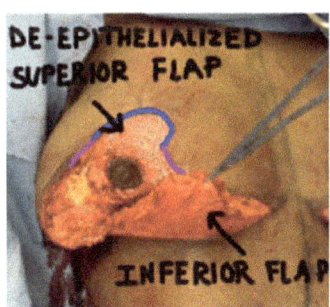
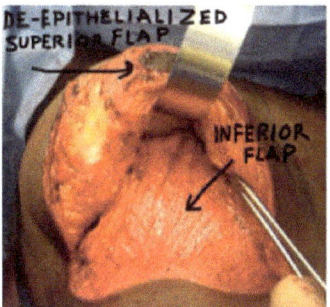
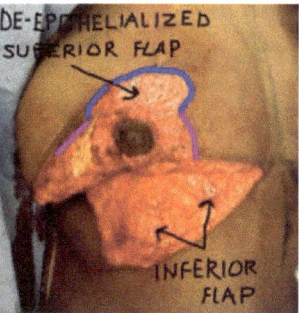

The resulting scar is anchor shaped as demonstrated in the first below.

She healed nicely, and the postoperative results below show breasts with a more aesthetically pleasing shape. She was quite happy with this result, as was I.

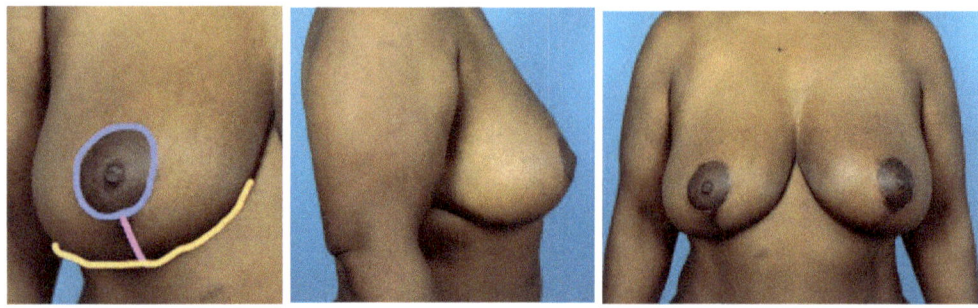

The following case is very illustrative because of the pre-existing small horizontal scar on the upper abdomen of this patient "Margie." This scar allows us to see the dramatic uplifting of the breast relative to that fixed mark. I performed this mastopexy with a Wise pattern and a de-epithelialized superior- medial pedicle. So, the scar closure is again anchor-shaped. She has healed with relatively inconspicuous scars. The lift has been quite useful, and I was delighted. Also, the patient was happy with the result.

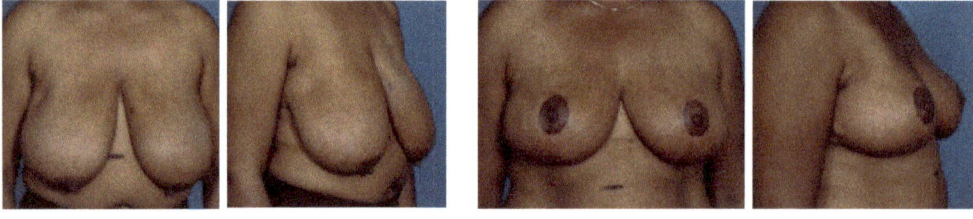

Below, "Janet" liked her breast size but not the sagging and downward position of her nipples.

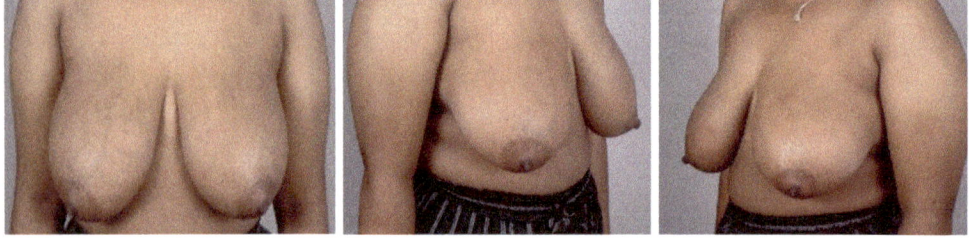

I performed a mastopexy with a superior based pedicle. She was pleased with her improved postoperative shape, as shown below.

The Healing Mission of Plastic Surgery

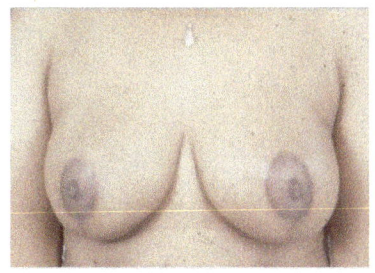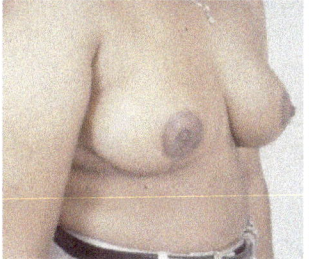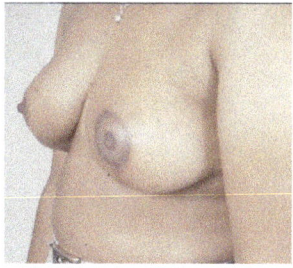

"Marcie," pictured below, wanted to keep her breast size but desired a more youthful look. I performed a mastopexy with an inferior pedicle technique. Her preoperative and postoperative photographs are below.

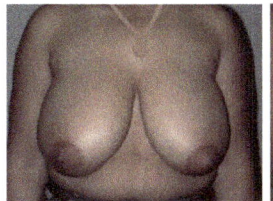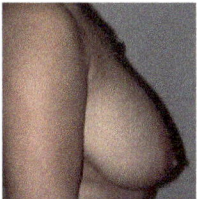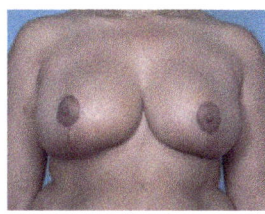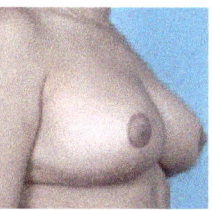

I used a superior based pedicle for nipple relocation in "Debra's" mastopexy to give her a more youthful appearance.

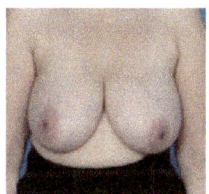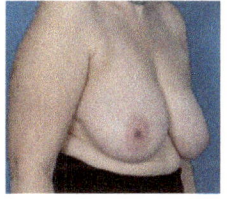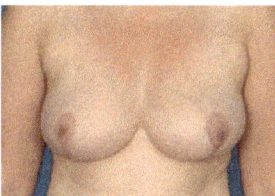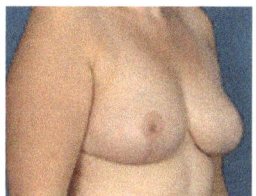

I performed an inferior based nipple pedicle procedure for "Trudy" whose pre and postoperative photos are below. She wanted to lift her breasts without losing significant volume. Her before and after pictures are below.

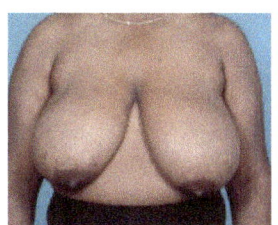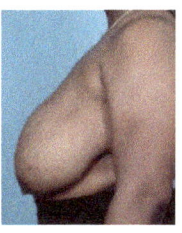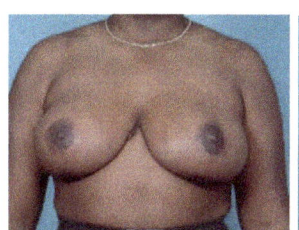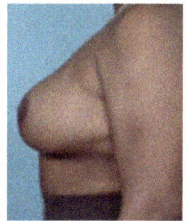

Augmentation – mastopexy

Another standard aesthetic breast procedure is augmentation - mastopexy, which combines breast enlargement with a silicone implant, and a breast lift. Some surgeons routinely do this problematic procedure in two stages rather than one step. Some do the augmentation first, followed a few months later by mastopexy. Or it can be done the other way around with a mastopexy first, followed a few months later by augmentation with an implant. Most of the time, I preferred to do a one-stage augmentation - mastopexy.

I figure even if a revision is needed because of the more complex nature of the combined procedure, it likely would only take one additional operation. The following case is an example of a one-stage augmentation - mastopexy procedure with a silicone gel implant placed beneath the breast tissue on top of the chest muscles.

The patient illustrated below, "Darlene" wanted both more abundant and more youthful breasts. The breast lift would require leaving her with an anchor-shaped scar pattern. While augmenting the size of her breasts would require a silicone gel breast implant. I performed both of these procedures for her at the same time. She was satisfied with her results.

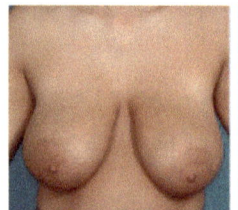 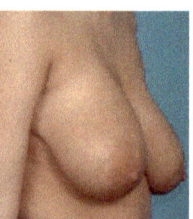 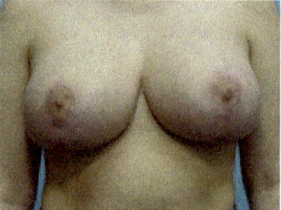 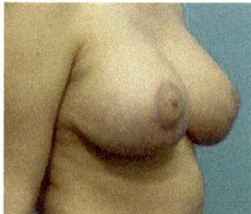

Asymmetric Breasts

Still another area breast plastic surgery is that for asymmetry of the breasts. This problem lends itself to similar corrective techniques as that for breast reduction, mastopexy, and sometimes augmentation.

"Viviana," pictured below, illustrates both asymmetry and significant breast ptosis (sagging). I treated her minor breast asymmetry and ptosis with a superior pedicle, wise pattern with a resultant anchor-shaped scar pattern. I excised a small amount of breast tissue from the left breast.

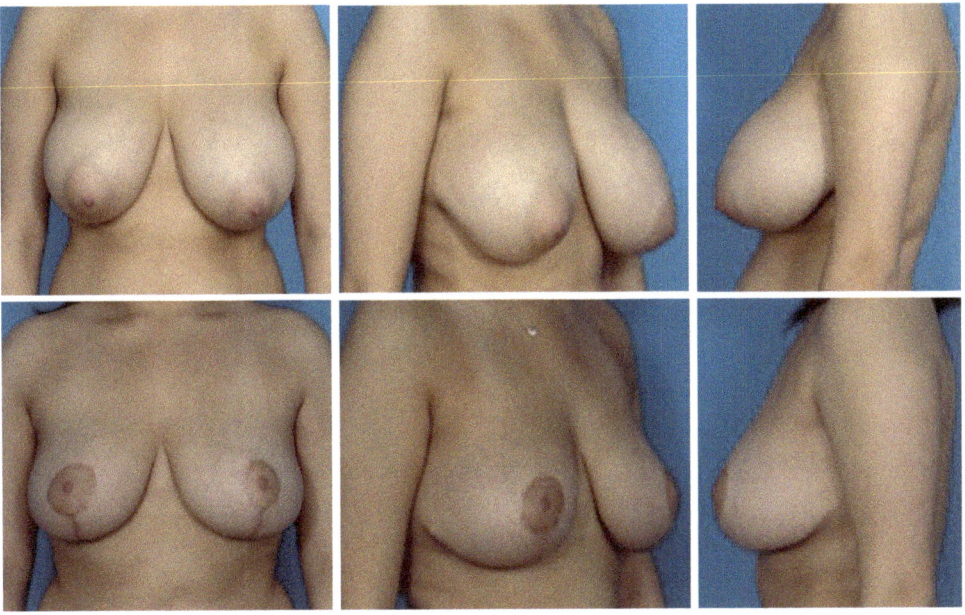

Cosmetic otoplasty

I described some of the technical details of otoplasty surgery are in Chapter 4.

The teenager below "Ruthie" claimed that her ears "stuck out too much," and she received ribbing about it from her friends. She liked to wear her hair up and knew her ears stood out even from behind. I excised some of each concha to reposition the ears closer to the mastoid with sutures.

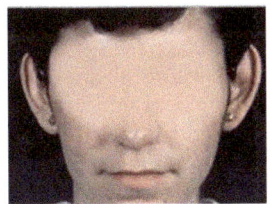 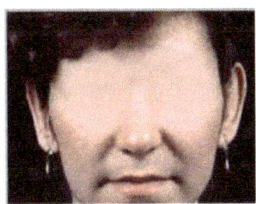 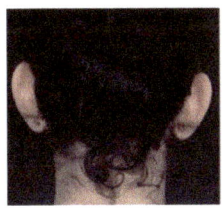 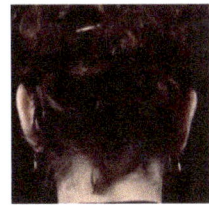

"Stephanie" below had some asymmetric prominence of the ears. The right ear problem was quite mild, while the left ear is more involved, and it is positioned lower than the right ear. I made the anti- helical fold on the left more pronounced by suturing and also reduced the concha of both ears.

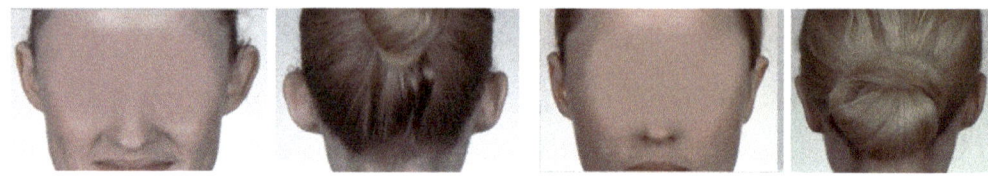

The patient below "Jason" had the standard procedures as described earlier. Below are his pre-and postoperative photos

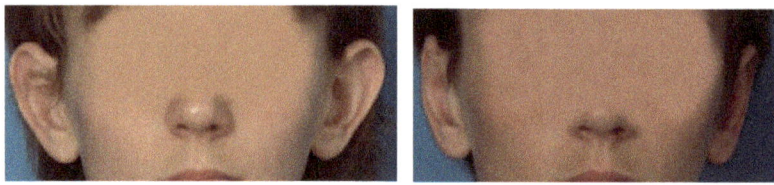

"This child below, "Margaret," had standard pin back otoplasty procedures. Her pre-and postop photos are above.

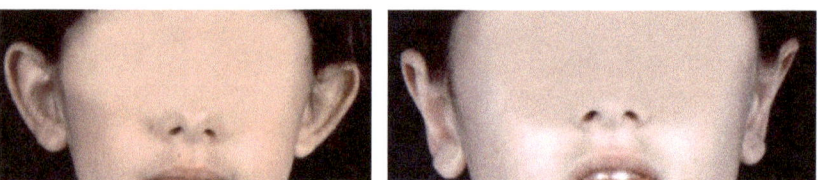

This adult patient below, "Franklin," had standard pin back otoplasty procedures with the result shown. Again, even though he had attained middle age, he still sought to improve his self-image by having his ears made less prominent with surgery.

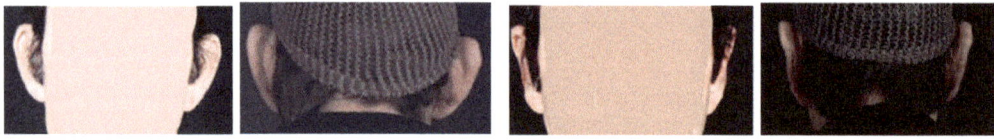

Rhinoplasty

Rhinoplasty was one of the operations I loved doing the most. Rhinoplasty is one of the most complicated surgeries done by plastic surgeons. ENT (ear nose and throat) surgeons can do excellent rhinoplasties. There are many practicing plastic surgeons who completed ENT residency training before beginning training in plastic surgery. That was my background; I first did an ENT residency and then a plastic surgery residency before going into practice. When one considers rhinoplasty, such a double-boarded plastic surgeon is exceptionally well qualified.

In the three drawings below, I pointed out the main anatomical features needed to understand rhinoplasty. I have drawn and labeled illustrations of the nasal bones, the upper lateral cartilages, the alar cartilages, and the cartilaginous nasal septum below.

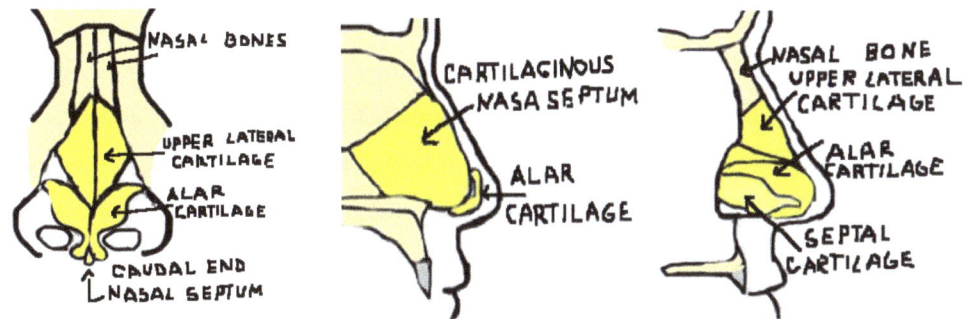

"Alicia," pictured below, complained that her nose was too large and the tip was too broad and flat.

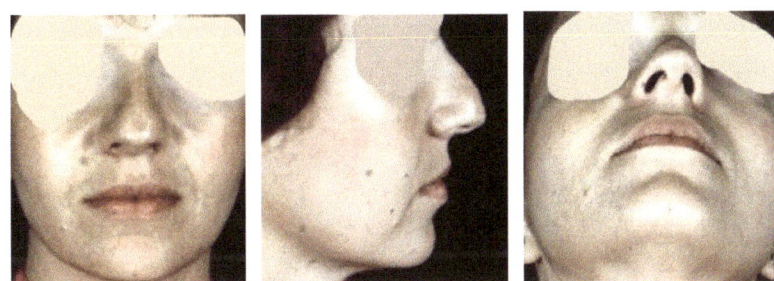

The three drawings below diagrammatically illustrate the surgery done for her. The cartilaginous structures of the nose are in yellow. The red presents areas of removal of the nasal cartilage and sometimes bone. Green represents cartilage grafts, added to alter contour. In her operation, I removed (red) cartilage and bone from the bridge of the nose and a portion of the nasal tip cartilages. I added a tip graft (green) by reshaping some of the septal cartilage, which I removed as removed in the central drawing(red). The grey dotted lines represent osteotomies of the nasal bone usually done to narrow or reshape them if I remove a large hump. All the following case examples use the same drawings and color keys to explain the details of the rhinoplasty.

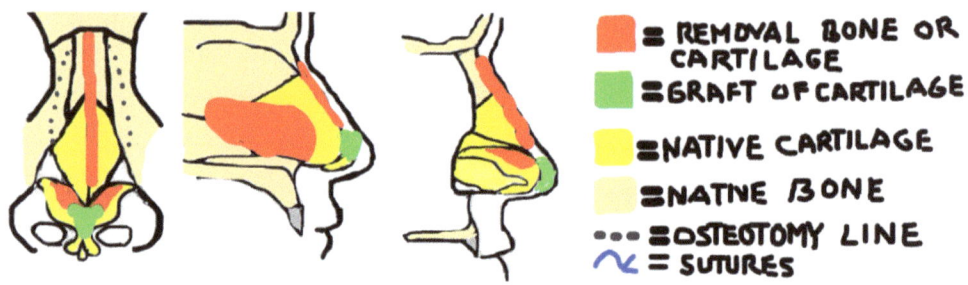

The photos below show her postoperative result with a straight bridge and a narrower nasal tip.

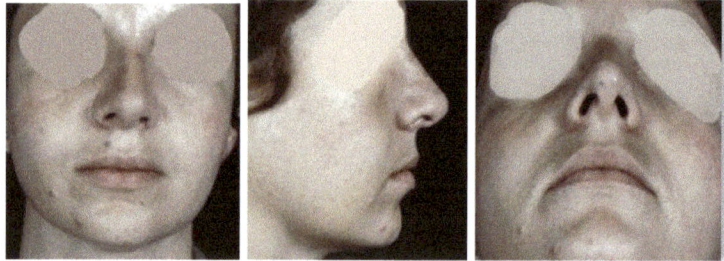

The patient below "Juliet" was a beautiful young woman who disliked her nose because of the prominent hump and the somewhat wide nasal tip. I performed a somewhat traditional rhinoplasty on her. I removed the nasal hump by cutting away upper lateral and septal cartilage and filing down some of the nasal bone. I also thinned the nasal tip by removing some cartilage from the upper (cephalic) edge of the alar cartilages and sutured the nasal tip domes together (blue). The drawings show the procedure diagrammatically. Again, red indicates cartilage or bone removal.

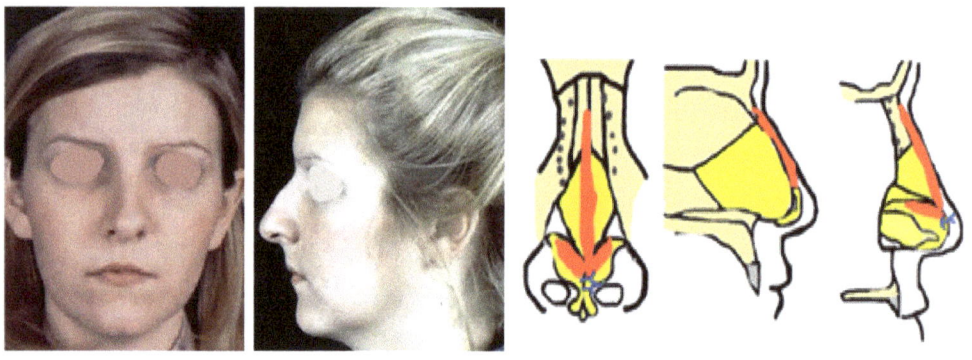

Her postoperative result with a narrower tip and a straighter nasal dorsum is below. She was pleased with the result.

The Healing Mission of Plastic Surgery

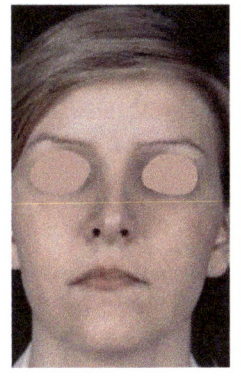
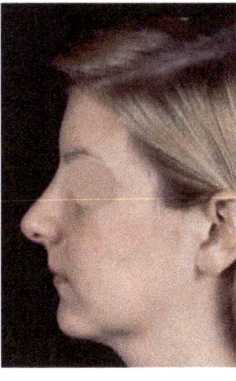

"Barbara" below had a large cartilaginous and bony removed, the nasal bones narrowed, and the tip refined by the removal of the portion of the tip cartilage. The preoperative photo, surgical diagram, and postop result are below.

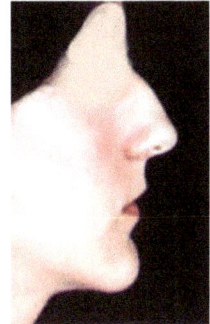
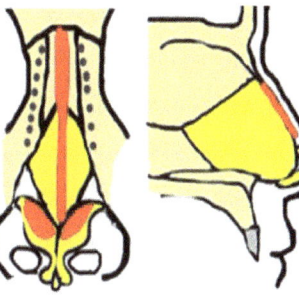
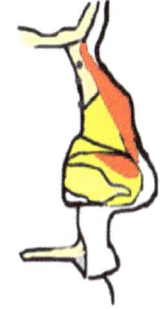
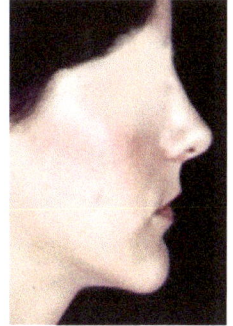

"Alianna" shown below had a lovely nose but wanted some subtle refinement. She particularly wished to have a straight profile

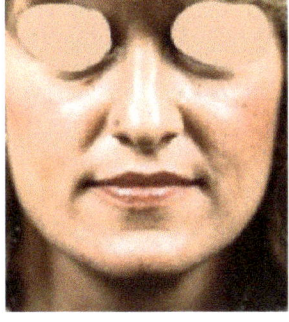
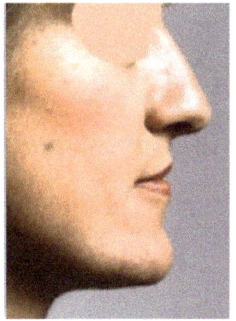

I removed a small amount of cartilage from the bridge and the nasal tip to obtain the result shown below.

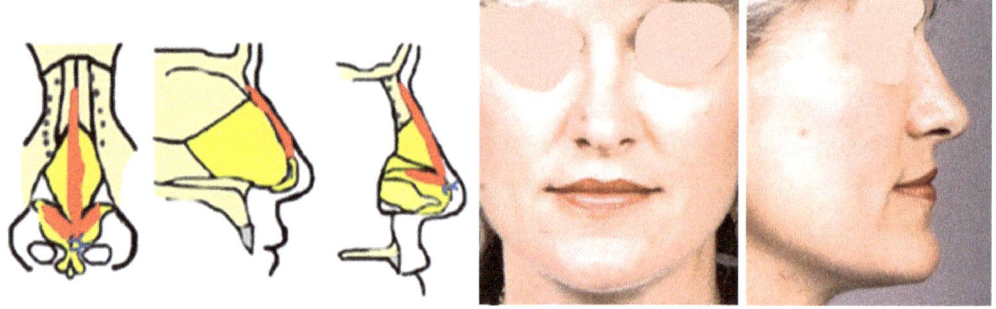

"Leon" was unhappy with his large nose, which he felt was disproportionate to his other facial features. I removed bone and cartilage from the bridge, in-fractured the nasal bones, and slightly reduced the nasal tip cartilages as in the diagram.

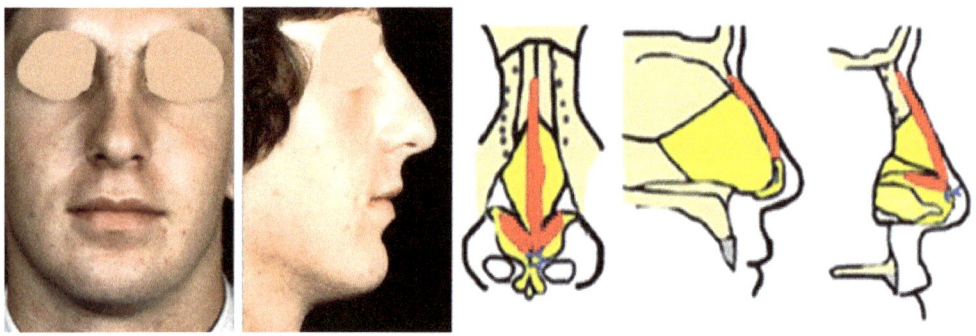

His postoperative results are below.

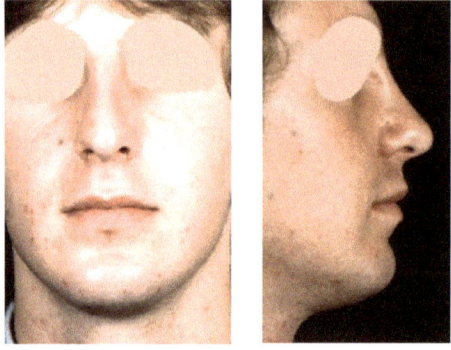

"Bridget," below, was displeased with the large hump on her nose. I removed the dorsal hump and refined the tip cartilages slightly. I did perform an in-fracture of the nasal bones because of the hump removal.

The Healing Mission of Plastic Surgery

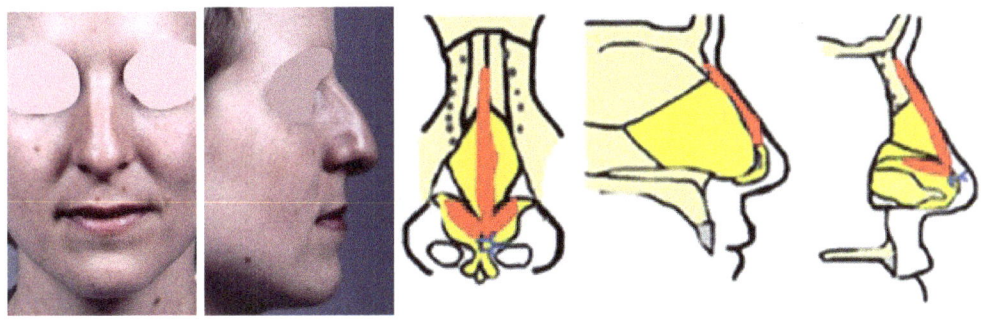

Postoperative photos are below.

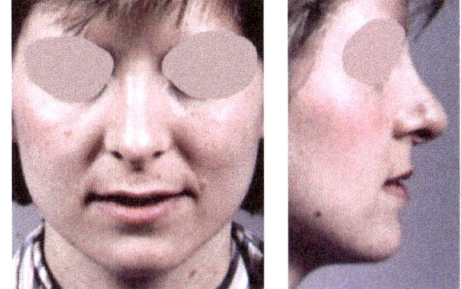

"Mia," below disliked her convex nasal dorsum and wanted better tip definition and projection. I performed a cartilage graft to obtain more tip projection and reduced the bridge a small amount to make it straight on the profile, as demonstrated in the drawing below.

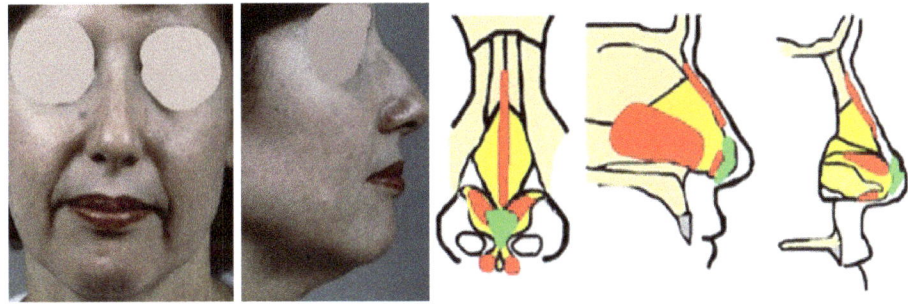

Below are "Mia's" postoperative photos.

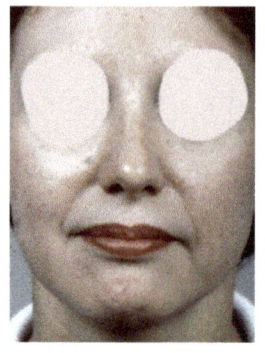 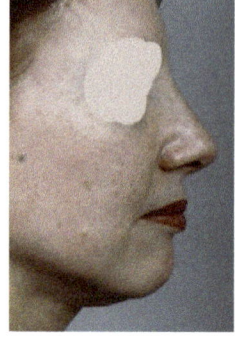

"Sophia" wanted a little smaller nose that was straighter on profile rather than convex. I took a small amount of cartilage and bone from the dorsum, removed some tip cartilage, and sutured the tip cartilage domes together to define the tip better.

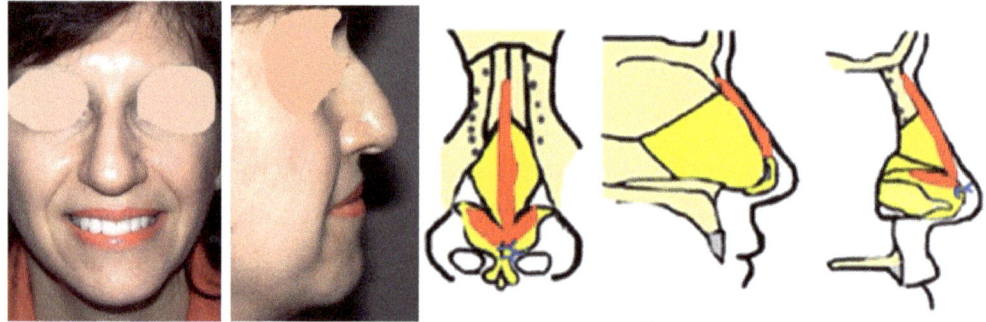

Postoperative photos of "Sophia" are below.

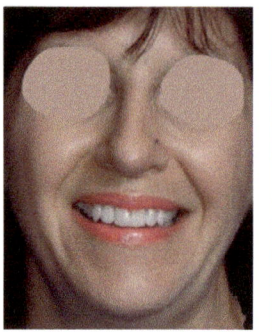 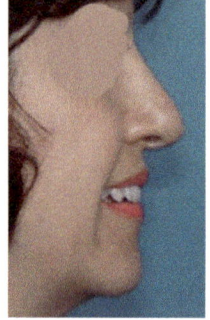

"Cynthia," complained of a prominent hump on her nose and lack of nasal tip definition. The preoperative photographs are shown below with the surgical diagram. As shown in red, she had cartilage and bone removed from the bridge of the nose, and the cephalic edge of the tip cartilages removed. I created more tip definitions with a nasal tip graft, shown in green

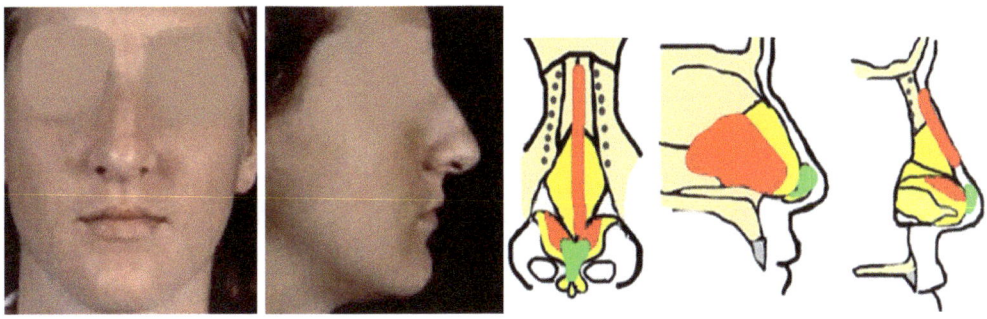

Her postoperative photographs are below.

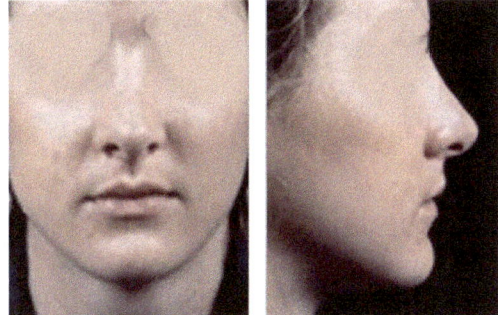

"Luke" pictured below wanted both a smaller nose and to improve his breathing through his nose. I did a reduction of the cartilaginous and bony bridge and a minor trimming of the tip cartilages with suturing of their domes together and in-fracture of the nasal bones. I relieved the nasal obstruction by excision of offending septal cartilage.

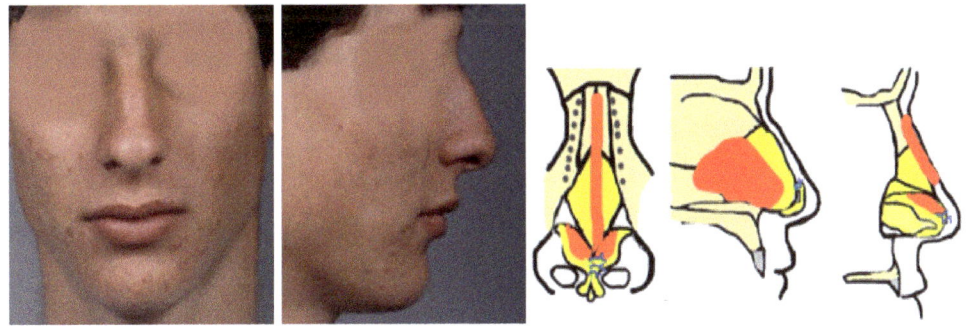

"Luke's postoperative result is shown below.

The Healing Mission of Plastic Surgery

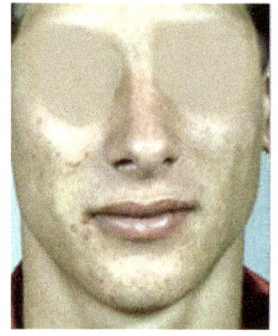
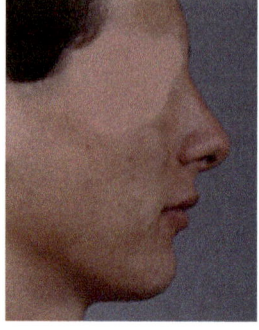

"Pricilla," pictured below at always wanted to have a smaller nose. She disliked the hump and finally decided that she would go through with a rhinoplasty to try to obtain a nose, which would make her happier.

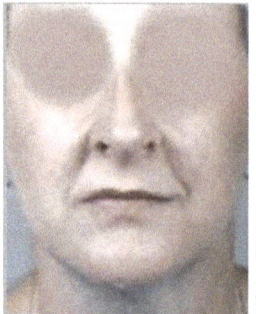
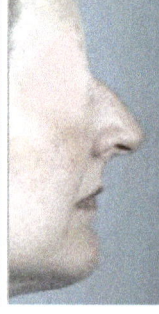
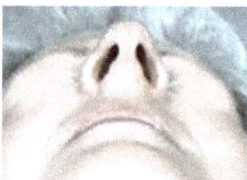

As shown in the surgical diagram below, she had a reduction of the bridge (dorsum) with the removal of cartilaginous and bony tissue. She also had trimming of the tip cartilage and suturing of their domes together.

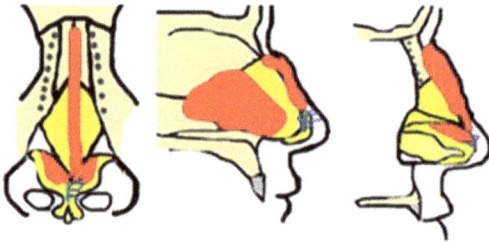

The postoperative results below show improvement, especially in her profile, thereby boosting her self-image.

The Healing Mission of Plastic Surgery

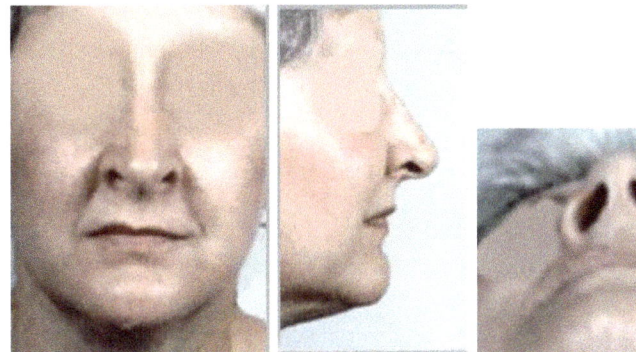

"Kathleen," pictured below, had difficulty breathing through her nose on the right side. She also wanted a small amount the bridge of the nose taken down and to have the nasal tip refined. In the middle preoperative pictured below, the caudal end of the deviated septum protrudes into the patient's right nostril.

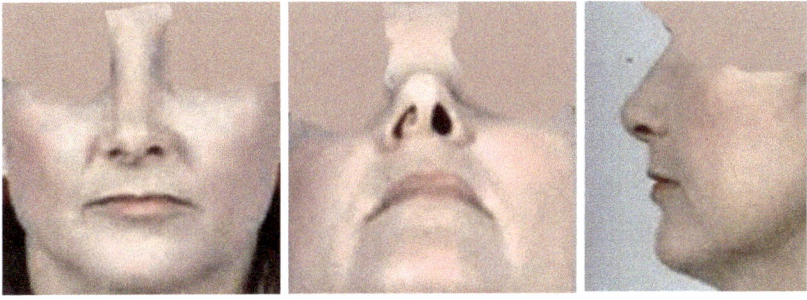

The drawings below show I removed a small amount of the bridge of the nose, and I refined the nasal tip cartilages. The central drawing shows I straightened the nasal septum and removed a portion of its caudal end

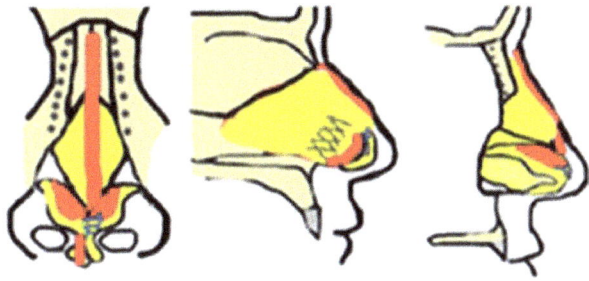

The post-operative results show mild improvement in the profile but a substantial improvement in the front view, especially from below because I straightened the caudal end of the nasal septum making the nostrils symmetrical.

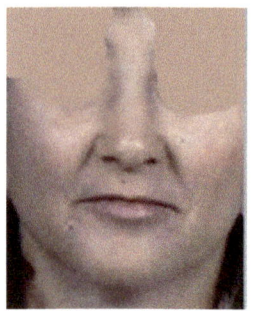 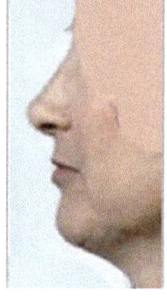 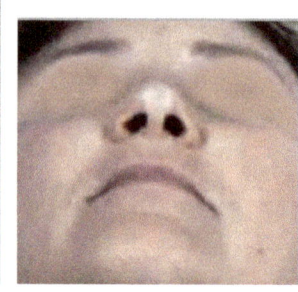

The patient below "Maureen" had had a rhinoplasty with which she was not satisfied. She especially disliked the very pointed nature of the nasal tip.

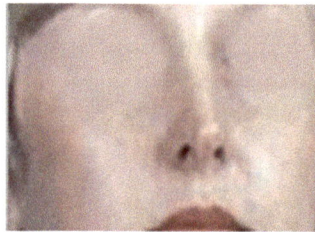 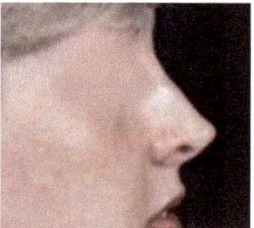

As represented in the drawings below, I took some cartilage from the nasal septum as grafts (green). Often a tip graft is used to make the tip appeared narrower; however, in this case, I used the tip graft to blunt the tip making it less pointed. I also inserted a very small dorsal graft.

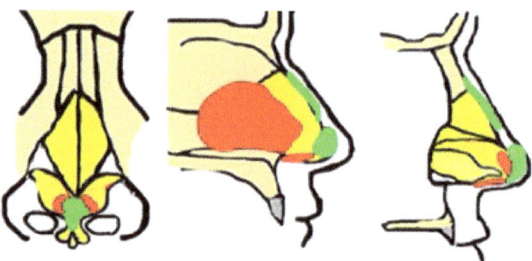

The postoperative views below show the nose to appear more natural. These changes satisfied her expectations.

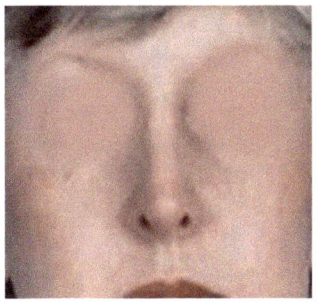
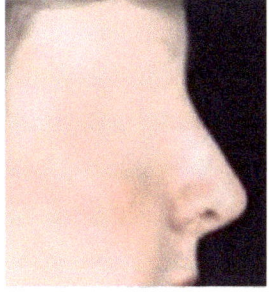

"John" pictured below wanted a smaller nose but did not want to lose his ethnic identity.

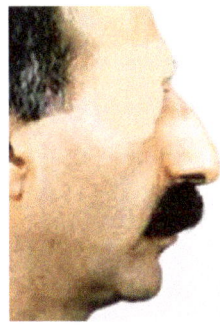
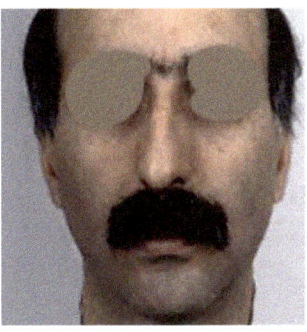

I performed a minor reduction rhinoplasty for him, as demonstrated in the drawings below.

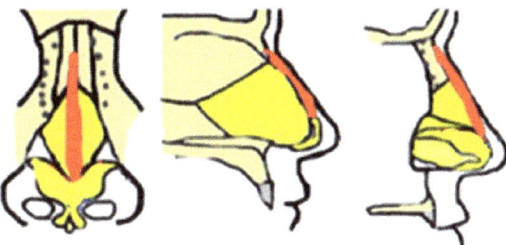

His postoperative photos are below.

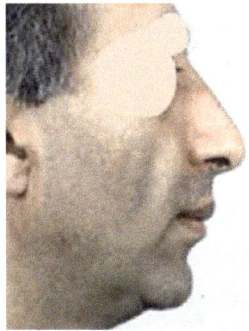
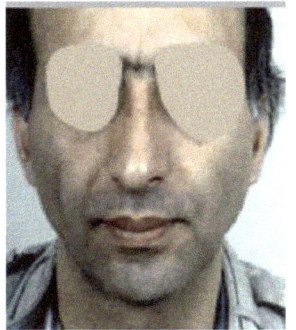

"Wanda" below, complained her nose was too large, the tip too full, and the columella much too broad.

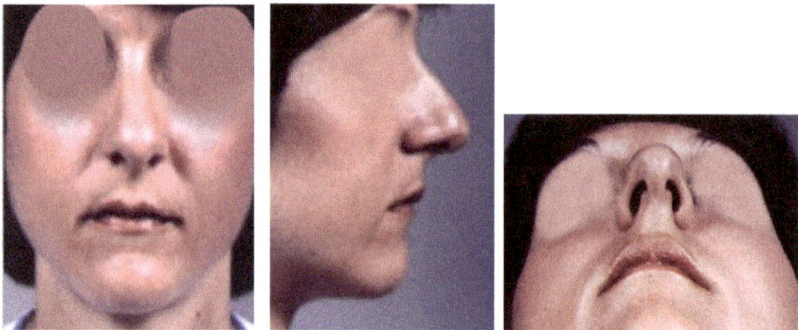

The diagrams below illustrate the surgery I did for her. I removed cartilage from the nasal tip and added a cartilage graft from the septum to better define the tip. I excised a portion of the cartilaginous and bony bridge to make the nose smaller. I cut out a small part of the caudal end of the nasal septum to shorten the nose. Also, to narrow the extremely wide columella, I removed the" feet" of the alar cartilage.

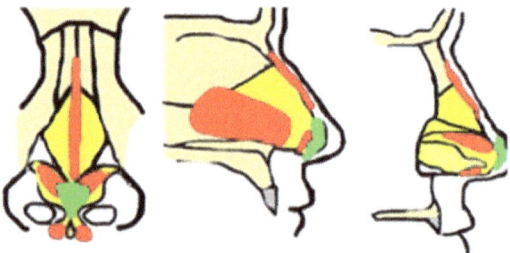

Her postoperative photos below show a smaller nose with a more normal appearing columella separating the nostrils.

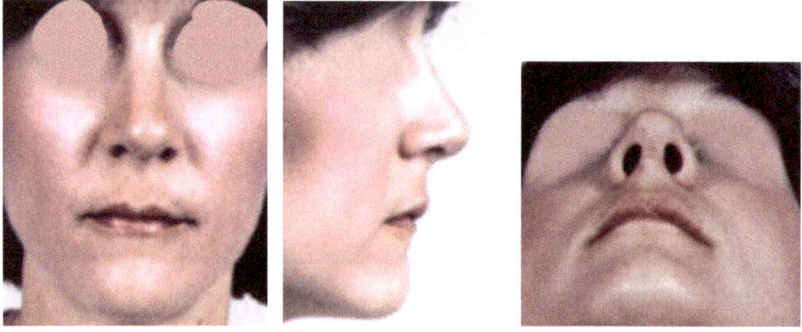

"Sarah," whose preoperative photographs are below, disliked the large convex nasal hump.

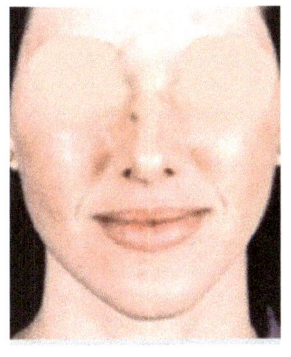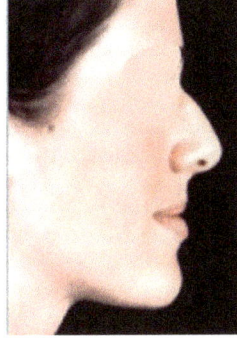

As shown in the diagrams below, she had a large amount of nasal cartilage and some bone removed from the nasal bridge. The nasal bones need to be fractured and narrowed to compensate for this. I also trimmed the cephalic portion of the nasal tip cartilages.

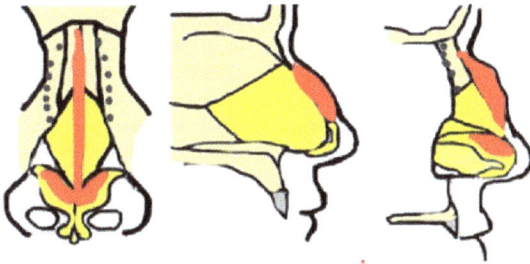

Her postoperative photos are below. She was happy that her appearance was more like the self- image she desired.

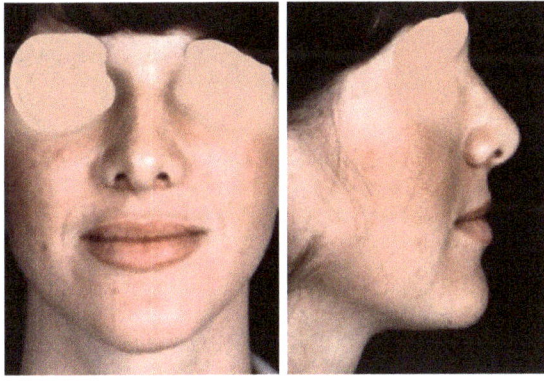

"Cindy," below, wanted more definition of the nasal tip, and her nose made a slightly smaller.

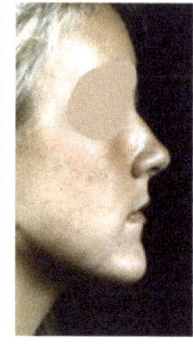

As shown in the diagrams below, I trimmed the cephalic edges of the nasal tip cartilages and placed a small nasal tip graft made from the alar trimmings. Postoperative photos are below. "Cindy" was pleased with the narrowing of the nasal tip.

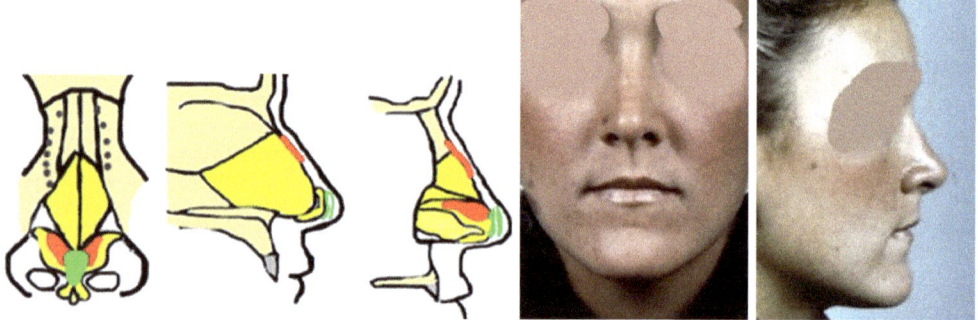

"Michaela" was bothered by the small hump on her nasal bridge.

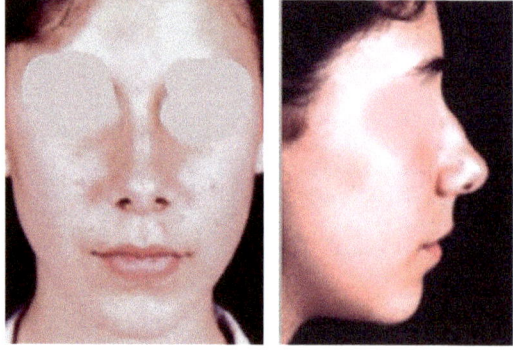

The diagrams below illustrate the removal of bone and cartilage from the bridge of the nose, fracturing to narrow the nasal bones, trimming the nasal tip cartilages, and placement of a tip graft made from the cartilaginous nasal hump. Her postoperative photos below show her final result. She was happy to be rid of the hump.

The Healing Mission of Plastic Surgery

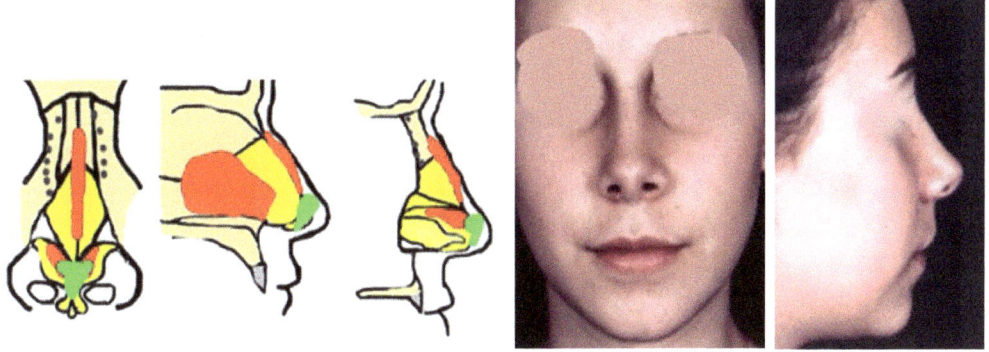

"Angelina" below had an unusually narrow, long, crooked, and plunging nasal tip, which she did not like.

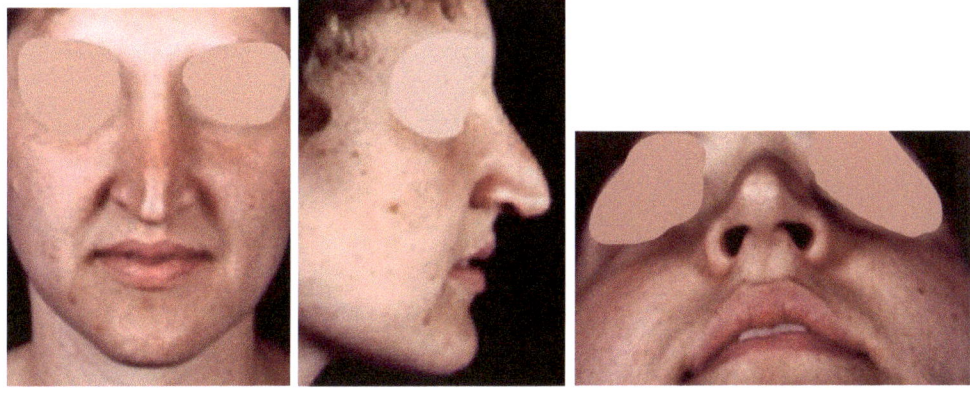

The diagrams below represent the surgery I performed. The operation consisted of removal of a small amount of cartilage from the bridge of the nose and placement of cartilaginous grafts (green) in the nasal tip and columella. These grafts lifted and supported the nasal tip, making it less pointed.

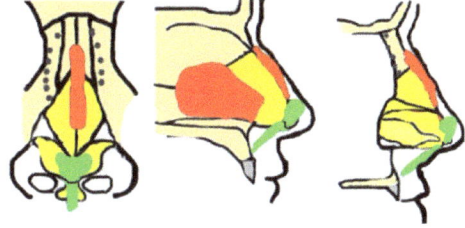

She was pleased with her postoperative transformation, shown below.

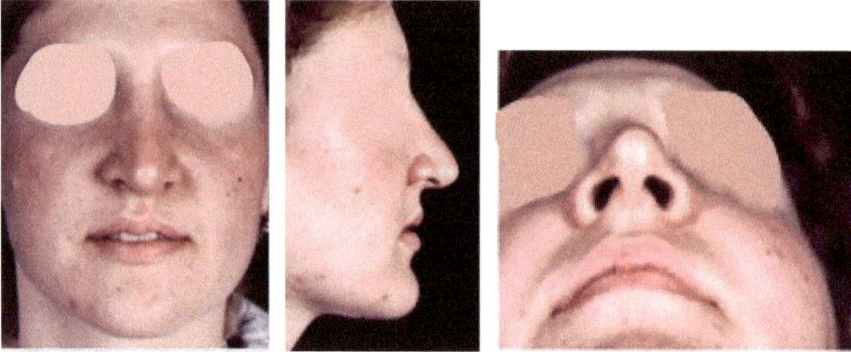

"Mary," shown below, wanted to have her nose little smaller with less convexity to the bridge. She also complained of the wide base of the columella.

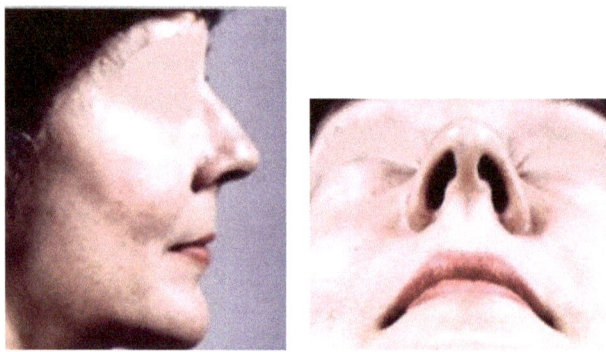

As indicated in the diagrams below, I removed a small amount of nasal bridge and trimmed the cephalic portion of the tip cartilages. Also, I removed the" feet" of the alar cartilages to narrow the lower part of the columella. Her postoperative result is below.

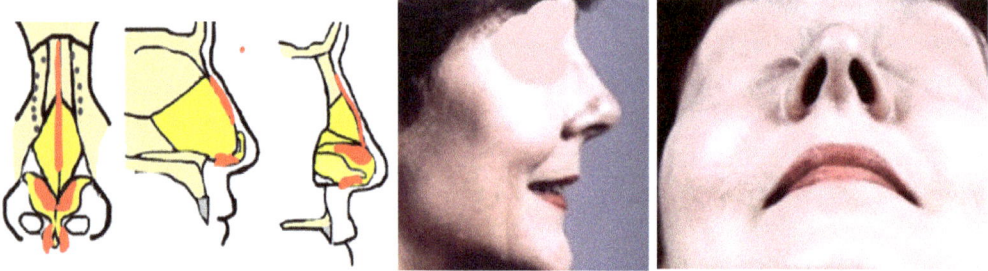

"Bobbie," below, did not like her nose. She felt it was large, and the nasal tip was too plunging. She wanted a smaller nose with a straight profile and an uplifted tip.

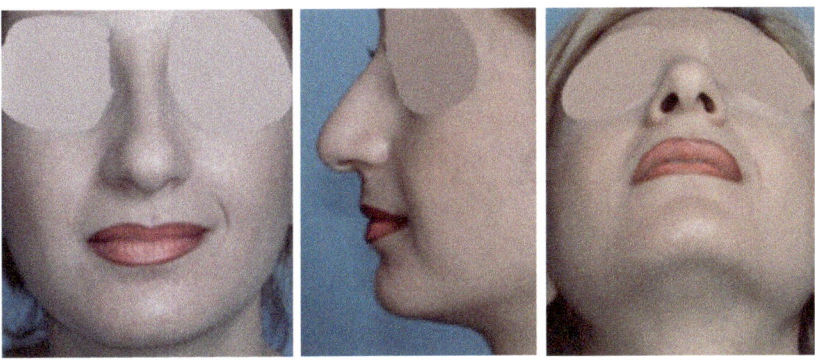

The diagram below indicates I removed the dorsal hump from the bridge, trimmed the tip cartilages, and placed cartilage grafts, harvested from the septum, on the tip, and in the columella.

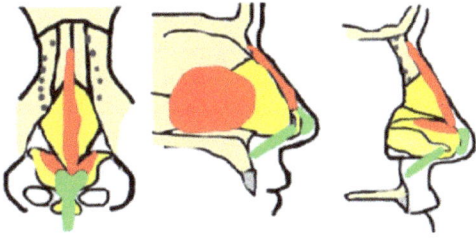

Her postoperative results show an uplifted tip and a straight bridge.

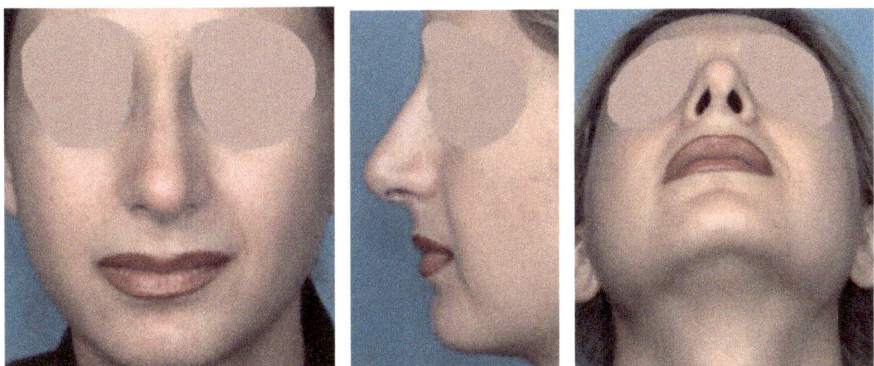

"Wolfgang," shown below, had broken his nose several times. The caudal septum deviated into the right nostril. As mentioned in the chapter on self-image, a crooked nose from trauma may give the person an undeserved pugilistic aura.

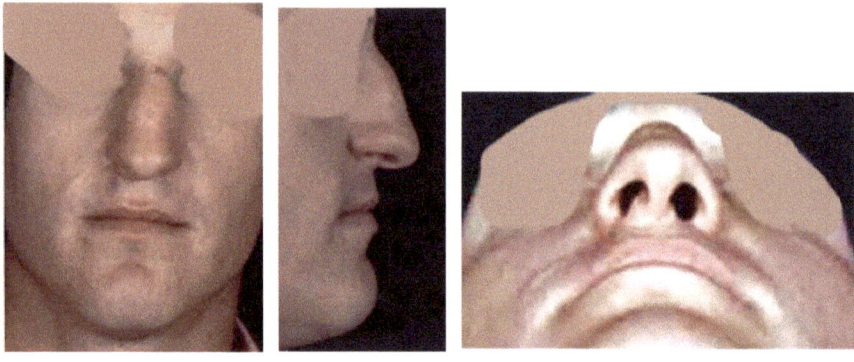

His rhinoplasty included harvesting nasal septum for cartilage grafts, which I used to define and support the nasal tip and to augment the bridge of the nose, which previous trauma had depressed. I also straightened the caudal septum.

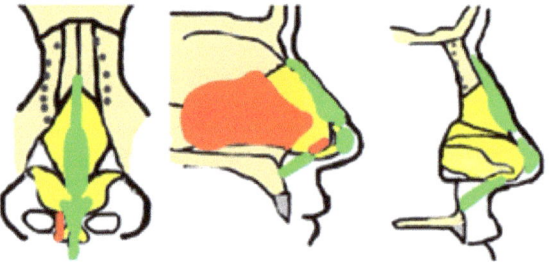

His postoperative photographs below show the improvement he received, especially in the worm's eye view and his profile.

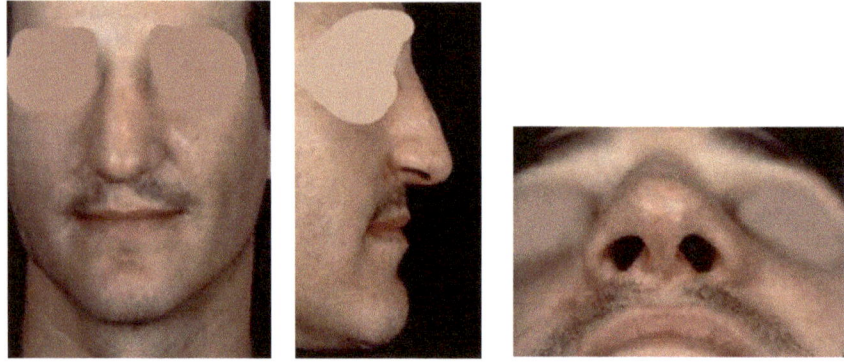

Everything does not always turn out as we plan with rhinoplasty. One patient, "Dorothy" comes to mind. She saw me because she wanted to have a rhinoplasty to get rid of a large hump on her nose. She also had a weak chin, which we also discussed augmenting with an implant. Our preoperative rapport seemed ok but was not particularly friendly. I performed the reduction rhinoplasty and chin implant under general anesthesia. The procedures appeared to go well. However, on the one-week postoperative visit, when I removed the nasal splint and the tape around her chin, she had a small bump from the nasal bone fracture on one side. This complication, called a rocker effect, occurs when an unintended attached segment of the nasal process of the frontal bone causes a relative prominence. The osteotomy caused a fracture that included more bone superiorly than expected. So, pushing the nasal bone fracture medially to narrow the nose, the upper portion paradoxically moves laterally.

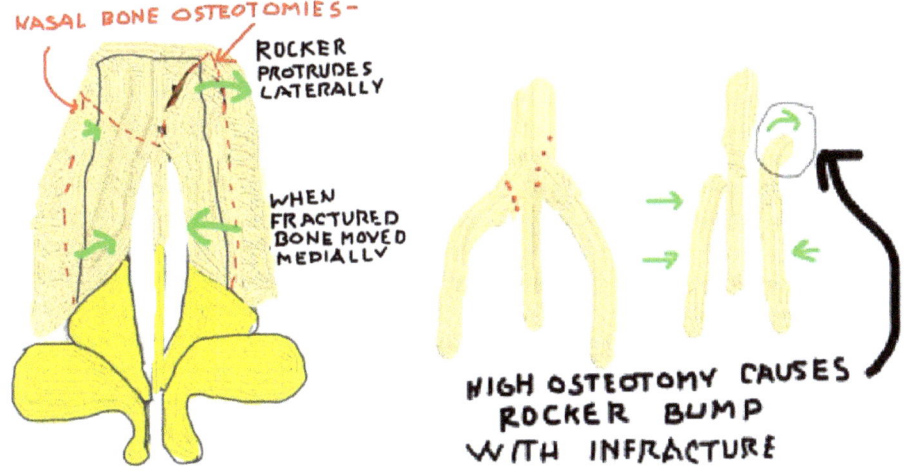

Usually, if this happened, I would recognize it and correct it during the rhinoplasty. "Dorothy" was naturally unhappy, having a bump on one side of her nose as was I. Additionally, she complained that her chin was now too prominent. What rapport we did have quickly vanished.

I felt like the chin position and prominence were right and that she would adjust her perception with a little time. I discussed a revision of the rhinoplasty with her. I felt terrible that she had this complication. I saw her back a couple of times and offered to revise the rhinoplasty with no surgical fee. She decided she did not want me to operate upon her but did want a revision. To accommodate her wishes, I arranged for her to see my partner, who offered to revise her rhinoplasty free of a surgical charge as a favor to me. She accepted. However, on a second office visit, their rapport fell apart, and he decided he would not operate upon her. I think her unfriendly attitude did not serve her well. I don't know what she did regarding a revision after that. As President Lincoln said, quoting poet John Lydgate: "You can please some of the people all the time, you can please all of the people some of the time, but you can't please all of the people all of the time."

Chin augmentation

"Julianna" pictured below wanted a rhinoplasty to make her nose smaller and more attractive. Upon analyzing her profile, I felt she would benefit from the augmentation of her chin. Profile -plasty is one area in cosmetic surgery where I sometimes voluntarily suggested additional surgery when the patient only had a rhinoplasty in mind. With prospective rhinoplasty patients, I took a lateral photo and printed it on regular paper so that I could draw on the back of the picture while placing it on a lighted slide file desktop. So, on the reverse of the photograph, I outlined what things might look like if I reduce the size of the nose, for example, or we augmented the chin.

I made clear there was no guarantee of a specific result, which is impossible. Today there are computer systems that can alter images with much more sophistication. Again, it is incumbent on the plastic surgeon not to promise a particular result or to present an example that would be very difficult to obtain. As technology has improved, disclaimers become even more critical.

"Julianna's" preoperative photos are below.

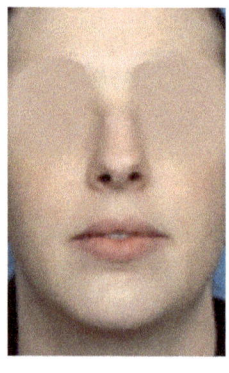 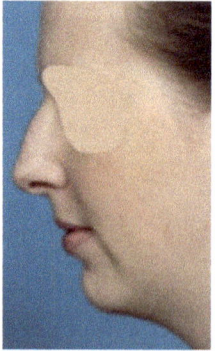

The altered photograph below was a representation of what we hoped to obtain surgically for "Julianna." The operation is also schematically represented below. I removed the hump on the bridge of the nose, reduce the nasal tip cartilages, in- fractured the nasal bones, and refined the tip with a small cartilaginous graft. I also inserted a small chin implant.

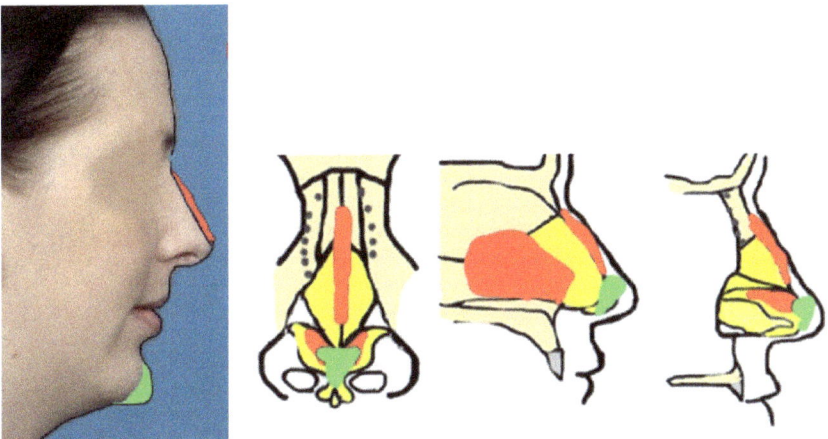

Postoperative photographs are below. A few weeks after surgery, she suffered a laceration to the nose, which she had sutured in an urgent care center. That scar had not yet faded when I took her postoperative pictures

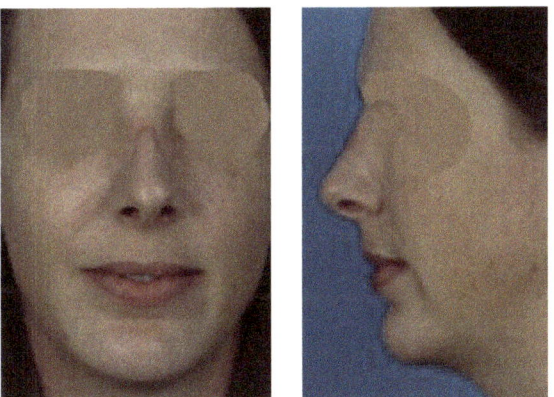

"Annamarie," pictured below, was unhappy with the size of her nose. She was also amenable to the use of a small implant to augment the chin to effect a more attractive profile.

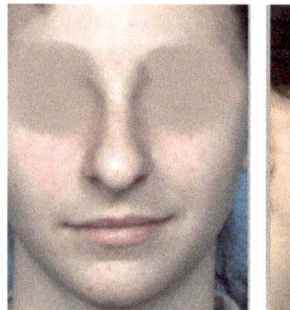 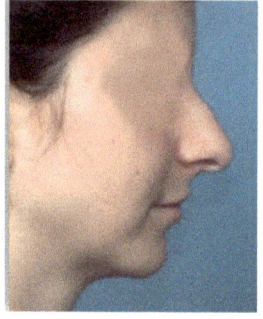 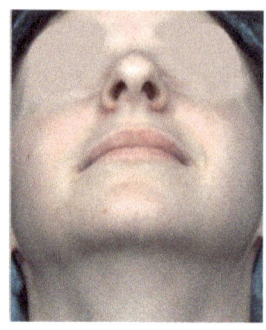

This surgery included harvesting cartilage from the nasal septum for tip and columella grafts. I removed the cephalic portion of the alar cartilages to narrow the tip. The tip graft helped to refined the nasal tip, and the columella strut graft added support to lift the tip.

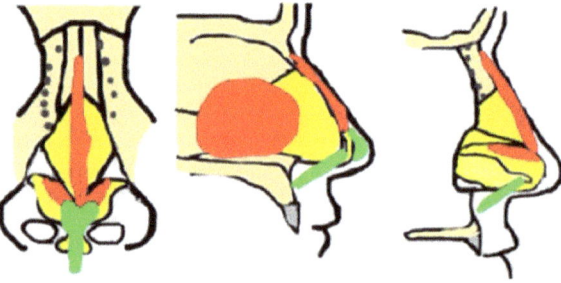

Her postoperative photographs, after septorhinoplasty and chin implant placement, are shown below

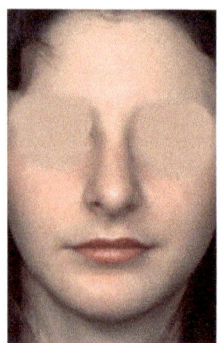 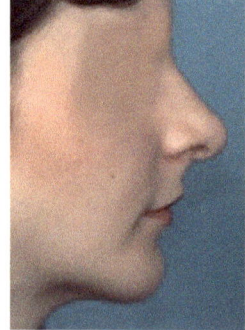 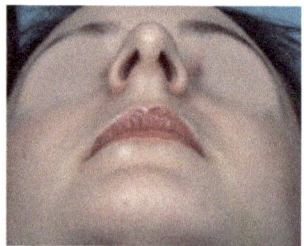

"Caroline," shown below, had a moderate-sized chin implant placed, which makes her profile view more youthful.

The Healing Mission of Plastic Surgery

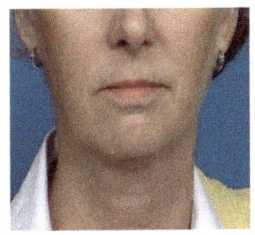 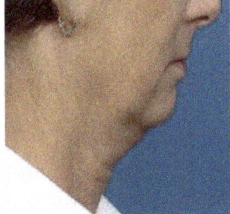 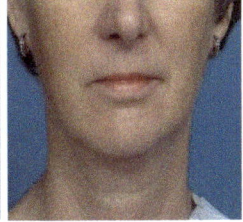 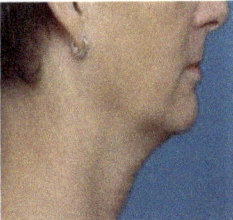

Pictured below, "Alexandria" wanted a less prominent nose. She was also amenable to alteration of her profile. Because of the shape of her chin and the amount of advancement needed, I recommended a genioplasty (structural alteration of the chin itself) instead of a chin implant. I performed this case with my resident surgeon Dr. Mike Lypka.

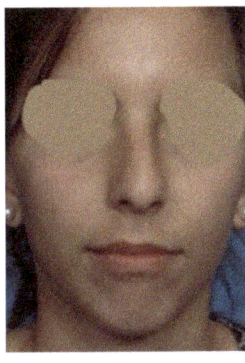 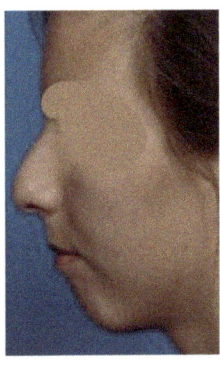

The surgical diagrams below represent a small amount of removal together with a cartilage graft of the tip and a columella strut graft to support the tip. I did an osteotomy of the chin, sliding the bony fragments forward to give more projection for the mentum. The chin bone(mentum) was secured in its new position with a titanium plate and screws, as shown below.

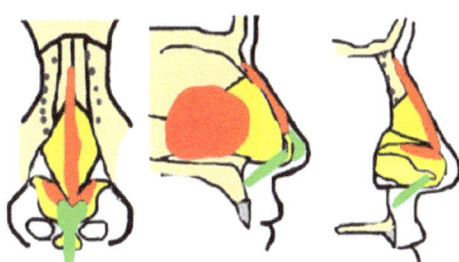 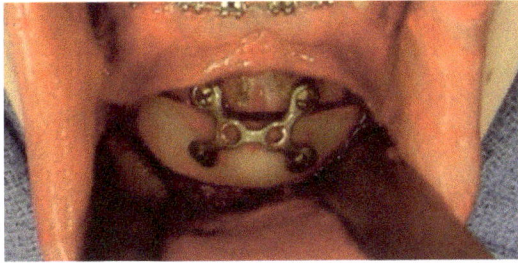

Her postoperative photos are below.

729

The Healing Mission of Plastic Surgery

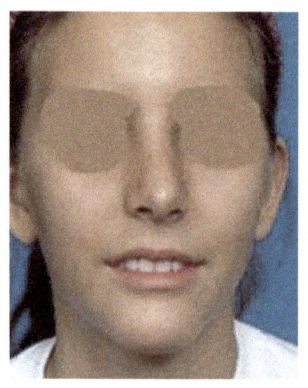
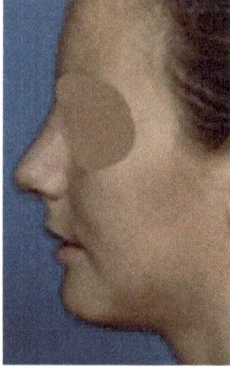

Structural facial alterations

Polyethylene implant to the angle of the jaw

This patient below, "Fred," sought help because he was unhappy with the appearance of his jaw, especially the lack of definition at the angle. After a discussion with him, I felt he had realistic ambitions. I believed that a synthetic polyethylene implant placed through the mouth to the angle of the jaw would be beneficial. The first two photos are preoperative. The third photo diagrammatically shows the approximate size and area of the implant, which was placed directly against the jaw bone from an incision in the mouth. The last two photos are after the placement of the polyethylene jaw angle implant. The postoperative views, especially the oblique one, show the sharper definition of the angle of the jaw below the left ear.

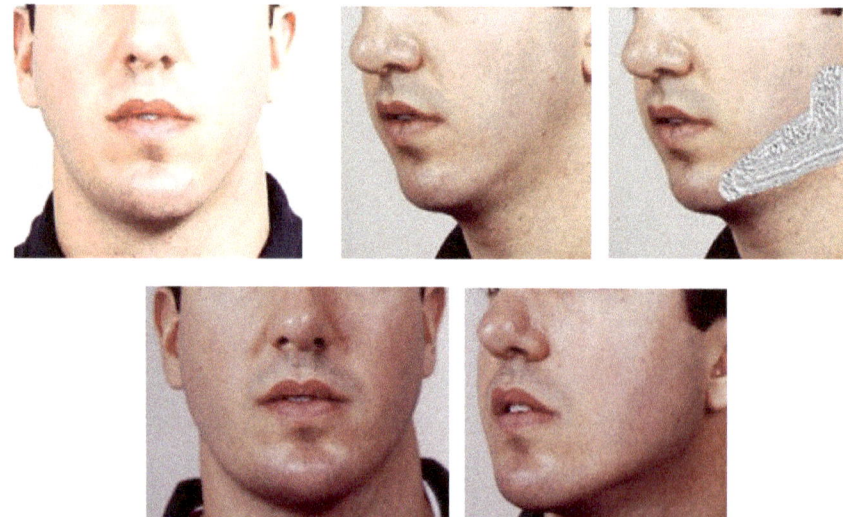

Genioplasty

In contrast to chin augmentation with a synthetic implant, a genioplasty usually refers to the alteration of the chin shape by directly advancing the bone or changing the chin bone in some other way. Genioplasty can be a powerful tool for the plastic surgeon to improve the patient's profile.

The young lady pictured below wanted to look better. After I evaluated her, I thought she could benefit from shortening the midface (like I did for "Amy" in chapter one). I also recommended a jumping genioplasty to improve her lower face profile. After explaining that a Le Fort I osteotomy was necessary to shorten the face, she declined that surgery. However, he did agree to a genioplasty. The first photographs below show the preoperative condition with the chin, both vertically long and deficient in anterior protection.

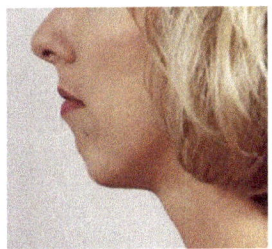
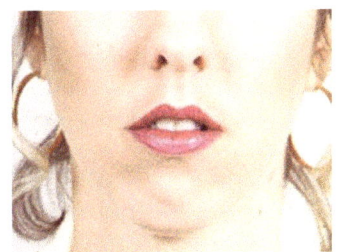

The diagrams below represent chin repositioning, both anteriorly and superiorly. I used the titanium plate with screws to hold the mentum in its new position after the osteotomy.

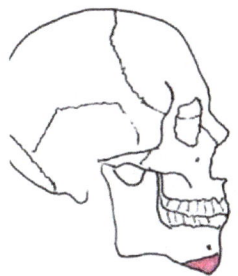
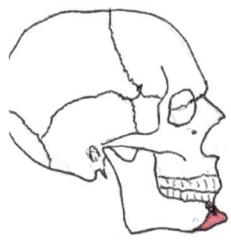
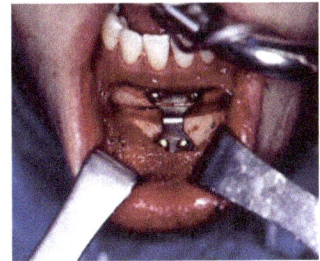

The final two photos show her postoperative result a few months later.

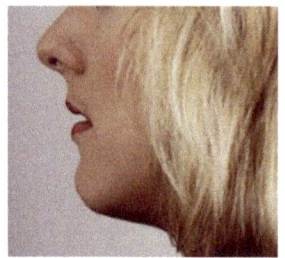 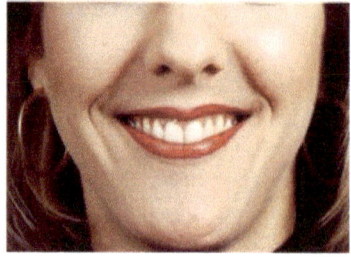

"Darlene" also benefited from a genioplasty to advance and vertically shorten the chin. I did a reduction rhinoplasty in conjunction with her genioplasty. Her before and after pictures are below.

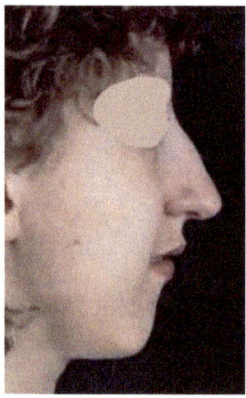 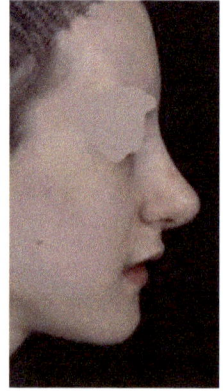

The patient below Maggie" had a chin which lacked projection and was vertically in excess. She also had a gummy smile and skinny lips

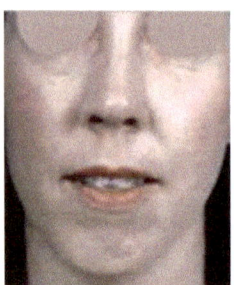 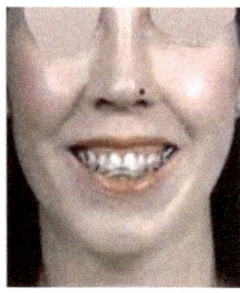 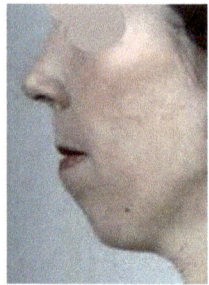

I performed an osteotomy of her chin and advanced it forward and upward. I also augmented her upper lip by turning tissue from inside downward and, at the same time, cutting some of the muscle that elevates the lip. These maneuvers corrected her gummy smile and gave her a better-proportioned profile. Her postoperative photos are below.

The Healing Mission of Plastic Surgery

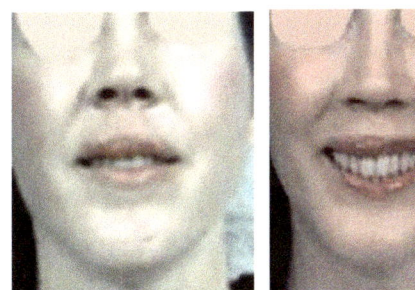
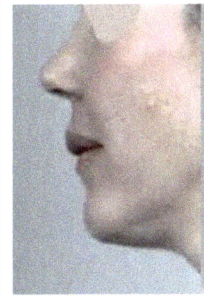

"Luanne" was displeased with her prognathic lower jaw. She also requested a rhinoplasty to make her nose a little smaller. I performed a vertical mandibular osteotomy, sliding the anterior jaw backward so that the posterior part of that anterior segment underlapped the posterior portion. I also made two cuts in the chin bone to remove a wedge(red) to make it less prominent.

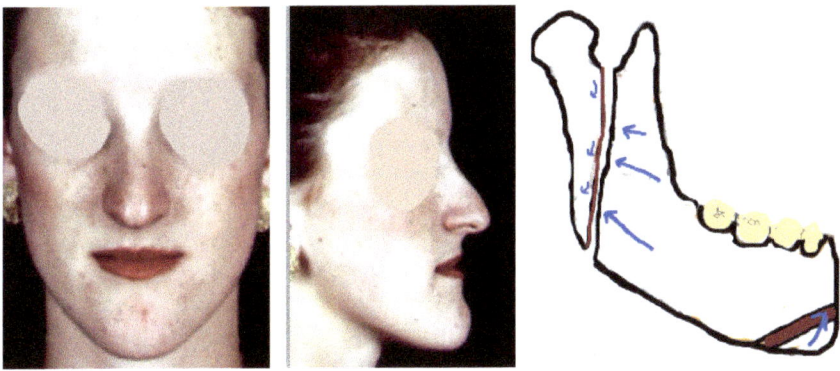

The drawing below shows the overlapping jaw bone segments secured with wire sutures(green). I reduced the mentum by the removal of a wedge of bone and then wired (green) the chin in its new position. The intraoperative photo on the right shows the chin bone secured. The "braces like" arch bar on the mandibular teeth will be used with another on the upper teeth to lock her bite into place for a few weeks with elastic bands.

The Healing Mission of Plastic Surgery

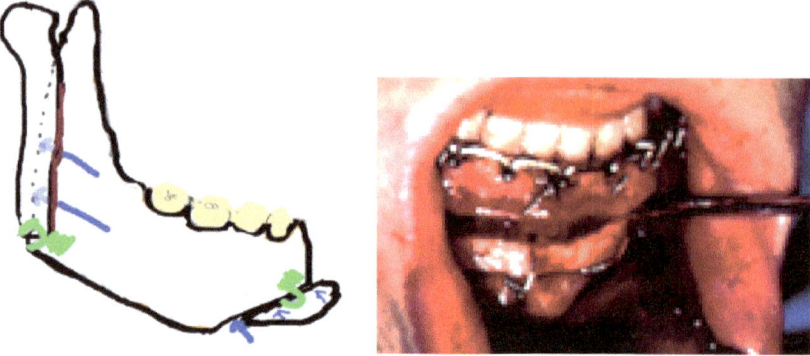

Her postoperative photos are below. In her case, she was not troubled by difficulties with mastication. However, it would not be unusual for eating and chewing problems to exist with similar prognathism. In those instances, I would do the mandibular surgery also to improve the bite and function of the jaws.

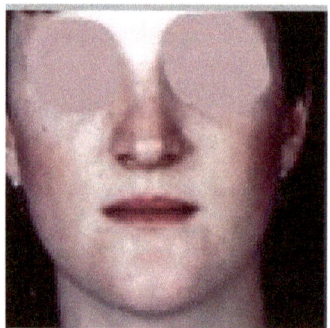 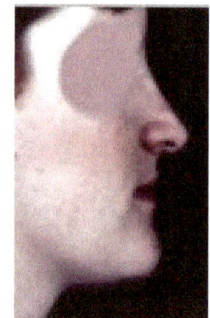

Chapter 17

Development of Plastic Surgery

The profession changed in many ways during my plastic surgery career. Many of the changes have been very productive, and some have greatly improved the quality of care that we can give our patients. Other changes have not been so positive.

Ethics

Advertising

When my practice began, physicians rarely advertised. The code of ethics of the American Medical Association, starting in 1847, forbade advertising by physicians. Beginning in 1975 Federal Trade Commission, under the guise of restraint of trade, strong-armed the medical professional societies to allow advertising by doctors. I doubt anyone today believes that the purported benefits of better and cheaper medical care occurred by this change. Advertisements now permeate the medical field like any commercial endeavor. Not the best start for a doctor-patient relationship.

Thus medicine, once the epitome of professions, by betraying its right to mandate ethical principles has allowed itself to degenerate into a trade. Some of the worst abuses relate to plastic surgery. Many doctors have misleading self - aggrandizing advertisements. Some practitioners insinuate they are plastic surgeons, when they may be a general surgeon, emergency medicine doctor, or even a general practitioner with no surgical training. The traditional doctor-patient relationship has been severely compromised, as has the ethics of all the medical societies. I quit my membership in the American Medical Association many decades ago because of its stance on abortion. So much for the Hippocratic oath.

CPT codes

When I began my practice, there was no universal coding method for the various procedures and operations we performed. When I did insurance-related procedures such as emergency room care, I would take into account the time involved, the complexity of the activity, and create a charge that I felt was appropriate for my patient. At that time, insurance companies and physicians use what was called "usual and customary fees." We occasionally had disputes with the insurance companies about these fees, but for the most part, from my standpoint, at work quite smoothly.

Of course, there was occasionally an outlier miscreant who billed exorbitantly. The local county medical society, Harris County Medical Society, tried to call out examples of such rapacious behavior. Beginning, about 1980, we were obliged to use the CPT coding system, which had been developed by the American Medical Association in the 1960s and 70s. This system characterized various surgical procedures by code and assigned a relative value number to each operation.

At first, because this caused me to itemize the multiple procedures I might have done in a complicated case, my fees increased for a while. As insurance companies began to be the controllers of access to patients, they were able to use these relative value codes to ratchet the fees down over time significantly. From my point of view, the physicians were basically at the mercy of the insurance companies. The individual physician could not hold out against large insurance companies over fees. Organized medicine, including the AMA, was impotent in my view. The CPT codes and relative value numbers are universally utilized by Medicare and all insurance companies today and therefore are indispensable for all physicians.

Cell phones

Cell phones were not around when I began to practice. We did have beepers that would beep and show a digital display of the phone number, which was calling. I used to keep a cache of quarters in my pocket so that if I got beeped on my way home from the hospital, I would have coins to call back from a payphone. I knew the location of the payphones on my daily commute and their likely locations throughout the city. Today we hardly can find a payphone anywhere in the city because of the sea change of ubiquitous cell phones.

Cell phones (when encrypted) can be useful in remote communication between a resident, who may be seeing a patient in the emergency room, on the hospital floor, or in the neonatal intensive care unit, and his or her faculty or staff physician. For example, the resident can send a photo display of an injury or wound or congenital problem and receive direction on taking care of those issues. So just like they have improved general communication, they have been a convenient modernization for medicine.

911

When I began practice in 1978, there was no 911 in Houston. An 82.5 % favorable referendum vote established the Greater Harris County 911 Emergency Network. It is hard to imagine how chaotic things would be without this service. I find irony in that I would call 911 for help if a patient collapsed in my office. For this program, the local governments get all of my praise!

Digital photography

Another tremendous technological advance that came about after I began practice is digital photography. I sometimes reviewed some of the oldest records of my uncle Dr. Thomas Cronin' and his original partner Dr. Brauer from the late 1940 and 1950s. They were black and white photographs printed on photographic paper and stored in photo albums. Below are several picture albums filled with their early plastic surgery cases. Note the first album uses the old terminology for cleft lip, which is not politically correct; surgeons do not use it today.

The Healing Mission of Plastic Surgery

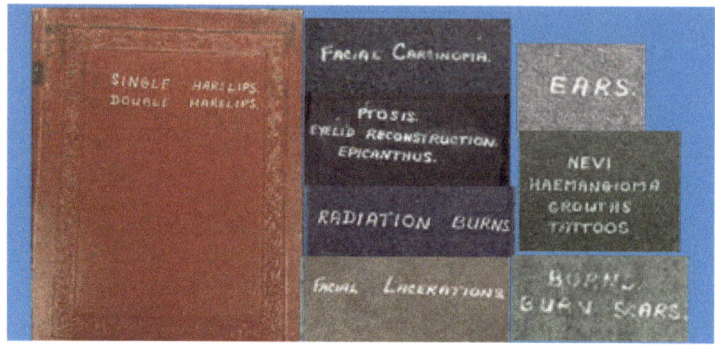

The following are a few photos from Dr. Thomas Cronin's picture books. The first shows a child with a bilateral cleft lip. He obtained a very nice result for her. The next case shown is of a child with a giant black congenital nevus on the left side of the face. The last picture shows the final result after concatenation of partial excisions of the lesion and advancement of surrounding healthy tissue

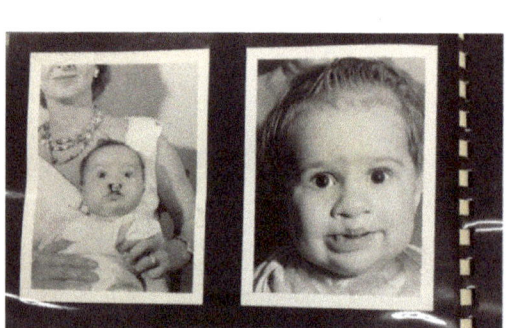 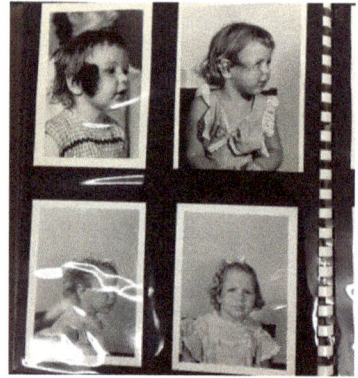

For presentation purposes, they had big glass slides. A particular projector could produce images on a screen. Dr. Tomas Cronin used wooded boxes like those below to file the fragile glass slides.

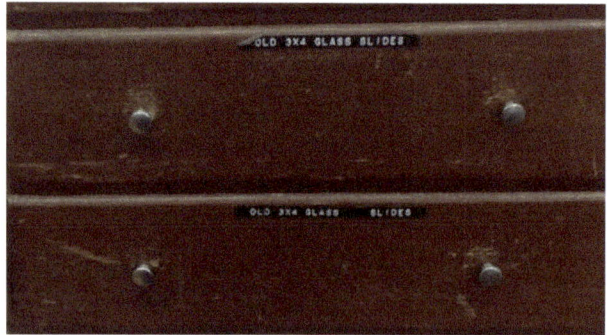 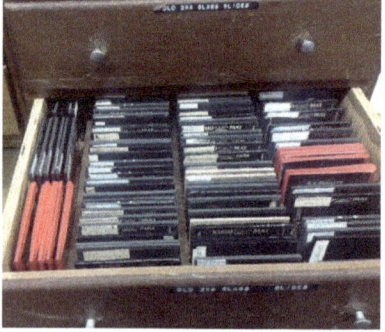

The Healing Mission of Plastic Surgery

I show a couple of examples of these clinical glass slides below. The first clinical slide is of a nasal reconstruction after the excision of a carcinoma. The second is of a pinback otoplasty for prominent ears.

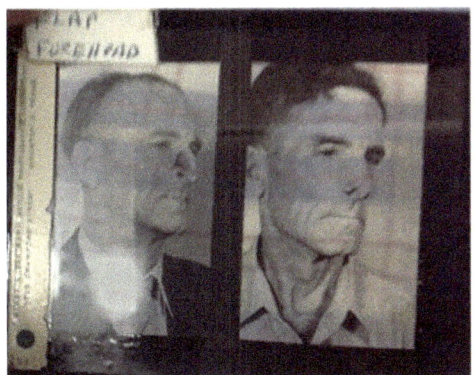 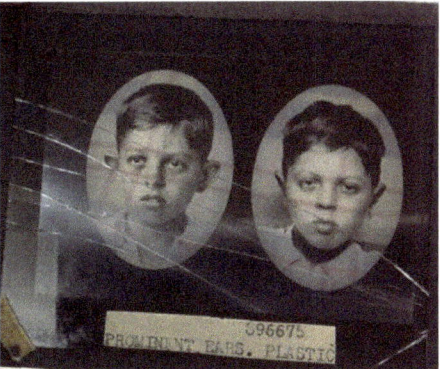

The drawing below on the glass slide is of a cleft palate repair technique developed by Dr. Thomas Cronin.

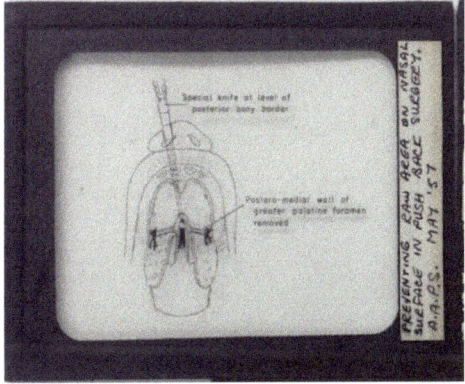

Dr. Brauer told me about a visit he made to a plastic surgery meeting in London early in his career. I assume this was in the late 1950s. He said they had just begun using 35mm color film for clinical cases. He showed a 35 mm slide presentation of a cleft lip repair. He showed close-up color photos of the child's lip pre-and post-op. Dr. Brauer did beautiful cleft lip repairs, but he thought the ovation he got when he put these photos up was as much for the beautiful color photos, which were unprecedented until that time. It was customary for the British doctors to not only clap but to stomp their feet and make a racket as a sign of approval.

The Healing Mission of Plastic Surgery

When I began my training in plastic surgery, we used 35mm color film and 35 mm slide carousel projectors for presentations. I remember several times during a national meeting; a slide show was interrupted because a single slide got stuck in the carousel, and someone would have to reset the slide manually. On a couple of occasions, I witnessed someone dropping a slide carousel and slides spilling out on the floor in disarray, which was probably every presenter's nightmare.

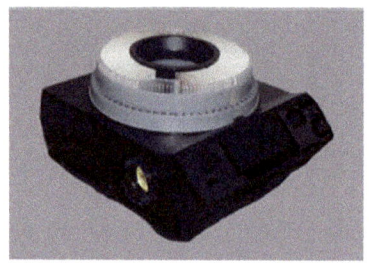 

As a resident in the Cronin and Brauer residency program at St. Joseph Hospital, I was responsible for occasionally giving a slide presentation. I made use of the photographic darkroom in the office. To make words slides, I would have to type the message on paper, then photograph it. The photos we took in the ER and the operating room were sometimes disappointing because they were unknowingly out of focus, etc. I would take the camera to the darkroom, remove the film, use a cookbook method of development with various containers and solutions. I would then hang the roll of film up to dry. Following this, I would cut the 35mm film and insinuate it into either paper or plastic slide holders.

To help organize a 35mm slide talk, we had a large plastic desktop viewing board lit through from underneath. We would place all the slides on the lit surface and could move them around manually to put them in the order we wanted before placing them in the slide carousel. Later I did enjoy telling new residents, preparing presentations, about how we used to have to "walk miles through the snow to go to school" as it were.

One can very quickly appreciate the technological revolution digital photography represented. Now images are immediately available. If it is out of focus, another can replace it immediately. We can manipulate digital pictures with ease on computer programs designed for slide type presentations. Such simple things as cropping of an image are no longer a production. Now presentations might easily include video as well as still pictures.

From the standpoint of medical records and cataloging patient photographs, the difference is like night and day. We used to have large cabinets filled with 35mm slides. Digital photography took over halfway through my medical career. Often, we would need to go back to our 35mm slide files and scan those files and turn them into digital images so that we might include those in computer "slide" presentations. Many of the images used in this book were initially 35mm slides that I have digitalized. Some loss of quality can occur in this process. I do envy our new surgeons who have been able to utilize digital photography from the beginning of their careers. Now instead of lugging around slide carousels, one can keep almost an unlimited number of presentations on one flash drive.

Titanium Plates and Screws

Before we had titanium microplates and screws, we used stainless steel wires to secure bony fragments in trauma, craniofacial, reconstructive, and orthognathic cases. For example, the surgeon used stainless steel wires in the supraorbital reconstruction below, as you see. He first drilled a hole through each adjacent bony segment, then passed a wire ligature through the drill holes and twisted the wire to secure the bones. It is like twisting a thin wire with a little paper on it to secure a plastic wrap on a loaf of bread.

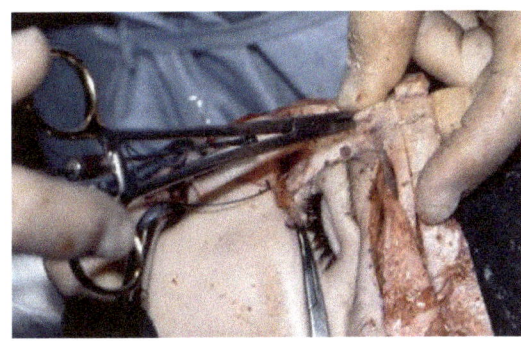
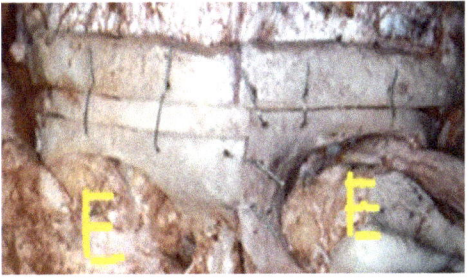

Titanium microplates and screws demonstrate the stabilization of the fragments of the plastic models below after osteotomies (or after fractures).

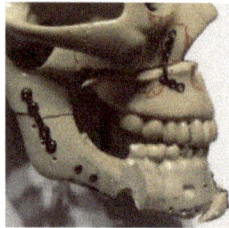 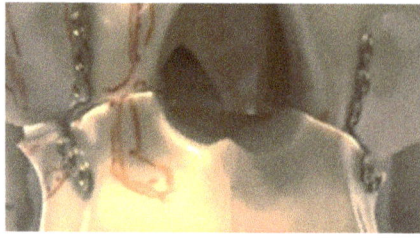 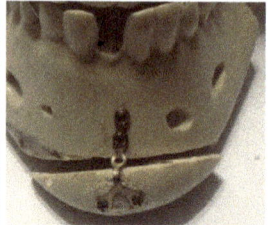

The patient below "Alfred" had a "blowout" fracture of the orbital floor. Surgeons do orbital floor reconstructions with various materials such as Teflon, silicone, titanium mesh, and bone grafts from the patient. Titanium mesh has been a beneficial nonreactive implant but sometimes was a little difficult to insert because of the "stickiness" of the cut edges of the implant created by customization of the implant for the individual case. Orbital floor implants are now available with porous polyethylene-coated titanium mesh. These implants are still easy to insert after cutting them to shape.

In "Alfred's" case, I reconstructed the orbital floor on the left side with a. customized porous polyethylene-coated/titanium orbital floor implant. Taking the actual shape of the orbital floor and its defect into account, I altered the implant by cutting it to the desired shape. The drawing I made below simulates the customized form. After I inserted the implant, I folded the anterior uncoated portion of the implant over the inferior orbital rim. I secured it with titanium screws, as shown in the middle picture below. The postoperative photo shows the patient's ability to look upward, which indicates the repair of the floor was successful, and the patient had no entrapment of soft tissue into the maxillary sinus below the eye, which might cause restriction of eyeball movement.

The Healing Mission of Plastic Surgery

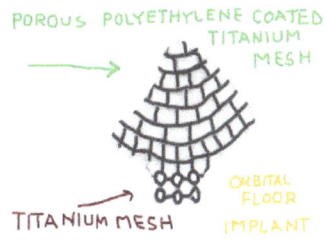
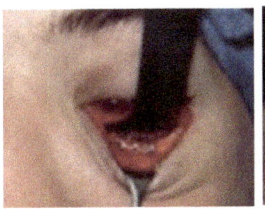
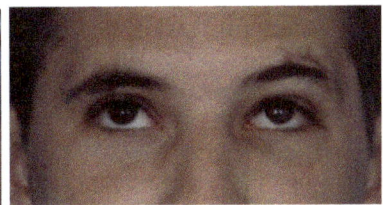

The elderly patient below was involved in a severe motor vehicle accident and suffered extensive facial fractures. She also had a fractured neck but had no spinal cord damage. She was a lovely lady who maintained an upbeat attitude throughout her treatment. The surgery did necessitate my doing a tracheostomy, which remained in place for several weeks. I reconstructed her by placing the fragments back into position and securing them with titanium plates and screws. The first photo shows plates on the left inferior orbital rim and the nasal bones.

The next view under the upper lip shows the titanium plates fixing the maxilla. The third shows a micro titanium plate on the nasal bones. Before the availability of these titanium plates and screws, this kind of surgery would need to be done by drilling small holes and placing wires between the various bony fragments and twisting the wires to hold the pieces in place. The final postoperative picture shows the satisfactory structure of the facial bones.

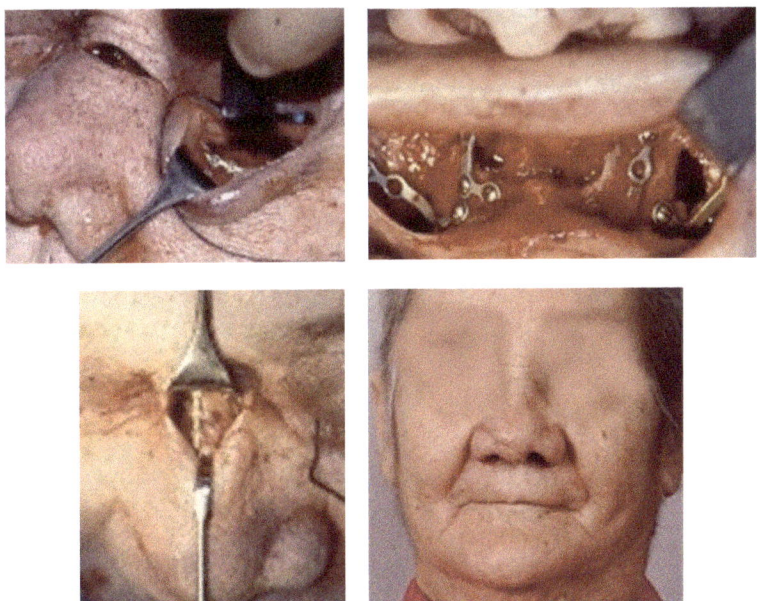

Osseointegrated implants

Another significant advance in the care of patients has occurred primarily because of the work of a Swedish physician Per-Ingvar Branemark. In 1952, Per-Ingvar Branemark, when trying to remove a titanium implant from a rabbit after a blood flow experiment, serendipitously observed that the implant had integrated so thoroughly with the bone he could not remove it. He saw the potential for beneficial use in humans and devoted his career to this endeavor, which has been transformational in both dentistry and medicine.

He introduced the term Osseointegration to indicate the relationship between titanium implants and living bone. Surface oxidation of titanium implants forms titanium O2. This reaction allows the direct connection between bone and a load-carrying implant. The implications are tremendous. He presented his work in 1982, which caused a paradigm shift in the dental as well as the extraoral implant world. Beginning in 1965 with his first dental implant, the concept of osseointegrated implants has spread from calvarium to calcaneus(heel). We are all now familiar with the wonderful dental implant technology available. These advances have also provided significant help to the dental health of large numbers of cleft palate patients, trauma patients, and many affected by oral cancer extirpation. As in the drawing below, dental implants can be as functional as natural teeth.

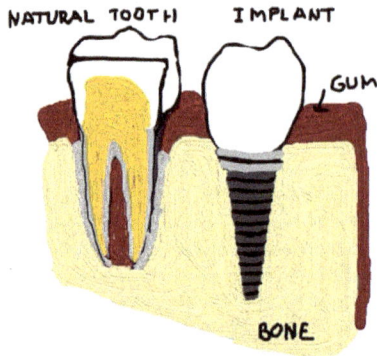

Osseointegration has also caused a quantum change in extraoral implantology. Extraoral osseointegrated implants fasten prosthesis such as external ears (see below left), and those of partial facial features for patients who are not candidates for standard plastic surgery techniques; previously they would have to be secured with glue as in the patient on the right below

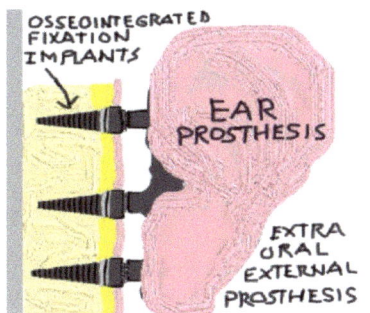 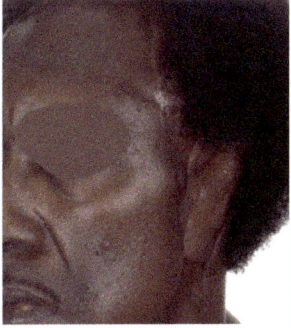 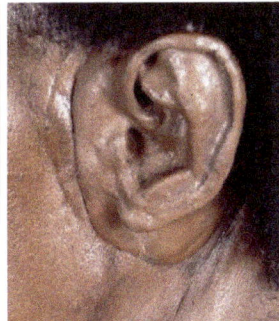

Osseointegrated implant fixation can be used for the fixation of orthopedic limb prostheses.

Lasers

"Laser" originated as an acronym for "light amplification by stimulated emission of radiation." My generation did not grow up using lasers, which began in 1958. Now we have the application of lasers throughout our daily life. We have laser printers, laser pointers for presentations, laser range finders for golf and other uses, various laser cutting devices in industry, laser barcode scanners, laser scanning microscopy, and different laser energy weapons for the military. Lasers for medical purposes were coming out when I began practice in 1978. That year the Cronin Brauer and Biggs practice bought one of the first argon lasers in Houston to use for treating hemangiomas and other skin lesions. The manufacturers promoted it as almost magic.

It certainly did not live up to its hyped expectations. The rep showed us that the laser beam would leave a piece of white paper alone but burn up black typed areas. That first laser was somewhat of a monster. It was about as large as a residential refrigerator, and it was water-cooled to prevent it from overheating. At that time, our office was on the 22nd floor of a large medical office building. If we were using the laser and someone flush a toilet on our floor, a fault light would come on, and the laser stopped functioning. That first laser was not very different from using electrocautery on the lesions we treated.

Lasers have come a long way since then. They have been especially beneficial in many medical areas, particularly ophthalmology and for angioplasties in vascular surgery. Plastic surgeons use lasers for treating benign skin lesions such as hemangiomas but also precancerous and cancerous skin lesions. They have also become much better for cosmetic skin rejuvenation and removal of tattoos. Lasers promoted to replace the traditional scalpel or electrosurgical instruments for ordinary surgeries have not succeeded. It seems that over the last 30 years periodically, another "breakthrough" laser was introduced, which was supposed to remove a scar, birthmarks, spider veins, varicose veins, wrinkles, etc. without leaving any scars or doing any damage.

Not wanting to be a Luddite, I attended more than a handful of instructional courses on new lasers. However, I was disappointed repeatedly by new lasers, not living up to the manufacturer's promotions. Therefore, I gradually pulled away from using lasers. As mentioned before, lasers can be quite useful for skin resurfacing, removal of tattoos, and some birthmarks.

However, some older techniques, i.e., chemical peels and dermabrasion, are effective and much cheaper.

Smoking

I have a recollection of attending an autopsy in medical school of a recently deceased chronic heavy smoker. The pathologist displayed the lung tissue turned black from the years of smoking. However, immediately after completion of the autopsy, the pathologist pulled out a cigarette, lit it, and took a big drag??

My mother was a three-pack a day smoker for several decades. I remember when I was a relatively small child, she would let me lite up her next cigarette so that there would be no hiatus between smokes. She later gave up smoking, but it was too late, and she was on continuous oxygen for the last ten years of her life. When I first began attending medical meetings, the auditoriums would be smoke-filled. A few years later, the lecture halls divided, one side for smoking and the other smoke-free. We began to see advertisements that said: "100,000 doctors have quit smoking". Next, smoking was eliminated from the lecture rooms and restricted to the lobbies. Finally, smoking became completely prohibited from medical meetings. It seems like organized medicine was only a little ahead of the general public.

Business computers

When I was a resident in 1977, the Cronin Brauer Biggs Clinic had no computers. The office used paper ledger cards for each patient transaction. The clinic hired a consultant who recommended switching to a computer system. So, one day, I think it was three, office computer "experts" arrived with 5 or 6 desktop monitors and the accompanying computers. They set things up and began the instruction of the office personnel. The process was to take about ten days to get any bugs out and to get the user training done.

Three months later, never having a satisfactory working situation, we fired the experts and the computers removed! Can you imagine something like that today? It was quite a while later before we consulted another company that installed a business system for the clinic without much fanfare. However, for a few months, we used duplicate systems, paper, and computers. When the clinic dissolved in 1988, and Dr. Cohen and I set up our practice, we debated whether to have both paper and computer business systems. We decide by that time that the computer systems were reliable enough to go it alone. We never had much trouble with it. Now there are computer systems that take care of business transactions, patient records, integrate photos with files, and that allows the sophisticated analysis of groups of similar cases, etc.

Muscle and myo-cutaneous flaps

Before muscle, myo-cutaneous flaps and free flaps random flaps were "walked" from one location to another. For example, the surgeon might suture a random flap from the abdomen to the wrist. Then after several weeks, to allow the wrist to supply blood flow to the flap, the surgeon would disconnect the flap from the abdomen while left connected to the wrist. The flap was then moved down and connected to the foot, as in the photo below. After a few more weeks, the flap was disconnected from the wrist and left on foot, which was the original wound defect to be repaired. The wrist would then be free again. This concatenation of steps could take months to complete!

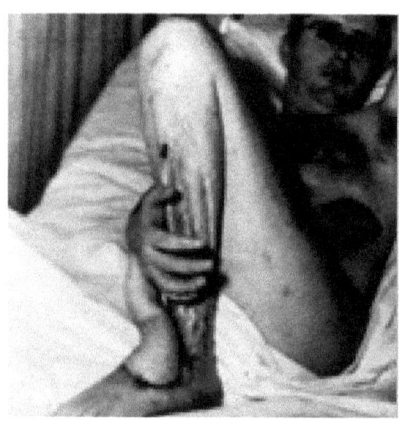

When I began training in plastic surgery, muscle and myo-cutaneous flaps were starting to show up in the literature. Courses were set up in various parts of the country to teach practicing plastic surgeons these new techniques. Every month in the major plastic surgery journals, there were presentations of new muscle and myo-cutaneous flaps for various applications. It was an exhilarating time to learn plastic surgery. I discussed the workings of these flaps in chapter 4 of the art and science of plastic surgery. And many examples are present throughout this book.

Micro -Surgery and Free Tissue Transfer

Microsurgery began in plastic surgery in the late 1970s. It was not yet standard treatment when I started to practice but reported as unusual or unique cases. Microsurgery enabled the better repair of nerve lacerations and repair of smaller nerves such as digital nerves. Microsurgery also allows the repair of small blood vessels for salvaging, de-vascularized, or amputated parts might by repairing the lacerated small blood vessels. For example, my partner Ben Cohen, ahead of the standard of care, had participated in a re-plantation of a severed penis during his residency at Massachusetts General Hospital in 1976.

Microvascular free tissue transfer is a procedure that allows tissue to be moved from one part of the body to another by including vascular pedicles (artery and vein) with the tissue and then anastomosing those pedicles into vessels at the recipient site so that blood supply would be available again for that tissue

The first photo below shows a microscopic repair of a digital nerve at the base of the finger. The second photograph shows the anastomosis of a digital artery to re-vascularize an injured little finger. The third photo below shows a free myo-cutaneous flap from its undersurface. The skin portion is faced down. The vascular pedicle enters the muscle from the left. There are a small muscle portion and a more substantial subcutaneous fat and skin paddle. The blood supply comes through the vascular pedicle to the muscle and then through the flesh via perforators to the subcutaneous tissue and skin. The plastic surgeon can move the whole flap to a distant part of the body and anastomose the pedicle to recipient vessels to re-establish blood supply to the flap. I discuss this type of flap in Chapter 4, the Art and Science of Plastic Surgery.

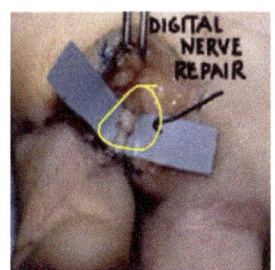 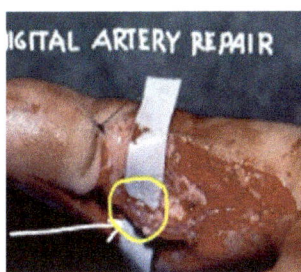 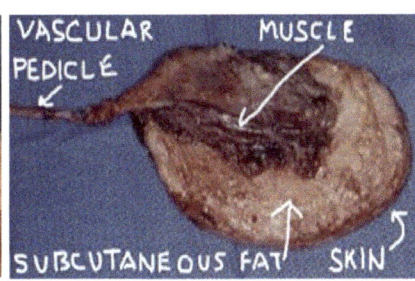

The case shown below of "Carlos" was a reconstruction of a traumatic injury involving the mandible and soft tissue of the lower face and neck. In this case, a septocutaneous flap, a scapular flap, was taken from the

back and transferred to replace lost tissue of the lower face and neck. In this case, the vascular pedicle from the flap was anastomosed to the external carotid artery to re-establish its blood supply. I discussed in more detail this type of flap in Chapter 4.

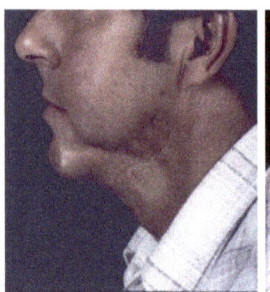 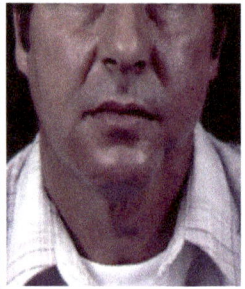 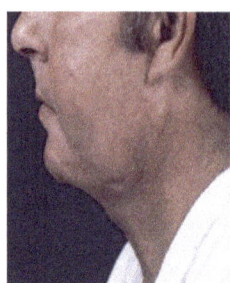 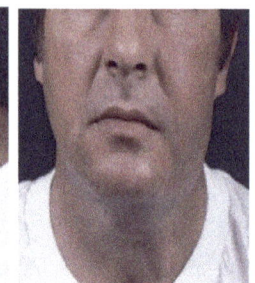

Tissue expansion

There was one article reporting post auricular tissue expansion with a rubber balloon for coverage in a cartilage ear reconstruction case as early as 1957 by Neuman. However, this article went virtually unnoticed. Working separately, Radovan and Austad were developing silicone tissue expanders about 1975. Radovan popularized tissue expansion for breast reconstruction in 1983. Silicone balloon tissue expansion with the later exchange for a conventional breast implant is probably the most common reconstructive method post-mastectomy today. Tissue expansion is used all over the body and has particular use in scalp reconstruction.

"Alice" was a young adult who was concerned with a large scar of her arm. Many years before, she had had melanoma, the dangerous malignant skin cancer. She had the tumor removed with wide excision, including a good deal of surrounding healthy tissue. The wound closure required a large skin graft to the upper arm. The graft was very conspicuous, and she was self-conscious about this. People were always asking her what happened, which reminded her of the malignant tumor. She came to me to see if there was a way to get rid of the graft scar.

The Healing Mission of Plastic Surgery

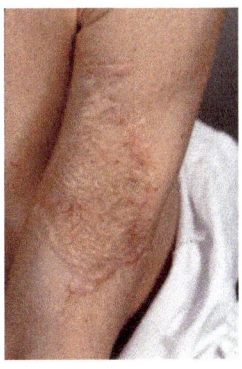

At that time, the new procedure of tissue expansion was in its infancy. Tissue expansion was popularized by Radovan for breast reconstruction and subsequently used all over the body. "Alice's" problems seemed amenable to this technique. After discussing this new technique with her and obtaining her consent, I took her to the operating room. I made an incision at the junction of the adjacent healthy skin. Through this incision, I made a pocket in which I inserted a tissue expander balloon and closed the incision.

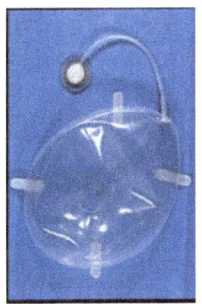 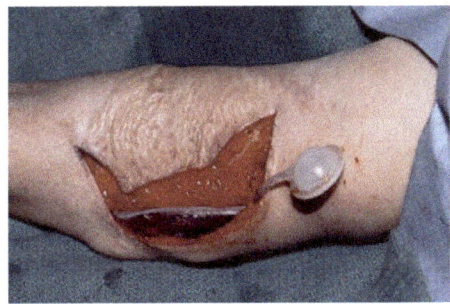

After a couple of weeks of healing, I began the expansion to stretch the healthy adjacent skin. I injected saline into the remote port to the expander balloon weekly for about four to five weeks. Eventually, "Alice's" forearm looked like Popeye, the sailor man's arm. After several weeks I removed the expander and was able to excise the entire skin graft and close the wound with this newly created excess skin adjacent to the skin graft. Although she still had a linear scar of the arm, she was much happier and less self-conscious of her appearance because of this plastic surgery. The early postoperative picture shown here is before the scar had a chance to mature, fade, and blend with the surrounding skin.

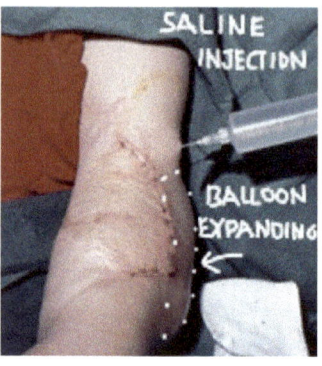 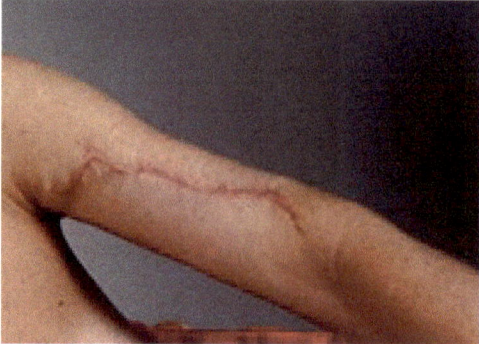

Endoscopic surgery, robotic surgery

The endoscope was not used in plastic surgery when I began to practice. The gynecologists used the endoscope routinely by the 1970s. When video magnification and projection of images started in the early 1980s, endoscopic surgery became integrated into general surgery and was soon used regularly, especially for gallbladder and appendix surgery.

Chow popularized endoscopic carpal tunnel release beginning in 1989. By 1990 plastic surgeons were using the endoscope for cosmetic surgery such as endoscopic forehead lifts. Before the endoscope, we did forehead lifts through a coronal incision in the scalp, which went from ear to ear. So, the endoscope offered the possibility of cosmetic improvement through minimal incisions. I wrote a paper on using the endoscope for the removal of forehead lesions such as lipomas and osteotomies. I showed examples in chapter 5.

With the onset of robotic surgery, the future holds the possibility of various endoscopic operations with robotic control. Harvesting of latissimus muscle- only flaps are now sometimes done with robotic surgery.

Liposuction & Fat Grafting

Although there were reports of liposuction as early as the 1920s, the modern methods of liposuction became widespread about 1982. A French surgeon Dr. Illouz presented his approach, which was a suction-assisted method using cannulas to remove fat. This technique rapidly became popular. The Cronin Brauer and Biggs clinic helped demonstrate this technique in a teaching conference in Houston in 1986. The method became more popular after we learned to control the bleeding by injection of dilute solutions of epinephrine throughout the fatty tissue, which we would then suction. This "wet technique" continues to be the mainstay for most plastic surgeons. Many variations exist, such as ultrasonic liposuction, power-assisted liposuction, and others.

One of the most common areas of liposuction in females is the lateral thigs. The following two, somewhat subtle, cases illustrate removal of mild tissue fullness from the lateral thighs

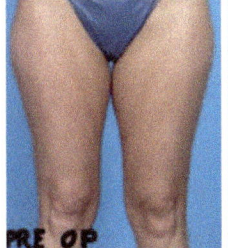 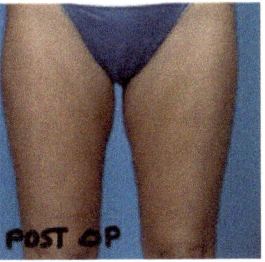 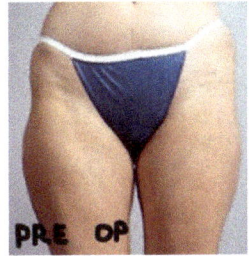 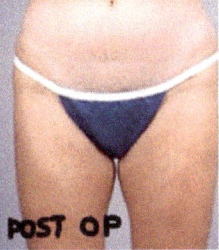

In the following third patient had more significant circumferential liposuction of the thighs.

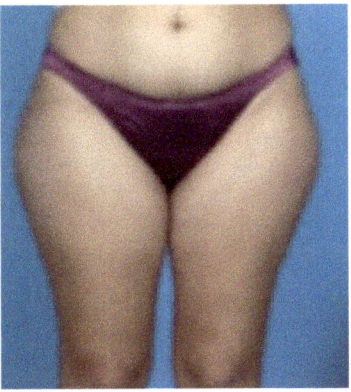 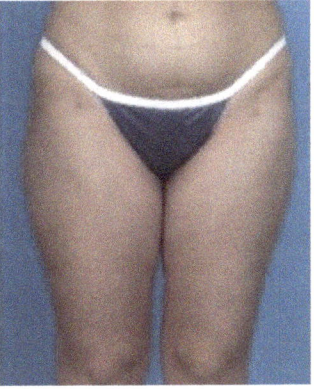

The patient below, "Thomas," wanted some improvement in his neck contour but was not ready for a facelift or some other open procedure such as a platysma-plasty. Therefore, I did liposuction only of the neck and was able to obtain some neck contour improvement, as shown in the photos.

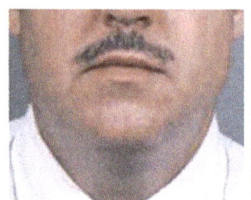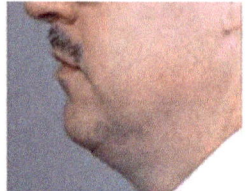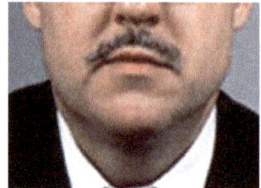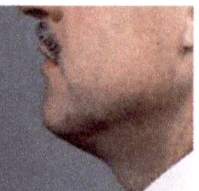

Fat Grafting

Fat removed with liposuction was soon being injected to fill various defects. Eventually, fat injection became typical for facial rejuvenation, especially around the nasolabial folds. I also found it useful for minor depressions in breast reconstruction cases. "Felicity" was the first patient upon whom I performed fat grafting by needle injection. She had a 2cm depression on one buttock from an injection several years previously. There was a significant divot, perhaps because of infection and necrosis of subcutaneous fat. I discussed the possible benefit of fat grafting by injection.

I told her it would be the first time I did the procedure, and she said it would be the first time for her also! Under local anesthesia as an office procedure, I aspirated about double the fat I thought I would need. I decanted it in a syringe to eliminate blood and serum. I injected the defect, and it had an immediate effect. I did overcorrect by probably 30% or so, leaving a slight bulge where there had been the depression. Within two weeks, it looked quite level. I was fortunate enough to see her back a couple of years later for another issue and was quite happy to find the correction had maintained itself.

Fat grafting has been quite beneficial for small secondary defects in breast reconstruction cases. Somewhat coincidentally, it seems that fat grafting beneath radiated chest wall skin in some of my breast reconstruction cases has caused an improvement in the quality of that irradiated skin. Some postulate that this improvement comes about because of stem cells that are present in the injected fat.

Mohs surgery

It seems to me there is a strange mystique about Mohs Surgery, even among physicians. This topic maybe a little bit of a diversion from developments of plastic surgery, but I think it is related and of interest. Mohs surgery was developed by the American physician Frederick Mohs in 1938. He began to use the technique routinely in his practice in 1940. The method consisted of first applying dichloroacetic acid to the area of suspected cancer on the patient so that he could scrape away the surface keratin. He then used a zinc chloride paste to "fix" the tissue in situ while maintaining the cellular structure for microscopic study.

However, this process usually took several hours, and the paste was quite painful. A benefit was, once "fixed," Dr. Mohs could remove the tissue without it bleeding. He removed or shaved the lesion with a saucer-shaped excision of the fixed tissue. Dr. Mohs then prepared slides for the frozen section microscopic examination. Another hallmark of Dr. Mohs's technique was the careful mapping of the lesion so that a notation of the location from which each microscopic slide originated existed.

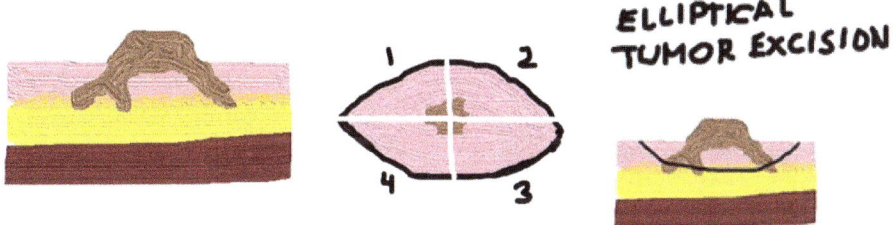

A cardinal factor in the Mohs micrographic technique is CCPDMA, the gold standard, which stands for Complete Circumferential Peripheral and Deep Margin Assessment. Histological slides come from tangential cuts at the margins of the excision peripherally and deep. If the specimens examined microscopically are not free of tumor, the whole process is repeated, for the affected areas only, until the margins are free. I have illustrated this process below. My first two drawings below show a tumor(brown) excised as a saucer-shaped specimen. The removal did not get all of the cancer from the underside of sections marked 3 and 4.

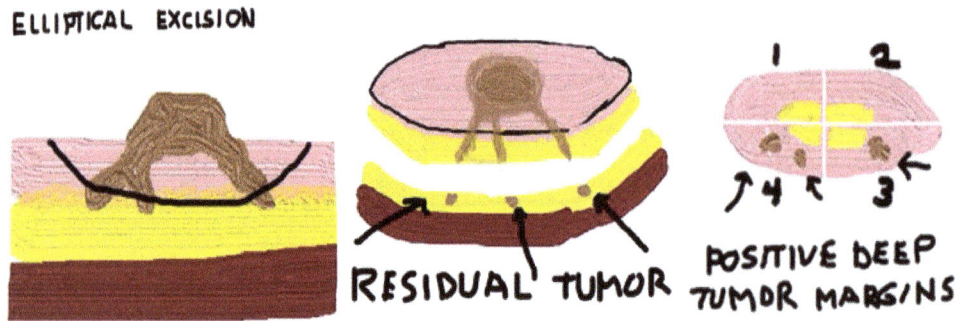

Therefore, additional specimens are needed, but only from sections 4 and 3. As shown below, the new samples again show positive for cancer.

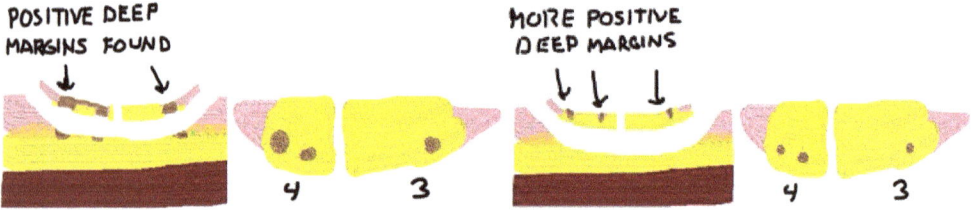

So, the operator takes additional deep slices from sections 4 and 3. In this example, they are free of tumor.

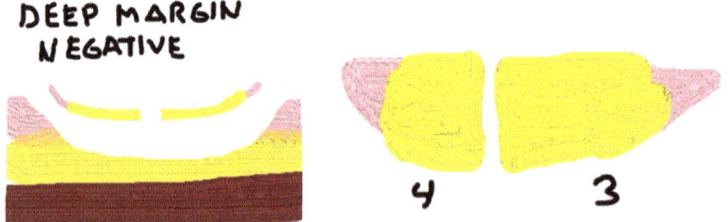

As you can appreciate, if the process needs repeating several times, the treatment could take days to complete. Mohs original technique was known as chemosurgery. Later by 1970, the process had evolved; standard fresh tissue immediate frozen sections replaced the abandoned chemo component. Now the operator could complete most cases within a few hours. Correspondingly, the official name became Mohs Micrographic Surgery in 1985.

What is the place of Mohs micrographic surgery? Mohs fresh frozen section method utilizing serial tangential excisions is notably suitable for sclerosing basal cell carcinomas and recurrent BCC and squamous cell carcinomas. It may also be desirable for extensive primary lesions with ill-defined borders or lesions with nerve infiltration.

However, Mohs micrographic surgery has some significant drawbacks. It is still very time consuming and expensive, and complex reconstructions may need to be delayed. For many routine discrete lesions in less critical areas of loose skin, the technique is unnecessary. Simple elliptical excisions with regular frozen section checks of the margins by a pathologist have a cure rate in the high 90% level. Discrete lesions on the trunk or extremities often can be removed with the standard delayed pathological examination in which the report comes back in a few days.

In the more critical head and neck area, one might ask what the difference between Mohs micrographic surgery and routine excision with frozen section examination of the tissue by a pathologist is? Well, that depends on two aspects, the oriented mapping of the lesion and the angle and location of the microscopic cuts for slides. If an elliptical excision of carcinoma is done and sent to the pathologist who then only examines a few bread loaf cuts for microscopic slides, the chance of getting a false negative report is significant because there was not CCPDMA. My drawing below demonstrates an example of the failure of the bread loaf method with a false negative result.

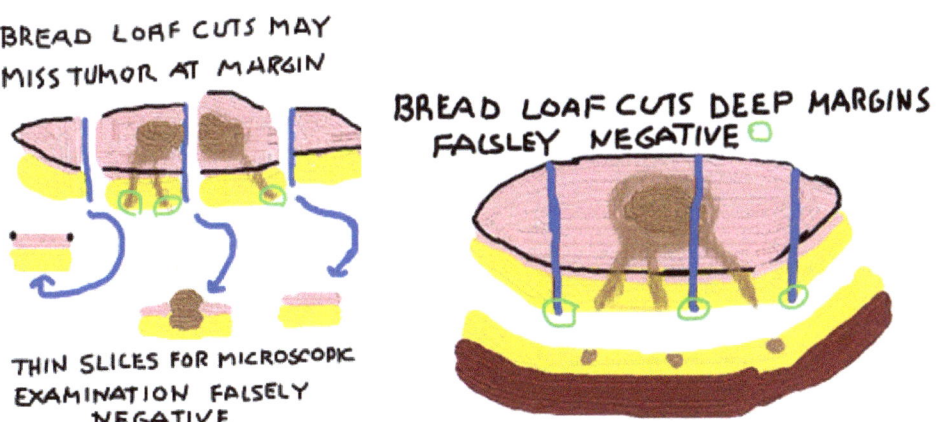

However, there are alternatives to the above bread loaf method. The pathologist and surgeon can utilize CCPDMA by mapping the ellipse and subdividing the surgical specimen into small units for frozen sections.

The identified units are then mounted with the peripheral and deep sides respectively facing the cutting surface so that the microscopic slides produced will represent the outer margin of the excised specimen.

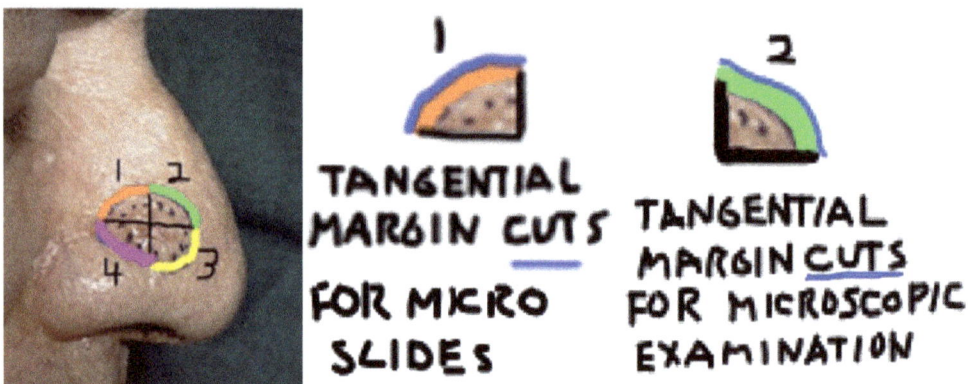

This method of CCPDMA with surgeon and pathologist allows for histological verification independent of the surgeon. Also, the reconstructive surgeon can immediately repair complex defects. No specialized training is necessary by the surgeon or pathologist to institute this technique. Drs. Menesi, Buchel, and Hayakawa have promoted this method.

Stem cells

Stem cells are individual cells that the surgeon can harvest from multiple sources such as umbilical cord blood, the umbilical cord itself, from aspirated fat, and other sources. Another ethically compromised source is human embryos. Some scientists felt like embryonic stem cells would be more efficacious for treating various diseases than those from other sources. However, as of this time, the opposite seems to be the case. Embryonic stem cells have cured no disorders. On the other hand, adult stem cells have been crucial in saving many lives. Adult stem cell therapy can cure sickle cell anemia. The ethically compromised and controversial use of embryonic stem cells seems unnecessary, unrewarding, and divisive. So far, in the field of plastic surgery, stem cells via fat grafting have been used as I mentioned above in treating radiation damage skin in the process of breast reconstruction.

The Healing Mission of Plastic Surgery

"Clarissa," below left, had a right partial mastectomy with radiation. She was unhappy with this result and came to see me asking for further reconstruction. I did bilateral mastopexies and augmented the right upper lateral breast with fat grafting from the abdomen. The fat grafting filled out the depression of the lateral aspect of the right breast. The fat graft seemed to improve the quality of the irradiated skin, but it is difficult to appreciate in this post-op result on the right below.

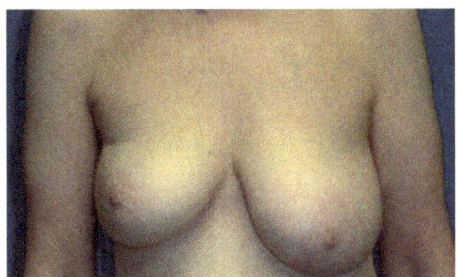
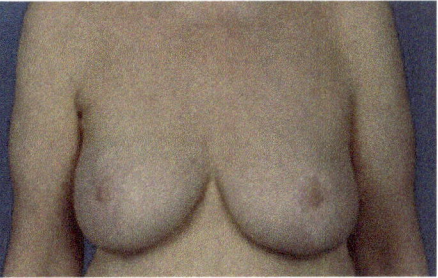

Wound Vac

Wound VAC (the vacuum-assisted closure) therapy, commonly known as negative pressure wound therapy, had a place in medicine as early as Roman times when practitioners would give direct suction by mouth to open traumatic wounds. Later, glass dome-shaped coping vessels drew out excess fluid. These methods fell out of favor in medical practice. Negative pressure wound therapy was reintroduced into common plastic surgery practice by Dr. Louis Argenta in the 1990s. By applying controlled negative pressure or a vacuum through a special sponge in the wound, new vascularity and tissue development can occur, allowing wounds to heal more rapidly.

VAC has become one of the most commonly used methods of wound closure. The United States military has extensively used it for battlefield casualties as well as for civilian injuries. VAC in a real paradigm shift in the treatment of challenging wounds. It is one of the most significant advances in plastic surgery in the last 50 years. Surgeons use VAC in combination with almost all other wound closure methods at times. The illustrations below show a sponge in the wound and an attached suction pump creating negative pressure. Polyurethane sealing tape prevents loss of the negative pressure. These devices may be short term or for chronic use.

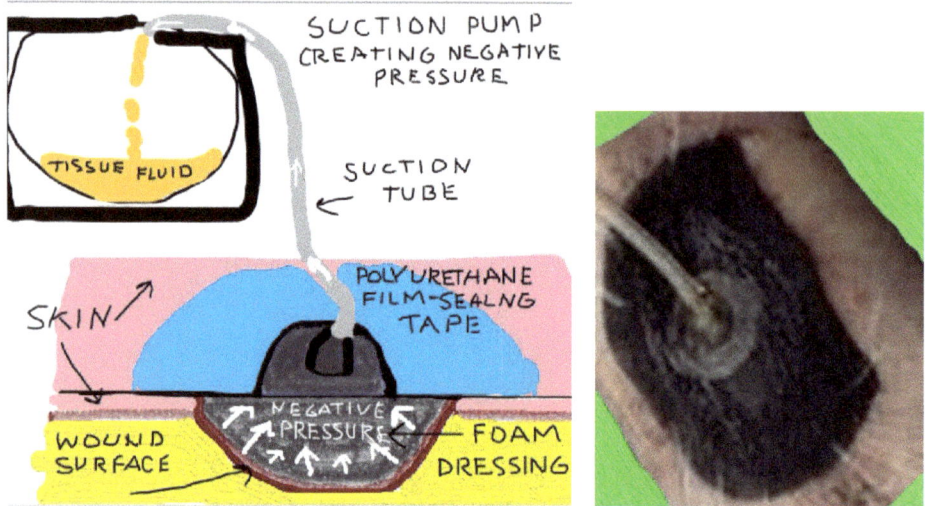

Hyperbaric oxygen therapy

Although the origins of hyperbaric oxygen therapy go back to the 17th century, it was only in the early 20th century that it was utilized effectively for treatment of the effects of diving accidents as decompression therapy. Beginning in the 1960's it was used for treating clostridial gas gangrene infections and carbon dioxide poisoning. When I was in residency training, hyperbaric oxygen was touted as adjunctive therapy for various conditions like diabetic ulcers, failing surgical flaps, and infections. Our hospital did not have a hyperbaric chamber when I was in training.

Like so many innovations, it is often difficult to know the rightful place of hyperbaric oxygen therapy. It has been particularly challenging to evaluate the evidence for its efficacy. However, slowly over many years, it has gradually become more accepted as a legitimate modality. I only occasionally prescribed this for my patients. It might help a patient with insufficient blood flow to a flap or recently manipulated segment of tissue that otherwise would necrose. Now most hospitals have such units. Medicare has approved it for numerous conditions. Many outpatient facilities and even spas have chambers. So, it seems like it has become an integral part of mainstream medical practice. I never saw many advantages for any of my patients.

Dermal matrix products

Various helpful dermal matrix products became available and had multiple uses in plastic surgery. I have used these products as sheets in breast surgery cases for "sling" support. The patient below "Monica" had breast augmentation elsewhere, which was complicated by severe implant descent, as shown below.

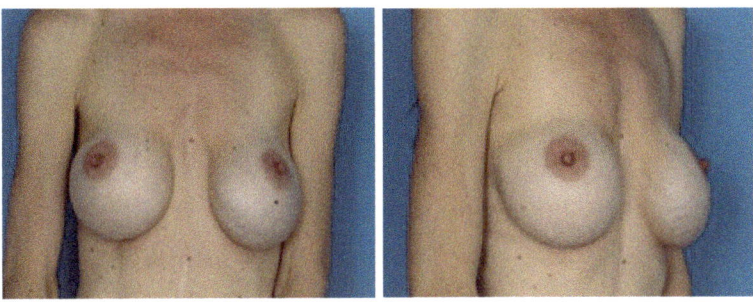

I performed a revision, which included a sling of dermal matrix sewn to the pectoralis major muscle to define the new breast implant pocket inferior margin. The matrix helped to hold new implants in the proper position. Her postoperative results are below. "Monica" was delighted with the revision surgery.

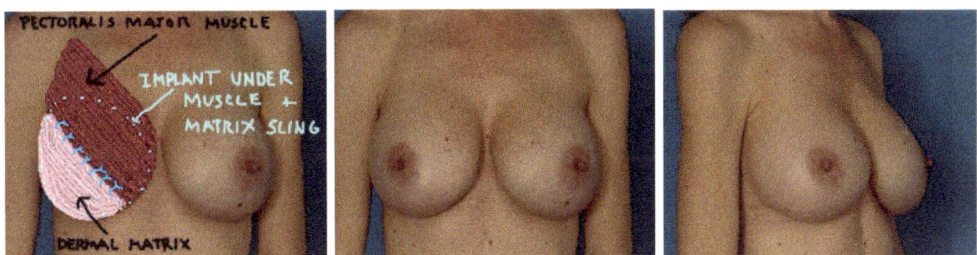

The dermal matrix may be helpful in the prevention of contracture, especially in refractory breast implant cases.

CAD and 3-D printing

Computer-aided design has recently become routinely available for orthognathic surgery. The surgeon can consult with specialized computer software companies that provide help in the planning of orthognathic procedures. Cone-beam x-ray data allows the fabrication of intermediate and final acrylic splints and even pre-bent surgical titanium hardware plates. Computer-aided designed custom implants using 3-D printing (the additive manufacturing process) are available for cranial and other reconstructive uses. There have already been some reports of 3-D printing of living tissue. What the future of 3-D printing holes regarding the production of flesh and blood replacement parts and vital organs is almost unimaginable!

DNA and the human genome.

Between its beginning in 1990 and its completion on April 14, 2001, the world's largest collaborative biological project mapped all human genes. The benefits are potentially unlimited. DNA will help us understand diseases, biological mutations, cancer, evolution, etc. I am jealous of the benefit future generations may attain from advances through the further study and application of the human genome. I believe physicians will be able to serve their patients in ways unimaginable now.

Tattoo

Initially, I used split-thickness skin grafts for areola reconstruction. For example, I would use upper inner thigh skin that was a little darker than the rest of the skin. When available, areola from the opposite breast has been a good source for a graft. Later the use of tattoo became quite common. As in the example below of a keyhole nipple reconstruction that I tattooed

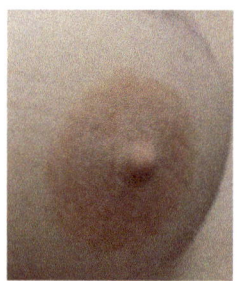

More recently, I have seen results from professional tattoo artists that even mimic the projection of the nipple! So, there has been advancement even in this ancient art.

Distraction osteogenesis

Modern techniques of bone elongation date to the work of a Russian orthopedic surgeon named Illizarov beginning during WWII and after. He designed an apparatus for lengthening long bones after traumatic injury. He cut the bony cortex while preserving most of the periosteum. Then with the aid of an external fixator, he would separate the bones slightly, and the bone would grow to fill the gap at a relatively uniform rate. Repeating the distraction at the speed of bone growth, he could significantly elongate the bone.

This process was a significant advance for certain types of injury. Dr. Joseph McCarty reported using this principle for lengthening the mandible in 1992. It is now used all over the body in specific instances. I used this principle in "Pete's" case in chapter 2.

Hair Transplantation

In 1971, when I was an intern in Kansas City, I assisted a plastic surgical resident at Kansas City General Hospital to do a massive hair transplant operation, for male pattern baldness, with 4mm punch grafts for harvesting. He operated under general anesthesia. I was not at all impressed with this procedure for several reasons. It was too bloody. The results from such large punch grafts had an unnatural cobblestone appearance.

However, over the next few decades, the procedures were much refined through the adaption of smaller and smaller grafts and only a mini-stab incision for the recipient area. With improved cosmetic results, hair transplantation for male pattern baldness has become extremely popular. Micrografts and minigrafts with as little as one to three hair follicles have transformed the outcomes, so that very natural results are routine.

This follicular unit concept has brought about some variations in the surgery. Surgeons abandoned the large punch grafts and began harvesting posterior scalp strip grafts, which they cut under magnification into small grafts of a few hairs (FU). Now some practitioners use micro punches to collect follicular units. Some even use robotic hair transfer techniques with a camera and robotic arms to assist the surgeon!

The vast majority of hair transplantation cases are for male pattern baldness. Still, these new techniques have made it available and more reliable for other indications such as female baldness, post-trauma hair loss, and after scalp surgery or for loss of sideburn or temporal hair after a facelift. A unique indication for hair transplantation is the adult male patient post bilateral lip repair, which has robust facial hair growth. Usually, the complete bilateral lip has no hair growth in the philtrum. A five o'clock shadow or a mustache will leave the philtrum appearing abnormally bare. I have sent a couple of such patients to my plastic surgery colleague, Dr. Alfonso Barrera, who is an expert at hair transplantation to match the philtrum to the lateral upper lip segments with excellent results.

Evidence-based medicine

Evidence-based medicine began with a group of Canadian clinical epidemiologists at Mc Master University under the leadership of David Sackett. Their first article was in the Canadian Medical Journal in 1981. One of Sackett's associates, Gordon Guyatt, coined the phrase "evidence-based medicine." A readership poll of the British Medical Journal reported in January 2007 that evidence-based medicine was the seventh most crucial milestone shaping modern medicine. They only judged discoveries such as antibiotics, immunization, sanitation, and radiology as more significant.

As a physician and indeed, as a plastic surgeon, I always tried to incorporate into my practice the latest scientific medical data that might be applicable to help my patients. However, it has only been in the last few years that the term evidence-based medicine has come to the forefront.

Evidence-based medicine is defined as a conscientious approach to medical practice that uses the current best evidence, integrating clinical experience and research information, and applying this to individual patient values and preferences for optimal care. Various pyramids representing a hierarchy of medical evidence illustrate the weight that is given to sources of information. I have composed an example below. The quality of the data increases as one goes from the base to the top of the pyramid. As one gets towards the top of the pyramid, the research information has been filtered by critical appraisal.

I believe most physicians can analyze data presented to them in research articles and medical papers. Meta-analysis examines data from several independent studies on the same topic. Systemic reviews collect and summarize all empirical evidence that fits the named criteria. The ability of individual physicians to filter such information must vary considerably.

In this modern era of the surgeon - patient shared decision making, the time-honored industrial concept of continuous quality improvement is a long-overdue paradigm shift. The basic principles are to integrate evidence gathering with clinical experience, which is then implemented with the understanding and approval of patients. Outcomes must then be analyzed and compared with current research results. Scientific Data and facts must take precedence over mere tradition and even expert opinion; on the one hand, however plastic surgery perhaps more than any other surgical field is also an art.

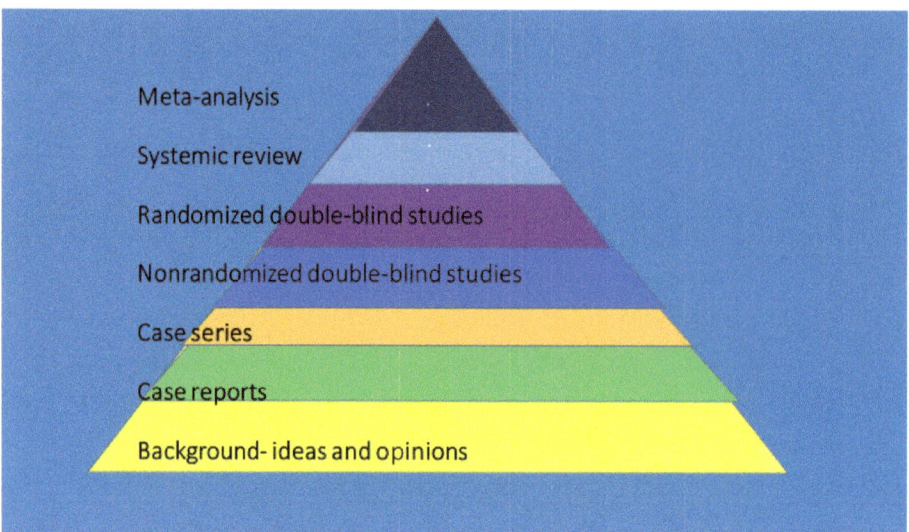

Chapter 18

Cancer- Retirement - Legacy

My Cancer

About three-thirty on the morning of Monday, March 21, 2016, I woke up with severe pain in my abdomen. I had been having some pain in the abdomen for a few days, which I had interpreted as a pulled muscle from some recent physical activity. But now I instinctively knew this was something significant. I gently rolled out of bed and began dressing because I knew I needed to go to the emergency room at the hospital. I thought that I most likely had appendicitis. As I finished my preparations to leave, my wife was still asleep. She looked so peaceful; I decided not to wake her.

I drove myself downtown and populated several rosaries with all the Hail Mary's that that I recited silently. When I arrived, I parked in my usual parking area in the hospital parking garage. The emergency room was on the ground floor of that building. I went to the reception desk, and told the clerk who I was and why I was there. I was given a wheelchair and quickly taken to one of the bays in the emergency room. The nurse asked me to take my clothes off and put on a hospital gown and lay down on the hospital emergency room bed.

I waited only a few minutes before Dr. Stepaniac came in and did a cursory examination. I knew him as he had been working in our emergency department for many years. He said he would have an IV started and see to it that I was given something for pain. He said he would contact Dr. Wallace, a good friend and colleague of mine, with whom I had operated and collaborated on many surgical cases. Dr. Stepaniac gave me an injection for pain right away. I waited a while for the nurse to return to insert an IV.

After 45 minutes or so, a transport tech whom I frequently saw in the hospital greeted me by name and took me to the radiology department for a cat scan of the abdomen. The logistics of getting off the stretcher to the cat scan and back was not complicated but a little uncomfortable. The scan only took a few minutes. I was then taken back to the same bay in the emergency department.

Now, as I was lying in my emergency room bed waiting for the general surgery consultation, I called my wife on my cell phone and woke her up about 6 AM. I told her where I was; she said she would get dressed and come down to the hospital right away. By this time, the pain medication had had some effect, and although I was still in some pain, it was not severe. I had been in the hospital for a couple of hours or so.

When Candy arrived in the emergency department, I was happy to see her. Of course, she was a little miffed that I'd driven myself to the hospital. She helped to make me more comfortable, finding extra pillows, etc.

A couple of general surgery residents who I had seen a couple of times around the hospital came in, introduced themselves, and examined me. They didn't seem to be too impressed. My pain tolerance is probably average, but because I had gotten a pain shot when I first came to the emergency department, perhaps I did not react very much to their probing. The residents were also noncommittal from their review of the cat scan. Time passed slowly as Candy and I waited in the emergency bay. Finally, about noon, Dr. Wallace came and examined me. He said the radiologist did see something on the CAT scan and thought I had acute appendicitis. He said that as soon as an operating room was available, he would take me to surgery, so I was to stay in the ER until then rather than go to a hospital patient room first.

It was late afternoon when another transporter with whom I was familiar took me up to the holding area outside of surgery, an area of the hospital which I visited on almost a daily basis. There, I saw some additional familiar friendly faces of nurses with whom I frequently worked. Father Tran, one of the hospital chaplains, graciously came and gave me the last rites.

I was readied for surgery and provided some additional preoperative medication. In my mind, I heard myself silently reciting a final *Pater Noster* and *Ave Maria*. My preoperative "cocktail" began kicking in, and I was woozy as I rolled on the gurney through the halls into the operating area. I meekly waved at a couple of well-known faces, who looked concerned but gave a cheery smile and hello. A nurse anesthetist I knew and trusted wheeled me into operating room number 14, an operating room that I had frequented as surgeon hundreds of times and as recently as a few days prior.

This time I had a more profound appreciation of being in a Catholic hospital, because of the crucifix on the wall representing *Coram Deo*, than any time before. It was a little bit like a dream, then "nothing" for a while.

The next thing I remember was slowly waking up and hearing several voices around me. As I lay there with my eyes closed, I felt the irritation of the anesthetic tube in my mouth and throat. Someone said, "Do you want it out?" Of course, I couldn't say anything but did try to nod in the affirmative.

My daughter-in-law, who was an RN at St. Joseph Hospital, was there and, according to my wife, handed me a paper and pen, and with my eyes still half-closed, I wrote something like: "Out damned spot, out" making a confused literary reference. My recollection is pretty vague. When the anesthesiologist removed the breathing tube, I opened my eyes and saw several people around me, including my wife. I was a little groggy but appreciated only a dull pain in my abdomen.

I soon recognized that I was in the intensive care unit, a familiar section of the hospital. Someone asked how I felt and did I have any pain. I said I didn't have much pain. Things were a little blurry, and I was still somewhat befuddled. I really can't quite remember who all was in the room; I remember my wife Candy was there. After a little conversation, I realized it was Wednesday and that I had spent Monday night and all of Tuesday intubated under sedation in the intensive care unit. I still sometimes joke about "whatever happened to Tuesday," No Tuesday with Morrie.

My wife and I had planned to go to New York the week following my illness. We were to spend a few days there before flying to the Holy Land for a pilgrimage we had been planning for several years. At this point, I erroneously thought that maybe we would still be able to make that trip. Robert Burns' poem *To a Mouse* came to mind, "The best laid schemes of mice and men often go awry." I soon found out that, because of the amount of infection in my abdomen, Dr. Wallace had left the skin and subcutaneous wound packed open with the skin edges about 4 inches apart. Of course, this would delay healing by several weeks.

At this point, I assumed I had had a ruptured appendix and peritonitis. Strangely, I don't remember exactly how I learned; I not only had a ruptured appendix and peritonitis but, more importantly, cancer of the appendix with four positive lymph nodes.

I spent a couple of days in the intensive care unit. My wife or one of my children was with me most of the time when I was awake. I also had many other visitors, including my practice partner Dr. Benjamin Cohen, Dr. Don Collins, Dr. Bruce Smith, Dr. Berkeley Powell, and several other medical colleagues. Father Chris, a Dominican priest from the nearby Holy Rosary parish church, came to see me. He was a friend of one of my daughters who told him about me.

While in the intensive care unit, I did have an IV pain pump, which I appreciated. After a couple of days, I moved from the ICU to a regular room in the hospital. For a few more days, I still had a nasogastric tube through the nose into the stomach. After a nurse pulled the tube out, ouch, I was placed on a liquid diet. I was comfortable except when the residents came to change and repack the open wound. I would try to anticipate that and use the pain pump right before that. However, after a few days, Dr. Wallace discontinued the pain pump. Because I did not have much baseline pain, I used only plain Tylenol from that point forward. I did not use any oral narcotics.

I slept somewhat fitfully. I silently repeated my night prayers, usually the rosary, perhaps like counting sheep, which did give me great comfort. I interspersed Our Father's and Hail Mary's with one of my favorite prayers. *Angus Dei qui tollis pecata mundu miserere nobis, Angus Dei qui tollis pecata mundi miserere nobis, Angus Dei qui tollis pecata mundi, donna nobis pacem* was like rhythmic musical therapy even in actual silence.

After a few days, I learned about the pathology report. As I mentioned before, I can't remember who told me. The report indicated four positive nodes out of 17 nodes removed with the surgical specimen. The primary tumor was an adenocarcinoma of the base of the appendix. My tumor was a T4 an N2a, stage IIIC cancer. The five-year survival rate for stage IIIC cancer of the appendix is about 50%.

At first, I had a bedside commode, which I needed help getting to because of frequent diarrhea. After a couple of days, the physical therapist started coming by once or twice a day to teach me to use a walker. With the help of a walker and the nurse, I began to get up to the bathroom frequently. I later started walking in the halls aided by the therapist. I was weak and shaky at first, but gradually I got the hang of using the walker.

Several things were bothering me. One was I was having a lot of diarrhea without much control. Another, the open wound dressing changes were quite uncomfortable. The central part of my abdomen had an elliptical opening and, although Dr. Wallace had closed the fascia, the edges of the skin were about 4 inches apart centrally. The length of the wound was probably about 10 inches. The residents would come in and pull gauze from the wound and replace it.

The idea was the bandage would stick to the wound and clean the surface when changed. Infection and cancer had contaminated the surgical site (my abdomen) because of the ruptured appendix. I eventually talked the residents into using some Silvadene cream in the wound to cut down on the bacteria while eliminating a lot of the pain of dressing changes caused by the gauze sticking to the wound surface.

For a while, it seemed like all I did was sleep and eat a minimal liquid diet, which the dietician gradually increased to soft foods. I began to walk up and down the halls of my hospital floor with the walker by myself. At first, I didn't want to read anything, although usually, I like to read a lot.

I realized that because of the tumor rupture and peritonitis, I would've died if I had not been fortunate enough to be in such good hands at the hospital. Indeed, if I had lived at an earlier age before modern medicine, I would have already been dead. So, being no "Miniver Cheevy," as in Edwin Arlington Robinson's poem, I was happy I was "born too late" for romantic medieval times.

As I became stronger, I was able to eat a soft diet. With the help of the physical therapist, I was able to graduate from a walker to a cane. I was grateful to be in St Joseph Hospital, where, as a twelve year -old I had spent six weeks in traction for a fractured femur received from playing football.

Over the ensuing half-century, the hospital retained much of its religious character. I was glad there was still a crucifix in my hospital room. As a child, I would get a visit from one of the nuns almost every day. Now I had compassionate care from everyone I encountered. But now the nurses and caregivers might be from practically anywhere in the world, Ireland to the Philippines. I noted a particular caring nurse from the middle east was Muslim.

Just as had been the case as a child, I was privileged to have the opportunity to receive holy communion almost every day because of volunteer extraordinary Eucharistic ministers. In my somewhat distraught mental state at that time, the reception of the *Panis Angelicus* was reassuring, consoling, and alleviated much of my distress. It also made me further appreciate my wife, who distributed communion at St Joseph for many years. She had several interesting stories about her experiences, such as taking communion to priests or nuns whom she knew or praying with patients who had been away from the church for a while but appreciated the opportunity her ministry provided.

It was only after several days recovering from surgery in the hospital that I had a pertinent and consequential discussion with Dr. Wallace, my oncologic general surgeon. He felt that I had had a proper cancer operation. Although I had four positive nodes, there were 13 surrounding negative nodes. He advised me that I needed to have chemotherapy, which should begin soon. He left me the impression that if I had chemo, I had somewhat better than a 50% five-year survival chance, and if I didn't receive chemotherapy, I would have slightly less than a 50% five-year survival rate.

To facilitate the administration of chemotherapy, he recommended I have an access port in my left subclavian vein. Therefore, I went to the operating room for a small procedure to insert the port. This minor procedure was uneventful, and I had almost no pain at the site. However, a day or two later, my left forearm swelled to about double its usual size.

My forearm looked like Popeye, the sailor man's arm, but it was painless. My wife was the one who first noticed this swelling, and we called it to the attention of my doctors. They sent me back to the imaging department for scans, which demonstrated a subclavian vein thrombosis. Because of that, I began taking the anticoagulant Eliquis orally, which was effective as the swelling started to subside within a few days and was almost gone ten days later. At that point, I was ready to go home. Arrangements were made for daily home nursing care to help change the dressings. My internist Dr. Holmes set up an appointment for me with a medical oncologist he recommended, Dr. Pandya.

After a total of about two weeks, I went home and began sleeping in my own bed again. I was still having a lot of diarrhea but was able to control it. I was allowed to start to eat a regular diet. I started walking with the help of my cane on the sidewalk in front of my house. Over a few days, I was able to walk pretty much the full length of the block and back. I felt like I was recovering very nicely.

The visiting home nurse, who was quite young, was pleasant and professional. I doubted that she had ever seen a wound left open like mine. Together we daily changed the dressing of the abdominal wound, and gradually I began to see some progress in its closure. The natural history of this type of wound was the skin edges would pull themselves progressively together by the healing process over a few weeks; it would seem very slow at first and then build up to a crescendo over the last week or so.

So about 3 ½ weeks after my surgery, I went to see Dr. Pandya, a medical oncologist in a large group oncology practice. He was very thorough and personable. He did not hesitate to recommend that I undergo chemotherapy. He said, because of the type of tumor, the ruptured, cancerous appendix, and the four positive lymph nodes, I needed chemo.

He told me there were three drugs used for this problem, and I would need to have two of them simultaneously. One was oxaliplatin, a platinum-based drug that was given intravenously over a few hours once a treatment cycle. Another drug was 5-FU (five fluorouracil), which he could provide intravenously once a treatment cycle. An alternative to 5-FU was an oral medication Xeloda (capecitabine), which he could provide for the same effect as 5-FU.

He recommended a series of 12 chemotherapy treatments, which included the platinum drug administered over a few hours intravenously and four Xeloda pills twice a day for two weeks. I would then wait another week and repeat the same regimen for a total of 12 treatments. He explained that I was likely to have considerable nausea and potentially vomiting from the medications. He prescribed several oral antiemetic medicines and also a promethazine topical gel medicine that I could place on the volar surface of my wrist for "breakthrough" nausea.

After the initial consultation with my oncologist and his recommendation, I decided that I would retire and devote my efforts to getting well and spending time with my wife and family.

I began the first treatment around April 15, 2016. The intravenous platinum drug, given over about a three-hour in the infusion room at the medical oncology practice, did not seem to have too much immediate effect. Nor did the oral medication. However, within a day or so, many different things happened.

One interesting phenomenon was cold sensitivity to touch. I could not tolerate holding a cold item retrieved from the refrigerator as there was an annoying, uncomfortable, almost electrical sensation in my hands. I also began to get constant numbness and tingling in my hands and feet. Eventually, I had peeling of the skin of my palms and lost my fingerprints. My cell phone would no longer recognize my index finger to unlock! My 70-year-old skin had many sun damage keratoses. These began to slough off like they might've done if I used 5-FU topical medicine, which I had often prescribed to my elderly patients with sun-damaged skin. Also, I noticed losing some of my hair when using a comb.

Another annoying side effect was that everything I tried to eat tasted bad. It was not just neutral or bland, but it was a negative taste. I sometimes described eating various foods was like eating contaminated cardboard. I kept experimenting with different foods to try to come up with something I could tolerate.

Everything also seemed to run right through me quickly. After a while, it seemed I could only tolerate crackers or toast or some soups. Then, on top of that, I started to become nauseated by whatever I did eat. I also began to have some small painful ulcers in my mouth. Dr. Pandya warned me about this and gave me a special mouth wash, which helped a little bit.

Over about 12 days, things seem to get worse and worse progressively. I had significant diarrhea multiple times per day. I began to feel quite weak. Up to that point, although nauseated, the oral antiemetics had worked. However, I finally began to experience breakthrough nausea, about which the doctor had warned me. Now I needed to place the topical gel on my wrists as well. The gel mostly kept me from vomiting, but not from feeling very sick.

Each morning and evening, I took four Xeloda pills. On the 14th and last day of the treatment cycle, I confess, I took only three of the Xeloda pills and threw the last one away in some silly act of defiance. Because I was feeling so poorly, at my wife's urging, we arranged to have my follow-up visit with Dr. Pandya earlier than planned. The scheduled appointment was to assess my condition for starting the second course of chemotherapy.

By the day of my visit, I felt like I was dying. My wife drove me to the doctor's office; it was with some difficulty, and with the help of my cane that I was able to get to the doctor's office. The lab tech drew some blood, which showed anemia and an electrolyte imbalance. When he saw me, Dr. Pandya was quite concerned with my fragile condition. He felt I was having a rare extreme reaction to the Xeloda. He arranged for admission that day to St. Joseph Hospital. I sincerely believe that if I had stayed home, I would not have lasted another day or two but would've died in my sleep!

I was admitted directly to my room in St. Joseph Hospital. After an initial assessment, the hospitalist placed me on a regimen of total parenteral nutrition. That is, I was given IV nutrition through the access port, which I already had for the IV chemotherapy. During that hospitalization, a nutritionist tried to help me with oral intake. I was able to ingest some high-protein liquid shakes such as Ensure. It was indeed a struggle as all food tasted terrible. I continue to be plagued with diarrhea, as everything I consumed orally ran right through me.

My gastroenterologist recommended oral probiotics, but nothing seemed to help. It was a struggle for a while to get up to a bedside commode. Not to mention the kind efforts the nurses went through to get me to the bathroom to have a shower. Again, I noticed a beautiful crucifix on the wall of my hospital room, and with the frequent visits from my wife, family, and friends, I felt like I was *Coram Deo*.

With improved IV nutrition, I gradually got better. I felt like the TPN was lifesaving. After a few days, I began to walk, with assistance from the physical therapist, in the hospital hallways, demoted to a walker again. I felt very grateful for my doctors at St. Joseph Hospital. I remember that one of my medical colleagues, Dr. John Bertini, gave me a book by Father Benedict Groeschel. It was entitled *Arise from Darkness._* I found it consoling, and it tended to put things in perspective when I began to feel sorry for myself. Two whole weeks of TPN were needed to build up my strength enough to go home. So, this was the second time the doctors and nurses at St. Joseph Hospital saved my life.

After another week at home, I went back to see my oncologist Dr. Pandya. He said he had had only one previous patient with such an abnormally severe reaction to Xeloda. Apparently, the Xeloda completely sloughed my intestinal tract lining so that I was not absorbing any nutrition. If he had asked me to repeat the same chemotherapy regimen, I would've refused. As it was, Dr. Pandya recommended we delay a few more weeks and then not use any more Xeloda, but again use the platinum drug IV and substitute IV 5 -FU for the Xeloda in the next chemotherapy treatment. IV 5- FU was the same medicine that I might have started on instead of the Xeloda in the first place.

While at home, I again started walking on the front sidewalk in my neighborhood first with the walker then, after several days with my cane. I was gradually getting a little stronger but still had symptoms such as diarrhea, cold intolerance, numbness and tingling of my hands and feet, and food intolerance.

A few weeks later, when it was time for the second chemotherapy treatment, I was understandably a little apprehensive. I received the entire treatment in the same office infusion area, where I had received the oxaliplatin portion of my first chemo regimen. This large room had numerous lounge chairs surrounded by IV poles. I came into the room picked out a chair near a window with a view of the Texas Medical Center and of the Shriners Hospital for Children, where for the past few years, I had been doing my cleft lip and palate surgeries. I received the two IV medications over a few hours. There were about 20 stations for chemotherapy in that large room.

Over the next several months, I would see some of the same people coming back who were also receiving their chemotherapy. My wife came with me and sat in the infusion area and read a book. I would usually either read a book are play chess on my iPad. If I needed to urinate because of all the IV fluid, I could disconnect one of the wires and then take the IV pole with the infusion medicine on it and walk myself to the nearby restroom in the infusion area.

This second chemotherapy treatment didn't cause any significant immediate reaction other than feeling slightly lightheaded when it was time to get up and walk out. With this new regimen, I was to receive treatments every two weeks instead of every three weeks. I began to feel worse four or five days after this second treatment. I continued to have diarrhea, and nausea returned but not to the degree that I had previously. The anti-nausea medicines worked fine. I was taking multiple vitamins, probiotics, and nutritional protein shakes. I continue to struggle to find other foods that I could eat. Oddly enough, for a while, it seemed like only smoked salmon with cream cheese on toast was tolerable. Otherwise, some soups were manageable.

The treatment under this new regimen was not fun, but it was nothing like the initial treatment. I began to think that perhaps it would be smooth sailing for the rest of my therapy. I saw the sky as red but must have confused morning for the evening because there was one more unusual episode to endure.

My wife's sister and brother-in-law invited us to go to a matinee performance at the Alley Theater in downtown Houston on Candy's birthday, June 26, 2016. That day I had not felt very well. After the play, we walked next door to have dinner at Biaporretti's Italian restaurant. Some of the items on the menu sounded good. I ordered a veal dish. Hope springs eternal. However, as usual, it tasted terrible, and I ate only a small portion. In fact, in the middle of the meal, I began to get antsy and felt like I wanted to go home and go to bed.

After the dinner, my wife's brother-in-law drove us back, and I felt even a little worse as we said goodbye to them, and I walked in the front door with the aid of my cane. I immediately went to bed. Within an hour or so, I started violently throwing up and was miserable. I felt like I was a reasonable patient enduring pain but that I was a crummy patient experiencing nausea, vomiting, or dizziness. While my wife was in another room phoning my internist, I was unable to even walk to the bathroom to throw up. I rolled out of bed and crawled to the bathroom to throw up in the toilet.

My internist friend advised my wife to have me use some of the breakthrough anti-nausea medicine, which I did, to no apparent benefit. I knew something was severely abnormal again, and I needed to get to the hospital. My wife called one of our sons, Chris, who came and drove us down to the emergency room at St. Joseph Hospital. On the way, I silently repeated *Kyrie Eleison* over and over as I was feeling so terrible. There was almost no traffic, so we arrived at the emergency entrance in about 20 minutes. I was placed in a wheelchair and quickly admitted through the ER and evaluated by the hospitalist doctor.

Laboratory work showed that I had a very severe deficiency of magnesium. I received magnesium intravenously, and within 24 hours, I felt 100% better. After an additional day of IV magnesium, I was able to be discharged home with oral magnesium supplements. I was impressed by how replenishing my magnesium could have such a dramatic and rapid effect on my well-being. I consider this the third time that the doctors and nurses at St. Joseph Hospital saved my life.

As I mentioned earlier, with the advice of my oncologist, my wife and I decided we needed to devote our full-time to my healing and recovery. So, I decided to retire. My wife and I also decided to downsize and buy a house Katy Texas, which would place us closer to several of our children, three of whom lived in Katy, a suburb of Houston. So, on October 1, 2016, we moved into a community called Heritage Grand, which is part of a vast development known as Cinco Ranch.

This move occurred while I was still engaged in my chemotherapy. The move made things easier for my wife and me as our children were able to give us a lot of support during this trying time of my cancer treatment. We found that this move has been very favorable. We have many friendly neighbors and a close-by clubhouse in which there are numerous community activities, dinners, periodic entertaining productions, and pastimes such as ping-pong, chess, billiards, etc.

Over the next several months, I completed a total of 12 chemotherapy treatments. A couple of times, the infusions had to be delayed a week or two because of a low blood count. I received some Neulasta on a few occasions, which helped to counteract the low blood count and helped prevent infection. I lost about 50 pounds during the treatments. Perhaps, fortunately, I was significantly overweight when everything started. I finally finished my last treatment and "rang the bell" in the chemotherapy treatment room at the end of January 2017, about ten months after my cancer surgery and diagnosis, with cheering optimistic nurses celebrating while my wife took the pictures.

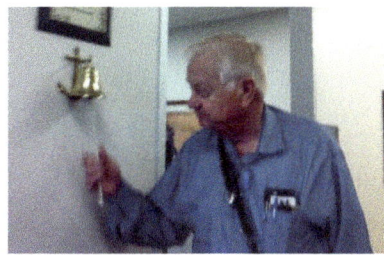 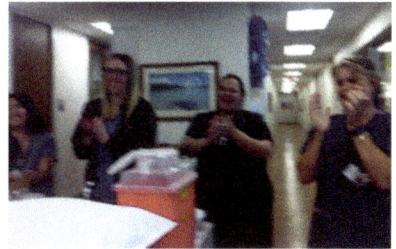

I reflected hopefully on John Donne's meditation, "No man hath affliction enough, that is not matured and ripened by it, and made fit for God by that affliction." I can only hope!

Slowly, over about 6 to 8 months after the completion of chemotherapy, my taste gradually came back to normal. My skin stopped peeling soon after I finished therapy. I never came close to losing all my hair; it only thinned out and turned white during the treatment. Over about a year, my hair thickened a bit, and I think at least a hint of red returned. My wife disputes that. The neuropathy irritation and numbness gradually improved in my hands, but as of this writing in 2020 continues to be significant in my feet, maybe even worse. For a few months during my therapy, I took gabapentin for neuropathy. It never seemed to make much difference; so, I stopped it. I suppose I was lucky that my neuropathy has not painful but only annoying.

Legacy

As I continued my recovery, I was fortunate and proud to be invited to the 2017 Texas Society of Plastic Surgeons Annual Meeting to give a presentation on my 38 years of plastic surgery practice. I titled my slide presentation The Healing Mission of Plastic Surgery. The Texas society of plastic surgeons was organized in 1953 and had its first meeting in 1955 with 14 founding members. I was fortunate to have known seven of those founding members: Truman Blocker, Bromley Freeman, Raymond Brauer, Thomas D. Cronin, Byron Hardy, Robert J. wise, and Stephen R. Lewis.

Two of these men, Dr. Thomas Cronin and Dr. Raymond Brauer, were my primary mentors in plastic surgery. They gave me priceless training, experience, and advice about plastic surgery. I reminded my audience that the Texas Society of Plastic Surgeons' purpose is "to benefit society by advancing the art and science of plastic and reconstructive surgery through promoting the highest standards in all aspects of the profession as well as to provide the public with information about plastic and reconstructive surgery." I pointed out that the Texas Society of Plastic Surgeons' "Raison d' etre" is synonymous with the healing mission of plastic surgery and that all of the plastic surgeons in attendance are part of this work.

Plastic surgeons are part of the healing mission of plastic surgery not because of various mission trips that might be associated with or because of their participation in plastic surgery outreach programs like the D Tag tattoo removal program. Instead, by its very nature, plastic surgery is a healing mission. Helping the child with protruding ears or the elderly patient with sagging upper eyelid is, with a woman with small breasts or the woman with overly large painful breasts, is part of the mission. Treating traumatic injuries of the face, body, or hands, or congenital deformities or tumors or the effects of tumors, are all part of the healing mission of plastic surgery.

With recovery and retirement, my wife Candy and I have been able to do some traveling. Finally, in November of 2018, we were able to fulfill our plans to visit the Holy Land, which had been interrupted by my illness. We went with an Equestrian Order of the Holy Sepulcher group led by a former pastor of ours. It was a beautiful, spiritually enlightening trip seeing the places Jesus walked, worked miracles, died, and rose from the dead. I now understand why Pope Paul VI said the Holy Land was the "fifth gospel."

A remarkable aspect has been the expanded meaning of the biblical references in the readings at Sunday Mass. Frequently my wife and I turn to each other when there is a reference to a place in the Holy Land where Jesus preached. We rejoice that we had physically visited that site. In a real way, our pilgrimage gave us a "fifth gospel" that further illuminates the actual gospels.

June 14, 2019, we celebrated our 50th wedding anniversary with a beautiful Mass at St Anne Church, where we were married. "O my love is like a red red rose ….". Robert Burns is one of my favorite poets. We were very appreciative that the celebrant was Fr. Drew Wood, who was a classmate of mine at St Thomas High School in Houston. Also, a priest from the high school, Fr. Belish, came and concelebrated the Mass. We had a party following at the high school with about 150 people attending. We had the picture below taken with our eight children, their spouses, and our grandchildren. We were able to get twenty-five of our twenty - eight, grandchildren, and all but one of our children's spouses in the picture below. What a blessing.

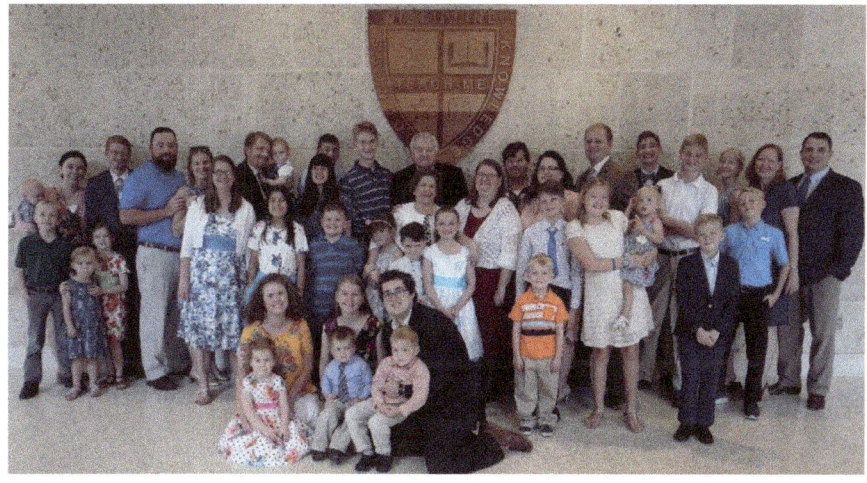

Since my unexpected and sooner than anticipated retirement, my operating days are over. I have taken my interest in plastic surgery in a new direction. By telling my professional story in this book, I hope to be of service to those of the curious general public who might be interested in this fascinating field of medicine. I am reminded of the famous last line from Milton's sonnet *When I Consider How My Light Is Spent*, "They also serve who only stand and wait.

When I look back on my career, I feel lucky and blessed to have practice during a time of exciting innovations and new techniques in plastic surgery. I was fortunate to be able to benefit many of my patients with some of these advances. It was my honor to help educate and train many plastic surgery residents, especially from St. Joseph Hospital/Houston Methodist, but also the University of Texas Health Science Center Houston and the University of Texas Medical Branch Galveston. I am very proud of this.

There are two programs I directed, which are dear to me. One is Operation San Jose, which I discuss in chapter 11. The other is the Cronin and Brauer Cleft Palate Clinic, which I discuss in Chapter 7. With the support from the Thomas Cronin Endowment at Christus Foundation for Healthcare, the Cronin and Brauer Cleft Palate Clinic, which I directed from its beginning in 1987 to 2014, seems to be flourishing. In 2014 I arranged for it to merged with the cleft palate program at Shriners Hospital for Children Houston. It continues as the Cronin and Brauer Cleft Lip and Palate Clinic at Shriners Hospital for Children Houston, currently under the direction of Dr. Stephen Blackwell, an accomplished cleft surgeon.

Operation San Jose Project, the cleft lip and palate outreach mission program I began in 1983, continues under the able direction of my former resident Dr. Michael Lipka of Kansas City. The Christus Foundation for HealthCare also supports OSJ. I am proud that I have arranged for both programs to continue following my retirement.

As I complete this memoir, I contemplate, as Qoheleth in Ecclesiastes, both "For everything, there is a season, and a time for every matter under heaven," and ultimately, "Vanity of vanity, all is vanity." Thank you for reading my book.

Chronological Bibliography

Ecclesiastes 1:1-1

Tagliacozzi. *De Curtorum Chirurgia per Insitionem, 1597*

Sabattini P. . Rinoplastica e Cheiliplastica Operate Sopra un Solo Individuo. *Bull SciMed(Bologna)* 1838; 10:387

Henry Alford, Ed. *The works of John Donne*, Vol. W. III London: John Parker, 1839. 574-5839

Bernard C. Cancer de la Levre Inferieur Opere par un Procede Nouveau. Bull Soc Chir Paris. 1853; 3:357-60.

Margaret Wolfe Hungerford, *Molly Bawn* Dublin 1878

Abbé R. A new plastic operation for the relief of deformity due to double harelip. *Med Rec.* 1898; 53:477.

Santayana, George. *The Life of Reason: Reason in Common Sense.* Scribner's, 1905: p284

Hughes WL. A new method for rebuilding a lower lid: report of a case. Arch Ophthalmol. 1937; 17:1008–1017.

Mohs FE Chemosurgery, a Microscopically Controlled Method of Cancer Excision. Arch Surgery 42: 279-295 1941

Cronin T D, The Cross - Finger Flap – A New Method of Repair, American Surgeon, May 1951, vol. XVII

Cronin T D Syndactyly: Results of Zig-Zag Incision to Prevent Postoperative Contracture, Plastic, and Reconstructive Surgery, Vol. I No.6, Dec.1956

Mohs, Frederic Edward (1956). *Chemosurgery in cancer, gangrene, and infections: featuring a new method for the microscopically controlled excision of cancer.* Springfield, Ill: Thomas.

Cronin T. D. Management of the Bilateral Cleft Lip with Protruding Premaxilla Amer. Journ. Surgery Vol 92, Dec. 1956

Pope Pius XII, "Discourse of His Holiness Pius XII to the Participants of the 10th National Congress of the Italian Society of Plastic Surgery," October 4th, 1958.

Maltz, Maxwell Psycho-Cybernetics Simon and Schuster 1969

Cronin TD, Gerow FG. Augmentation mammaplasty: A new natural feel prosthesis. *Transactions of the Third International Congress of Plastic Surgery.* Amsterdam: Excerpta Medica Foundation, 1964:41-9.

Cronin T D, Guthrie T, Herr D, Experiences in the Surgical Correction of Hypospadius. American Journal of Surgery vol. 110 November 1965

Cronin T D: Use of Hair Bearing Punch Grafts for Partial Traumatic Loss of scalp Plast. Reconstr. Surg. 42: 446-449, 1968

Cronin TD, Biggs TM. The T-Z-plasty for the male "turkey gobbler" neck. Plast Reconstr Surg 1971; 47:534-538.

McKissock PK. Reduction mammaplasty with a vertical dermal flap. Plast Reconstr Surg. 1972; 49:245–252)

Brauer R O, Retropharyngeal Implantation of Silicone Gel Pillows for Velopharyngeal Incompetence, Plastic and Reconstructive Surgery 1973, Vol. 51, No 3

Tord Skoog, *Plastic surgery: new methods and refinements*, Philadelphia: Saunders, 1974

Karapandiz M. Reconstruction of lip defects py local arterial flaps. Br. J Plast Surg. 1976; 27:93-97

Thomas Thompson, *Blood, and Money*, New York: Doubleday 1976

Mallard, D. Ralph, *Cleft Craft: The Evolution of its Surgery*, Little Brown 1976

Courtiss EH, Goldwyn RM. Reduction mammaplasty by the inferior pedicle technique Plast Reconstr Surg. 1977 Apr;59(4):500-7.

Biggs T.M., Upton J., Cronin T.D. Texas Medicine. Jan. 1978 Vil. 74, No. 1: 53-58

Cronin, E.D.: Soft tissue injuries of the face. The Medical Journal of St. Joseph Hospital. Vol. 13, pp 45-51, March 1978.

Cronin, T.D., Cronin, E.D.: Reconstruction of the breast following mastectomy for malignancy. *Breast Disease, Proceedings of an International Symposium*. New Orleans, LA. May 1978. Grune & Stratton, Inc., New York, NY. pp 279-293, 1979.

Cronin, T.D., Cronin, E.D.: Reconstruction of the breast after mastectomy. Surgical Rounds. Port Washington, NY. Vol 2:11, p 12, November 1979.

Cronin, T.D., Cronin, E.D.: Reconstruction of the breast without additional skin or muscle flaps. Clinics in Plastic Surgery. W.B. Saunders Co., Philadelphia, PA. Vol 6:1, pp 47-55, January 1979.

Foucher G., Henderson H P., Maneau M., Merle M., Braun F M., Distal digital replantation. International Journal of Microsurgery 3, 1981, p 265-270.

Cronin, T.D., Cronin, E.D.: Nipple areola reconstruction. *Post-Mastectomy Reconstruction*. T. Grant & L. Vasconez. Williams and Wilkins Co., Baltimore, MD. Chapter 10, pp 131-147, 1981.

Sackett D. How to read clinical journals: I. why to read them and how to start reading them critically, *Can Med Assoc J* 1981: 1245:555-558

Cronin, T.D., Cronin, E.D.: Thoracoepigastric flap. *Post-Mastectomy Reconstruction*. T. Gant & L. Vasconez. Williams and Wilkins Co., Baltimore, MD. Chapter 7, pp 91-100, 1981.

Biggs, T.M., Cronin, E.D.: Technical aspects of the latissimus dorsi myocutaneous flap in breast reconstruction. Annals of Plastic Surgery. 6:5, pp 381-188, May 1981.

John M. Goin, M.D., Marcia Kraft Goin M.D., *Changing the Body - Psychological Effects of Plastic Surgery*, Williams, and Wilkins Co. Baltimore 1981.

Cronin, E.D., Cronin, T.D.: Breast reconstruction after modified radical and radical mastectomy. *Operative Surgery.* Butterworths. Kent, England. pp 316-324, 1982.

Cronin, E.D., Romero, R.: Augmentation mammaplasty. *Operative Surgery.* Butterworth. Kent, England. pp 325-331, 1982.

Hartrampf, C. R., Scheflan, M., and Black, P. W. Breast reconstruction with a transverse abdominal island flap. Plast. Reconstr. Surg. 69: 216, 1982.

Brown, P.W. Less than ten: Surgeons with amputated fingers (J Hand Surg Am 1982 Jan;7(1):31-7.

Austad E D, A self- inflating tissue expander Plast Reconstr Surg. 1982 Nov. 70(5): 588- 94.

Cohen, B.E., Cronin, E.D.: An innervated cross finger flap for fingertip reconstruction. Plastic and Reconstructive Surgery. 72:5, p 688, 1983.

Radovan C. Tissue expansion in soft tissue reconstruction Plast Reconstr Surg. 1984 Oct; 74(4):482-92.

Dos Santos L F. The Vascular anatomy and dissection of the free scapular flap Plas Reconstr Surg. 1984 April. 73(4);599-604.

Cohen, B.E., Cronin, E.D.: Breast reconstruction with the latissimus dorsi musculocutaneous flap. Clinics in Plastic Surgery. 11:2, pp 287-302, April 1984.

Cronin, E.D., Wright Jr., R.M.: Breast reconstruction after mastectomy. The Medical Journal of St. Joseph Hospital. 18:3, p 129, September 1983.

Cronin, E.D., Romero, R.: An unusual approach to a case of breast asymmetry. Annals of Plastic Surgery. 12:5, pp 461-465, May 1984.

Cronin, E.D., Humphreys, D.A., Ruiz-Razura, A., "Nipple Reconstruction: The S Flap." Plastic and Reconstructive Surgery. 81 (5): 783-787, 1985.

Furlow LT. Cleft palate repair by double opposing Z-plasty. Plast Reconstr Surg. 1986; 78:724–736.

Cronin, T.D., Cronin, E.D.: Nipple areolar reconstruction update. Gant, T. & Vasconez, L. (Eds.). *Post-Mastectomy Reconstruction.* 2nd edition, chapter 15, Williams & Wilkins Co., Baltimore, MD, 1987, pp 181-204.

Cronin, T.D., Cronin, E.D.: Thoraco-epigastric flap update. T. Gant & L. Vasconez (Eds.) *Post-Mastectomy Reconstruction.* 2nd edition, chapter 10, Williams & Wilkins Co., Baltimore, MD, 1987, pp 115-124.

Cronin, E.D., Humphreys, D.A., Ruiz-Razura, A.: Nipple reconstruction: The S flap. Plastic Reconstructive Surgery. Volume 81, No. 5, pp 783-787.

Cronin, T.D., Cronin, E.D., Roper, P.: Bilateral clefts. McCarthy, J. (Ed.), *Plastic Surgery*, Vol. 4, W. B. Saunders, Philadelphia, 1989, pp 2653-2722.

Ilizarov GA (1989a) The tension-stress effect on the genesis and growth of tissues. Part I. The influence of stability of fixation and soft-tissue preservation. Clin Orthop Relat Res 238:249–281.

Ilizarov GA (1989b) The tension-stress effect on the genesis and growth of tissues: part II. The influence of the rate and frequency of distraction. Clin Orthop Relat Res 239:263–285.

Chow, J Endoscopic release of the carpal ligament: A new technique for carpal tunnel syndrome. Arthroscopy. 1989, 5: 19-24.

Cronin, T.D., Cronin, E.D., Denkler, K.A.: Correction of secondary unilateral and bilateral nasal deformities. In Bardach, J. & Morris, H.L. (Eds.). *Multidisciplinary Management of Cleft Lip and Palate.* W. B. Saunders, Philadelphia, 1990, pp 264-273.

Cronin, T. D., Cronin, E. D.: Transverse Thoracoepigastric Skin Flap. *Grabb's Encyclopedia of Flaps III.* Little Brown and Company, Boston, Toronto, London, 1990, section 3B-289.

Ramirez OM, Ruas E, Dellon AL "Components separation" method for closure of abdominal-wall defects: an anatomic and clinical study Plast Reconstr Surg 1990: 86:519.

Guyatt, G. Evidence-based medicine *Ann Intern Med* 1991;149Supp); A-16.

Stanley Applebaum: *Poems and Songs: by Robert Burns*. Ed. Dover Publications 1991

McCarthy Joseph G. M.D.; Schreiber, Jonathan M.D.; Karp, Nolan M.D.; Thorne, Charles H. M.D.; Grayson, Barry H. D.M.D. Lengthening of the Human Mandible by Gradual Distraction. Plastic and Reconstructive Surgery: January 1992 - Volume 89 - Issue 1 - p 1-8

Cronin, E. D., Sozer, S. O., Biggs, T. M., "The Use of the TRAM Flap After Abdominoplasty" Annals of Plastic Surgery. Little Brown and Company, Boston, Massachusetts, Vol. 35, No. 4, 409-412, 1995.

Cronin, E. D., Haber, J. L, "A New Technique of Dermabrasion for Traumatic Tattoos." Annals of Plastic Surgery. Little Brown and Company, Boston, Massachusetts, April 1996, Vol. 36, No. 4:401-402.

Cronin, E. D., Cohen, B. E., Biggs, T. M., Collins, D. R: "Assessment and Longevity of the Silicone Gel Breast Implant." Plast. Reconstr. Surg. Vol. 99(6) pp 1597-1601, 1997.

Edward Arlington Robinson, *Selected Poems* by Penguin 1997. Edited by Scott Donaldson

Kenneth L. Mattox Editor, *The History of Surgery in Houston.*, Eakin Press 1998

Fr. Benedict J. Groeschel. *Arise from Darkness: What to Do When Life Doesn't Make Sense* Ignatius Press 1995

Barrera A: Hair Transplantation- Micrograft and Minigraft Mega-session. Aesthetic Plastic Surgery Journal 17:165-169 1997

Argenta LC, Morykwas MJ. Vacuum-assisted closure: a new method for wound control and treatment: clinical experience. Ann Plast Surg. 1997;38(6):563–577.

Marvin Zindler, March 1st, 2000 KPRC TV channel Houston "Dr. Cronin is one of the finest plastic surgeons in the country".

Cronin, E.D., Ruiz-Razura, A., Navarro, C.E.: "Creating Long-Term Benefits in Cleft Lip and Palate Volunteer Missions." Plast. Reconstr. Surg. 105:195-201, 2000.

Biggs TM, Steely RL. (2000) The male neck and T-Z-plasty: 28 years later. Aesthetic Surg J. 1: 31-34.

Cronin, E.D., Jabor, M.A.: "Bilateral Cleft Lip and Palate and Limb Deformities: A Presentation of Amniotic Band Sequence?" Journal of Craniofacial Surgery. 2000; 11:388-393.

Cronin, E.D., Ruiz-Razura, A., Livingston, C.K., Katzen, J.T.: "Endoscopic Approach for the Resection of Forehead Masses." Plast. Reconstr. Surg. 105:2459-2463 June 2000.

Cronin, E.D., Jabor, M., Shayani, P: "Cleft Palate Lateral Synechia Syndrome: Case Report with Review of Literature." Plast. Reconstr. Surg. Vol. 108, October 2001.

Barrera, Alfonso. *Hair Transplantation: The Art of Micrografting and Minigrafting,* St. Louis: Quality Medical Publishing 2002

Cronin, E.D., Williams, J.L., Roesel, J., Shayani, P.: "Short Stay Following Cleft Palate Surgery". Plast. Reconstr. Surg. Vol 108(4):838-840. September 2001.

Cronin, E.D., Shayani, P, Jabor, M.: A New Technique of Dermabrasion for Traumatic Tattoos. In: Harahap, M. ed. *Innovative Techniques in Skin Surgery.* Marcel Dekker, Inc.,

New York. 2002:521-525.

Cronin, E.D.: Discussion—Outpatient Cleft Lip Repair. Plast. Reconstr. Surg. August 2003.

Cronin, E.D., Weinrach, J.C., Smith, B.K., Collins, Jr., D.R., Cohen, B.E.: "Preventing Seroma in the Latissimus Dorsi Flap Donor Site with Fibrin Sealant." Annals of Plastic Surgery; July 2004- Volume 53-Issue 1-p 12-16.

Cronin, E.D., Rafols, Francisco J. M.D., Shayani Payam M.D., JD, Al-Haj, Iman MD. Primary Cleft Nasal Repair the Composite V-Y Flap with Extended Mucosal Tab. Annals of Plastic Surgery. Volume 52, Number 2, August 2004.

Fisher D M. Unilateral cleft lip repair: an anatomical subunit approximation technique. Plast Reconstr Surg. 2005 Jul;116(1):61-71.

Kamerow, D. BJM.2007;334:0-a Milestones, tombstones, and sex education.

McCord CD, Seify H, Codner MA, Trans blepharoplasty ptosis repair: three-step technique. Plast Reconstr Surg. 2007 Sep 15;120(4):1037-44.

S. Anthony Wolfe M.D, *A man from Herrick: The Life and Work of Paul Tessier, M.D., Father of Craniofacial Surgery*. Lulu.com, United Kingdom (2012).

Menesi W, Buchel EW, and Hayakawa T J Plastic Surgery (Oakv.) 2014 Autumn; 22(3):179-182

Praise for Dr. Ernest Cronin and The Healing Mission of Plastic Surgery

"Enlightening, memorable, professional, this amazing book has it all. Do read this unusual personal story of the healing journey of a life spent as a plastic surgeon." - Donna R Fox Ph.D., Speech Pathologist, Fellow of American Speech-Language-Hearing Association and Professor Emeritus University of Houston

"It is a great honor and a pleasure for me to recommend this fascinating book highly. It chronologically summarizes his professional career in the field of Plastic and Reconstructive Surgery, witnessing and participating in significant advances in the specialty throughout four decades. Dr. Ernest Cronin is a generous humanitarian who has improved countless patients' lives and mentored many plastic surgeons, including me." - Alfonso Barrera M. D. Clinical Assistant Professor Baylor College of Medicine and author of *Hair Transplantation. The Art of Follicular Unit Micro and Minigrafting*.

"Like a great conductor, Dr. Ernest Cronin masterfully orchestrated the sequence and tempo of every surgery. Every action served a purpose---he wasted no motion. His technical savvy, coupled with his kindness and compassion, made him the best surgeon with whom I ever worked." - Henry Mentz, MD, F.A.C.S. Aesthetic Center for Plastic Surgery. Awarded - Best Plastic Surgeon of the Year for US 2016-20 by Medical Livewire, A.I., Global 100, M&A, Leading Advisor, The Global Venture.

"Over three decades ago, I met a seemingly simple, quiet, unassuming individual. I quickly appreciated how privileged I was to be in the presence of greatness. In Dr. Ernest Cronin's *Healing Mission of Plastic Surgery*, a skilled, compassionate sagacious surgeon, sage, philosopher, and friend provides an honest glimpse into the life of a living legend" – plastic surgeon Gary Branfman M. D., F.A.C.S.

"One word for this book – SENSATIONAL - a gem! - great experience, excellent surgical results, clear explanations, good artwork, and all presented in a simple conversational way. I feel as if every resident should read it. The book presents a huge experience in plastic surgery as a real *healing mission*." - Thomas Biggs M. D. Clinical Professor Plastic Surgery Baylor College of Medicine, ICON of the American Association of Plastic Surgeons, Former President of the International Society of Aesthetic Plastic Surgery

"Dr. Cronin is one of the finest plastic surgeons in the country." Marvin Zindler, KPRC TV Personality Houston March 1st, 2000.

Dr. Ernest C. Cronin, a true legend in International Plastic Surgery, has graced our literature with *The Healing Mission of Plastic Surgery*… his experiences, successes, and failures, philosophies, and dedication to his craft of plastic surgery. Woven through the fabric of this wonderful treatise are the threads of Dr. Cronin's kindness and generosity, passion for his mission, conceptual brilliance, and surgical skills. *The Healing Mission of Plastic Surgery* is beautifully illustrated with Dr. Cronin's photos and diagrams, many personally embellished for instructional purposes! - Donald H. Parks BA, MD, FRCS(C), F.A.C.S., Professor of Surgery, McGovern Medical School, University of Texas Health Science Center at Houston, Chief, Division of Plastic Surgery (Retired)

www.ingramcontent.com/pod-product-compliance
Ingram Content Group UK Ltd.
Pitfield, Milton Keynes, MK11 3LW, UK
UKHW060216240426
12048UKWH00030BB/1698